D0890221

Health Informatics

(formerly Computers in Health Care)

Kathryn J. Hannah Marion J. Ball
Series Editors

Health Informatics Series
(formerly Computers in Health Care)

Series Editors
Kathryn J. Hannah   Marion J. Ball

Dental Informatics
Integrating Technology into the Dental Environment
L.M. Abbey and J. Zimmerman

Ethics and Information Technology
A Case-Based Approach to a Health Care System in Transition
J.G. Anderson and K.W. Goodman

Aspects of the Computer-Based Patient Record
M.J. Ball and M.F. Collen

Performance Improvement Through Information Management
Health Care's Bridge to Success
M.J. Ball and J.V. Douglas

Strategies and Technologies for Healthcare Information
Theory into Practice
M.J. Ball, J.V. Douglas, and D.E. Garets

Nursing Informatics
Where Caring and Technology Meet, Third Edition
M.J. Ball, K.J. Hannah, S.K. Newbold, and J.V. Douglas

Healthcare Information Management Systems
A Practical Guide, Second Edition
M.J. Ball, D.W. Simborg, J.W. Albright, and J.V. Douglas

Healthcare Information Management Systems
Cases, Strategies, and Solutions, Third Edition
M.J. Ball, C.A. Weaver, and J.M. Kiel

Clinical Decision Support Systems
Theory and Practice
E.S. Berner

Strategy and Architecture of Health Care Information Systems
M.K. Bourke

Information Networks for Community Health
P.F. Brennan, S.J. Schneider, and E. Tornquist

Informatics for the Clinical Laboratory
A Practical Guide
D.F. Cowan

(continued after index)

Marion J. Ball
Charlotte A. Weaver   Joan M. Kiel
Editors

Healthcare Information Management Systems

Cases, Strategies, and Solutions

Third Edition

With 64 Figures

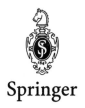

Springer

Marion J. Ball, EdD
Vice President
Clinical Informatics Strategies
Healthlink Incorporated
Baltimore, MD
and
Adjunct Professor
Johns Hopkins University
School of Nursing
Baltimore, MD
USA

Charlotte A. Weaver
CNO and Vice President of
    Patient Care Systems
Cerner Corporation
Kansas City, MO
USA

Joan M. Kiel, PhD, MPA, MPhil
Chairman, Department of
    Health Management
    Systems
John G. Rangos, Sr., School
    of Health Sciences
Duquesne University
Pittsburgh, PA
USA

Series Editors:

Kathryn J. Hannah, PhD, RN
President, HECS, Inc.
and
Professor (ADJ)
Department of Community
    Health Sciences
Faculty of Medicine
The University of Calgary
Calgary, Alberta
Canada

Marion J. Ball, EdD
Vice President
Clinical Information Strategies
Healthlink Incorporated
Baltimore, MD
and
Adjunct Professor
Johns Hopkins University
School of Nursing
Baltimore, MD
USA

Library of Congress Cataloging-in-Publication Data
Healthcare information management systems: cases, strategies, and solutions/Marion Ball . . . [et al.],
    [editors].—3rd ed.
        p.   ;   cm.—(Health informatics series)
    Includes bibliographical references and index.
    ISBN 0-387-40805-3 (alk. paper)
    1. Health services administration—Data processing.   2. Information storage and retrieval
systems—Medical care.   I. Ball, Marion J.   II. Health informatics.
    [DNLM: 1. Health Facilities—organization & administration.   2. Management
Information Systems. WX 26.5 H4345 2003]
    RA394.H45 2003
    362.1′068—dc22
                                                                                        2003065727

ISBN 0-387-40805-3   Printed on acid-free paper.

Printed in the United States of America.   (MP/MVY)

9 8 7 6 5 4 3 2

Springer-Verlag is a part of *Springer Science+Business Media*

springeronline.com

To my beloved husband, Dr. John Charles Ball, to our children, Charles, Elizabeth, Michael, and Debbie, and to our grandchildren, Alexis, Alex, Mike, Ryan, and Erica.

Marion J. Ball

To my mother and father, Betty and Richard Weaver, who raised the nine of us against all odds, and to my son, Kevin, who remains my best project.

Charlotte A. Weaver

To Thomas D. Kiel, MD
Joan M. Kiel

Foreword I

It has often been stated that the hospital and its associated information system is the most complex organizational structure created by people. Therefore, it should not come as any surprise that the implementation of successful healthcare information management systems has lagged commercial, banking, and other nonhealthcare information systems.

Computer-based systems for the management of healthcare information began in the 1960s. During the past four decades, the requirements for healthcare information management systems have continually changed due to frequent major advances in medical technology and the vicissitudes of healthcare legislation. Important changes in medical technology and in healthcare legislation require flexible information management systems that can provide timely and appropriate enhancements.

There is little question that efficient information management systems are essential for the provision of modern, high-quality, cost-effective patient care. High-quality care requires online, clinical decision support for the physician while entering medical orders that are not only consistent with up-to-date, evidence-based, clinical-practice guidelines, but that also minimize the occurrence of drug–drug interactions and medication errors. Cost-effective patient care requires ready access to patient record data whenever and wherever needed by the healthcare professionals. Satisfying all such requirements is possible only with computer-based patient records. Cost-effective care cannot be supported by paper-based patient records that often contain illegible notes and are very time consuming for the physician who needs to search for relevant past data in the bulky paper chart of a long-term patient with a chronic disease.

The implementation of a healthcare information management system is further complicated by the intensive training required of its user healthcare professionals to change their habits and behavior. Users of the system must be frequently retrained to exploit new system enhancements to survive in an increasingly competitive healthcare environment. However, since most healthcare professionals are now computer literate, and most physicians now use computers in their offices, the acceptance of a healthcare information system is less of a problem now than it was a decade ago.

Based on my personal experience since the 1960s with healthcare information management systems, I believe the experiences and wisdom of experts from some of the most advanced systems in the world, which are contained in the third edition of this very practical guide, will be of inestimable help to anyone involved in implementing a new healthcare information management system or in operating an existing system.

Morris F. Collen, MD
Director Emeritus, Division of Research
Kaiser Permanente Medical Care Program
Oakland, California

Foreword II

Marion J. Ball, Charlotte A. Weaver, and Joan M. Kiel present to us a book that is a chronicle of numerous recent Information Technology (IT) success stories, a roadmap for continued development, and a vehicle for knowledge sharing that will benefit future IT implementations.

This compilation provides a snapshot of the state of health care IT today. The book's diverse collection of industry insights and strategic analyses combines with many domestic and international case studies to connect the interrelated threads—revealing how each element is tied to the complex tapestry of health care.

This book is also about the future, in two distinct ways. First, it contains forward-thinking accounts of where today's advancements are heading and where the next great opportunities lie. It provides a vision of health care's future, with progressive phases characterized by increasing connectedness, responsiveness, and collaboration.

On a second, more valuable level, this book provides a vehicle for knowledge sharing and continuous improvement that organizations will use to cultivate a new generation of success stories. It shares not only results, but also descriptions of *how* those results were achieved. This book gives you many detailed accounts of real change in real organizations. In doing so, it reveals the various detours and roadblocks along the road that start with IT systems and end in organizational transformation.

When viewed as a whole, certain common threads emerge from the collection of individual submissions. Among them:

- A recognition of the universal value of planning.
- An emphasis on the management of human factors, not just the technology.
- A persistent focus on the customer as a guide for decisions.
- An understanding that true transformation goes beyond the automation of existing processes:

The healthcare leaders who contributed to this book have done more than advance the cause of IT in their organizations. They have taken a vital extra step by sharing their stories for the benefit of the greater healthcare community. Now, we may all learn their lessons, build on their progress, and move closer to our common vision. So, as it helps us *see* a transformed future for health care, this book actually helps us *create* a future of better care through technology.

Judith R. Faulkner
Chief Executive Officer
Epic Systems Corporation

Series Preface

This series is directed to healthcare professionals who are leading the transformation of health care by using information and knowledge to advance the quality of patient care. Launched in 1988 as Computers in Health Care, the series offers a broad range of titles: some are addressed to specific professions such as nursing, medicine, and health administration; others to special areas of practice such as trauma and radiology. Still other books in the series focus on interdisciplinary issues, such as the computer-based patient record, electronic health records, and networked healthcare systems.

Renamed Health Informatics in 1998 to reflect the rapid evolution in the discipline now known as health informatics, the series continues to add titles that contribute to the evolution of the field. In the series, eminent experts, serving as editors or authors, offer their accounts of innovation in health informatics. Increasingly, these accounts go beyond hardware and software to address the role of information in influencing the transformation of healthcare delivery systems around the world. The series also increasingly focuses on "peopleware" and the organizational, behavioral, and societal changes that accompany the diffusion of information technology in health services environments.

These changes will shape health services in the new millennium. By making full and creative use of the technology to tame data and to transform information, health informatics will foster the development of the knowledge age in health care. As coeditors, we pledge to support our professional colleagues and the series readers as they share the advances in the emerging and exciting field of health informatics.

Kathryn J. Hannah
Marion J. Ball

Preface

It has been nine years since publication of the Second Edition of *Healthcare Information Management Systems: A Practical Guide*. In computer time, nine years is six lifetimes of computers, given that computers are replaced every 18 months. Not only has the technology itself changed, but so have the economics of computing, the planning process of system implementation, and the human–computer interaction. On the healthcare side, change has been omnipresent with events such as the Health Insurance Portability and Accountability Act (HIPAA), cost-based proposals such as Medicare reform, the development of strategies for disease management, and managed care reform. When one considers changes that have occurred in the integration of information technology and health care, more wonders appear—the use of personal digital assistants to track patient progress, online patient registration, electronic medical records that patients can access from home, technology as an enabler to quality health care, and healthcare providers who work in a paperless environment. So comparing this edition to the second one, only six chapter topics are based on the same concepts. In a sense, this is the first edition of an entire new philosophy of healthcare computing. But given the dynamics of the current healthcare environment, it will enjoy the same success of the first two editions, if not more.

In the past nine years, new roles have emerged in healthcare computing. No longer is the chief information officer the only player. In today's healthcare environment, other team members have made their appearances, such as the nurse informatician, compliance officer, health information administrator, medical technology officer, security officer, network developer, multimedia coordinator, project manager, technology planner, systems analyst, and the future of health informatics—the student—and the faculties that build that future. All these essential players will benefit from this book. In addition, in recognition of the global character of health care, this book also conveys an international flavor with case studies taken from several corners of the world.

Think about what is involved in either upgrading your present healthcare information systems or embarking on an initiative to explore new technologies. First, you need to develop a plan, perhaps with the help of consultants, and devise a strategy to exercise that plan. In doing so, you can talk to those who have accomplished something similar, either in your country or abroad, and you can review case studies that tie theory to practice. Your journey may not be without obstacles; thus, those who have come before you can provide tried and true lessons from which to learn. This is the premise of Section 1, Chapters 1 to 6. Section 2, Chapters 7 to 11, recognizes that the plan is well underway, but that it must exist within an organizational structure. This section discusses how the organization readies itself for change. It must consider organizational politics, ethics, decision factors, culture, and change agents. Without a thorough analysis of these factors, the healthcare information management system will not ingrain itself into the organization, and, thus, optimal benefits will not be realized. Given this book's theory to practice approach, you will be taken precisely through the steps needed to accomplish this. And this is done in Section 3, through the eyes and minds of those who have lived the experience—the Chief Information Officers and their staffs. Chapters 12 through 22 in this section, convey the "worker bee's" perspective in terms of what it actually takes to transform an organization via information technology and what is actually involved in managing implementation. At times the scenarios may seem futuristic, but these experiences are actually happening, and the dissemination and duplication of sophisticated healthcare information systems is a reality. The reader will notice, however, that are no guarantees or promises of success; rather, one must be daring to confront and overcome obstacles, politics, and culture.

As the book progresses to Section 4, you will become immersed in the utilization and consequences of information technology across the continuum of care. HIPAA, outcomes management, the electronic health record, patient safety, medical errors, pharmacy delivery systems, and so on will showcase just how technology is an enabler in health care. Although the content of the whole book revolves around the patient as the center, this section, in particular, takes a patient-centric approach in portraying the patient as the driver in the utilization of technology. No one who uses this book will walk away a naysayer. In fact, the enthusiasm exuded by these examples is so infectious, both on a domestic and on an international level, that one is tempted to run and start the process of transformation. But wait—Section 5 takes you even further into the future, but with technologies that are, literally, just around the corner. Soon telehealth, evidence-based medicine, Web-enabled medicine, and public health surveillance will become commonplace.

Author-contributors to this book lived their individual chapters, thus making this book highly readable and applicable. This book will become for you a "how to" guide, a technology manual, a planning tool, and so much more as you take on a role in creating a new future for health care. We hope that you will enjoy this book—not only reading it, but also putting into practice information technology as an enabler of quality health care.

Marion J. Ball
Charlotte A. Weaver
Joan M. Kiel

Acknowledgments

The idea for this book emerged out of a need to showcase the rapid changes that are occurring in healthcare information systems today. As you can imagine, the field is rich not only with savvy information technologies and case studies, but more importantly with the people behind them. There are many stories that help us share the wonders of this technology. The Third Edition of this volume captures some of the best, and we thank the following people for helping us bring them to you.

Our greatest thanks go to Nhora Cortes-Comerer, a consulting editor in the field of healthcare informatics, who was extraordinarily supportive through all phases of this project. Her advice and guidance contributed significantly to the overall content and development of this book. Without her dedication, this book would not have been possible.

We would also like to thank our colleagues in our respective professional communities for their support and contributions, in particular, Ivo Nelson, President of Healthlink Incorporated; Dave Garets, Senior Vice President of Healthlink Incorporated; Neal Patterson, CEO of Cerner Corporation; Peter Valotta and Julie Smith of Duquesne University; and Dan Swain.

A resounding thank you also goes out to all the authors and coauthors of the many chapters in this book for their cooperation and commitment in telling the story of healthcare information candidly and professionally.

Many of our colleagues behind the scenes also contributed their time, ideas, and creativity. We are indebted to Dana Sellers, Melinda Costin, Karen Knecht, Andra Granek, Ken O'Quinn, and Amanda LeBlanc of Healthlink Incorporated, and April Martin, Russ Pedersen, Karen Colston, Ann Wurster, Marikay Menard, and Amanda Hurd of Cerner Corporation.

We also want to thank Michelle Schmitt and Laura Gillan DiZerega of Springer-Verlag for their support of the Health Informatics Series and of this volume. A very special note of appreciation goes to Kathryn J. Hannah, who as coeditor of the Springer-Verlag Health Informatics Series, is a constant source of moral support.

Marion J. Ball
Charlotte A. Weaver
Joan M. Kiel

Contents

SECTION 1   PLANNING AND DEVELOPING AN IT STRATEGY

SECTION 2   PREPARING FOR ORGANIZATIONAL CHANGE

SECTION 3   TRANSFORMATION: MAKING IT HAPPEN

SECTION 4   PATIENT-CENTERED TECHNOLOGIES

SECTION 5   OUTLOOK ON FUTURE TECHNOLOGIES

Contributors

Y. Nor Akma, MD, MHA
Deputy Director, Selayang Hospital, Selangor, Malaysia

James G. Anderson, PhD
Professor of Medical Sociology, Co-Director Rural Center for AIDS/STD Prevention, Department of Sociology & Anthropology, Purdue University, West Lafayette, IN, USA

Warren J. Armitage, MBA
General Manager, Strategy and Information, Uniting Healthcare; Director, IT Strategy for Uniting Care, Milton Q, Australia

Ron M. Aryel, MD, MBA
Consultant, Del Rey Technologies, Santa Monica, CA, USA

John W. Bachman, MD
Consultant, Department of Family Medicine, Mayo Clinic; Professor of Family Medicine, Mayo Medical School, Rochester, MN, USA

Marion J. Ball, EdD
Vice President, Clinical Informatics Strategies, Healthlink Incorporated, Baltimore, MD, USA

Edward N. Barthell
Vice President, Infinity Healthcare, Mequon, WI, USA

Beverly Bell, RN, BS, HMA, CPHIMS
Vice President, Healthlink Incorporated, Westerville, OH , USA

Eta S. Berner, EdD
Professor, Health Informatics, Department of Health Services Administration School of Health Related Professions, University of Alabama at Birmingham, Birmingham, AL, USA

Kathryn Bingman
Vice President and General Manager, Cerner Corporation; President, Cerner IQHealth, Kansas City, MO, USA (kbingman@cerner.com)

BERNADETTE BISKUP, RN, MSN
Interim CIO, University of Illinois at Chicago Medical Center, Chicago IL, USA

PIERRE BOIRON, PhD
Chief Engineer, Laboratory and Imaging Systems, Medical Informatics Department, Georges Pompidou University Hospital, Paris, France

DAVID BRADSHAW
Vice President and CIO, Memorial Hermann Healthcare System, Houston, TX, USA

JENNIFER ALLAN BROWNE, RN, BC
Clinical Informatics Coordinator, Methodist Healthcare System, San Antonio, TX, USA

ROBERT J. CAMPBELL, BA, MLS, EdD
Assistant Professor, Department of Health Management Systems, John G. Rangos, Sr., School of Health Science, Duquesne University, Pittsburgh, PA, USA

KRISTINE M. CERCHIARA
Vice President and CIO, The Jewish Home and Hospital Lifecare System, New York, NY, USA

BETTY L. CHANG, DNSc, FNP-C, FAAN
Professor, University of California Los Angeles School of Nursing, Los Angeles, CA, USA

BILL W. CHILDS
Senior Executive, Eclipsys Corporation, Evergreen, CO, USA

NHORA CORTES-COMERER, BA
Independent Consultant, New York, NY, USA

PATRICE DEGOULET, MD, PhD
CIO, Georges Pompidou University Hospital and Cochair of the Public Health and Medical Informatics Department at the Broussais Faculty of Medicine, Paris, France

ELISABETH DELBECKE, RN
Head, Education and Training Programme, Medical Informatics Department, Georges Pompidou University Hospital, Paris, France

JEREMY U. ESPINO, MD
National Library of Medicine Postdoctoral Fellow, RODS Laboratory, Center for Biomedical Informatics, University of Pittsburgh School of Medicine, Pittsburgh, PA, USA

GARY EVANS
President and CEO, Hiawatha Broadband Communications, Inc., Winona, MN, USA

DAVE GARETS, BS
Executive Vice President, Healthlink Incorporated, Snohomish, WA, USA

SURESH GUNASEKARAN
Consultant, Healthlink Incorporated, Houston, TX, USA

PAUL HALL, MD
Former Project Leader, Computerized Patient Record Project, Serafimer Hospital;
Private Practice, Stockholm, Sweden

BETSY S. HERSHER, BA
President, Hersher Associates, Ltd., Northbrook, IL, USA

TONYA HONGSERMEIER, MD, MBA
Corporate Manager, Clinical Knowledge Management and Decision Support, Partners
HealthCare System, Wellesley, MA, USA

JOHN HUMMEL, BS
CIO, Vice President Information Services, Sutter Health, Sacramento, CA, USA

JOAN M. KIEL, PHD, MPA, MPHIL
Chairman, Department of Health Management Systems, John G. Rangos, Sr., School
of Health Science, Duquesne University, Pittsburgh, PA, USA

KATHLEEN COVERT KIMMEL, RN, MHA, CHE
Director, Clinical Information Systems, Catholic Health Initiatives, Louisville, CO,
USA

KAREN L. KNECHT, RN, BSN
Vice President, Advisory/Benefits Realization, Healthlink Incorporated, Houston, TX,
USA

ED KOPETSKY, MS
Executive Vice President, Healthlink Incorporated, Houston, TX, USA

KLAUS A. KUHN, DR. MED.
Professor and Director, Institute of Medical Informatics, and CIO, Philipps-University
Marburg Medical Center, Marburg, Germany

TONYA LA LANDE
Graduate Assistant, Health Informatics Program, Department of Health
Services Administration, School of Health Related Professions, University of Alabama
at Birmingham, Birmingham, AL, USA

CRAIG S. LEDBETTER, RN, BSIS
Manager, Product Development, Misys Healthcare Systems, San Bernardino, CA,
USA

ANNE LEMAISTRE, MD
Medical Director, Information Services, Seton Healthcare Network, Austin, TX,
USA

KEITH J. LIVINGSTON, BBA
Chief Information Officer, ThedaCare, Appleton, WI, USA

NANCY M. LORENZI, PhD
Professor of Biomedical Informatics and Assistant Vice Chancellor for Health Affairs, Vanderbilt University Medical Center, Nashville, TN, USA

GEORGE D. LUNDBERG, MD, ScD
Editor, Medscape General Medicine; Special HealthCare Advisor to the Chair and CEO of WebMD, Los Gatos, CA, USA (glundberg@medscapeinc.com)

PATRICIA L. LUNDBERG, PhD
Associate Professor and Executive Director of the Center for Cultural Discovery and Learning at Indiana University Northwest, Los Gatos, CA, USA

LISE MARIN, MD
Vice Director of the Information Systems Program at the Hospital Informatics Department, Georges Pompidou University Hospital, Paris, France

LEE MARLEY, MHA
Chief Information Officer, Vice President of Technology Assessment, Mills-Peninsula Health Services, A Sutter Health Affiliate, Burlingame, CA, USA

MARY ETTA MILLS, RN, ScD, CNAA, FAAN
Associate Professor of Nursing Informatics and Administration; Assistant Dean for Graduate Studies at the University of Maryland School of Nursing, Baltimore, MD, USA

NEAL L. PATTERSON, MBA
Cofounder, Chairman, Chief Executive Officer, Cerner Corporation, Kansas City, MO, USA

VELMA L. PAYNE, MS, MBA
CIO, OB/GYN Partner, LLC, Pittsburgh, PA, USA

MARVIN PEMBER, MM
Executive Vice President and CFO, Clarian Health Partners, Indianapolis, IN, USA

HANS PETERSON, MD
Former Director, Department of Medical Informatics, Stockholm Health Care Administration and former Senior Medical Adviser to the Swedish Institute for Health Services Development, Stockholm, Sweden

ROBERT J. PICKTON, MBA
Senior Vice President and CEO, Baylor Health Care System, Dallas, TX, USA

ROBERT T. RILEY
Former President, Riley Associates, Nashville, TN, USA

JEFFREY S. ROSE, MD
Vice President and Chief Medical Officer, Cerner Corporation, Kansas City, MO, USA

HADIS ROSNAH, MD, MHP
Director of Telehealth, Ministry of Health, Malaysia

ROBERT A. SCHWYN, MBA
Vice President, Information Services, Children's Hospital, Columbus, OH, USA

FRANCES C. SEEHAUSEN, BSN, MBA
Independent Consultant, Lewisville, NC, USA

JOYCE SENSMEIER, MS, RN, BC, CPHIMS
Director of Professional Services, Healthcare Information and Management Systems
Society (HIMSS), Chicago, IL, USA

ROGER H. SHANNON, MD, FACR, FACMI
Health System Consultant, Belgrade, ME, USA

JOHN S. SILVA, MD
Chief Architect, Silva Consulting Services, Eldersburg, MD, USA

PETER L. STEERE, MBA, RPH
Assistant Professor, Healthcare Administration, Massachusetts College of Pharmacy
and Health Sciences, Boston, MA, USA

DONALD M. STEINWACHS, PhD
Professor and Chair, Department of Health Policy and Management, Johns Hopkins
School of Public Health, Baltimore, MD, USA

NANCY STODDARD, RN, BSN, MBA
Director, Clinical Information Systems, The Jewish Home and Hospital Lifecare
System, New York, NY, USA

ANN C. SULLIVAN, MBA
Senior Vice President and CIO, Maimonides Medical Center, Brooklyn, NY, USA

DARINDA E. SUTTON, RNC, MSN
Director of Clinical Systems, UPMC Health System, Pittsburgh, PA, USA

FU-CHIANG TSUI, PhD
Assistant Research Professor of Medicine and Associate Director, RODS Laboratory,
Center for Biomedical Informatics, University of Pittsburgh, Pittsburgh, PA, USA

MICHAEL M. WAGNER, MD, PhD
Associate Professor of Medicine and Intelligent Systems and Director of the RODS
Laboratory at the Center for Biomedical Informatics, University of Pittsburgh,
Pittsburgh, PA, USA

CHARLOTTE A. WEAVER, RN, MSPH, PhD
CNO and Vice President of Patient Care Systems, Cerner Corporation, Kansas City,
MO, USA

ALLEN R. WENNER, MD
Content Designer, Primetime Medical Software, University of South Carolina School
of Medicine at Columbia, Columbia, SC, USA

TIMOTHY R. ZOPH, BS, MS, MBA
CIO and Vice President, Information Services, Northwestern Memorial Hospital,
Chicago, IL, USA

MOHAMAD AZRIN ZUBIR, MD, MSc, IT
CIO, Selayang Hospital, Selangor, Malaysia

Section 1
Planning and Developing
an IT Strategy

Section Introduction

The title of Chapter 1 in this section, "The Mission of Information Technology in Health Care: Creating a System That Cares" by Neal L. Patterson, the CEO of the Cerner Corporation, can almost be the title for this entire book, or, at least, for this first section. Patterson's chapter serves as the umbrella for the state of the industry of the health information management field. New stakeholders, the rise of consumerism, and the promise of technology are creating the need to continually reexamine how health care is delivered.

As this first section progresses, the framework for planning and developing an organization's information technology strategy is presented. The entire book utilizes an approach that takes the reader from theory to practice. In this section, Chapters 2 and 3 explore issues related to strategic planning, decision making, and the role of consultants in facilitating the process. The theory to practice route of implementing information systems is bombarded with obstacles and confounding issues, of which the book presents creative solutions. Based on this, Chapters 4, 5, and 6 showcase two domestic cases—the first, an integrated health delivery network, the second, a health system rated as one of the best in the United States—and an international case, Sweden. The chapter on Clarian Health System elaborates the utilization of the strategic planning process, mission development, and community outreach to reach its goals. The chapter on the Swedish healthcare system focuses on how government agencies facilitate the strategic planning process with a key element of having input from the citizens. It also brings us valuable information on an issue of major import to health care today, the development of a lifelong electronic health record. This entire section gives promise to all those embarking on information technology changes in their organizations.

1
The Mission of IT in Health Care: Creating a System That Cares

NEAL L. PATTERSON

Information technology is still the best hope for the future of health care. It has unique abilities to shape organizations, automate processes, and create and sustain relationships.

Public concern about the quality and safety of healthcare delivery reached an unparalleled high in the closing days of the 1990s. The patient safety movement that had been growing slowly all decade exploded in November 1999 when the Institute of Medicine of the National Academy of Sciences released a compelling and controversial report claiming that between 44,000 and 98,000 Americans die each year as a result of preventable medical errors [1]. Implicit in the name of the report, *To Err Is Human: Building a Safer Health System*, was the message that we have only one alternative. No matter how much we strive for perfection, it is our nature as human beings to make mistakes. The only way to eradicate inevitable, understandable human errors is to construct a healthcare environment that systematically eliminates threats to our safety.

Concern over alarming deficiencies in safety remains at the forefront of health care today, but any close examination reveals an industry stressed by other systemic issues. Fragmentation of care, escalating costs, significant waste of resources, incoherent incentives, an aging and discontented workforce, inequalities in access, lack of investment capital, and a general lack of preparedness for the future: these are the issues that have kept health care a topic of political debate for more than five decades. Solutions to most of these problems are on a scale that cannot be addressed by individual organizations. Yet without change, the current health system is probably not sustainable for future generations.

Every participant in health care feels the effect of these burdens. As the major bankrollers for the health care of an aging baby boom generation, federal and state governments cry out for relief from widespread inefficiencies and safety hazards. Employer-provided health plans, which replaced group insurance health plans several decades ago, failed to "manage care" during the past decade and now struggle to find sustainable business models in the face of escalating consumer expectations. Corporations strain under the competitive obligation to supply an expensive benefit for employ-

Neal L. Patterson, MBA, is Cofounder, Chairman, and Chief Executive Officer of the Cerner Corporation in Kansas City, MO.

ees. The same company that *advocates* for its workers' safety in the health system in one meeting may *arbitrate* with its workers over healthcare costs in the next. General Electric is a member of the Leapfrog Group for Patient Safety, a coalition of companies that use their combined spending power to invent better patient safety practices [2]. Yet GE is also the company whose labor unions staged a 2-day walkout in January 2003 in a clash over which party would absorb the pain of annually repeating double-digit increases in healthcare costs [3]. This strike was but the opening salvo in what is sure to be a bitter war in years to come if healthcare costs continue to escalate [4].

The health system burden does not merely rest with governments and corporations. On the front line, doctors, nurses, and medical technicians—all historical heroes of medicine—are torn between their original calling to heal people and the increasingly bureaucratic tasks that are now part of their jobs. Executives of healthcare provider organizations are overloaded by the tacit responsibility to act as society's safety net by serving patient populations regardless of their ability to pay. Last, but never least, the consumers of health care also shoulder this burden. These are *the people*, our communities, who come to the system expecting a modern-day miracle, but many times leave frightened, frustrated, and furious that no one seems to be able to break down the silos of information and let the best care come forth. They are our brothers, our sisters, our mothers, our children, our best friends, and ourselves—for the healthcare dilemma is an astonishingly personal crisis.

A New Future for Health Care

So what role can information technology (IT) play amid this array of problems? One obvious, but unsatisfactory, answer is that IT already plays a *reactive* role, responding to the status quo; or as someone once said, "paving the cow paths" with software that reinforces a tangle of negative trends rather than constructing new highways through the wilderness. Bad or simply shortsighted software and platforms already support the infrastructure of much of today's health system. But like the system they support, these reactive IT offerings are fragmented, inefficient, ill-equipped for the future, and, in some cases, more likely to aggravate rather than mitigate risks to the person receiving quality care. Frighteningly, not only did our last generation of IT "solutions" automate the existing silos, they further crystallized many of their negative attributes as well.

The more promising answer is that IT is still the best hope for creating a new future for health care. It is the implied answer in *To Err Is Human*. Information technology has unique abilities to shape organizations, automate processes, and create and sustain relationships. When the right vision and principles guide the creation and use of new IT architectures, key elements in the healthcare crisis will be addressed—and hopefully are being addressed even now. Transformation of health care will occur when these powerful new architectures are deployed to reconstruct our current health system. Achieving this transformation will require amazing focus on the right vision.

That is not to say that this is an easy or even straightforward proposition. This book is about information technology in health care. Taken separately, each half of this topic warrants a level of complexity that fills libraries and consumes careers. To be engaged on either side of this equation is to grapple with a vast, dynamic, and stimulating domain. To stand at the *intersection* of health care and information technology, however, is to recognize the challenge of a lifetime and potentially the opportunity of the new millennium.

Luckily, each of us has adequate motivation to envision this change and see it through. The incentives are inside the thresholds of our homes, possibly within the confines of our own genome. We are motivated to reshape the health system for our loved ones and ourselves. If we put our preconceptions about healthcare delivery aside, the direction of transformation is not difficult to imagine. As we examine the problems and pressures, the solutions become clear. To attend to the basic human desire to be healthy, vibrant, and alive is to serve human dignity. This is a powerful market driver that will never evaporate.

This chapter is broken into three segments. It begins by surveying the current healthcare landscape, examining the inherent complexity of the health system and exposing five adverse conditions that must be eliminated. The second broad segment looks at the forces that are working to compel a transformation. The third and final segment asserts that information technology is elemental to creating a system that cares, and it lays out the fundamental rules that should guide our efforts in this area.

Disintegration of Trust in the Current Environment

Transformation implies an unmistakable change from one state to another. Those who wish to transform health care must understand the current state but never permit that understanding to limit their vision of what health care can be. At the start of the new millennium, the typical metropolitan healthcare delivery system in the United States consists of a patchwork of numerous independent organizations. Physician practices and acute/tertiary care hospitals are fragments at the center. These in turn are surrounded by even more fragmented organizations that provide diagnostic and therapeutic procedures. Home health care and long-term care organizations are coupled loosely from the perimeter.

Former Kaiser Permanente CEO Dr. David Lawrence best described the dire consequences of this fragmentation in an address before the National Press Club in 1999:

Almost all medical care in the United States is delivered in a fragmented, disorganized manner. In such situations, the patient, sometimes working with his or her primary care physician, must assemble the resources required to provide support . . . the hospital, the nursing home, the home health agency, the health education services, the hospice, etc. This is especially difficult for patients with chronic conditions and seriously impairs efforts to deliver effective preventive services that reduce the likelihood of death or disability [5].

A related fragmentation occurs when clinicians or departments fail to collaborate or sometimes even to communicate with one another regarding a person's care. *Millennium Health Imperative: Prescribed Pathways for an Industry on the Critical List*, a report about the healthcare industry published by Cerner and its cosponsor *Modern Healthcare* magazine in June 2001, describes professional factors that reinforce this effect:

Health care is arguably the most balkanized industry in the United States. Our workers tend to function in departmental silos, minimizing the opportunity for cross-functional utilization. Further, professional certification bodies tend to reinforce such separation [6].

This "silo" effect is aggravated by the fact that elements of data collected during individual visits to various specialists often reside in completely separate physical or electronic locations.

Years after he had already become a leading thinker on the subject of quality in health care, Don Berwick, M.D., became an eyewitness to the fragmentation in the system when his own wife became ill:

When Ann Berwick was hospitalized in 1999 with symptoms of a rare autoimmune disorder of the spinal cord, she fell victim to many of the flaws in the U.S. health-care system. Mrs. Berwick was scheduled for immediate treatment with a crucial drug. But even though she was gravely ill, she didn't get the first dose for 60 hours. Again and again, as new doctors got involved in the case, they repeated orders for other drugs that had already been tried unsuccessfully. Hospital staff gathered Mrs. Berwick's vital data, such as blood counts, body temperature and weight, in a disorganized way. And, on three occasions, they left her frightened and alone on a gurney late at night in a hospital subbasement. "Nothing I could do . . . made any difference," recalls her husband, Donald Berwick, a Harvard-trained physician. "It nearly drove me mad."

For Dr. Berwick, it was an eye-opening experience. Eight years earlier, he had founded a non-profit institute bent on improving the quality of medical care in the U.S. "Before, I was concerned," he told a gathering of 2500 medical professionals a few months after his wife's hospitalization. "Now, I have been radicalized" [7].

As Dr. Berwick's account of his wife's experience illustrates, sometimes the person at the center of fragmented care becomes painfully aware that the pieces do not add up to a rational or compassionate whole.

As if a broken-up system of care were not enough of a challenge, the current state of healthcare delivery is also greatly influenced by our human inability to integrate and internalize the large amount of scientific knowledge we create as a race. Simply stated, we can't keep up with ourselves. David Lawrence commented on how this inability to stay current affects the health system:

Physicians and other health professionals must try to keep up with a barrage of new care approaches appearing in a medical literature that expands at a rate of an estimated 1000 articles daily. Though specialty societies provide continuing education and recertification, it is generally accepted that more than half of practicing physicians do not use currently available scientific evidence in their care for patients [7].

This inability to assimilate new knowledge into medical practice may have always existed, but it is spotlighted as never before because of a shift in public awareness caused by the Internet. In a speech to a group of biogenetic executives, Dr. William Neaves, CEO of The Stowers Institute for Medical Research and past dean of the University of Texas Southwestern Medical Center at Dallas, drew an elegant analogy between this modern-day shift and one from the past:

Physicians must prepare for an exponential increase in the mass of medically relevant new information that patients will expect their doctors to master. And patients' expectations grow every day as they rely on the Internet to educate themselves about the latest medical advances. Physicians in the Postgenome Era confront a challenge similar to that experienced by priests during the Reformation.

Prior to the Reformation, priests in medieval Europe enjoyed a monopoly on religious knowledge. Dissemination of the holy word relied on an inefficient, labor-intensive technology. Generating a single copy of the Bible consumed at least a full year of effort by a well-trained and highly skilled scribe wielding a goose quill over vellum sheets. Only the Church possessed enough wealth to sustain the transmission of biblical knowledge from one generation of the priesthood to the next. Ordinary people were ignorant of the written word residing in scarce and inaccessible Bibles. Only ordained priests had direct access to a Bible, and laypeople depended on them to reveal its contents. Priests occupied positions of trust, prestige, and power. In pre-Reformation Europe, it was good to be a priest.

In the second half of the 15th century, a technological breakthrough sowed the seeds of a revolution in the way people acquired information. Gutenberg invented the moveable-type printing press and mass-produced Bibles, an act that triggered many unintended and unimagined consequences. One of them was the Reformation, which shook the foundations of the Church and changed forever the relationship between the priesthood and laypeople.

By the end of the 16th century, ordinary people could own a Bible and read for themselves what was in it. For example, Proverbs 24:5, "vir sapiens fortis est et vir doctus robustus et validus," articulates the concept that knowledge is power. The knowledge monopoly of the priesthood disintegrated, and survivors had to find new ways to add value to the lives of their parishioners. In post-Reformation Europe, it became much harder for priests to know more than their congregations.

Fast-forward 500 years to the second half of the 20th century and consider the parallel between the priesthood during the Reformation and the medical profession as it enters the Postgenome Era. Formerly ignorant patients are being empowered by a new technology that gives ordinary people access to the latest medical information. This time it is the Internet rather than the printing press, but the threat posed to professional hegemony is the same [8].

When a person's level of knowledge collides with a significant difference in what a provider practices, the effect can be similar to the one felt with fragmentation. Unnerved and uncertain, the person feels abandoned by the system and forced into a piecemeal form of self-guided care. For some people, this is empowerment; for too many others, it is an unwanted and potentially dangerous burden.

Health Care's Inherent Complexity

The fragmentation and simultaneous explosion of knowledge in the health system create a complexity that makes it difficult to think about solving problems in a traditional way. There is no single point of authority to "fix" the problem. Paul Plsek's appendix to a second Institute of Medicine report, published in 2001, *Crossing the Quality Chasm: A New Health System for the 21st Century*, advocates using the science of complexity theory (cousin of chaos theory) to explore the healthcare crisis. Rather than thinking of the U.S. health system as an elaborate but ultimately definable mechanical system, Plsek invites us to see it as a "complex adaptive system":

A distinction can also be made between systems that are largely mechanical in nature and those that are naturally adaptive.... In mechanical systems, we can know and predict in great detail what each of the parts will do in response to a given stimulus. Thus, it is possible to study and predict in great detail what the system will do in a variety of circumstances. Complex mechanical systems rarely exhibit surprising, emergent behavior. When they do—for example, an airplane explosion or computer network crash—experts study the phenomenon in detail to design surprise out of future systems.

In complex adaptive systems (CAS), on the other hand, the "parts" (in the case of the U.S. healthcare system, this includes human beings) have the freedom and ability to respond to stimuli in many different and fundamentally unpredictable ways. For this reason, emergent, surprising, creative behavior is a real possibility. Such behavior can be for better or for worse; that is, it can manifest itself as either innovation or error [9, p. 310].

This theoretical framework helps us understand health care as a naturally adaptive system that is acted upon by many agents (the fragments, if you will). These agents include, but are not limited to, government policy, health plans, healthcare delivery organizations, IT companies, researchers, corporations, provider organizations, specialties, individual physicians and caregivers, communities and people. These agents act in self-interest and respond to one another freely, producing all the while an ever-changing array of advancements *and* problems. By thinking of the health system as a complex adaptive system, it is easy to understand how we have arrived where we are today.

Complexity theory paints a picture of constant and seemingly unmanageable change. What hope is there, then, of transforming the system? Fortunately, according to Plsek, the same theoretical framework that gives us such an overwhelming perspective also gives us the expectation that to "design" radical change into the system is not as difficult as we might think. Plsek observes, "A somewhat surprising finding from research on [complex adaptive systems] is that relatively simple rules can lead to complex, emergent, innovative system behavior" [9, p. 315]. In addition, he notes, "experience in the fields of creativity and innovation suggests that changing these underlying rules might result in great innovation" [9, pp. 316–317]. Applying that reasoning to health care, Plsek makes a critical observation about how to design a better system:

It is more helpful to think like a farmer than an engineer or architect in designing a healthcare system. Engineers and architects need to design every detail of a system. This approach is possible because the responses of the component parts are mechanical and, therefore, predictable. In contrast, the farmer knows that he or she can do only so much. The farmer uses knowledge and evidence from past experience, and desires an optimum crop. However, in the end, the farmer simply creates the conditions under which a good crop is possible [9, pp. 314–315].

In this context, designing a system refers to the overall health system rather than to a specific IT system, but it stands to reason that the implications for healthcare IT are the same. To transform the current health system, designers of healthcare IT must seek to change the unfavorable conditions under which healthcare delivery is currently failing to thrive.

Paradoxes: Adverse Conditions in the Current Climate of Care

To get the best yield and ultimately transform health care, there are five negative conditions that must be eliminated: errors, variance, waste, delays, and friction. These are menaces that threaten to nullify the benefits delivered by modern health care. They assault the prime directive that is the distillation of the physician's Hippocratic oath—to first do no harm—and it is time for these contradictions to go.

Preventable Errors

Ask any doctor, nurse, or pharmacist to state the five "rights" of medication administration, and chances are that you will hear, without hesitation, "Right patient, right drug, right dose, right route, and right time." Virtually every degreed clinician can recite this mantra as though Moses carried it down from the mountain on stone tablets. Why is it, then, that a study of 36 institutions published in 2002 by the *Archives of Internal Medicine* reports that medication errors occur in nearly one of five doses given in the typical hospital, and that 7 percent of these errors have the potential to harm the person they are intending to aid? The study's conclusion estimates that the typical 300-bed facility sees more than 40 potentially harmful medication errors a day [10]. Wrong patient, wrong drug, wrong dose, wrong route, and wrong time: these are all scenarios that can and do happen, in addition to a host of other medication-related errors.

The annual cost associated with treating *preventable* adverse drug events to a 700-bed teaching hospital has been estimated to be $2.8 million [11]. This estimate does not include the costs of injuries to patients or malpractice. If the estimate holds true across the U.S., according to the same research, the national cost of preventable adverse drug events is $2 billion [11]. The true cost of errors is inestimable, however, when we consider that human lives are involved.

The same Institute of Medicine report that shocked the nation with the implication that between 44,000 and 98,000 Americans die each year from preventable medical errors offers an answer in its title as to why such errors occur: *To Err Is Human*. The report encourages a departure from the old mindset of blame:

> Even apparently single events or errors are due most often to the convergence of multiple contributing factors. Blaming an individual does not change these factors and the same error is likely to recur. Preventing errors and improving safety for patients requires a systems approach in order to modify the conditions that contribute to errors. People working in health care are among the most educated and dedicated workforce in any industry. The problem is not bad people; the problem is that the system needs to be made safer [1, p. 49].

So long as we depend on humans to routinely do the right thing, we will have errors. Humans are very good at many things, but routine precision is not one of them. Today's health system relies on human memory to be accurate 100 percent of the time. Yet memories are imperfect and subject to many influences, including the amount of sleep we got last night, other things competing for our attention, our state of mind—*Are we grieving? Did our spouse leave us today?*—and not the least of which are our age and how long we have been out of school. Practicing memory-based medicine creates an environment where errors are certain to occur.

Inappropriate Variance

Except for identical twins (or perhaps clones), each of us is biologically unique on this earth. This makes a certain amount of variance implicit in the practice of medicine. In the context of care, however, we are ultimately more similar than we are different. The variance that occurs in the quality of care, and the changing degree to which the best science is used at the point of care, are inappropriate types of variance. This undesired variance is a quiet counterpart to the errors that persist in the current health system. While variance may be an even more consequential problem, it may never capture public attention as the topic of errors already has because it requires an understanding of statistics (not a popular course) and an implicit understanding of what is being measured, which requires understanding an "outcome."

Examples of inappropriate variance in health care are not hard to find. *Millennium Health Imperative* points to three relatively well-known studies [12]:

> [A] recent study demonstrated that a paltry 21% of eligible heart attack patients received beta blockers that, according to established care guidelines, could reduce the risk of a subsequent heart attack; the patients who did not receive the beta blockers experienced a 75% higher death rate than those who did [13]. Another study estimated the percentage of eligible beta blocker recipients to be 49%, still a shockingly low percentage [14].
>
> In a second example, assessments of breast cancer care reveal the underuse of mammography to detect cancer early and the underuse of radiation therapy and chemotherapy after surgery, despite published guidelines for care; the consequences include reduced survival or compromised quality of life [15].
>
> Astonishing—and clinically unexplainable—variation in care exists, heavily influenced by the capacity of the local health system and local physicians' practice patterns rather than by medical need. For example, angioplasty rates exhibit more than a six-fold variation across the country—from 2.3 procedures for every 1,000 Medicare patients in Buffalo, NY to 14.1 per 1,000 in Stockton, CA [16].

Somewhat surprisingly, variance also exists within nationalized systems of health care. In Canada, both the length of time a person waits to receive surgery and the method of determining who is in most urgent need of surgery varies from province to province. The waiting time for coronary bypass surgery ranges from an average of 6 weeks in Ontario to 52 weeks in Newfoundland [17]. Across the United States and the world, the standard of care varies, even though the science is the same and the biology is the same.

Another type of variance that has special significance for the information age is a variance in the way we record information. For example, clinicians in one wing of a hospital might use the term "heart attack" whereas "myocardial infarction" is used in another. As more and more healthcare organizations adopt electronic medical records, this lack of standardization diminishes the usefulness of data in the record.

Underreporting of disease statistics and error is another type of variance that occurs within the health system. A review of available research by the Agency for Healthcare Research and Quality shows a serious trend toward underreporting:

Studies of medical services suggest that only 1.5% of all adverse events result in an incident report and only 6% of adverse drug events are identified through traditional incident reporting or a telephone hotline. The American College of Surgeons estimates that incident reports generally capture only 5–30% of adverse events. A study of a general surgery service showed that only 20% of complications on a surgical service ever resulted in discussion at Morbidity and Mortality rounds [18].

Cerner's own data from a pilot of its *HealthSentry*™ biosurveillance system confirm that underreporting is also an issue at the community level. Infectious disease data electronically collected from 22 healthcare facilities in the Kansas City area over a 200-day period of time demonstrated underreporting in 14 diseases for which reporting was required by the local health department. The traditional method of reporting failed to account for 81 percent of hepatitis C cases, 43 percent of Lyme disease cases, and 74 percent of Chlamydia cases detected by the *HealthSentry* system. For a complete list of diseases included in the study and their outcomes, see Table 1.1. Overall, the number of cases of infectious disease reported to the health department were significantly lower than the number detected by the biosurveillance system [19].

TABLE 1.1. *HealthSentry*™ Biosurveillance System Pilot Data.

Infectious Disease for Which Reporting was Required	Percentage of Cases Unreported by Conventional Means
Campylobacteriosis	41%
Chlamydia	74%
E. coli 0157:H7	67%
Giardiasis	92%*
Gonorrhea	49%
Hepatitis B	43%
Hepatitis C	81%
Influenza	38%
Invasive *Haemophilus influenzae*	50%
Invasive Streptococcal infections	13%
Lyme disease	43%
Salmonellosis	30%
Shigellosis	33%
Syphilis	81%

* Giardiasis was added/removed from the reportable list, hence confusion on whether its reporting was required.

If this level of underreporting is routine for community-acquired infectious diseases, what must it be for medical errors? No health professional would ever be "blamed" for a community-acquired infectious disease, and no possibility for litigation exists. If this amount of underreporting is common when there is no fear of reprisal, what must it be for preventable medical errors, when denial, shame, or fear might hold someone back? Underreporting variance makes it impossible to know the true incidence of medical errors that occur in the system. If this seems like a purely academic point, consider what we lose when information is not reported. Accountability decreases, and we lose the ability to detect data trends that could lead to increased safety in the future.

Finally, a growing body of evidence, highlighted in an Institute of Medicine report entitled *Unequal Treatment*, suggests that a shameful type of variance may exist in the way our health system treats—or fails to treat—minorities. The reporting committee examined new and past research in an attempt to compare the health system treatment of minorities to that of nonminorities. Even after correcting the results for factors involving differences in insurance coverage or ability to pay, the evidence spoke to the fact that racial and ethnic disparities exist in health care and are associated with worse health outcomes [20]. At its heart, the problem of "inappropriate variance" is really just a new way to talk about an old problem, that of inequality. Our health system will not be fixed until this variance is eliminated. Every person who comes to our health system must be treated with the same standard of care.

Waste

Healthcare delivery today is replete with examples of waste. Sometimes this waste is as obvious and thoughtless as the overconsumption of a clearly identifiable resource or raw material. Other times, waste is as subtle as failing to take advantage of a new process or opportunity that has the potential to free human time, effort, or knowledge. *Millennium Health Imperative* offers the following examples of widespread inefficiency in our health system:

- The necessity for duplicating processes such as information collection, patient registration, and scheduling permeates administrative mechanisms.
- Redundant tests and physician visits characterize the structure of care.
- Resources are often quickly and unthinkingly deployed to heroic, high-cost (and litigiously safer) interventions, while ongoing prevention and health promotion activities are underfunded, uncoordinated, or even ignored [6, pp. 24–25].

On a personal level, why are we resigned to telling our allergies, family histories of illness, and personal health history to each link in our circle of care, or to repeat tests because the results have not yet arrived or were done by one of our other physicians? Is it too much to ask the health system we entrust with our lives to at least pretend to know who we are?

The healthcare industry is commonly perceived as a "laggard," failing to invest in information technologies at the same rate as other industries [21]. In an age of automation, it should surprise us that very few hospitals and physician practices have adopted computerized physician order entry (CPOE) solutions, even though effective CPOE solutions give many qualitative and quantitative returns on initial investment [22, 23]. The most sophisticated of these solutions not only eliminate dangerous handwritten prescriptions, but also provide interactive decision support, drug interaction checking, evidence-based alerts, and access to the person's medication profile and laboratory results. In a hospital setting, fully integrated CPOE solutions eliminate the wasteful and potentially dangerous practice of transcribing or reentering physicians' orders in other departments, and allow changes to orders to be recognized instantaneously across all departments, extending as far as the nurse's electronic Medication Administration Record and even the IV pump that sits at the person's bedside. Adoption of CPOE is not an overnight undertaking; it requires advance planning, process change, and cultural leadership within the adopting organization to be successful [24]. Despite the careful planning required, the failure to adopt CPOE at a quicker rate can only be viewed as a waste of opportunity to achieve better health outcomes through technology.

Perhaps the least exposed source of waste is the failure to routinely measure outcomes of care and reapply that knowledge at the point of care, creating a fundamental feedback loop that would correct many issues. A publication of the Office of Quality Management at the University of Medicine & Dentistry of New Jersey offers insight into this preventable waste:

Citing that "we have allowed the public to proceed on the dangerous and expensive assumption that more is better," the U.S. Preventive Services Task Force (USPSTF) reviewed the scientific evidence of over 6000 journals and papers for and against 200 clinical preventive practices. It found that few practices, even the most common ones, were based on scientific evidence. Ineffective use of tests, procedures, drugs and office visits are known to drive up the cost of care. According to USPSTF, the system is not designed to distinguish between needed services and wasteful ones. Group Health Care Cooperative of Puget Sound decided to reduce demand when it discovered overuse of Prostate-Specific Antigen (PSA) test. Through carefully applied patient education, clinical guidelines, outcomes research and feedback, they were able to report that the incidence of misusing PSAs had been reduced from 80 percent to 3 percent [25].

Even in this positive example of waste reduction, there still is room for improvement. Further efficiency could be gained if the guidelines above were data-driven, rather than paper-based, and were referenced and enforced electronically.

Delays

Delays are a fact of life in health care. This is reflected in the design of the doctor's office, where the first thing inside the door is—what else?—the waiting room. Delays are a constituent in some of the most common annoyances and most feared scenarios in health care today.

Delays of access can occur when a person requests same-day care, tries to schedule a visit, and finds that no appointment times have been held open for this purpose. If specialty care is required, additional delays occur due to the referral process, especially in managed care or in countries with publicly administered health care. In the payment layer, manual confirmation of eligibility adds even further delay to accessing care. In some countries, "wait lists" are the norm. In March 2003, the number of people waiting to receive operations in the United Kingdom dropped to just below 1 million for the first time in over 10 years [26].

Once access is gained, the practice of paper-based medicine within a fragmented system proves a major source of everyday delay. Consider the unnecessary and dangerous delay of having to wait for a single paper chart to arrive back in an ICU when an electronic version *could* be accessed from any workstation or PDA in the hospital instead. Or what about the delay involved in locating and transferring radiology films or test results that *could* instead be accessed by a mouse click?

Some delays directly interfere with care; these represent some of the worst-case scenarios in health care. A study of 605 preventable medication errors revealed that 43 percent of these errors were attributed to delayed doses or medications given at the wrong time, including potential adverse drug events such as administering insulin almost 3 hours late [27].

Delays in the diagnosis of chronic and acute conditions eliminate the chance to make life-altering therapeutic decisions. Delayed diagnosis and control of chronic hypertension can lead to cardiovascular disease [28]. The tragic failure to diagnose breast cancer in a timely manner is the leading cause of medical malpractice lawsuits in the U.S. [29].

In the post-9-11, post-anthrax-scare world, delays in disease outbreak detection take on new significance. SARS, anthrax, smallpox, "mad cow," West Nile—whether purposeful or simply pathogenic, these infectious diseases threaten our common public health and security. Unnecessary delays in detecting disease epidemics could prove deadly on a higher level than anything we have collectively known.

Friction

It is generally accepted that more than 20 percent of the cost of health care is consumed in administration of the system, which would be almost $300 billion in the U.S. alone. Most of these resources are consumed in connecting fragments of the system together and provide little added value. In his 1999 address to the National Press Club, mentioned earlier, David Lawrence made these observations about the friction in the system:

Imagine, for example, dealing with 111,000 pages of rules, regulations, guidelines, and protocols, as we must with Medicare. Contrast this with the 12,000 pages needed to clarify IRS requirements. Or consider what it means to meet the expectations of over 100 state and national regulatory, licensing, and accreditation entities, as we do in Kaiser Permanente. Or think about tracking and responding to over 2000 separate pieces of state and federal health care legislation as KP is doing this year [5].

The effects of friction inside the care process were also quantified in a PricewaterhouseCoopers study on the effects of Medicaid paperwork. For every hour a nurse spent caring for a Medicaid patient, another 36 minutes was required to fill out regulatory paperwork. And in the emergency room, where the science of delivering efficient care takes on almost religious significance, the friction was even worse—1 hour of ER care time was repaid by a full hour of paperwork [30]. At Cerner, we spend $300 per person each year shuffling paperwork to process insurance claims for 4800 associates. This has an undesired effect of delaying payment to providers, potentially driving up costs in the future. Friction is the drag in the system that has nothing to do with providing care.

Forces Compelling a Transformation

Errors, variance, waste, delays, and friction are contradictory to the central aims of health care. From a purely analytical perspective, it is clear that health care must be transformed if it is to fulfill its mission. IT holds the promise of being the primary agent of this change. But what are the forces intrinsic and extrinsic to the "complex adaptive system" that will compel it to change?

One of the conclusions of Cerner's *Millennium Health Imperative*, which was the result of a multiyear think-tank endeavor that included two sponsoring organizations and 11 healthcare executives, was that "the industry is being driven by underlying forces toward an all-encompassing strategic shift—an 'inflection point'—potentially culminating in a new system that can function appropriately and efficiently and can achieve true excellence in the provision of safe, effective care" [p. 3]. The report identified and described five forces converging on the health system: demographics, consumerism, biological breakthroughs, information technology, and public mandate. These five forces do not represent *what* will be transformed in the future of healthcare delivery (the negative conditions) or *how* transformation will occur, but they do explain *why* health care is being forced to change. The following five descriptions have been excerpted from *Millennium Health Imperative* with permission from Cerner and *Modern Healthcare*:

Force No. 1: Demographics

The largest demographic cohort in history—the baby boom generation—is reaching the age when health care needs to grow exponentially. At the same time, high healthcare consumption generally is forcing most government- and employer-funded plans to the brink of bankruptcy. The need to serve and finance the aging population is forcing a reassessment of the structure of the U.S. healthcare system and is a forefront topic on virtually every governmental, corporate, and community agenda.

Force No. 2: Consumerism

As is true in all aspects of 21st century life, individuals are demanding the right to manage their own health care and to participate in decision-making regarding choice of providers and treatment alternatives. The Internet alone is fueling a sense of consumer enlightenment that is overhauling every aspect of human interaction regarding medical care, destroying previous hallowed traditions. Enhanced consumer access to medical information is also allowing consumers greater potential for self-care, in terms of both prevention and management of acute and chronic conditions. And consumer demand for greater choice has prompted plans to offer increasingly broad provider panels in order to stay competitive. New healthcare structures must accommodate the needs and desires of consumers, empowering them to participate in decisions regarding their care and coverage and conferring accountability for their healthcare choices.

Force No. 3: Biological Breakthroughs

The Human Genome Project, which reached initial completion in 2000 by both the private sector and the federal government, will revolutionize the fields of prevention, diagnosis, and treatment as genetic mapping creates the means to predetermine and either avoid or postpone many diseases. This will, in turn, create an explosion of new knowledge that will increase the appetite of the empowered consumer. In addition, the move to minimally invasive medicine is already impacting capital and facility factors, and discoveries from cloning experiments, protein investigations and accelerated applications from combinatorial chemistry will make many current treatment protocols obsolete. Any healthcare provider wishing to survive must quickly adapt to accommodate and incorporate new scientific discoveries, eliminating obsolete methods of treatment and harnessing new methods of diagnosing and treating disease.

Force No. 4: Information Technology

Today's fundamental information technology trends are as profound as the fundamental scientific trends that led to the great surges in medical knowledge at the beginning of the 20th century. It is astounding how little the industry truly uses information technology today beyond financial transaction processing. Soon, information technology will envelop health care just as it has other industries, driven by the convergence of computing technologies with communications technologies, increased focus on improving both quality of care and the process of care delivery, and implementation of the electronic patient record. ... At the same time, the Internet will facilitate consumer demand for a more responsive healthcare sector, which will be monitored for all to see. The healthcare sector must speed the adoption of new information technology the way virtually all other industries have done, and, in the process, vastly improve the safety, quality and cost-effectiveness of care.

Force No. 5: Public Mandate

Public awareness of the healthcare industry's shortcomings has increased along with the corresponding news media coverage. In daily newspapers across the country, headlines ring out, exposing the issues: "Snared In HMO Hell" (The Tampa Tribune, 5/6/99); "Overdose by Pharmacy Blamed in Boy's Death" (The Washington Post, 6/10/00); "Ensuring the Care You Get Isn't Botched is Up to You" (The LA Times, 12/20/99). Television news magazines have covered medical malfeasance in lurid detail, as in a recent Dateline NBC story entitled "Routine Surgery?" The Institute of Medicine reports have further fueled the growing public outcry for fundamental change in the nation's health system. The formation of the Leapfrog Group, an alliance of heavy-hitting U.S. businesses that believe in leveraging their health plan purchasing power to protect patient safety, is but one response to the public consternation over health care [6, pp. 15–17].

While all five forces mentioned in *Millennium Health Imperative* represent *reasons* the transformation will occur in the 21st century, only one force also represents the *means* by which the transformation will occur. Visionary IT architectures remain the real vehicle for transformation.

Confidence in IT as the Agent of Transformation

Many advocates of healthcare quality reform initiatives are taking note of information technology's unique position in the landscape of change. The Leapfrog Group, for example, asks its members to favor plans that give access to hospitals with CPOE systems in practice [31]. The powerful assembly of health reformers known as the Jackson Hole Group, previously responsible for ideas that launched the "managed care" movement in the 1970s and the "managed competition" debate in the early 1990s, reconvened in 2002 with a consumer-oriented agenda that identifies information technology as a key component of healthcare reform. A *Wall Street Journal* columnist who attended the group's 2002 meeting described the IT-powered plan of Jackson Hole Group's founder, Dr. Paul Ellwood, in a September 2002, *Wall Street Journal* article:

At the center of Mr. Ellwood's ambitious new proposal is a voluntary system of electronic medical records that would be transportable over the Internet, but owned and controlled by individual patients. Instead of "being secreted away in files in innumerable physicians' offices and hospital record rooms," Dr. Ellwood says, each person's lifetime medical history, or "personal health journal"—from blood tests to drug allergies to insurance data—would be compiled in one record. Patients could make it available to any health-care provider [32].

Furthermore, the 2001 IOM report *Crossing the Quality Chasm* devotes an entire chapter to information technology's potential role in improving the quality of care. The reporting body asserts that IT can effect improvement in *six of six* recommended areas of quality improvement laid out by the Advisory Commission on Consumer Protection and Quality in the Health Care Industry [33]. A 2002 follow-up IOM report, *Fostering Rapid Advances in Health Care: Learning from System Demonstrations*, recommends implementing numerous community-based, connectivity-enhancing IT "demonstration projects" as a way to evaluate potential solutions to national healthcare crises in the United States [34].

Simple Rules to Guide the Transformation

Complexity theory tells us that simple rule changes can have far-reaching effects on the behavior of a complex adaptive system, and that the actions of one agent can have great impact on the entire system. There is reason to believe, then, that by making intentional changes to the underlying rules of healthcare information technology, *all* of health care can be transformed. These implications might have a paralyzing effect on the timid, but they shouldn't. Plsek explains that one of the beauties of the theory of complex adaptive systems (CAS) is that it provides a freedom to act that comes from embracing the unknowable:

Because the parts of a CAS are adaptable and embedded within a unique context, every change within a CAS can stimulate other changes that we could not expect. This approach to system design can never provide the assurance that is possible in a mechanical system. This is the nature of CAS. Therefore, rather than agonizing over plans, the goal is to generate a "good enough plan" and begin to observe what happens. Then, modifications can occur in an evolutionary fashion [9, p. 317].

The invitation to action is clear. The question merely remains as to what the simple rule changes should be. This is where the real vision resides. Fortunately, we are fundamentally motivated by factors close to home. What do we want health care to look like in the future for our children? What do we want it to look like in our old age? Because we all desire dignity and respect for life, the shape of these rules is not difficult to imagine.

1. Build Healthcare IT Architecture Around the Person

Every system architecture has three inherent models: process, data, and information. Many times, these models are poorly expressed and are really just an accumulation of decisions made by system architects, analysts, and programmers. *The person*—not any enterprise—must be at the center of these architectural models. Note that this entity is always *the person* and never *the patient*. *Patient* should never be used as a noun, for it is dehumanizing. Patients are sick, vulnerable, and dependent. *The person* wants to be healthy and independent. Moreover, the word *patient* fails to acknowledge the lifetime of care the transformed health system will provide.

In the current fragmented health system, *patient* is used as a descriptor for an encounter-based relationship that exists between two dates on a calendar. Typically, data are captured from within the parameters of those two dates—say, for an injury or a procedure—rather than within the continuous context of a lifetime. But when does an episode of diabetes end? And after being diagnosed with cancer, when does that episode end? After giving birth to a new life, when does the episode end? The answer is never in a person's lifetime.

Expand the processes beyond the boundary of a single enterprise or organization. Design the data about the person's health and medical problems to be controlled and managed well beyond the encounter. Make the information relevant to an entire lifetime. "Defrag" time.

2. Automate the Process: Eliminate the Paper-Based Record

Eliminate the paper-based medical record—totally. In doing so, a number of indirect objectives will be realized. First, most of the major processes of care delivery will be automated and streamlined, including administrative workflows that will speed access to the system. Next, most of these workflows will be defined much more holistically by modeling the human roles within health care. Finally, the most dangerous medical device will be rendered useless—without any paper, *the pen* will be retired.

Enabling all medical decisions to be made online allows for the possibility that all medical decisions will be made with the most recent medical science available. Also, automating the reporting functions of a department or organization will increase the regulatory compliance that may prevent a disease outbreak or aid the discovery of the next best practice.

3. Connect the Person—from Living Room to Operating Room

Only rarely today do we "institutionalize" a person to deal with his or her medical problems. We still hospitalize a person, but we wait until the acuity and severity of the disease justifies this level of care, and we dismiss the person as soon as possible. In a population full of chronic conditions, the majority of care is delivered outside of a single "enterprise" and is instead delivered by the person or family from home.

Create a lifelong secure personal health record that can be maintained from home, over the Internet. Such a record is an extension of the electronic medical record. It *is* the electronic medical record, accessible at home. It is also automatic. Each interaction with a physician, nurse, pharmacist, laboratory, or technician in the various inpatient, outpatient, home health, public health, and long-term care facilities will contribute something to the personal health record. Allergies, medications, tests, treatments, images, and immunizations will all be here. More importantly, between checkups, each glucose test, each blood pressure reading, each fact and figure relating to the management of a chronic condition or disease recovery will be entered here and can be reviewed by whomever the person chooses. The person has complete control of this private and secure record.

4. Structure, Store, and Study the Information: Make Every Event a Learnable Moment

Every year, month, day, and minute, medically relevant information is carefully collected and recorded. Sometimes this is the result of highly structured research projects, but more often it is the by-product of the care process and is used only for the improvement of the individual encounter or for reporting to a specific interest. When this information is virtually entombed in paper and film (or worse, segmented into a multitude of dead-end electronic data silos), it fails to become part of the collective result of learning we call knowledge. Symptoms, demographic data, diagnoses, procedures, observations, attempted protocols, reasons for overriding common processes, costs, preferences, and outcomes—beneficial and adverse—are all in jeopardy of being lost forever. This waste can be rectified if the potential knowledge is structured, stored, and studied in a way that makes sense. The purpose of this rule is to make sure no opportunity is lost in the future because of an inability to access the information we collected today.

First, structure the information in a way that is useful for future discovery. Capture the specific context, decision, result, and outcome, and preserve them in such a way that they can be rerelated to one another. Build a capacity for measurement into the system. Use universal nomenclatures (or aliases tied to nomenclatures) so that coded outcomes can be compared between different medical specialties, organizations, communities, and countries. Second, store the information in a way that is usable. Integrate the architecture so that redundant (and possibly differing) repositories of data are eliminated. In cases where differing or older data sources are pooled, synchronize the information so that it is ready for analytics. Capture every outcome, and store it in such a way that it can be accessed in the future. Third, study the information that is captured by the system. Mine the data using queries, reports, and summaries designed to reveal outcomes and trends. Compare the information to past data, and that of peer organizations and the rest of the world. In doing so, transform raw information into knowledge.

5. *Close the Loop: Implement Evidence-Based Medicine*

The goal of this rule is to embed access to science inside the core of information technology, making memory-based medicine a thing of the past. To do so, it is necessary to bring referential, empirical, and specific clinical information and content to the point of care to support clinicians' decisions about diagnoses and treatment. Start by establishing sources of referential knowledge and exposing these sources at the points where they are critically needed. Fortify this bedrock of knowledge with an underlying but seldom-seen capability to interrupt action through rules, reminders, and alerts. On the exposed level, seek always to minimize interruptions through the use of order sets, dynamic pathways, and intuitive workflows modeled after human experiences. Likewise, format human interfaces and drug labels to eliminate common but deadly mistakes such as decimal error. Give clinicians access to predictive data in support of outcomes analysis. At all times, mesh scientific excellence with convenience so that knowledge is created only at the precise moment when it is needed. Finally, continually reap the benefit of available benchmark data by generating new content, rules and pathways that will improve clinical and financial outcomes in the future.

The Reintegration of Trust

Basic human dignity is a permanent need, a market driver that will never go away. The five rules outlined above provide the basis for transforming health care in response to this need. In the transformed health system, *the person* will take the rightful place at the center, eliminating the effects of fragmentation and providing a platform of *shared care. The person* will have control of his or her own lifelong personal health record. The data in the personal health record will be the by-product of an efficient system of care and health management where all *avoidable errors, variance, waste, and delays* are eliminated. It will be a *frictionless* system, primarily digital at the center, where core clinical, operational, and management processes are completely automated and paperless. The best scientific evidence available at the moment of decision will guide all clinical decisions. Every decision will provide a *learnable event* from which outcomes are measured and studied. Empirical outcomes will be measured with a universal nomenclature and structure, and then compared to other outcomes realized from within the same organizations, same communities, same countries, and the world to create a continuous discovery of best practice. Most of the friction from non-value-added processes (think insurance claims) will be eliminated, releasing huge capital—estimated to be more than 20 percent of the current spending—for investments in infrastructure. Eliminating errors and variance will contribute another 10 to 20 percent. The phenomenon of unequal treatment will be greatly reduced, and the critical gap between the discovery of best practice and its application will be closed. The natural end result will be that both *the people receiving care* and *the people providing care* will regain confidence in the system.

Is this a vision worth pursuing? Without a doubt. Are powerful IT architectures going to be the lever by which the transformation is attempted? Also doubtless. The environment for widespread adoption of IT as a platform to practice medicine has never been better. Healthcare delivery organizations are facing an increasing set of issues that can only be solved with an effective IT strategy. The expanding capability of fundamental IT platforms and specifically the improvements in healthcare architectures and applications make these solutions more appealing. The attitudes of the major players—primarily healthcare boards of directors, CEOs, doctors, nurses, and the person (patient)—have all changed drastically as information technology has been used with more frequency in their daily lives. Expectations have risen significantly. Moreover, governments and employers are increasingly asking for and expecting a digital health system.

Information technology is uniquely situated as a platform from which to experiment with the kind of simple rule changes that have the potential to transform health care. Once the rules are put into place and the beginnings of a transformation are observed, information technology will also have the necessary ability and agility to continue to tweak and refine the vision in response to the changing needs of the complex adaptive system.

Computers are the only tools by which a vast amount of human knowledge and insight can be collected and reapplied to the world. The microprocessor has won. It is everywhere, being used anytime, anywhere, in anything. Healthcare delivery is no exception. We should take care, however, lest our confidence in the broad potential of IT lulls us into a sense of inevitable victory. This is the right time to remember a proverb from the dawn of the computing age: Garbage In, Garbage Out. The power of information technology is wasted without intelligent design. Inadequately conceived, reactive IT platforms will never transform health care. But passionately conceived, intelligently designed IT architectures just might. The vision must be in everything we do.

References

1. Committee on Quality of Health Care in America, Institute of Medicine. In: Kohn LT, Corrigan JM, Donaldson MS, editors. To err is human: building a safer health system. Washington, DC: National Academy Press; 2000. p. 31.
2. The Leapfrog Group for Patient Safety. About Us [Web Page]. Accessed May 15, 2003, from http://www.leapfroggroup.org/about2.htm.
3. Herper M. GE strike sounds health care alarm. Forbes 2002 Jan 14. Accessed January 21, 2003, from http://www.forbes.com/2003/01/14/cx_mh_0114ge.html.

4. McNeil Hamilton M. GE braces for strike as it lifts co-pays. Washington Post 2003 Jan; Sect E:01.
5. Lawrence D, Kaiser Permanente, speech given before the National Press Club on July 14, 1999. Is Medical Care Obsolete? Transcript retrieved November 15, 2002, from http://www.kaiserpermanente.org/newsroom/releases/speech.html.
6. Cerner Corporation and Modern Healthcare magazine. Millennium Health Imperative: Prescribed Pathways for an Industry on the Critical List. Publication 0324/2001, 2001 June 18. p. 42.
7. Wysocki B Jr. Doctor prescribes quality control for medicine's ills: Don Berwick leads crusade to replace many visits with e-mail, phone calls. The Wall Street Journal 2002 May 30. p. 1.
8. Neaves WB, Stowers Institute for Medical Research, speech given before the Association for Pathology Informatics' Clinical Information System/Life Sciences Roundtable, 2002 July. Transcript retrieved November 16, 2002, from the College of American Pathologists newsletter, CAP Today: http://www.cap.org/captoday/archive/2002/genome_roundtable_feature.html.
9. Plsek P. Appendix B: Redesigning health care with insights from the science of complex adaptive systems. In: Committee on Quality of Health Care in America, Institute of Medicine. Crossing the quality chasm: a new health system for the 21st century. Washington, DC: National Academy Press; 2001.
10. Barker K, Flynn E, Pepper G, et al. Medication errors observed in 36 health care facilities. Arch Intern Med 2002;162:1897–1903.
11. Bates D, Spell N, Cullen D, et al. The costs of adverse drug events in hospitalized patients. JAMA 1997;277(4):307–311.
12. Cerner Corporation and Modern Healthcare magazine; 2001. p. 5, 19.
13. Soumerai SB, McLaughlin TJ, Spiegelman D, et al. Adverse outcomes of under use of beta-blockers in elderly survivors of acute myocardial infarction. JAMA 1997;277:115–121.
14. Millenson ML. The battle for better healthcare. Cerner Report, January 2000.
15. National Cancer Policy Board, Institute of Medicine. National Research Council. Ensuring quality cancer care. Washington, DC: National Academy Press; 1999. p. 3.
16. The Dartmouth Atlas of Health Care in the United States, 1999.
17. The Fraser Institute. Waiting your turn: hospital waiting lists in Canada, 12th ed; 2002 Sept. p. 17.
18. Agency for Healthcare Research and Quality. Making health care safer: a critical analysis of patient safety practices. Chapter 4: Incidence reporting evidence report/technology assessment, No. 43.
19. Cerner's own data gathered from 22 healthcare facilities in the Kansas City, Missouri, area over a 200-day period in 2002.
20. Committee on Understanding and Eliminating Racial and Ethnic Disparities in Health Care, Institute of Medicine. Unequal treatment: confronting racial and ethnic disparities in health care. Washington, DC: National Academy Press; 2002. p. 1.
21. Gaudin S. IT spending is low in healthcare industry. Network World 2000 December 18.
22. Doolan DF, Bates DW. Computerized physician order entry systems in hospitals: mandates and incentives. Health Affairs 2002;21(4):180–188.
23. Center for Information Technology Leadership. The value of computerized provider order entry in ambulatory settings. Executive preview; 2003; p. 6–11.
24. Versel N. CPOE without culture change may increase drug errors. Modern Physician 2003 Feb 11. [Electronic Version.] Accessed May 2, 2003, from http://www.modernphysician.com/printwindow.cms?newsId=507&pageType=news. Note: Article is a report of David Classen's CPOE address at HIMSS 2003.
25. Department of Planning, University of Medicine & Dentistry of New Jersey. Quality Corner, Winter 1998 [Web Page]. Accessed November 15, 2002 from http://www.umdnj.edu/qualityweb/qualitycorner/qcwinter98.htm.
26. Reuters Health. UK Hospital waiting list drops below one million; 2003 May 16. [Electronic Version.] Accessed May 21, 2003, from MedScape http://www.medscape.com/viewarticle/455681.

27. Barker KN, Flynn EA, Pepper GA, et al. Medication errors observed in 36 health care facilities. Arch Intern Med 2002;162:1897–1903.
28. Kannel WB. Blood pressure as a cardiovascular risk factor: prevention and treatment. JAMA 1996;275:1571–1576.
29. Physician Insurers Association of America: Breast Cancer Study. Washington, DC: Physician Insurers Association of America; 1995.
30. American Hospital Association and PricewaterhouseCoopers, Inc. Patients or paperwork: the regulatory burden facing America's hospitals. Chicago: American Hospital Association; 2001.
31. The Leapfrog Group for Patient Safety. Purchasing Principles [Web Page]. Accessed May 29, 2003, from http://www.leapfroggroup.org/purchase1.htm.
32. Landro L. Not so new health group pursues new reform idea. The Wall Street Journal 2002 September 29.
33. Committee on Quality of Health Care in America, Institute of Medicine. Crossing the quality chasm: a new health system for the 21st century. Washington, DC: National Academy Press; 2001. p. 164.
34. Committee on Rapid Advance Demonstration Projects, Institute of Medicine. Fostering rapid advances in health care: learning from system demonstrations. Washington, DC: National Academy Press; 2002. p. 1.

2
Managing the IT Strategic Planning Process

SURESH GUNASEKARAN and DAVE GARETS

The ultimate goal of IT strategic planning is to provide a broad and stable vision of how IT contributes to the long-term success of the organization.

The modern healthcare organization (HCO) is critically dependent on information technology (IT) to accomplish its many administrative and clinical functions. The Information Services (IS) department is now one of the largest internal service organizations in an HCO, supporting the use of IT by all employees and maintaining essential scheduling, billing, and clinical systems that enable the modern healthcare enterprise. Accordingly, IT strategic planning has become a critical part of most HCO corporate planning activities.

The current pressures and mandates on the industry to adopt information technologies as a process of enhancing patient safety and complying with HIIPAA and other industry and legislative initiatives have caused IT to be moved even higher up on the strategic planning agenda. Information technologies are no longer just an item on an annual "wish" list of hardware and software. As the case histories in this book demonstrate, the planning and implementation of clinical and health information systems is now a critical integral part of the healthcare landscape.

This chapter addresses the IT strategic planning process and how it can be best facilitated to meet the robust and diverse IT needs of the modern healthcare enterprise. We specifically focus on managing competing priorities and personalities in a way to develop a holistic IT strategic planning process that best fits the healthcare organization and its business strategy. And finally, we present tools and frameworks to ensure that you can translate your IT strategic vision into operational reality.

IT Strategic Planning Overview

IT strategic planning comes in many shapes and forms depending on the kind of organizations performing it and for what reason. Some organizations perform IT strategic planning as part of an annual corporate or community process, others perform it

Suresh Gunasekaran is a Consultant with Healthlink Incorporated. Dave Garets, BS, is Executive Vice President of Healthlink Incorporated.

because of specific organizational events: change in leadership, mergers or acquisitions, perception of lack of IT value, etc. Regardless of the reason, organizations generally follow the high-level methodology detailed here. A typical IT strategic planning process consists of five major steps.

1. In the first step, the organization defines the strategic context—the strategic backdrop for which the IT strategic plan is being developed. During this phase, the organization identifies (1) why the planning is being conducted, (2) the desired outcomes of the IT strategic planning, and (3) clear executive understanding of the major business priorities at both the organizational and business unit level.

2. Complementary to this phase is a study of current-state IT realities: How effective is the current IT environment and how well does it support current business needs? During this step, the organization takes inventory of its overall IT staff (whether they report to the IS organization or are part of a business unit), assesses the effectiveness of its applications and infrastructure, and identifies vulnerabilities, as well as areas for operational improvement. After the completion of the first two steps, the organization should have a clear understanding of business priorities and the current effectiveness of IT in support of the business.

3. This sets the stage for developing a compelling and unique future-state vision of IT for the organization. Normally, this involves the collaboration of multiple department heads and members of senior management to think about the long-term contributions of IT to the business strategy, specifically, finding areas of focus for IT investments. During this phase, intangible factors, such as corporate culture (what kind of IT innovation would fit our culture?), receptivity to change (how likely are our physicians and staff to accept new technology?), and quality of current IT vendor relationships (how supportive is our IT vendor in developing new products that support our vision?), are taken into account.

4. In this step, strategy options are developed and evaluated in an effort to find the appropriate strategic path to ensure that the IT vision is realized. During this phase, high-level budgets, major IT projects, and vendor product strategies are evaluated in an effort to determine the most viable blueprint for strategy success.

5. The final step is all too often neglected or altogether forgotten after a long and hard planning cycle. Formalizing the strategic plan into an actionable strategy document with budget and project details occurs during this phase. A communication document is developed to inform managers and employees alike of the strategic vision and plan. Most importantly, the executive team facilitates the operationalization of the strategic plan by creating and deploying a strategy implementation plan. It is during the strategy implementation process that specific project leaders are selected, major IT projects are tasked, necessary funds are allocated, and milestones and metrics are established to monitor progress. In addition, areas of organizational reengineering are identified, strategies to align incentives and reward good outcomes are developed, and opportunities to foster organizational ownership are established.

This chapter is largely devoted to successfully managing the latter three steps in the strategic planning process: developing a vision, formulating a strategy, and implementation. Woven into one objective, it would read: To develop, through executive consensus, a compelling long-term vision of a business strategy that is IT supporting which can be successfully implemented by your healthcare organization.

Building the Strategic Planning Team

Creating a comprehensive and sophisticated long-term IT vision during the strategic planning process can be a daunting task, and one of the factors that either facilitates or hinders this process begins with the development and management of the strategic planning team. Quite often, the strategic planning team has very diverse levels of IT understanding, competing business priorities, and a whole host of "below the surface" political agendas. Given this backdrop, it can be quite daunting for the IT leadership to facilitate this group while remaining objective (maintaining the entire group's trust) and effective (maintaining the entire group's interest). IT leadership should drive team consensus by focusing on the basics: building a strong strategic planning team, validating the organizational mission and vision, and defining realistic "guardrails" (boundaries) for the planning process.

One CIO recently remarked, "I can tell you whether strategic planning efforts are going to succeed at an organization simply based on knowing who is on the strategic planning committee." This CIO is right: without a balanced and representative strategic planning team with a very specific charter and support from executive leadership, strategic planning success is impossible. There are several critical success factors in development of the team:

- *Representative Microcosm.* Ensure that representation on the committee is a representative reflection of the customers that IT supports within the organization. Be sure to include representation from potential customers that do not currently take advantage of IT resources.
- *Multiple Levels of Management.* It is important that multiple levels of management are represented on the committee. Clearly for purposes of meeting facilitation, the strategic planning team should not grow beyond 10 to 12 members; however, it is important to engage department heads, executive management, and potentially, board members in the team.
- *External Perspective.* One of the greatest challenges in strategic planning facilitation is getting members of the team to look beyond the four walls of the organization for perspective on what is going in the healthcare IT industry and how IT can contribute to business results outside of current operations. External speakers (CIOs, consultants, and vendors) can be quite useful in providing this perspective.
- *Even Mix of Business Leadership and IT Champions.* It is crucial to balance participation of key business customers with "IT champions," those within your organization who have sophisticated understanding of how IT can improve business and clinical performance. However, a team composed solely of IT champions will not be effective because the rank and file of managers, employees, and physicians might consider the group not to be representative of the level of computer literacy of the organization and therefore to be overly optimistic about the role of IT in achieving business goals. It is important to include "leaders" of the various constituencies of the HCO regardless of their IT literacy.
- *Clear Charter and Executive Support.* A committee is only as powerful as its charter. Ensure that there is a clear, written mandate with executive and board level support so that the planning team can be empowered by the mandate. All too often strategic planning teams flounder because of perceived lack of authority or changing committee charter.

Focusing the Team on a Shared Mission and Vision

It is important to drive team consensus during the IT strategic planning process. To ensure that this can be accomplished, every team member must "start" planning from the same point of reference. The IT strategic planner should initiate the process with a review of the team charter and a mandate of support from the executive leadership. This should then be followed by a review of work accomplished during Steps 1 and 2 of the planning process. This will guarantee that everyone has a clear understanding of why the committee has been established and what it is supposed to accomplish. Further, the review of Steps 1 and 2 will provide a common understanding of where business needs to be headed and where IT is today.

It is equally important to review the organization's mission and vision with the team before commencing discussion of the future of IT. Basic questions, such as who are the customers, how important are research and education to the mission, and what level of community support the organization provides, help cast solid focus for IT planning.

Regardless of the next-generation functionalities of many computer-based patient record application suites, it is important that the strategic planning team understand that "we are a 250-bed community hospital whose primary mission is to serve as many patients in need as efficiently as possible." Placing the organizational mission first, allows the group to start from a point of direction and agreement; it further allows the group to look beyond the way IT is applied today and really question how well IT holistically supports the mission. "If we are an academic medical center, and our three-part mission is clinical service, teaching, and research, why is IT only focused on clinical service?" This starting point also repositions the focus of strategic planning on what the organization needs to succeed as opposed to what new toys vendors are offering this season.

Developing Planning "Guardrails"

Another critical success factor during the strategic planning process is defining the "guardrails" that will ensure that we stay on track during our vision development. Another way of thinking of guardrails is identifying your planning limits: what you cannot change about your organization or IT situation during the strategic planning process. In a perfect world, we could commence a truly "blue-sky" approach to IT development with only our business strategies and the latest vendor products and technologies on the table. However, most often, we are planning for a resource constrained healthcare enterprise with limitations. These limitations take many different forms:

- Budget limitations.
- Staff skill sets and capabilities.
- Existing product vendor relationships.
- Level of executive/board support for IT initiatives.
- Corporate culture.

These limitations should be above discussion: they should be fairly obvious to the members of the committee and the rationale for their inclusion should be fairly self-evident. Once these limitations are identified, a set of guardrails that is positioned as opportunities should be formally established within the planning team. There are a variety of "types" of guardrails. Common types include Executive, Financial, Operational, Cultural, and Technical. A sample set of guardrails is presented in Table 2.1.

TABLE 2.1. Sample strategic planning guardrails.

Guardrail type	Guardrail example
Financial	Available noncommitted IT budget for the upcoming year is $6.2 million.
Operational	New cancer center is being constructed on campus that will require IT investment.
Operational	The CPOE implementation that was initiated last year must be supported and continued.
Cultural	Physician leadership is strongly committed to Epic solutions for ambulatory setting.
Executive	Board of Directors requires a major focus on enterprise patient safety initiatives.
Technical	The majority of IS staff are skilled in mainframe platforms and desktop support.
Technical	The majority of applications in the hospital are from McKesson.

Evaluating Alternatives: Taking a Holistic Approach

Once the future state IT vision is developed (typically in the form of major IT priorities), then the work of evaluating strategic alternatives to achieve that vision begins. It is usually during this step when business unit priorities and personal politics dominate as various different organizational members try to impose their agendas on the process. As an IT strategic planner, it is essential that a holistic perspective that encompasses overall organizational goals be maintained, lest it descend into numerous competing concerns with no means of comparative evaluation. First, it is important that alternatives are in fact developed and fairly evaluated to a relevant level of detail. Each alternative should be assigned to a different team member who is tasked with researching necessary details and making a presentation to the committee with three major areas of focus: the business value of the alternative, the potential organizational impact of the alternative, and the technology risk associated with the investment. We discuss these three areas in greater detail in the following sections.

Determining the Business Case

Determining the business return on investment (ROI) of IT initiatives has returned as an industry hot-button once again. There are multiple ways to evaluate the return on investment of a proposed IT initiative, but largely they fall into three main categories: financial ROI, operational ROI, and clinical quality ROI. Although ultimately the driver of ROI analysis has been to understand when and how the financial investment associated with IT can be recouped, it must be noted that there are many "returns" that are not solely financial: improving patient safety, improving customer satisfaction, improving staff productivity, and improving employee satisfaction/retention, etc. Some of the major metrics used in determining the business ROI of IT initiatives:

- Cost savings.
- Cost avoidance.
- Improved staff productivity.
- Clinical quality improvement/medical outcome improvement.
- Reduced cycle time.
- Improved process accuracy.

- Improved customer (physician/patient) satisfaction.
- Improved employee satisfaction.

Regardless of the metric utilized, it is important that a realistic pro forma estimate of business value be developed with major forecast assumptions. Although projecting these business returns is hardly an exact science, the exercise of developing the projections will serve the organization well during strategy implementation. Furthermore, team members should be encouraged to provide business ROI analysis utilizing business metrics that are regularly used in business management at your organization.

Assessing Organizational Impact

After performing a business case analysis, an organizational impact analysis should be performed to assess the feasibility of implementing the alternative within your organization. Quite often, strategic planners get "disconnected" from operations during the planning process; this step allows for a serious "reality check" within your organization. It is important that strategic planning staff take time to elicit feedback from relevant operational staff and line managers when performing this analysis. Prior to these interactions, a communication document should be developed explaining the strategic planning process and the purpose of these meetings so as to not needlessly cause anxiety and confusion among staff members.

Several variables should be analyzed during the organizational impact analysis. We discuss several of the major variables below, but each organization should select the variables that are most relevant to the current situation. Common variables include:

- *Workload Analysis.* Assess the current and projected workload of staff that will be involved or directly affected by change in technology strategy; this includes staff both within and beyond the IS department. Assess the ability of these staff members to accommodate new tasks or responsibilities resulting from a strategic change.
- *Workflow Analysis.* Understand the way that business is conducted currently within affected business units, and assess whether changes to IT strategy will cause major disruptions to these existing workflows. Specifically, identify targets for business process reengineering and retraining of existing staff members.
- *Affected Cross-Departmental Dependencies.* Most of the departments within a hospital system work closely with other departments. It is important to identify the "cascading" effect of changes in IT strategy on other departments. For instance, a change to the medical records documentation strategy could have significant impact on coding efforts in the business office and chart requests on the unit floors.
- *Downstream Budget and Staff Implications.* In addition to the cross-departmental implications, further budget and staff implications should be analyzed to ascertain whether changes in IT strategy may require additional budget or staff expenditures in other business units. For example, implementation of a point-of-care charge posting billing system could require additional staff on unit floors.
- *Cultural Barriers.* Most organizations exhibit a moderate to healthy resistance to change as staff members are ordinarily vested in organizational policies and procedures. However, over time this investment in "doing the work" a certain way can lead to a corporate culture resistant to cross-department collaboration and reorganization of core processes.

Technology Risk Assessment

The final step of alternative evaluation involves a detailed technology risk assessment to understand the technology implications of the IT strategy alternatives. The overall goals of the risk assessment are to understand the technology feasibility of strategic alternatives while understanding long-term cost and operational implications. Although the level of detail of the assessment can be largely determined by available time and data, relevant vendor research should be at the center of the assessment. Common aspects of a technology risk assessment include:

- *Infrastructure Assessment.* Availability, level of hardware replacement, operating systems management, bandwidth, storage and backup, disaster readiness, and recovery procedures.
- *Applications Assessment.* Product life cycle evaluation, enterprise application integration strategy, user interface design, vendor support strategy, new system implementation costs, and total cost of ownership.
- *Sourcing Assessment.* Skill-mix analysis, availability of development and implementation resources, project management capabilities, and outsourcing analysis.

Strategic Decision Making: Everyone Leaves a Winner

The hallmark of a successful strategic making process is a clear consensus-driven strategic decision that is owned by not only the strategic planning team but also by the organization as a whole. In many cases, after months of excellent planning and due diligence, organizational clarity is lost as factions are unable to reach consensus on a viable IT strategy for the organization. There are usually several reasons for this state of failure:

- *Lack of Clarity Around Business Strategy.* Many organizations struggle in IT strategy development because there is no single shared understanding of the overall business strategy, and often business planning assumptions have not been documented. For instance, there is no clear understanding of whether the health system's major growth strategy is expanded payer contracting, development of specialty health networks, or expansion of bed capacity.
- *Inability to Respect Planning Guardrails.* Some strategic planning teams are not mindful of the guardrails and spend much of their time trying to change these guardrails during the planning process. For example, trying to expand the available IT budget during the planning process is often a remarkable distraction and diverts attention away from how to optimize the utilization of available IT funding. Trying to change an operational guardrail can be equally challenging: attempting to convince physician leadership to accept a centralized financial application can be politically challenging if it was decided during the project initiation that such issues would not be considered.
- *Overly Focused on One IT initiative.* The most common mistake made during the strategic planning process is to focus IT strategy development around one very specific IT initiative (i.e., implementing a computer-based patient record system, outsourcing desktop support, etc.). Focus on one initiative rather than overall business strategy is not only myopic, but it also conditions the organization to think more tactically about their IT investments (and view them as purchases) as opposed to viewing IT investments holistically (in support of a business strategy).
- *Lack of Shared Understanding as to the Role of IT.* Simply stated, organizations struggle to understand the primary and secondary functions of IT within the enter-

prise. Is the goal of IT to replace paper forms with computer forms? Is it to give clinicians better tools to drive care delivery or tools to document care that was provided? Over the long term, successful IT strategies provide an easily communicated message as to the role of IT in supporting health system operations.

As an IT strategic planner, one of the single most effective ways to ensure organization clarity during the planning process is through skillful management of the members of the strategic planning team. It is crucial that the different members of the planning team (each selected specifically to represent various constituencies of the enterprise) gain ownership of the process as well as a shared understanding of the role of IT in supporting the business strategy. There are several useful techniques in facilitating the process. All begin with a clear definition of whose role it is to effect change during various stages of planning:

- *Health system executives determine areas of focus and success criteria.* The executive leadership team (ELT) must provide a clear focus to IT planning efforts by defining the scope and nature of contribution of IT in business strategy. For instance, is the health system primarily focused on using IT to submit claims and ensure timely billing or will the organization rely on IT to drive improvement in clinical quality? The ELT should further define how "success" will be measured in these areas of focus: A/R days, clinical quality outcomes, patient satisfaction, revenue growth, etc.
- *Business unit leaders deliver business value and operational excellence.* Although business unit leaders (BULs) should be provided with the opportunity to contribute to development of corporate business strategy, they should be primarily focused on delivering business value to the organization through operational excellence. That said, the business units are responsible for quality improvement and development of new products and services, as well as improved staff development and productivity. During the planning process, BULs should own all business initiatives (including the IT enablers) and provide detailed project plans around these efforts.
- *IS department delivers reliable technological innovation in support of business performance.* The IS department is ultimately an internal service organization. It typically does not decide where to focus its efforts or force operational improvements; rather, it supports the work of business units at both the executive and operational level. Most modern IS departments are measured along two performance criteria: level of reliability (how reliable are our systems?) and level of technological performance (do our systems meet our needs?). During the planning process, the CIO and IS organization should own IT reliability and performance improvements.

Once these roles are defined, the IT strategic planner must ensure that each team member, based on job orientation (executive, business unit, or IT), stays focused on their critical tasks. Typically, planning teams are undermined by team members who overstep their bounds or conversely do not meet the basic requirements of what is expected of them. One common challenge is when IT leadership attempts to dictate business priorities: the hospital should focus on patient safety because we "know" that IT systems, when properly implemented, can dramatically reduce medical errors. Though IT should participate in discussions of these efforts, enterprise patient safety efforts will only succeed if championed by clinical, compliance, and business leadership. On the other hand, when IT is not perceived as being reliable (the billing system is constantly "going down"), the credibility of the IT leadership is severely undermined when participating in the development of new technology strategies.

Clear role definition is a critical success factor in strategic decision making, but roles should not be used as boundaries to prevent collaboration among team members. In fact, collaboration should be actively encouraged during the planning process. Team trust should also be actively encouraged. Everyone should understand that although one unified team is working together to improve the organization, each team member has different skills and competencies that he or she to brings to bear during plan development. Ultimately, if everyone contributes value, everyone can benefit from the process and own the result.

Strategic Imperative: Creating an Operational Reality

Many organizations incorrectly conclude that development of a strategic plan is the final step in strategic planning. This could not be further from the truth. Strategic planning is in fact a continuous never-ending process with phases cycling between strategy development and strategy implementation. The primary goal of strategy implementation is to create a fit between the newly developed IT strategy and the way that business is conducted within the health system. Many organizations struggle to make this correlation between the IT vision and operational reality, and this places many strategic plans on the shelf only to be rapidly forgotten. There are many challenges to strategy implementation:

- *Too Many Managerial Activities, Too Few Managers.* Implementing new technology strategies can be particularly taxing on health system business and IT managers who typically already have very full workloads. Implementation or optimization of IT systems can often require more management resources than are currently available.
- *Both People and Technology Management Skills Required.* The challenge of successful IT strategy implementation in today's healthcare environment is that health systems require sophisticated leaders with both people and IT management skills to lead strategy implementation efforts. These leaders must have the skills and experience to interact with both business unit leaders and technology vendors to succeed in their roles.
- *Politics and Control Issues.* As with any major strategic change, reporting structures and departmental relationships will be affected by new technology and business processes, and often cultural barriers can derail strategy implementation before it even begins. The most famous examples in the healthcare IT industry of this phenomenon are found in the area of physician compliance with IT policies.
- *Too Many Plans/Too Few Plans.* Quite often, health systems have too many strategic plans that detail high-level ideas of where the system should be headed, but too few detailed plans that help manage the numerous competing priorities within the organization. Many hospitals and health systems have decided to focus on patient safety, revenue cycle management, and supply chain management at the same time with no details on how to manage these competing resource priorities.

To avoid these challenges, healthcare organizations must build a strategy implementation plan in coordination with the development of the IT strategic plan. The implementation plan will present the relevant details to make the IT vision a sustainable long-term reality.

Defining the Strategy Implementation Process

The task of strategy implementation largely has two goals: developing a viable IT roadmap for improvement and a framework for measuring progress toward this vision. Although IT strategies will vary drastically given the unique situations of healthcare organizations, the strategy implementation process typically consists of five steps that are detailed in Table 2.2.

Building Strategy Implementation Structure

Strategy implementation should begin with a clear communication of the IT strategy to the enterprise from executive management. This will convey to the organization the role of IT and its focus in support of the business strategy. Once the strategy has been communicated, a formal strategy implementation structure should be built. This broadly involves three major tasks:

- Selecting the right people.
- Developing the appropriate core competencies.
- Aligning organizational structures.

Selecting the right people is a crucial management competency that is particularly important during strategy implementation. The strategy implementation process is typically a time of great change within the organization, and identifying managers that can help lead this change is crucial to overall success. Identifying the right people involves looking both within the current management structure as well as examining qualified external candidates. Staff members who understand the operational realities of the work involved should be recruited so that they can maintain credibility with business unit staff. Moreover, appoint managers with prior project management experience in relevant IT spaces and key leadership positions. Often, the most valuable asset can be a project manager who has previously implemented the relevant application or is knowledgeable in the necessary business process engineering.

For instance, one large integrated delivery system in the Midwest recently pursued a very comprehensive revenue cycle performance improvement project. To manage this process, they selected two different project managers. They selected a former McKesson project manager to handle the implementation of their Healthquest financial application, and they promoted a former business office manager to help lead orga-

TABLE 2.2. Five-step strategy implementation process.

Step	Description
1. Building strategy implementation structure	HCO develops a capable leadership team with dedicated time and support to implement IT vision.
2. Resource allocation	HCO guarantees budget and staffing resources to manage and perform strategy implementation.
3. Implementing IT-enabled strategic initiatives	HCO implements a set of prioritized IT-enabled strategic initiatives to support business strategy.
4. Quality management/improvement	HCO establishes business metrics to monitor progress toward preset goals and effect continuous improvement.
5. Incentive alignment	HCO establishes incentive structure to reward management and staff efforts to meet business and IT goals.

nizational business process reengineering and training efforts. Balancing both business and IT expertise along with balancing internal promotion with external recruitment allowed this organization to make rapid technological progress while gradually effecting change management within the staff ranks.

In addition to selecting the right people, all organizations must develop specific IT core competencies within their IS departments to enable their business strategy. The specific core competency will vary based on IT strategy; however, it is important to develop a focused core competency. All too often, HCOs have rushed to embrace a "best-of-breed" strategy in application implementation. This has led to the recruitment and retention of numerous generalist IT staff members who can handle work with a large number of vendor solutions. Although this approach often leaves the average IS department with a highly capable generalist staff that can guarantee application reliability and availability, the group does not have the technical or process competencies to offer true IT innovation in specific areas of focus for the health system (patient safety, supply chain management, etc.). For example, numerous HCOs are currently investing in physician order entry systems; however, for the most part, until now these organizations have taken a very siloed approach to their computerized patient record (CPR) environment. This leaves a large competency vacuum: they would like to have strong patient safety competencies that they do not currently enjoy. Over time, they must recruit staff, invest in vendor systems, and effect organizational business process reengineering to truly get value out of their physician order entry systems.

Finally, regardless of the specific core competency that is selected, each major IT strategic initiative must be aligned with a specific unit on the organization chart to improve accountability and to ensure proper focus. All too often, strategic initiatives that are not clearly owned by one or more specific business units fail, as there is not the requisite ownership and discipline to ensure implementation success. Quite often, a matrix reporting structure with representation from both IT and business units can provide an effective balance in the delivery of projects.

Resource Allocation

Without a doubt, timely resource allocation is crucial to strategy implementation. In the modern health system IS department, the normal state of affairs has far too many demands on far too few available resources. The resource allocation process not only should serve to finalize budgets but should also serve as a resource prioritization process to ensure that those initiatives that are most important to overall business strategy receive the majority of resources while other requests are recorded and prioritized based on availability. Moreover, multiyear resource projections should be finalized to ensure that once a project is initiated there will be adequate resources to guarantee completion. Specifically, resources that may be utilized by multiple projects (i.e., infrastructure specialists who would participate in both a clinical system implementation and HIPAA remediation efforts) should be analyzed to ensure that they will be available as necessary to support active projects. Each resource allocation should be tied to specific project plans with project milestones, resource estimates, and sourcing strategies (internal staff and external consultant/outsourcer use). This level of resource detail will allow for continuous monitoring through implementation.

Implementing IT-Enabled Strategic Initiatives

The heart of strategy implementation lies in the delivery of major IT-enabled business initiatives. During this process, there must be adequate collaboration and coordination between the business unit and the IS department to ensure that overall business benefits are realized. For the purposes of strategy implementation, communication of achievement of project milestones and business benefits realized is paramount. Obviously, there are also important implementation best practices discussed in subsequent chapters in this book.

Quality Management/Improvement

It is important that IS projects be measured against business metrics to ensure that business goals are being met and to understand where and how IT plays an integral role in operational improvement. This is easier said than done: the single greatest challenge within many healthcare enterprises is getting adequate business and clinical data on hospital operations. In some health systems this operation is already available and being used in specific areas to manage business units. However, there is still a tremendous void in the area of metrics to assess technology performance relative to business contribution. The most common technology metrics include total cost, application and infrastructure availability statistics, responsiveness of the help desk, and overall use of specific applications. Not a single one of these metrics provides a direct measure on the contribution of IT to business objectives.

In recent years, the first set of metrics that has begun to help manage the performance of technology is often called error reporting. These reports provide information on when a patient registration was incomplete, a claim was denied by the payer, or a charge was not entered with proper documentation. At this time, not all metrics provide useful and actionable information to empower managers. Often these metrics identify when a process has failed, but do not identify what step in the process specifically was errant, resulting in overall process failure. For instance, was the clinic's claim denied because the patient was not eligible for services or because it was coded incorrectly? Many of today's healthcare applications provide these metric-driven monitoring capabilities; others require improvement of out-of-box functionalities.

Incentive Alignment

Regardless of approach, healthcare organizations must identify business operations metrics and use technology to both monitor and improve departmental performance against these metrics. It is also important to have the appropriate metrics in the hands of the right person in the enterprise. The billing clerk requires different reports to improve his or her performance as compared to the CFO. Finally, incentives should be aligned by tying compensation rewards to improvements in these operational metrics. Although this requires significant refinement of the metrics, it is this form of incentive alignment that ultimately guarantees sustainability in the strategic improvement.

Conclusion

The ultimate goal of any IT strategic planning process is to provide a broad and stable vision of how IT can provide a measurable contribution to the long-term success of an organization. The plan must be sophisticated enough to not simply justify a single application purchase or to get an annual budget approved, but rather to have the depth of vision to paint a clear picture of what the contributions of technology will be both 3 years and 5 years from now. All too often, healthcare organizations make a significant error by falsely setting expectations that technology investment will change business behavior overnight. These expectations are rarely met and plant a seed of resistance toward IT-enabled change in the executive team and the user community.

In fact, there is a significant lag between implementation of a technology and the achievement of top-line business benefit. This is driven by the fact that enterprise change can never be driven by changing technology alone; it must be joined by corresponding improvements in business processes and cultural changes in the way that users utilize these new systems and procedures. Most often, successful technology change will have a steady grassroots business effect on the enterprise. For this reason, one must build not only the strategic plan, but also the implementation to ensure that goals can be reached.

The IT strategic planning process should not be done at one moment in time and put on the shelf. Rather, it should be continuously tested and revisited and modified for changing business environments and new technologies. The IT strategic planning process should be used to facilitate discussions both within and across business units as to operations improvements and new business strategies. The true measure of an IT strategic plan is not whether it has all the answers, but whether it is focused on the most important questions.

3
Strategies in Consulting for the 21st Century

Bill W. Childs

As healthcare information explodes and new information systems evolve, consultants are strategically positioned to help balance quality and cost.

Health Care, the Space

Health care is big business. Hovering between 13 and 14 percent of the Gross Domestic Product, national healthcare expenditures are projected to cost about $1.5 trillion in 2003. The U.S. government picked up about 32 percent of this tab in 2000, underscoring why it has such an important say in the practice of medicine, the delivery of health care, and cost reimbursement. Another significant indicator of the rate of growth in health care is Medicare spending, which stood at $3.2 billion in 1967, and today, 36 years later, has risen to $150 billion. In Fiscal Year 2002, the Department of Health and Human Services handled more than 900 million claims. In short, health care is big business. I am not sure we have an accurate number for information systems (IS) spending, but estimates run between 1 and 3 percent of total healthcare spending. Healthcare delivery systems are, of course, a subset of this group, and IS spending for these systems is expected to be $20 billion in 2003.

The Challenge for Consulting

Let us consider, for a moment, the phenomenon of information explosion and its role in health care (Figure 3.1). Doubling of information is now occurring so quickly that scientists who keep track of these figures are often at a loss to say how frequently it is occurring. In medicine, according to a statement by the Chairman of the American Medical Association in 1990, the knowledge base was doubling every 3 to 5 years. Physicians and nurses have been able to manage this information overload for well more than 50 years by concentrating on the specific details of medicine through specialization. Today both physicians and nurses specialize, subspecialize, and even subsubspecialize. Larry Weed, MD, is fond of saying that "with specialization, we know more and more about less and less, until one day we will know everything about nothing."

Bill W. Childs is Senior Executive at the Eclipsys Corporation.

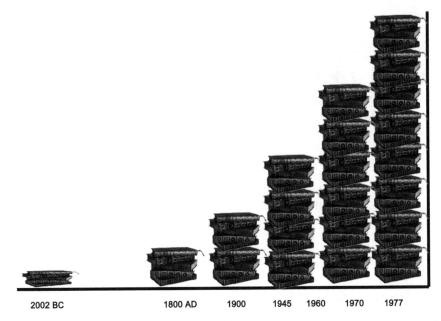

FIGURE 3.1. Since the beginning of recorded information, information moved fairly slowly until about 1800 A.D. when the rate of information growth began to accelerate. Today information doubles at such an alarming rate that only computers are capable of managing this information explosion.

Several years ago, in an editorial in *Healthcare Informatics* magazine, I suggested that to deal with this information overload, we would need to adopt a new paradigm in information technology, which I called "Just-in-Time-Knowledge." The takeoff was obviously from the concept of "Just-in-Time-Inventory," with the premise that there is too much to know, and it would be better if we knew the facts just as we needed them. The trend to develop knowledge-based systems that provide clinical decision support at the point of care is an indication that clearly we are headed toward that paradigm.

While these technologies promise to make some aspects of information explosion more manageable, they arrive at a time of other complicating factors in the delivery of health care. Chief among these is the ratcheting down of reimbursements in the face of ever-expanding new technologies and procedures that promise to enhance quality, yet none of which represent cost savings (Figure 3.2). This problem of balancing cost and quality has been and continues to be a thorn in the side of U.S. health care. Any consultant with the knowledge and ability to come up with a system that addresses these issues and that is properly conceived, designed, built, integrated, and managed would be worth his or her weight in gold.

Potential for Growth

It is difficult to ascertain the actual number of consultants in the healthcare information systems marketplace today, but to arrive at a fair number, one should consider all the various providers, payers, vendors, and government entities that use consultants. A number of experts in this area have proposed estimates that range from 5000 to 15,000 FTE consultants working in health care in 2002. At an average of $100,000 per year in billable hours, we can deduce the cost of consultants to the overall healthcare industry to be in the range of $500 million to $1.5 billion. Although, this is a broad range, both numbers are significant when one considers that every single consultant and other "hangers-on to healthcare" have to be figured into every pill dispensed, surgery performed, and diagnosis rendered.

Consulting in health care recently took a big hit in billable hours with the completion of Y2K assignments. Before this nonevent, there was literally a consultant in every niche of the healthcare marketplace. My own firm, for example, went from annual revenues of about $10 million in 1999 to $4 million in 2000. It was a difficult time for many. Surely, most consultants were not engaged in Y2K issues, but other projects took a backseat to this would-be crisis. A lot of dollars set aside to do many other things were used up in 1999. But what is the state of consulting today, and will this be a growth market again as it was in the last decade of the 20th century?

Consulting firms are actually seeing growth this past year and projecting it into the future. Other firms also expecting growth include the traditional product/systems vendors. There are seven basic reasons why consulting will increase over the next several years:

1. An increasing demand for healthcare services.
2. Our ongoing information explosion.
3. The ever-increasing technological explosion.
4. The growing complexity of medicine and delivery systems.

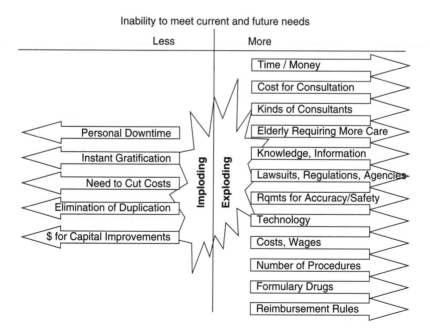

FIGURE 3.2. In the 21st century we face many opposing needs/forces: less time and fewer dollars at a time when we need better and more comprehensive health care and coverage for all. There is so much to do and so little time.

5. Our need and desire to deliver quality patient care.
6. Reduced staffs in our delivery systems due to cost constraints.
7. Increased governing agencies with changing rules and regulations.

The need to find ways to cut costs will also add to the demand for consultants. Consider the fact that almost all healthcare technological advances over the past 30 years have been cost increasing; these include, but are not limited to CAT scans, MRIs, NMRs, beta knives, hundreds of new procedures, and significant advances in drug therapy. Today we are being asked to do more and more with less and less because health care is perceived to cost too much in the United States and, indeed, throughout the world.

There is one rhetorical question, however: Where better to spend our money than on good health? If we could put spare parts in the body when old ones have worn out, make the blind see, cure cancer, diabetes, and heart disease, make the lame walk, and raise up the dead, who among us wouldn't spend the dollars to do it? Indeed, we are already doing many of these very things in hospitals across the nation. New hips, heart valves, corneas, bypasses, skin grafts, joints, cancer cures, transplants, limb lengthening, and the list goes on forever. Complex medicine and patient care are getting more complicated every single day. Does anyone need a knowledgeable consultant? Indeed, when these things were first attempted, a consultant was most likely involved.

Problems and Solutions

The problems in the consultant segment of the market are many and varied. Solutions to healthcare problems often come down to the eye and experience of the beholder— or of his or her consultant. In the past, consultants have attacked problems piecemeal due to budgets or powerful strongholds. We are also guilty of not having looked at some problems and solutions after major changes in the way that health care does business. Some areas that have changed include:

- A shift from fee-for-service to managed care reimbursement.
- A shift from inpatient care to ambulatory care for many services.
- Integration—movement from silos of care and information to continuums of care over multiple caregivers and locations, which creates the need for sharing information.
- A national realization that we can no longer accept 98,000 deaths in the U.S. every year from preventable medical errors.
- Realization that computerized physician order entry and comprehensive electronic medical records within healthcare information systems can make a positive difference in the quality and cost of healthcare delivery systems.

The above are but five examples of changes that are significantly affecting information systems and the delivery of health care.

Meeting Health Care's Needs

On the more positive side of the spectrum, consultants often bring market perspectives and best practices to your attention. In strategic assessments, they can ask the right questions that may focus or refocus priorities in your organization. They also bring strategy, process, systems, and tools to help implement systems and change. Most consulting firms also have access to knowledge bases and benchmarking tools. They bring methodologies, standards, and understanding of regulations that might be extremely important to your operation.

One of the most important areas where consultants make a contribution is when they bring knowledge that your organization does not possess. Difficult-to-find skill sets such as Microsoft, NET or clinical decision support are examples of these needs today. Tomorrow it will be something else. Efforts that are outside the scope of your current information system department's efforts may be another reason to bring in a consultant.

One place to consider bringing in a total outsourcing solution that assumes responsibility for all information systems activity is where it is difficult to attract and maintain good information systems support. Some providers find this to be the best way to proceed, even in large metropolitan areas where qualified help is readily available. It can be a way to effect positive change and off-load responsibility to a qualified organization. Often, clinical information systems vendors will provide substantially reduced prices on their software when coupled with an outsourcing agreement.

New Demands, New Opportunities

Pick up *USA Today*, turn on CNN, or have a conversation with coworkers around the water cooler or on the Internet. The news and conversation are replete with references to miracle cures from weight-reducing surgery to new hair growth to skin peels to limb-lengthening procedures. All represent relatively new healthcare costs and are in demand from health-savvy consumers. There are many more discoveries waiting to be introduced, and the costs are, in some cases, astronomical. Consultants will undoubtedly be asked to give their expert opinion on the practicality of these product lines "making it" in your healthcare delivery system. Major areas of need are related to:

- Strategic issues.
- System selection and implementation.
- Specific ancillary and specialty groups.
- Reimbursement maximization.
- Workflow improvement.
- Challenges to improve quality.
- System integration.
- Process improvement.
- Training.
- Outsourcing.

Consultants and Cost

An old joke about consultants was making the rounds a few years ago: When asked by a customer for the time, a good consultant borrowed the customer's watch and replied, "What time do you want it to be?" Unfortunately, sometimes this can be a true perception, because somewhere along the way, one has received some bad advice from a consultant. As a result, one ends up overlooking the hundreds of good things consultants have done.

Ten characteristics of good consultants:

1. They listen well and are good at making the right suggestions.
2. They have a successful track record at meeting customers' needs.

3. They are organized and capable of developing workable plans.
4. They can deal with a customer's organization at all levels.
5. They are capable of asking the right questions and persistent enough to get the right answers.
6. They have outstanding verbal and written presentation skills.
7. They have the resources to draw upon expertise that the customer or the consultant does not possess.
8. They have the ability to assimilate data into meaningful information.
9. They understand the "big picture" as well as the specific problem they are working on.
10. They recognize that time is money, and they are responsive to customer needs and limitations.

One important addition: They do not immediately waste time plotting an extension or proliferation of the services for which the customer has just contracted. There is time enough for that when the first job is done.

Consultants should represent a valuable return on investment fiscally, in terms of quality, and even intangibly. What price or cost can one place on the reduction of medication errors or the unnecessary death of 1 of the 98,000 patients every year? It is easy enough to add up the savings of reducing your A/R days by 5 every month, but what if your system was able to move managed care patients through your hospital 1 full day faster?

Consultants come in all shapes and sizes. The best often receive recognition from customers who purchase their services and receive a great return on their investment. A recent review of fees shows them to be all over the board. A small independent specialty consultant can charge as little as $50 per hour, while a major consulting firm under contract by a large HMO for a sizeable multiyear project involving a significant number of people can cost as little as $90 per hour. Usually, though, these fees range from $150 per hour to $300 per hour. On another scale, one might also expect to pay more than $2500 an hour for a senior tax partner due to the implications of a purchase/merger with another healthcare provider.

Balancing Opportunity, Cost, and Quality

At the rate of change that we are experiencing in medicine and within our healthcare delivery systems, opportunity abounds; indeed, it appears to be limitless in the foreseeable future. In 50 years time or maybe less, we have the potential to eliminate many of our killer and crippling diseases. Today, we have the capability to implement computerized physician order entry (CPOE) and electronic medical records (EMR) systems at 100 percent levels, seamlessly through all venues of care. Both of these technologies would give providers the ability to significantly reduce avoidable medical errors.

Consultants will play a major role in these ventures. But the journey is also replete with costs. Every new drug, every new instrument, and every new procedure represents a significant cost to us, as taxpayers. But with these triumphs will also come unprecedented and valuable knowledge and information. An essential principle to keep in mind is that the only systems that can and will save dollars are those that are well conceived, designed, built, implemented, and managed. If your organization has not yet arrived, a consultant with the right qualities and qualifications can help it get there.

4
Baylor Health Care: From Integrated Delivery Network to Organized Delivery System

ROBERT J. PICKTON and FRANCES C. SEEHAUSEN

The Integrated Delivery Networks of the 1990s are evolving into the Organized Delivery Systems of the 21st Century.

The delivery of health care in the 1990s was focused on a managed care approach, which emphasized wellness and preventive care, as well as the need for providers to survive in a capitated market. Integrated delivery systems (IDSs) emerged to replace hospital systems, and many IDSs strove to promote functional integration in response to these demands. As experience revealed, however, many organizations found their information systems to be "woefully inadequate." This recognition has led progressively to an evolution from systems focusing primarily on financial and operational functionality to Organized Delivery Systems (ODSs) that incorporate clinical requirements as well as a greater organizational vision and strategy.

Barriers to Integration

A study of 11 healthcare organizations in 1996, *Remaking Health Care in America: Building Organized Delivery Systems* (ODSs) [1], documented the many obstacles that healthcare organizations in the 1990s were encountering in their efforts to implement integrated systems. These included the following:

1. A lack of understanding of integration.
2. The inability to identify the key functions of integration.
3. A lack of commitment to the integration strategy on the part of operating units.
4. A continued focus on the operating unit, especially the hospital, rather than on the system as a whole.
5. A lack of geographic concentration of operating units.
6. A lack of trained personnel.
7. Inadequate information systems.

The study also went on to identify two major barriers to integration posed by information systems themselves:

Robert J. Pickton, MBA, is Senior Vice President and Chief Executive Officer of the Baylor Health Care System. Frances C. Seehausen, BSN, MBA, is an independent consultant.

1. Underdeveloped information systems that inhibited the development of physician systems and clinical integration.
2. The lack of agreement about what constitutes an information system.

Most organizations that participated in the study characterized their information systems as "woefully inadequate for their integration efforts." Few participants had developed patient identifiers, and none had an information system that could link the key actors in a patient episode of care—such as the primary care physician, home care, and hospital—or that could analyze treatment costs and outcomes. Relatively few were far along in assembling the pieces of an information system. In addition, there was no common definition of what the components of a "full-scale" system should be. Many operating units had the necessary data components (financial, administrative, and clinical), limited as they were, but the adoption and implementation of systemwide standards that would allow cross-unit comparison, exchange of data, and merging of data for cost-effectiveness and cost–benefit analysis remained elusive.

As health care entered the new century, information systems emerged with a black eye. The human and financial capital required to make healthcare information systems Year 2000 compliant slowed the key efforts toward system integration. Lost was the momentum built up around clinical integration. In addition, compliance with the Balanced Budget Act of 1997, which created budget shortfalls in many IDSs, caused energy to be redirected toward the implementation of immediate cost-cutting initiatives and reduced investments in information systems.

The Emergence of a New Vision

Within this context, the researchers revisited their 1996 study, now subtitled *The Evolution of Organized Delivery Systems* [2]. The updated survey indicated that it was most important to integrate "information systems along with financial management and operating policies . . . " Despite the obvious importance of information technology (IT), respondents still were not satisfied with progress made in that area. The study further elaborated on the major impediments to integration, despite the expenditure of millions, if not billions, of dollars:

1. No part of the information system was sufficiently developed to become an asset for physicians and clinical integration.
2. Continued lack of agreement about the design and scope of the information system continued to inhibit system integration.
3. Most IDSs in the study continued to characterize their information systems as inadequate.
4. Systems continued to lack a common patient identifier and failed to link key actors involved in a typical episode of patient care. Patient information that was essential for determining treatment cost and outcome was still missing.

Most researchers agreed that an integrated information system was both a key factor in the development of an ODS as well as a consequence of that development: improving information systems helps system integration, and system integration helps develop information systems. They also concluded that continued emphasis should be placed on developing clinical management information systems as the foundation for facilitating overall integration efforts. However, they advised, information system development must also be linked to a system's vision and strategies. The information system of an ODS should be designed around the needs of the various customers (community, patient caregivers, payers, external stakeholders) and incorporate relational data to link patients and providers across the continuum. Information system integration efforts should also focus on information that can be used for continued improvement.

Early Efforts at Baylor Health Care

The Baylor Health Care System (BHCS) was one of 11 IDSs across the United States that participated in the systematic study that served as the basis for *Remaking Health Care in America* [1, 2].

Baylor's tradition of caring began a century ago with the dream of the Reverend George W. Truett to establish a "great humanitarian hospital." Although the healthcare system was officially formed in 1981, Baylor University Medical Center (BUMC), the system's flagship hospital, opened its doors to patients in 1903. Today, the medical center is a major patient care, teaching, and research center in the Southwest.

BHCS, itself, is a network of 15 owned, leased, or affiliated hospitals, as well as primary care physician centers and practices, rehabilitation clinics, senior health centers, affiliated ambulatory surgical centers, and a research institute. As one of the largest private-sector employers in the Dallas-Fort Worth Metropolitan area, Baylor employs more than 14,000 people and has more than 2,800 physicians on its medical staff.

Early BUMC and BHCS efforts to develop and use information systems and technology followed the path taken by many other healthcare institutions. The tendency was to meet financial and operational needs first and to address patient care needs, quality of care, and system integration gradually. In the late 1990s and early 2000s, the emphasis changed to support clinical integration and to evaluate and improve the quality of patient care progressively. Services were also enhanced to support BHCS's diverse operations, the financial management of the system, and each operating unit.

As the organization gained more insight into the opportunities offered by IT in health care, leaders recognized the need for continued growth, improved planning, better measures of success, and opportunities for growth for key individuals in the organization.

Six Principles of High Performance

In 1995, IT managers recognized that physicians should play a vital role in the implementation of IT in health care. The role of chief medical information officer was added to the office of the chief information officer, and a formal strategic partnership was forged between Baylor Information Services (BIS) and the physician leadership.

Early in 1998, BIS adopted the six principles of high-performing IT, a set of principles published by Microsoft/McKinsey [3]:

1. To make IT a business-driven line item activity, not a technology-driven staff function.
2. To demand near-term business results from development efforts.
3. To make IT funding decisions like other business decisions—on the basis of value.
4. To drive constant year-to-year operational productivity improvements.

5. To drive simplicity and flexibility throughout the technology environment.
6. To build a business-smart IT organization and an IT-smart business organization.

Through the adoption of these principles and the aggressive measurement of progress toward goals, the BIS culture has become one committed to delivering the best technology to improve health care.

Organizing Around Core Competencies

BIS provides technical services in support of the strategic initiatives and ongoing operations of BHCS. BIS's services are organized around three core business competencies: technology, applications, and data management. This organization also supports a program management strategy that serves to form all three business competencies into customer-oriented direct accountability for project delivery. Two key cross-departmental areas provide systemwide strategies for customer service support and security. In addition, BIS also offers its customers convenient access to healthcare information through the use of Internet-based technology, as well as through a well-integrated, reliable, and secure networking system. BIS works diligently to ensure the integrity of hospital data, productivity, and efficiency, and ultimately creates standards for systems at all affiliated Baylor hospitals and business units. Figure 4.1 illustrates the BIS Organizational Structure of Corporate, Administrative, and Program functions.

Technology

Technology is a broad term that can blanket many areas, from program code to the latest handheld devices. For an IDS like Baylor, technology has been broken down into four clearly defined areas: networking and telecommunications, communications technology, e-strategy, and operation centers. Each of these areas is crucial to providing the service and information necessary for the care of patients and the support of the employees.

Networking and Telecommunications

Networking and telecommunications are responsible for providing the entire BHCS with voice, video, and data connectivity. This is not a simple task because the network consists of more than 20,000 data connections and spans more than 100 sites. BHCS maintains its own phone switch to support campuses in Dallas and Garland. This switch supplies service to more than 15,000 phones. Plans include integrating all Baylor hospital sites to a single switch. The Baylor fiberoptic network connects all the BHCS campuses, spanning the Dallas–Fort Worth metropolitan area. It operates with better than 99.999% availability, which is crucial when data are required at any time by caregivers making critical decisions concerning patient care. Key criteria in considering the design of the fiberoptic network include reliability, scalability, integration, and being standards-based and value-driven.

Communications Technology

Communications technology is responsible for the enablement of user interfaces, desktop/device management, access solutions, intranet/Internet infrastructure, mobile computing, messaging systems, and servers. The rapid changes in devices

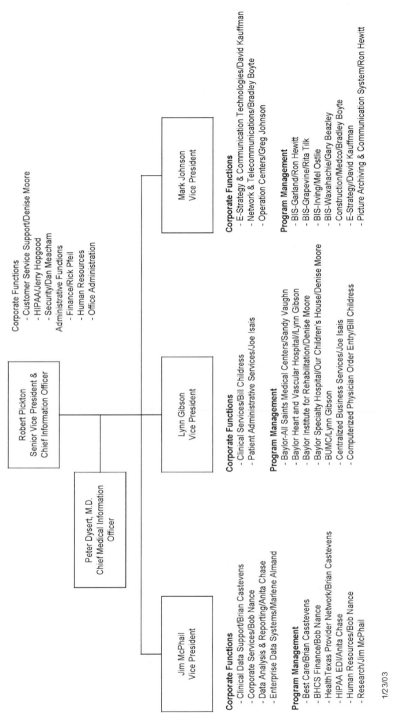

FIGURE 4.1. Baylor Information Services: Organizational Structure of Corporate, Administrative, and Program Functions.

have forced BHCS to support any number of devices that make information easily accessible.

With mobile computing, the user is no longer tied to stationary terminals. BHCS users are employing desktop PCs, notebook PCs, tablet PCs, personal digital assistants, and Blackberry devices through a wired or a wireless connection. Thus, creative solutions are needed for access technologies. Using the principle of keeping it simple and flexible, BHCS works to make access innovative and personalized, fitting the type of work the user performs. Access may be through a private wired Baylor fiberoptic network, a wireless Baylor network, remote access points such as Remote Access Solutions (RAS), a Secured Socket Layer (SSL), Internet connection, or an Internet Virtual Private Network (VPN) service. The right solution is vital to keeping information timely and communication flowing among Baylor employees, affiliated physicians, and varied stakeholders throughout North Texas.

E-Strategy

The e-strategy area is responsible for all Internet products. Both internal and external customers have access to the Web sites; therefore, a uniform look for the entire Baylor system enables users to trust the source of the data. The BIS e-strategy embraces three key areas: consumers, physicians, and enterprise stakeholders.

Consumers

The key objective of Baylor's consumer Web site is to drive business volume by providing content, interactivity, and calls-to-action that engage consumers and invite them to interact with Baylor. To attract consumers and convert them into patients, the Web site helps them get to know Baylor. BHCS provides timely clinical information to patients and consumers in a way that fits their lifestyle.

An average of 150,000 potential patients log on to BaylorHealth.com on a monthly basis. The site's utilization of Internet solutions increases consumer awareness, improves patient service interactions from a clinical and administrative perspective, and establishes greater patient satisfaction with Baylor. The key objective of Baylor's consumer Web site is met by using e-business solutions that focus on direct patient acquisition and retention.

Physicians

Perhaps one of the most challenging quests for any IDS is the ability to integrate all of the available clinical information and have it easily accessed by physicians. Recognizing this as one of the obstacles to becoming a fully integrated ODS, BIS made it a priority to develop portal products that support an aggregated information access point for physicians, employees, and patients. Figure 4.2 illustrates the Baylor Health Care System Portal.

Dr. Peter Dysert, BHCS's chief medical information officer, has said, "The World Wide Web is our best hope for speeding up or eliminating the costly and time-consuming transactions that add layers of waste and inefficiency." This concept dominated the selection of available technology that would allow physicians access to patient data. The result was "My Baylor," a portal based on the "My Yahoo" interface. The portal is defined as a single point of entry whereby a physician can access clinical information to benefit the delivery of care to his or her patients from anywhere at any time.

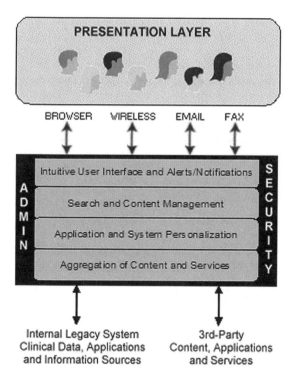

FIGURE 4.2. Baylor Health Care System's portal supports an aggregated information access point for physicians, employees, and patients.

Baylor's portal currently serves more than 2,500 clinical users and provides 24-hour-per-day access to important clinical data, such as fact sheets, lab results, radiology reports, pathology reports, transcribed reports, electrocardiograms, surgery schedules, numerous forms, and various internal publications relating to the healthcare system. This clinical information is presented in a secure and personalized format enabling physicians to see a "real-time" patient census, search for patient information, deputize other physicians and medical office staff to gain access to patient records, and manage preferences for automatic report delivery to e-mail or fax machine.

The Baylor physician portal represents a tool for the organization to create operational efficiencies around how patient information is entered, processed, captured, and presented. The near future holds a vision for Baylor to offer services such as computerized physician order entry and wireless dictation with automated, built-in "patient safety checkers" for drug orders and procedures, further extending and leveraging the investments Baylor has made in using technology to help solve real-world clinical business problems and improve patient care.

Enterprise

The enterprise portal is a critical component of Baylor's vision to become the most trusted source of healthcare information. With the combination of access to critical information from multiple data sources and the integration of wide-ranging enterprise applications, users have everything they need to perform needed tasks right at their fingertips. The enterprise portal offers a single point of access for critical internal data and resources, providing not just information but self-service capabilities, workflow processes, and even integrated application interfaces.

Baylor's enterprise portal enables employees, patients, board members, and business partners to communicate and interact directly over a secure, scalable, and reliable platform. By bringing together communications and collaboration tools, dynamic Internet content, Web services, legacy data sources, and enterprisewide applications, BIS provides Baylor with an enterprise portal that successfully empowers users' access to a central, personalized start page that includes everything they need to do their jobs, regardless of functional role or geography. Utilization of the enterprise portal allows users to fulfill their potential by becoming catalysts for improving health care and creating knowledge from information.

Operation Centers

The operations centers are not glamorous, but without them the very heart of technology would be arrested. They house the equipment, operations, and technical services staff, processes, and procedures that serve all BIS customers. The centers are expected to be available and operating 24 hours a day, 365 days a year. State-of-the-art monitoring tools are required in the command center, and upgrades are made as required to facilitate high-quality operations.

Applications

Almost all IDSs have applications that run the continuum from legacy to clinical to sophisticated monitoring systems. Each offers data about the patient, but it is the ability to integrate these sources and accept a standard for values that can transform data to information and then to knowledge. This is the major challenge of the ODS—making information accessible to the providers of multidimensional care provided in any episode of care.

In the 1990s, same-vendor solutions were recommended to standardize and make data easily and uniformly accessible to the entire user IDS community. As time, financial resources, and technology have shown, this is probably the least effective answer to transform the IDS into an ODS. The review of current systems and the selection of replacement systems or new systems must take into account the six principles stated at the beginning of this chapter.

For corporate services at BHCS, however, the single-vendor solution was beneficial. Accounting, fixed assets, material management, payroll, and treasury were all standardized. For clinical systems, on the other hand, multiple platforms and multiple vendors supply clinical systems for the collection and dissemination of patient data. The applications are selected with an eye to their functionality, their ability to improve clinical productivity, and a clear cost–benefit ratio. The "perfect" clinical application solution is not currently available to the healthcare community. The success of clinical data and the ability to provide it for an ODS rely on portal development, data management, and the ability to provide interfaces to the many sources of data.

With more and more specialized applications being made available to the healthcare community, and with users becoming more sophisticated about the latest technology, it is imperative to understand the business of the user community. IT must be a business-driven activity, one that aligns the strategies of BHCS with user needs while achieving efficiency through IT.

To support efforts to become an ODS with the aid of technology, a partnership is required between the systems champion, IT, users, and selected vendor to review and identify the significance of a new purchase, identify the benefits expected, and then be able to measure them.

The inabilities of healthcare vendors to offer fully integrated ("perfect") solutions with business models that are compelling to IDS have forced the adoption of multi-vendor solutions. We are, however, entering an exciting time. Several vendors have created viable products that fully integrate patient data across the full continuum of care. Implementation of this technology and toolset, coupled with process redesign and people training, give real hope to ODS management that systems will not only become "adequate" but also will realize the promise of becoming accelerators toward achieving integration.

Data Management

Critics of healthcare delivery systems claim that one of the systems' greatest weaknesses is the lack of information or the inability to access information in a timely manner. This drawback is not for lack of effort. There are many external drivers for better data and information, including efforts by the Joint Commission for Accreditation of Healthcare Organizations, the Leapfrog Group, the Institute of Medicine, the Centers for Medicare and Medicaid Services, the National Quality Forum, and state governments. While it is true that an overwhelming amount of paper data is collected, the challenge lies in capturing it in electronic format, standardizing it, storing it, and transforming it into meaningful information, which can lead to improved healthcare decisions. BHCS addressed this concern by creating an internal data management group within BIS.

The data management group is composed of three key areas: enterprise data systems, data analysis and reporting, and clinical data support. The three areas are aligned to provide strategic, analytical, and infrastructure services to ensure BHCS access to reliable, timely, and quality data when and where these are needed.

Enterprise Data Systems

The enterprise data systems area maintains the overall technical infrastructure for the data management group and ensures overall reliability and accessibility to quality data for customers. An enterprise data warehouse, which is a large repository of aggregated administrative data collected throughout BHCS, is also maintained. Various middleware tools are also utilized in this area, including interface engines and extraction, translation, and loading tools. These tools are utilized to move between data and between critical applications both in real-time and in batch mode. Database administration and development functions also reside in this area. Figure 4.3 illustrates the architecture for the data management infrastructure.

Data Analysis and Reporting

The data analysis and reporting area handles state discharge and reporting functions for BHCS, including data submission, data certification, and data analysis and reporting from submission, certification, and the state public use data files. Additional third-party data submissions are performed by this group, including core measures, or

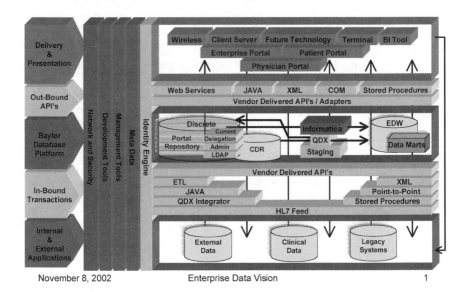

November 8, 2002   Enterprise Data Vision   1

FIGURE 4.3. The Enterprise Data Vision for BHCS, phase III, illustrates the architecture for the data management infrastructure.

ORYX, for the Joint Commission and administrative data for the Texas Health Association (THA) and others. This area also supports research, quality, education, and safety initiatives by performing data mining, reporting, and statistical analysis across a multitude of BHCS data sources. The function supports many reporting and analysis tools, including statistical packages and business intelligence.

Clinical Data Support

The clinical data support area is focused on supporting and managing clinical data initiatives. It provides clinical, project management, process design, and IT expertise. This skill set is applied to quality, research, education, and safety development projects. A significant amount of effort is placed on creating standards for data definitions, nomenclature, and processes. This area also ensures the quality, validity, and integrity of the resulting data. Without clinical data integrity and validity, the resulting information and knowledge desired by clinical users will always be called into question.

Program Management

While functional organization charts serve internal BIS communications and administrative needs well, customers of BIS services prefer, and frankly demand, a single point of contact when dealing with information services requests. The program management approach aligns BIS into a business-driven line activity. Each business unit management team and strategic business area has an accountable BIS management structure and single point of contact and accountability. Another example of how program management supports the organization has to do with acquisitions, new construction, reconstruction, and expansion. These are all part of any healthcare system today. Traditional organizational approaches spread the responsibility to local staff who frequently have varying degrees of expertise in these areas, in much the same way that architects and contractors often consider only the nuts and bolts of a building. Significant last-minute challenges and budget overruns can be avoided when IT oversight of all facilities is assigned to an individual within the IT organization. Cable, electrical, cooling, and storage requirements for technology are only a few of the areas with which this group can assist. This enhances the value of the organization, making it work toward the goal of becoming an ODS.

Customer Service Support

Averaging more than 700 calls a day, the customer service support center is designed to serve BIS customers by providing technical knowledge and assistance while offering the simplicity of a single point of contact. Customer service is the driving factor of this group, which has achieved an average first-call resolution rate of 85 percent. Investment in standard desktops and in automated support tools that allow call tracking, problem history, and resolution via local network and Web access have leveraged knowledge workers in this function. If an issue is not resolved on the first call, it is then triaged to customer service field support. This group is an essential component and provides professional, prompt, and proficient on-site technical assistance.

Security

IT security starts with understanding business needs, developing a strategy (security program) to address those needs, and then applying the current "best practices" (in alignment with the security program and business needs) to meet those needs. Specifically, without a security program architecture and a security policy, the organization cannot communicate or implement security expectations, let alone train employees. Thus, without the core security program, there is no compliance to security because there is nothing with which to comply.

There are four main "speed bumps" that may misalign any security program: lack of senior management support, unreasonable directives, lack of communication and involvement, and limited funding. Organizations may boast about their senior management sponsorship and dedicated security budgets; however, without user support and corporate culture support of security, the information security program will fail. One of the measures of success for a security strategy is the ability to implement reasonable and appropriate information security without impeding the quality of work. Information security implementation occurs through communication, user involvement, and awareness training.

A quick test of an information system security program involves asking two questions:

1. When was the last information security meeting that included members of finance, human resources, internal audit, corporate compliance, general council, marketing, and users?
2. Was it a reactionary meeting to discuss an incident, or was it a proactive meeting to discuss next year's business security plan?

The answers to these questions provide IT with a hint of the direction necessary to achieve information security.

Summary

A wise man said, "The more things change, the more they remain the same." Technology has evolved and made available to the world, especially to the healthcare industry, the tools to make a difference. Yet, despite all the advances in hardware, software, and available tools, the issues remain centered on the healthcare institution: managing the costs and benefits, linking information throughout a system and getting the support of the user community, while providing the best possible care for the patients. BHCS's strategy continues to reflect its tradition of caring, enabled by the complementary strategy of using technology as an accelerator to achieve the goals of the organization. Baylor Information Services has integrated the commitment to deliver the best technology, the best information, and the best user support it can while keeping costs reasonable. A key to helping BHCS evolve into an ODS will be to adhere to the six principles of high-performing IT and to meet the expectations of its customers, both inside and outside the system.

References

1. Shortell SM, Gillies RR, Anderson DA, Erickson KM, Mitchell JB. Remaking health care in America: building organized delivery systems. San Francisco: Jossey-Bass; 1996.
2. Shortell SM, Gillies RR, Anderson DA, Erickson KM, Mitchell JB. Remaking health care in America: the evolution of organized delivery systems, second edition. San Francisco: Jossey-Bass; 2000.
3. Dvorak RE, Holen E, Mark D, Meehan WF. Six principles of high-performance IT. The McKinsey Quarterly 1997; number 3.

5
Clarian Health: Clinical Excellence Through Quality and Patient Safety

Marvin Pember

> *Commitment to excellence and quality and patient safety initiatives have helped placed Clarian Health's hospitals among the top 205 in the nation.*

Commitment to Excellence

Clarian Health is a consolidated healthcare organization that united three premier organizations, Methodist Hospital, Indiana University Academic Medical Center, and Riley Hospital for Children, in 1996. These organizations have distinguished themselves in a variety of ways, including being recognized for advanced surgeries such as Indiana's first kidney, liver, heart, and bone marrow transplants. Committed to excellence in patient care, education, and research, Clarian Health hospitals are recognized as premier healthcare facilities in Indiana and the Midwest.

In a climate of consolidation pressures centering on cost, it is not unusual for a hospital's business imperatives to compete with core values related to patient care. Clarian's leadership, however, strategically and unanimously agreed to take a back-to-basics approach to achieve its stated mission of Clinical, Operational, Service, and Financial Excellence. Crucial to meeting these objectives has been the launching of quality and patient safety initiatives in support of clinical excellence. These initiatives encompass all major components of a successful program: advanced technologies to deliver clinical knowledge in the care process; evidence-based care provided at the point of care; process improvement; performance measures to monitor success; and restructuring to lead and support change. Clarian's mindset has been to go beyond regulatory compliance and assume responsibility for stimulating the passion and proactive leadership needed to achieve continuous process improvement focused on clinical excellence.

Confronting Quality Patient Safety Issues

Clarian's effort began in early 2001 when its executive team began to explore the quality and safety issues facing their organization, as well as other healthcare provider organizations throughout the United States. Among the issues examined was the over-

---

Marvin Pember, MM, is Executive Vice President and Chief Financial Officer of Clarian Health Partners.

and underutilization of healthcare services, as well as the prevalence of medical errors that directly affect the quality of our nation's health care. The Institute of Medicine report, in 1999, *To Err is Human: Building a Safer Health System*, published in 2000, has estimated the number of deaths per year due to medical errors to be between 44,000 and 98,000. The report cites medical errors as the fifth to eighth leading cause of death and claims that medical errors are responsible for more deaths per year than motor vehicle accidents, breast cancer, or AIDS. The report also totals the national cost of preventable adverse events at $17 to $29 billion [1].

Other factors that indirectly contribute to safety and quality include the growing complexity of medical science, the increase in chronic illnesses and the complexity of treating these illnesses, inappropriate variance in treatment, and the pressures of rising costs. The complexity of medical science, including biomedical, care treatment, and drug research has grown significantly during the past 5 to 10 years. This research has resulted in an exponential growth of medical knowledge. Generalists, specialists, nurses, and other clinicians have difficulty finding the most recent medical knowledge and staying current.

One of the advantages of increased medical science and technology is a longer life expectancy. As the elder population increases during the next 10 to 20 years, the need for health services will also increase. Thus the prevalence of chronic conditions will continue to add complexity to the provision of quality health care. Chronic conditions require consistent treatment plans over a longer period of time, the involvement of many different caregivers, and treatments tailored based on an individual patient's needs. Many physicians and caregivers have "individual" preferences on treatment plans and level of appropriate care. This treatment may or may not be based on the evidence produced by the research available. Although treatments may vary based on a patient's needs, inappropriate variance contributes to quality and patient safety issues.

Basing Excellence on Principles

Clarian recognizes that quality and safety are greatly affected when healthcare organizations have a shared mindset about the principles that guide the care process and take actions based on those principles. A second IOM report, *Crossing the Quality Chasm*, published in 2001, offers six principles that can be used by healthcare organizations to set goals and to create a culture focused on quality and safety [2]. These principles propose that care must be:

1. *Safe:* Patients must not be injured by care that is intended to help them.
2. *Effective:* Services should be based on scientific, evidence-based knowledge and provided to all those, and only those, who could benefit.
3. *Patient-centered:* Care provision needs to be respectful of and responsive to individual patient preferences, needs, and values.
4. *Timely:* Waiting and harmful delays must be reduced.
5. *Efficient:* Care provision must avoid waste, including the waste of equipment, supplies, ideas, and energy.
6. *Equitable:* Care provision must not vary in quality because of characteristics such as gender, ethnicity, geographic location, and socioeconomic status.

In recognition that technology and clinical knowledge, particularly when available at the point of care, also enhance quality and safety, the IOM report also delineated five key areas where automation and technology can contribute to improved health care [2]:

- Medical knowledge bases. Providing clinicians and consumers with better clinical evidence.
- Computer-aided decision support systems. Embedding knowledge tools in systems, and training clinicians to use those tools to better facilitate the use of evidence in making care decisions.
- Collection and sharing of clinical information. The automation of patient-specific clinical information is essential in managing the care of chronic conditions.
- Reduction in errors. Standardizing and automating decisions as well as helping identify the source of potential errors, such as adverse drug interactions.
- Enhanced patient and clinician communication. The use of the Web and other technologies to allow electronic communication and better access to health information.

Despite the cost pressures the industry is experiencing, Clarian believes economic resources must be allocated to advance quality care and patient safety. Clarian's administrative and clinical leadership also believes that quality and effective medicine will produce cost-effective medicine as a by-product. Shrinking hospital margins and a weak economy contribute to quality issues. Understaffing or lack of ability to focus resources to create effective processes add to the inability to make quality a focus in the provider environment. Since clinical decisions directly or indirectly drive costs, it is imperative that effective clinical decisions are made such that providers can effectively manage costs.

This conviction has prompted Clarian to implement enterprisewide systems integrating both clinical and financial information across three major facilities (Methodist Hospital, Indiana University Hospital, and Riley Hospital for Children) and all outpatient centers distributed throughout Indianapolis. The fully integrated health information system provides automated processing from the time the patient is registered and scheduled, throughout the acute and ambulatory care process, as well as ending with comprehensive financial management and billing for patient services. The expectation is that many efficiencies and reductions in error will be realized by a comprehensive clinical and financial solution.

In a comprehensive assessment of the market, Cerner had the only system with a new (built within the past 5 to 7 years) architectural platform that could meet the needs of seamless integration of clinical data, resulting in a true Electronic Medical Record. That technical capability was most significantly enhanced by their commitment to building a medical knowledge base that would be fully integrated with the technology platform, resulting in true delivery of the latest medical knowledge at the point of clinical decision making.

The Cerner systems being implemented include the provision of evidence-based care, Computerized Physician Order Entry (CPOE), online physician and nursing documentation, electronic medical record, and a variety of departmental systems. All ancillary and care departments will have access to a patient's single electronic medical record. A personal health record is also available via the Clarian Web site for all registered individuals. The automation of clinical decision support systems will enable the use of clinical best practices and automated workflow for clinical multidisciplinary teams. Computerized physician order entry integrated with the pharmacy solution provides comprehensive drug interaction checking and safety alerts for patient-specific conditions. These technologies will increase the timeliness and availability of information throughout the care process and across multidisciplinary teams throughout their facilities, resulting in a positive impact on quality and patient safety in Clarian's pursuit of Clinical Excellence.

Technology and Knowledge Based on Evidence

Clarian recognizes that clinical excellence cannot be achieved with technology alone; knowledge based on evidence must also be embedded in the technology and systems for use at the point of care. Too many organizations mistakenly think of the electronic medical record (EMR) itself as the goal; instead, the EMR should be considered a dramatic enabler on the path to achieving the real goal of delivering knowledge at the point of care. The knowledge used in the system should be recognized as the standard for clinical practice and aim for the highest quality and patient safety possible. The evidence is referenced online and acknowledges clinical leaders in various specialties, such as cardiology, transplant, orthopedics, and women's services. All members of the multidisciplinary team will have appropriate knowledge from the system, allowing each member to contribute to the team with the appropriate evidence for specific care plans. All benefits and outcomes also have baseline measurements to quantify the increase in quality and effectiveness of the overall organization.

Prioritizing Disease Areas

In a knowledge-based environment, knowledge is made available throughout the organization across both horizontal and vertical clinical processes. Horizontal processes include medication administration, regulatory requirements, ambulatory care, nursing care, and other general patient safety requirements that reach across all parts of the organization. These processes affect many caregivers and patients across more than one clinical center. Vertical processes focus on care provided in specific clinical centers, such as cardiology, women's health, neurology, or orthopedics. The clinical centers base their improvements on evidence-based medicine and improved care processes across the continuum of care.

One of the first steps in developing a knowledge-based environment is to create a framework based on prioritizing disease areas to be treated by clinical centers (Table 5.1). This process rates all disease areas according to three specific factors:

1. Performance improvement opportunity (case volume, potential avoidable days, potential avoidable deaths, avoidable readmission, etc.).
2. Impact potential from clinical knowledge available via research—is clinical evidence available in a specific disease area?
3. Leadership—are there specific clinical leaders and is the structure available to lead the care and technology redesign efforts?

The prioritization process rates highest those disease areas with the most potential clinical impact across the institution. The process is designed to drive clinical best practices, remove inappropriate variance, decrease adverse outcomes, increase patient safety, and leverage the current clinical leadership in the organization to promote change.

The knowledge framework was built by defining the care process for each of the prioritized disease areas. As an example, the care process for congestive heart failure (Figure 5.1) identifies clinical knowledge (noted as gray and black boxes) that can be used by physicians, nurses, other clinicians, or patients across all venues in the care process, including ambulatory, critical care, emergency, surgery, and acute medical care.

Upon identifying the required care process and its associated knowledge interactions, the team researched the evidence needed for that knowledge as well as the

TABLE 5.1. Creating a knowledge framework that prioritizes disease areas and rates highest those areas with most potential clinical impact.

Adult Prioritization Results

Cardiovascular
Acute myocardial infarction
Cardiac dysrhythmias
Cardiac interventions: PCI
Cardiac surgery: CABG
Cardiac surgery: values
Carotid endarterectomy
Heart failure
Hypertension
Major vascular procedures
Stable angina
Unstable angina

Pulmonary
Asthma
Chest procedure (thoracotomy)
COPD
Pneumonia (CAP/HAP)
Mechanical ventilation/tracheostomy

Orthopedics
Back and neck procedures except spinal fusion
Hip replacement
Knee replacement

Gastrointestinal
Esophagitis, gastroenteritis
Gallbladder and biliary tract disease
GI hemorrhage
Major abdominal procedure

Oncology
Bladder cancer
Chemotherapy
Lymphoma and leukemia
Prostate cancer
Testicular cancer

Women's Health
Cesarean section
Normal spontaneous vaginal delivery

Genitourinary
Acute renal failure

Infectious Disease
Fever of unknown origin
Sepsis
Urinary tract infection

Endocrine/Metabolic
Diabetes mellitus

Pediatric Prioritization Results
Cardiac surgery
Asthma
Bronchiolitis
Cystic fibrosis
Pulmonary infections/pneumonia
PICU ventilator mgmt
Diabetes/DKA
NICU: Prematurity
Fever

technology/system tools needed for using it. These technology/system tools include orders, order sets, alerts, reminders, structured clinical documentation, reference documentation, and patient education media. The resulting framework identified the venue, process flow, clinical knowledge to be used in the care process, associated evidence, and tools to be used for embedding the knowledge in the system. An example for cardiac surgery (CABG) is shown in Figure 5.2.

Building Blocks and Process for Change

In addition to technology and evidence-based knowledge as enablers for change, several other building blocks drive change throughout the Clarian organization. Chief among these is performance improvement and change management. Change cannot be sustained without the application of performance improvement techniques in the care process. Performance improvement is structured within Clarian in such a way that processes can be changed and enhanced on a continuous basis. Change management is also essential to the change process as well as building a culture of continuous learning.

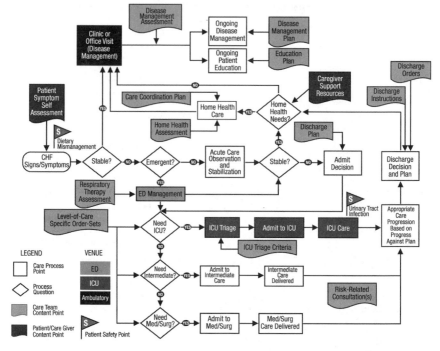

FIGURE 5.1. The knowledge framework is built by defining the care process for each of the prioritized disease areas. This is an example of the care process for congestive heart failure. The process identifies clinical knowledge (noted on the legend as Content Points) that can be used by physicians, nurses, other clinicians, or patients across all venues in the care process.

Content Guideline Cardiac Surgery CABG

Content Formats
PF = Power Form
PN = Power Note
FS = Flowsheet
O = Orders or Order Sets
CP = Clinical Pathways
RP = Report
DS = Decision Support
A = Alternative Mechanism
ST = Smart Template

Venue	Process	Clinical Process Flow	Discipline	Content Points	Content Format	Content Sources	Content Sources
Acute	Assess	Assess Person-RN: History	RN	Assessment Form	PF	ACC CABG Surgery Guidelines	Zynx Clinical Pathway Constructor
Acute	Assess	Assess Person-RN: Physical Exam	RN	RN Assessment Form	PF	ACC CABG Surgery Guidelines	Zynx Clinical Pathway Constructor
Acute	Plan Care	Initiate Interdisciplinary Clinical Pathway/Orders	RN/MD	Clinical Pathway	CP	ACC CABG Surgery Guidelines	Zynx Clinical Pathway Constructor
Acute	Deliver Care	Test at Point of Care	RN	Clinical Pathway	PF, CP, DS	ACC CABG Surgery Guidelines	Zynx Clinical Pathway Constructor
Acute	Assess	Assess Person-Physician: HPI	MD	Physician Admission History and Physical	PN	ACC CABG Surgery Guidelines	Zynx Clinical Pathway Constructor
Acute	Assess	Assess Person-Physician: PMHx	MD	Physician Admission History and Physical	PN	ACC CABG Surgery Guidelines	Zynx Clinical Pathway Constructor
Acute	Assess	Assess Person-Physician: Physical Exam	MD	Physician Admission History and Physical	PN	ACC CABG Surgery Guidelines	Zynx Clinical Pathway Constructor
Acute	Assess	Establish Working Diagnosis	MD	Physician Power Note	PN	ACC CABG Surgery Guidelines	Zynx Clinical Pathway Constructor
Acute	Assess	Stratify Risk	MD	Prognosis Assessment	PN, DS	ACC CABG Surgery Guidelines	Zynx Clinical Pathway Constructor
Acute	Plan Care	Order/Perform Diagnostic Evaluation	MD/Other	Clinical Pathway	PN, O, CP	ACC CABG Surgery Guidelines	Zynx Clinical Pathway Constructor
Acute	Assess	Review/Document Findings	MD/RN/Other	Physician Note and Nursing Note	PN, O, CP	ACC CABG Surgery Guidelines	Zynx Clinical Pathway Constructor

FIGURE 5.2. The framework for Cardiac Surgery (CABG) identifies the venue, process flow, and clinical knowledge to be used in the care process.

The ongoing change management and performance improvement process is known as the Clarian Knowledge-Driven Care process. It begins with an analysis of both the evidence-based knowledge and the actual care experience used in the organization. This knowledge is assembled and vetted with the appropriate clinical stakeholders. The knowledge is embedded in the software for testing and deployment. Performance measures and feedback are gathered as the care process and knowledge are used throughout the organization. Updates are made to the knowledge on a continuous basis as part of the learning organization model.

This process is only successful when the Clarian multidisciplinary teams are actively involved in the process. The Clarian clinical leadership, which includes nurse executives and physician executives/leaders, is instrumental in championing and leading the use of knowledge in the care process. Some factors that influence physician acceptance of knowledge-based care include:

- Its impact on the quality of patient care.
- Commitment of the clinical leadership.
- Influence of other physician champions.
- Recognition that use of the system makes life "easier."
- Engagement of the physician, by the system, as the leader and authority in the care of the patient.
- Ownership by the clinical team of the new care process(es).
- Creation of a culture, focused on Clinical Excellence, that is led by Physician and Nurse Executives.

Organizing for Quality Care

Clarian's Clinical Quality Program is led and managed by the Quality and Patient Care Committee. This Committee is directly accountable to the Clarian Board of Directors. Because clinical excellence is the heart of the Clarian mission, the Board of Directors is actively engaged in the sponsorship and ownership of the Clinical Quality Program. The Executive Leadership Team, Chief Medical Officer, Chief Medical Informatics Officer, and Vice President of Nursing Quality lead the multidisciplinary teams managing change in the line organization. All processes and departments throughout the organization are involved in the process, including laboratory, surgery, emergency, pharmacy, general patient care, critical care, medication management and safety, patient access, ambulatory, and physician processes (Figure 5.3).

Quality Steering Committee

The Quality Steering Committee is chartered with the leadership, direction, and coordination of Clarian's continuous process improvement efforts. Membership consists of physician executives, nurse executives, VP of Nursing Quality, and the Chief Medical Information Officer. The primary functions of the committee include:

- Medical staff quality oversight.
- Establishing mission and vision for quality and performance improvement.
- Developing a conceptual framework for quality and performance improvement.
- Providing guidelines for project prioritization matrix.
- Preparing metrics and report cards pertaining to quality of care for the Quality and Patient Care Committee of the Board.

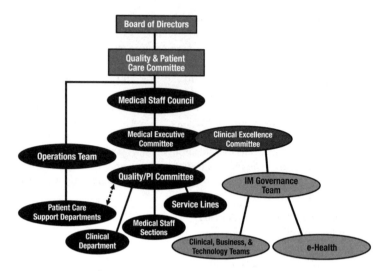

FIGURE 5.3. Clarian's Quality and Patient Care Committee heads the Clinical Quality Program and reports directly to the Board of Directors.

Clinical Practice Improvements

Clarian is focused on measuring both quality and patient safety in the organization. Clinical practice improvements are measured by adjusted length of stay, improved time to diagnostics, decreased adverse drug events, reduced complications, reduced mortality rates, and improved quality of life. Other improvements such as patient safety, patient satisfaction, regulatory compliance, supply management, and operative services are measured and monitored for increased operational efficiencies. Patient safety and patient satisfaction metrics include decreased falls, decreased adverse drug events, decreased ED wait times, timely bed placement, and patient satisfaction ratings. Operational efficiencies in supply management are measured by decreased product costs associated with consistent product usage, standardized products for specific treatment protocols, and availability of supplies. Operative services' metrics include decreased days in PACU, first case on-time starts, improved infection control, and standardized instrument management.

One example of the implementation of clinical practice improvement involves the redesign process for heart transplants. This process has the potential of improving the heart transplant survival rate to more than 85 percent, improving quality of life by increasing time at home, and reducing length of stay. Two programs will be implemented: (1) A fast-track protocol to improve efficiencies in time to transplant listing, and (2) pre-transplant home management program. The leadership personnel engaged in defining and managing the new program are a lead transplant surgeon, a transplant cardiologist, and a cardiac care center director. The heart transplant home maintenance program is planned to provide biweekly outpatient visits, increased communication and relationship with a home infusion nurse, increased communication and relationship with a home care nurse, laboratory markers, and a nutritional, exercise, and weight program. Outcomes are measured by in-home deaths, readmission to hospital before transplant admission, number of cardiac arrhythmias, morbidity/mortality, and patient/family satisfaction.

Leadership from Industry and Government

Many organizations are focused on promoting quality and safety in the industry. The leaders include various government, academic, and commercial organizations such as the Centers for Medicare and Medicaid Services, the Leapfrog Group, the Joint Commission on Accreditation of Healthcare Organizations (JCAHO), the Agency for Healthcare Quality and Research (AHQR), and the Risk Management Foundation of the Harvard Medical Institutions (RMF).

The Leapfrog Group, a coalition of some of the nation's major employers and purchasers of healthcare services, is one of the largest advocates for measures to improve patient safety. Leapfrog leverages its purchasing power by selecting healthcare service providers who are actively pursuing the application of information technologies to improve patient safety and enhance customer value [3]. The Leapfrog Group has focused its patient safety initiatives in three major technology areas: Computer Physician Order Entry, Evidence-based Hospital Referral, and ICU Physician Staffing.

JCAHO recently began the collection of clinical core measure sets for measuring safety and quality from providers in 2002. The program began with ORYX, which focused on the collection of statistics; however, the core measures program standardizes the data collected across all hospitals and providers. JCAHO has produced 6 National Patient Safety Goals and 11 recommendations to guide providers in achieving quality and safety in the care environment. The 6 safety goals are as follows: (1) to improve the accuracy of patient identification; (2) to improve effective communication among caregivers; (3) to improve the safety of using high-alert medications; (4) to eliminate wrong site, patient, or procedure surgery; (5) to improve safety of using infusion pumps; and (6) to improve the effectiveness of clinical alarm systems [4].

AHRQ, the Agency for Healthcare Research and Quality, has made substantial investments in patient safety and quality studies. Its mission is "to support research designed to improve the outcomes and quality of healthcare, reduce its costs, address patient safety and medical errors, and broaden access to effective services" [5]. AHRQ has a significant number of research projects and initiatives under way; several of the initiatives that specifically affect quality include outcomes measurement, quality indicators, and evidence-based medicine.

As can be seen, there are many organizations working on quality and safety. It is also appropriate to ask to what degree providers, themselves, are organizing to lead the efforts to influence quality and safety. Should healthcare providers be more aggressive in publishing quality indicators, gathering and synthesizing evidence, and defining best practice? Will the provider community wait to be driven by one or more of the external agencies or be more proactive in defining high quality and safe care for the communities they serve? The answers will become more evident as the drive to achieve quality care and patient safety continues.

Conclusion

Clarian has assumed responsibility for stimulating the passion and proactive leadership needed to achieve its goal of continuous process improvement focused on clinical excellence. Furthermore, it is committed to transcending a mindset of mere regulatory compliance. The Quality and Patient Safety initiatives it has implemented include all the components for a successful program: advanced technology, evidence-based medicine, process improvement, measures to monitor success, and a structure to lead and support change.

References

1. Kohn LT, Corrigan JM, Donaldson MS, editors. Committee on Quality Health Care in America, Institute of Medicine. To err is human: building a safer health system. Washington, DC: National Academy Press; 2000.
2. Committee on Quality of Healthcare in America, Institute of Medicine. Crossing the quality chasm: a new health system for the 21st century. Washington, DC: National Academy Press; 2001.
3. The Leapfrog Group, Patient Safety Initiatives to drive great leaps in patient safety. *www.leapfroggroup.org*, December 2001.
4. Joint Commission on Accreditation of Healthcare Organizations. www.JCAHO.org.
5. Quality Assessment and Research Findings. www.ahrq.gov.

6
INTERNATIONAL PERSPECTIVE
Sweden: The Evolution of Healthcare Information

HANS PETERSON and PAUL HALL

Sweden's long history in the collection and processing of medical information has allowed its systems to keep pace with evolving technology and changing healthcare requirements.

Sweden's Public Health System

Sweden is a unitary state with its political power being distributed among three layers: the central government, the regional governments, and the municipalities. Swedish citizens pay taxes to all three administrations.

The responsibility for formulating policy and standardized procedures has been retained by the central government, while the responsibility for the provision of health care is divested in the 17 county councils (local governments) and 3 regional administrations. Taking care of elderly people is the responsibility of the 280 municipalities.

With a national population of nearly 9 million people, it is clear that the average county cannot provide a full range of medical facilities. To overcome this problem, seven particular centers have been designated to provide a full range of services and the country is divided into seven corresponding health regions. Stockholm, the capital city, is one of these regional centers. Its catchment region is the county of Stockholm and the lightly populated island of Gotland. The total population of this area, less than 2 million people, is virtually 22 percent of the national population, and that makes Stockholm the most populous of the seven regions.

Each county or health region is responsible by law for providing all its residents with both outpatient and inpatient care for illness, injury, deformity, and childbirth, to the extent that they do not receive care from other sources. Private medical practice exists, and the State health insurance authorities reimburse patients for visits to private practitioners, but each county must offer similar services through hospital or outpatient facilities, and neighborhood outpatient centers have a salient and increasing role in this regard. The Swedish public health system is based upon compulsory state insurance.

Hans Peterson, MD, was Director of the Department of Medical Informatics at the greater Stockholm Health Care Administration from 1971 until his retirement in 1994. He then served as Senior Medical Adviser to the Swedish Institute for Health Services Development until 2001. Paul Hall, MD, was the project leader for the Computerized Patient Record project at the Serafimer Hospital, which started in 1962. He was at the Karolinska University Hospital from 1966 to 1974, when he went into private practice.

Every citizen more than 16 years of age pays for his or her insurance through state tax. Children are included in their parents' insurance. The patient pays a standard fee for hospital care, which was just over $1 per day in 1970 and has increased over the years to around $10 in 2001. The fee for ambulatory services was $3 around 1970, except for the university hospitals where it was 50 cents. This fee has also changed and in 2001 was around $15 for a visit to a general practitioner and $30 for a visit to a specialist. This fee also includes the cost for all tests and X-rays ordered during the visit. Furthermore, the patient is free to see any private physician of his or her choice and then be reimbursed from the insurance according to a fixed scale.

Personal Identification and Population Registration

Every Swedish national and every foreigner granted a residence permit of more than some minimum duration is assigned a permanent identification number. This number embeds the date of birth and a sequential number for all persons born on the same day and a check digit. In the beginning, the number was 11 digits, but it is 12 digits today. The 10th or 11th digit embeds the sex, using even numbers for females and odd numbers for males.

This form of personal identification was used before the introduction of computers and facilitated the identification of patients. The government used it for all purposes. It was also widely used for identification in official and nongovernmental processes, such as a driver's license, all insurance policies, bank accounts, and society memberships. Later the government terminated the use of the number for these purposes, although it is still used in health care in all parts of the healthcare system.

The use of the personal identification number has now been used in its present form for more than 40 years and is now widely accepted, although not without skepticism. In addition to this systematic numbering of residents and the registration of births, marriages, and deaths, there is a thorough system of recording the residents in each locality. The operation of this system, common vital statistics, the national cancer registry, the twin database, and other information rests with the central government. Thus, in conceiving a medical information system based on a central population database, the authorities had the advantage of a well-established scheme for identifying the population and for recording demographic changes.

Legislation

A very important principle in Sweden is the "Publicity Principle." This means that everyone has the right to see or have a copy of all information held by the government and its agencies. The actual law is the "Freedom of the Press" act. Because all information cannot be distributed, there is a second law, the "Security act," that lists all the exceptions. Both legislations date back to 1766. For health care, this means that the patient record is open for the patient to read and obtain a copy. There is one exception, and that is if the physician in charge states that to do so would obstruct the treatment of the patient. If the patient insists, he or she can complain to the National Board of Health and Social Security, which will make a decision. This rule makes it necessary for the treating staff to use care when documenting.

The first data act in Sweden was enacted in 1973 and regulates the different responsibilities that rest with organizations using computers to store and process data. The quality of the data can be checked by the person registered by requesting a printout of the information stored about him or her. If something is incorrect, the "Data Inspection Board" can instruct the person in charge to change or delete the data. Every Swede has the right once a year to ask for a printout of all information stored about him or her and get it free of charge.

In 1983 Sweden got its first "Patient Records Act," which among many other things states that any healthcare staff who examine or treat a patient are responsible for documenting the findings and the actions taken.

Early Initiatives in Education and Training

Training thousands of users to use the systems in a short amount of time and without interfering with daily work was a challenge that was overcome by having courses and training sessions at the different locations. The result of this approach, however, was not as expected. Many complaints about the system surfaced, which resulted in too much work for the programmers. In most cases, no problems with systems performance were found; the problem was that users had not learned how to use the system properly. Therefore, a procedure was introduced requiring staff to take an examination after they had taken the training course. Those who did not pass the exam were not given the password necessary to enter the systems, and they had to come back until they passed the exam. Complaints were reduced to a minimum, and this has become the normal procedure when implementing a new system. It has paid in the long run, even if some hospital administrators complain that it takes too much time away from their regular work.

A problem with the training of systems analysts and programmers also emerged. Initially, the vendor trained them, but in the early 1970s, interest in education and R&D in Medical Informatics began to grow in Sweden. A unique opportunity arose when the new Linköping University was founded in the late 1960s with Philosophical, Engineering, and Medical faculties (the Health University). A Biomedical Engineering Department was started in 1972 with full professor chairs in both Biomedical Engineering and Medical Informatics. Students came mainly from the engineering side, but organized cooperation between that department and the Health University made it possible to also give courses and/or lectures to medical students. The students were offered courses in basic cell biology, basic medicine (terminology, anatomy, physiology), biomedical engineering, and medical informatics. Laboratory applications of medical computing are taught mainly within the courses in biomedical engineering whereas clinical information systems, knowledge-based decision support, and image processing are included within the medical informatics courses [1].

After completing the offered courses, which consist of about 400 hours of scheduled study in biomedical engineering and medical informatics, the engineering students graduate as biomedical engineers, and most are sought after by hospitals to be in charge of Hospital Engineering or Information Technology (IT) departments or within industry. The medical students do not graduate as medical informaticians, but are well prepared for collaborative projects with informatics engineers to develop computer systems and programs in the healthcare area. Up to now, some 500 biomedical engineers and medical informaticians have graduated and have found work opportunities all over Sweden.

The success of these education efforts has been very important for the development and implementation of computer systems and tools for the Swedish Health Care system. Good medical informatics training has been in such demand by students that in 2000 the Karolinska Institute, together with the Royal Institute of Technology in Stockholm, initiated a program in medical informatics education. The program takes 3.5 years to complete and leads to a master's degree in medical informatics.

Nationwide Use of Stored Information

Sweden has collected hospital care information for many years and produced national statistics into yearbooks that have been available since the mid-19th century. This information consists only of yearly summaries and cannot be used for detailed research. Since 1958, however, detailed information has been stored in computers and made available to researchers. The content consists of patient identification, hospital, department, date for admission and discharge, diagnoses, and therapeutic procedures. Since 1970 it has also been mandatory to deliver this information in computer-readable form.

An example of a detailed national register is the National Cancer Register. This registration started out as voluntary, but since 1958 it became mandatory to report all cases of cancer incidents to the Register. The reports originate from all physicians responsible for in- and outpatient departments in both public and private hospitals. Hospital and forensic pathologists give independent compulsory reports for every cancer diagnosis made from surgical biopsies, cytological specimens, and autopsies. Reporting is also compulsory for pathologists in the private sector. The coding schemes used are the ICD-7 and ICD-9, and since 1993, also ICD O/2 and Snomed. Detailed information about the register and how it can be used can be found at http://www.sos.se/epc/english/cancerreg.htm.

Another example of storage is the national quality registers, which track about 50 different diagnoses. The main goal of these registers is to contribute to the improvement of quality care. Detailed information can be found at http://www.sos.se.

The use of all information, not only from these files but also from all information stored in the Swedish healthcare system, is free to all healthcare staff and researchers. The only administrative requirement is permission from the Board of Medical Ethics if identification of the patients is necessary. If the identity of individuals is to be made public, permission from all the patients is necessary.

Computer Applications in the Stockholm Region

Around the mid-1960s, Stockholm County operated 54 hospitals including 13 emergency hospitals, plus 28 other inpatient care facilities. These 82 county institutions provided nearly 9000 general beds, 6000 psychiatric beds, and more than 11,000 longer-term beds.

The hospital organization, at that time, was characterized by complex working conditions and rapid development. The diversification of medical care and the increasing number of specialties made it difficult to plan the patients' way through the hospitals. The patients' demands for personal treatment and personal attention were also getting more and more difficult to satisfy.

Systems development to address these issues started around 1965 and centered on "The Danderyd Project," a major new hospital facility that was being built in the northern suburb of Danderyd [2,3]. Although the project was primarily focused on one facility, from the outset its objectives encompassed countywide applicability and the fullest integration that was reasonable. In 1962 the county had decided to build a large (1600-bed) new university hospital at Huddinge, south of the city. In tune with the times, consideration was given to the widespread use of computers in the new hospital. This led to the decision to develop an integrated computer-based hospital information system for the Danderyd project, similar to many others being conceived elsewhere at that time.

It seemed obvious to the county that it would be beneficial to implement a computer system that would encompass all healthcare activities, as well as provide a tool for controlling and efficiently planning for the provision and use of healthcare resources. Though highly complex and widely disseminated, these activities must focus around the needs of the population, and so it was concluded that the basis for any system would be a central population database, easily and quickly accessible by many and varied users. Small systems, applicable to a single institution or a single application, would be acceptable as offspring of this central patient database. It was recognized, however, that although they might provide local value, they could not provide the broad benefits to be realized from a computer system used in a broader context. Maximum benefit was seen as being derived from integration. Starting with a central population database would allow all types of information and processes to be added in a rational way as dictated by requirements and opportunity. Starting with isolated applications, on the other hand, would require considerable coordination and make integration difficult.

The main goal of the system was to make it possible to continuously follow the morbidity and mortality of the total population in the region and to control the actual use of available resources. This made it possible, for the first time, to build a database that could be used as a rational basis for the long-term planning of medical care, because the system would record activities related to each patient at the hospitals, the primary care centers, and the other medical institutions. Input from the private sector is not seen as significant, since it is very small and does not have a crucial influence on statistics. Some of the basic information from the private sector is collected through the reimbursement system.

Specifications for the system required that it:

- Cover a complete region.
- Be based on a central population database.
- Be communications oriented.
- Be real-time oriented.
- Be function oriented.

As defined in 1970, the main goals of the system were:

- To supply physicians and nurses with patient information.
- To offer means for follow-up studies on individuals or groups of patients.
- To make possible short- and long-term planning on how to use available resources.
- To provide means for financial follow-up.
- To make possible comparison of costs and outcomes for different treatments of patients with specific diseases.

The Master Index

The heart of the system was the Master Index file, the first part of which consisted of census information about the population. Collecting this information would have meant an enormous amount of work had the basic information not already been available on computer-readable media. Since basic population data are registered and stored by the State Office for Census and Tax purposes, a copy of the information for the population in the Stockholm region was placed at disposal of the system. The data were then updated on a weekly basis until the time when an online connection was possible.

In addition to the personal ID number, census information contains the person's full name, address, gender, marriage status, number of children, occupation/profession, district, and parish. The second part contains information about allergies, adverse reactions to drugs, and a number of lifelong diseases such as diabetes, blood coagulation disorders, epilepsy, and pacemaker use. The third part contains information about previous inpatient visits, such as date and terms of admission and discharge, hospital, department and ward unit, diagnoses, and surgical and therapeutic procedures and X-rays. This information is automatically collected from the patient file that is opened at admissions and is kept active during the treatment period. It also contains information from all laboratories, referrals, waiting lists, and scheduled appointments [4].

The Master Index has been updated since 1969 and contains more than 30 years of information about all hospital admissions sorted by the personal identification number and is retrievable online. As of 2002, the Master Index was still on a central server.

Implementation of Application Modules

Implementation of the first version of the application modules for inpatient registration, waiting list, appointment scheduling, laboratory systems, and outpatient registration was realized during 1971–1976. During that time the system was centralized and communication was through telephone lines to terminals in the hospitals. The different laboratories were connected either directly or via a local computer. This setup gradually changed, and today is a wide area network connected to local area networks in the hospitals and numerous servers in the different departments and clinics.

Around 1990 all necessary application modules were in place, and the introduction of the new computerized patient record (CPR) became the main topic. As stated earlier, this development had already started in the mid-1960s. The definition of a CPR is strict in Sweden. All data about the patient except for images, analogue information, and sound tracks have to be included, which means that the patient history, the findings from physical examinations, and all results from laboratories and X-ray departments have to be included, otherwise the system is considered a patient administrative system or a hospital information system.

Systems Development at Karolinska Hospital

The Karolinska Institute, the medical university of Stockholm, enjoys worldwide prestige, and its associated hospital, the Karolinska Hospital (KS), has held a special position within the national health service, being one of the central government-operated hospitals. However, because its patients are overwhelmingly from Stockholm County, KS is essentially integrated into County operations.

In 1962 the National Office of Organization (NOOM) together with Serafimer hospital began an information systems experiment, which was later joined by KS in 1965. The intention was to study the possibilities of using data processing techniques in hospital procedures. One condition was that the systems developed should be designed for large as well as small hospitals. The objective was to set up a complete patient information system based on existing medical practices and established technical solutions and be geared primarily to certain central functions, particularly the planning required to coordinate various routines for processing a patient through the hospital and the patient record.

The project was based on certain generally defined and accepted ideas: treatment must be preceded by an investigation to illuminate and define the problems. Certain parts of this investigation can be done before the patient meets the physician, and the computer can be used for this work.

The KS project can be divided into three phases: before 1966, a preceding experimental stage at the Serafimer Hospital during 1962–1966; a real-life test, 1966–1969, at the medical development department at KS; and the final stage, 1969–1974, the evaluation phase [5,6].

The first phase was sponsored by an insurance company (Folksam), Sjura, and NOOM. The goal for this phase was to develop a CPR, independent of specialty and of in- and outpatient care. The basic idea was to follow the patient thorough the healthcare system, to rationalize the patient's path through the hospital, and to increase an effective use of resources.

The CPR was built in a Swedish computer (SAAB D 21). The versions of the programming efforts were called J = Journal = record and the applications were geared toward the patient's medical history, which is the most informative part of the record. Self-administered questionnaires were used for both in- and outpatients. Results of these activities were later published in a dissertation [7]. J1 was a fixed format structure, which turned out to be of limited value for clinical practice. The next version, J2, gave more flexibility as it could accept all values, free text and codes, but was still of limited value. The conclusion after several experiments was that there was no way to define and standardize a complete medical history or a record. The exception to this rule is for a defined group of patients. In this case it can be an excellent tool for followup and clinical research. The conclusion from the versions J1 to J4 was to build a flexible system (J5) designed for one patient over a lifetime.

When the development began at Karolinska Hospital in 1966, the CPR system was batch oriented. The experiences accumulated were that the patient should be followed during the treatment period, which made a scheduling and follow-up system necessary. An online system for these applications was developed and interlinked with the J5 system [8]. A hypothesis was that physicians should have less administrative work and a better presentation of, and easier access to, the data. Each patient was allocated to a treatment team consisting of a physician, a nurse, and a secretary. This organization facilitated contact for the patient with the team and for the team to distribute the work among the members in a more efficient way. All members of the team used the same record for documenting the data. From the beginning, the problem-oriented approach was accepted. All problems for the patient were defined and described, and an action plan was made up. The source-oriented information was presented in the regular way.

Several scientific research projects, scientific papers, and dissertations were published with data from the J5 system. One example is the computerized anesthetic patient record [9] where 70,000 anesthetic records were recorded and analyzed and no manual records were kept.

The evaluation period was divided into two parts, the first internal and the second external. To study and evaluate a computer system was, at that time, and still is, difficult. There was no good method to measure quality of patient care or quality of life. A serious attempt was made to evaluate the effects of the system and the following examples are an indicator of what was done.

The scheduling system made it possible to schedule up to 9 different consultations, examinations, or tests per day for a patient. In clinical practice, it was easy to schedule

4, compared with 2.2, which was the mean with a manual system. To make this system financially cost-effective, more than 50,000 patient visits per year were necessary. This number was easy to reach at a large hospital like Karolinska. The CPR system was cost-effective if the number of inpatients was 10,000 and outpatients 30,000 per year. The KS project was terminated in 1974.

The Computerized Patient Record

A patient record consists of all the documents that are created by different care providers or that are received in connection with the care of a patient. Usually there are many care providers involved in the care of a patient. It is, therefore, necessary to be able to take only part of the information and to document the findings. Traditionally, the patient record was a tool for subsequent documentation of actions already taken, but is used more and more as a planning instrument to steer and follow up the entire care process.

When a change is made to electronically stored patient records, the traditional patient record structure does not really exist any more. The screen representation can be rendered in a traditional way, but it can also appear in a customized desirable format. The data are accessed in different ways depending on the structure of the database. The functions of the CPR are too limited if the objectives are to facilitate carrying out the processes that we find in the framework of diagnostics, treatment, prognosis, and follow-up.

In 1994 the Swedish Institute for Health Services Development (Spri) and the Federation of the Swedish County Councils carried out a survey of computer-supported patient record systems that were available on the Swedish market. (These surveys have been carried out every year since 1988.) A total of 27 different CPRs were identified on the market. Of these, only 5 had greater distribution. The report also showed that more than 80 percent of the patient records used in primary care were CPRs, but that in hospitals only 5 percent were CPRs, according to the strict definition used in Sweden. The missing part in most of these latter systems was what is called the "bedside" part, which means medications, temperature, and nursing notes. In 2001, 95 percent of the records in primary care and 15 percent in hospital care were CPRs, but that latter figure is increasing rapidly.

In 1994, however, the situation was not acceptable, and the central government, together with the Federation of the Swedish County Councils, decided to initiate a project to describe the requirements for a computerized patient record. The project, which was funded by the central government, started in 1994 and was called "The Spri Study." The first results were presented in Swedish in late 1995 and in English in 1996. The final results were presented between 1998 and 1999.

The Spri Study

The Swedish Institute for Health Services Development, Spri, was originally founded in 1971 and was funded half by the central government and half by the Federation of the County Councils as an independent nonprofit institute. Spri is not an authority that draws up regulations, but it can give advice that is formulated in a general manner so that everyone may use it and is free to use it. Usually the advice given is followed and appreciated.

The Spri study, whose official name was "Computerized Information Related to the Health Care Sector," took place during the years 1995–1999. The result was 15 reports of which 3 were translated into English [10–12]. These reports are only available through the authors as Spri was closed at the end of 1999.

The objectives of the study were to achieve the following:

- A comprehensive list of requirements that should apply for all health documentation systems in health care, which meant requirements for the functionality of the patient record, and also requirements for the CPR to include support for follow-up of performance, costs, and the quality of care.
- Unified requirements for the supporting surrounding routines that are needed.

An important condition for the project was that it should concentrate on user requirements. An information system for health care consists of many other functions, such as application systems. These were described in special reports.

User participation in development has been a rule since the early 1970s, but for the first time this study had access to what were called "educated or experienced" users. About 700 users involved had used several systems or versions of systems before and knew the requirements. Some of them had also been involved in the development of the existing systems together with different vendors.

Processing Specifications and Functional Descriptions

A survey was sent out to all authorities dealing with health care, and more than 70 percent replied. The responses received were analyzed and divided into four groups: requirements for somatic care, for primary care, for psychiatric care, and requirements common to all types of care. The requirements in the respective groups were processed separately and divided into subgroups, such as user interface, confidentiality, and technical requirements. When the processing had been completed, seven 2-day seminars were held, with an average of 60 to 70 users in each group. At these seminars, agreement was reached on what requirements should be fulfilled before the implementation of the system. The common requirements were revised at all seminars. After the results of each seminar were compiled, the participants were allowed again to voice their opinion about the requirements. This allowed for comparison of the pattern of requirements that had emerged from the seminars. It showed that most of the requirements were common. It was also revealed that the requirements from the paramedical groups had not been presented clearly enough. A special round of requirement collection was held with almoners, physiotherapists, speech therapists, and dietitians providing input. Only a few requirements were added.

The compiled requirements were sent to more than 500 authorities, organizations, IT departments, IT coordinators, and participants in the seminars. Suggestions for changes were filed under each respective requirement, and apart from a few cases, it was possible to correct the requirements according to the opinions that had been received. To check the requirements once more, a 2-day seminar was arranged to review the revised version. After 3 years (1998) of use, both by customers for selecting a new system and by vendors to change their systems, a new revision was made. It was published in the Spri Report No. 477, "Introducing Computer-based Patient Records: Prerequisites and Requirements" [10].

The requirements are presented under the following headings: user interfaces, data capture, supportive functions, safety and confidentiality, output, communication, special requirements concerning psychiatric care, special requirements concerning paramedical groups, and record structure. This is presented in detail in "RAM-X. A Reference Architecture Supporting Process-oriented Health Care" [11].

Indicators to Define Quality of Care

It was impossible to agree on what indicators should be used to define quality of care, but agreement on the following was finally reached: quality indicators in health care apply both to structure and process. It is not only a question of results in the form of improvement but also a question of the staff's competence, reception of patients, the patient's understanding of the treatment result, etc.

Index Words as Structural Elements

The structure of the patient record has gradually been changed over the years and has been adapted to the increased requirements of availability and clarity of information, especially when considering the number of care providers who are involved in the care of the patient. In 1971 Spri presented a structure for the patient record, based on the usage of headings and subheadings commonly known as index words. This structure was widely adopted by Swedish healthcare professionals. Since 1971 different care categories and specialties have been developing their own index words on a lower level and practically adapted to their own specialty. When the CPR is introduced on a broader scale, however, it is necessary to have more coordination and communication. Index words used as structural elements become the key for communicating patient record data. It was, therefore, necessary to agree upon the definitions of the index words used, and this proved to be a difficult exercise. In the end, however, it was possible to come to agreement on the definition of the index words that are used in the Swedish CPR.

General Conclusions

Toward a Networking Knowledge Society

Spri has published a series of studies to investigate the limits and opportunities of the information society in health care. The results are summarized in Report No. 477 "Introducing Computer-Based Patient Records: Prerequisites and Requirements" (1998), from which this chapter is a summary [10].

The entry of computer technology in health care has been slow, partly due to conservatism and partly due to the immense complexity of health care in work routines as well as in organization. Until now, it has not been feasible to create overall and effective computer support for the multifaceted and varying activities of health care. To understand why this has been the case and why this will now change radically, it is necessary to understand what information technology means, including what it is, how IT is developed, and where it is headed. Without this basic understanding of the new concepts and the new patterns of thought that govern and distinguish IT today, discussions of IT unavoidably end in confusion.

Information technology has evolved beyond its status as an aid. Information technology is not about computers, it is about the networking of knowledge communities. The main reason healthcare professionals want computerized patient records is that they do not want to look for records. At the same time, they may complain about how difficult it is to make technologists and engineers understand health care. As a result, there is little understanding of the many suggestions for changes in such areas as work routines to fully realize the benefits of IT. The purpose of the systems of computer-supported healthcare documentation that have been available on the market, so far, has always been to computerize paper-based patient records in the most authentic-looking way possible and the ingrained work routines they represent. For example, some systems emulate sheets of paper, even including spiral bindings and tab dividers, lest anybody miss the paper-based patient records.

Developments are occurring so quickly on so many fronts that it is impossible to predict what information society will want in the future, and in what format. The challenge is to learn what fundamental values in health care are supported by IT and how they can contribute to its continued development. In short, the best way to anticipate the future is to learn as much as possible about the present.

One of the most important advances in IT is the development of object-oriented development methodology. Dividing tasks into independent parts known as "objects" and having these perform their tasks "without anybody watching" has resulted in a completely new view of how organizations work, as well as a revolution in the development of large complex software systems. IT increasingly governs how activities are conducted and organized. New technology breeds new forms of work, which in turn breeds new organizational forms. The differences between technological development in general and IT in particular are that IT manages information and, thus, "knowledge." To refer to IT as computer support in health care is no longer true. IT is not about computers but about globally interlinked collaborative information technology, which creates a networking knowledge society, applying Internet and intranet.

A New Paradigm

When a new paradigm arises, there is also a new epoch. Groundbreaking technology is often epoch making, but this is not always so. In 1776, in his book *The Wealth of Nations*, Adam Smith formulated the paradigm that forms the basis for industrial society, which we are now leaving to enter information society. All work should be divided up into primitive tasks, simple enough that any worker should be able to perform them with a minimum of training. This formed the basis for mass production. Adam Smith's paradigm must now yield to the paradigm that expresses the new information society. In general terms this means:

- Tailor-made solutions instead of mass production.
- Highly educated staff rather than unskilled labor.
- Individual responsibility and initiative, instead of industrial hierarchies.

The new paradigm for the information systems of health care entails progressing according to the following:

- From hierarchies to networking health care.
- From function-oriented to process-oriented health care.
- From fixed format patient records to functional and flexible patient records.

Trends in the Healthcare Organization

Changing to process-oriented thinking means changing the focus from function to product, that is, the end result that the patient receives and how this is best provided, rather than how each healthcare provider will function best. This view has emerged from IT, and especially from object-oriented methodology, which combines method and means. This methodology now permeates activity models as well as information models and software systems. In the traditional activity model, the organization is fitted to optimize functions (specialists). This does not necessarily produce an optimal organization as a whole, and the product—health care—may not be optimal in the eyes of the patient. Areas of decision and responsibility often extend beyond discrete functions. To optimize activities and performance, it is, therefore, necessary to consider the entire healthcare process from the patient's point of view, the product in case.

Although the current restructuring of health care was motivated by a lack of funds, it has often been justified in terms of theories about improving efficiency and achieving health care that is product focused, thus also patient focused. In the long run, the activity does not improve, and health care—the product—does not become any better. The primary reason for this failure can be traced to a deficient understanding of the basic process-oriented mode of thought that forms the basis for business process reengineering (BPR), and that also forms the foundation for modern IT. Most people are not process oriented. They focus instead on tasks, on individual tasks, on humans, on the surrounding structure—but not on processes. BPR, like object-oriented process thinking, is not about making small changes. It is about making radical change by means of thorough restructuring, which means completely forgetting about existing structures and working methods and inventing totally new ones.

Networking Health Care

Workflow redesign, by means of administrative programs and computer-supported healthcare documentation, can integrate and consolidate activities. The results that can be achieved through workflow technology become even greater when units merge, as initiatives all over the world demonstrate.

The driving force behind this kind of integration is primarily an idea of how an activity should be managed, not what specific results are desirable. New trends in management take hold rapidly. Still, there is no clear view of the intended results. The focus is primarily on management rules and only secondarily on the product. This is management by directives, not management by objectives. Under the latter, the product (objective) is healthcare services, as experienced by the patients, and not budgetary outcomes or organizational changes. The strong tradition of function-oriented activities discourages change, and occasionally function is only addressed when reorganizing and integrating. Nevertheless, it is never possible, whatever the activity, to disregard the product and consider only organization and working methods. It is rare to find patient benefits specifically included in planning or evaluation, certainly not as defined from the patient's point of view. This also explains why healthcare staff finds it difficult to accept new technology and organizational changes: they find it hard to understand the benefit to patients.

The New Computerized Patient Record

It has long been obvious that computerized patient records have real value for healthcare principals and providers, and that part of this lies in the ability to transfer patient data where these are needed. This is the problem that the new ways of communication try to solve. For the healthcare provider, patient data must be presented as one computerized record, even if the data may be scattered across a hospital, region, or country.

Typically, the healthcare provider requires only a subset of the data about the patient at each visit or consultation. By means of distributed object technology, these requirements can now be met.

The new CPR is a bold concept in the sense that the original data can be presented or formatted in different ways in different places, although the data have a common format when retrieved from different databases. Thus, distributed patient data are made available through references, such as hypertext links, and are accessed as needed by the healthcare provider. Object technology allows the user to retrieve parts of the records (such as single patient record items or patient record item complexes), in preference to the entire patient record, minimizing the data flow across the network. See "Ram-X. A Reference Architecture Supporting Process-oriented Health Care" [11]. In such networked systems, distributed transaction management and reference counting preserve and protect the data from contamination. In this way, full access and updating of patient records can be given to many different healthcare providers, simultaneously or at different times, without record items being overwritten or lost. Many of these functions and procedures are already specified. Although this requires that the database be continuously connected to all parts of the network for full data integrity to be preserved, large bandwidth (network speed) is not needed unless large amounts of imaging or video data are to be transmitted. Of course, an extensive data security infrastructure is needed to prevent patient data from getting into the wrong hands.

Summary of Practical Results

For the purpose of summarizing the Spri study, the conclusions were split up into four groups: purpose, user requirements, goals, and prerequisites.

Purpose:

- To support high-quality health care with high-quality information processing.
- To produce administrative statistics about production, quality of care, cost, and staff.
- To allow individual clinical follow-up and research.

Functional user requirements:

- The system must support daily work with the patients.
- The system must support process-oriented healthcare delivery.
- Communication must be possible both inside and outside the healthcare unit.
- A common structure/architecture and a common terminology must be used to the extent possible.

The goals for a modern healthcare information system should be:

- To build local modular application systems that support process-oriented health care. These modules must be so small that they can be used in different applications, have a standard interface, and are easy to replace.
- The modules must be able to communicate within the system but also be a part of the "total" system.

Prerequisites:

- A standardized overall structure/architecture.
- An agreed-upon terminology.
- Rules for communication, security, and safety.
- Agreement on patient identification.
- Electronic addresses to all units and users.

The healthcare delivery system is also changing over time. Following up on costs was not important in Sweden in the 1970s, but it is now, which means that tools for follow-up on costs and quality of care are important. The change from function- to process-oriented care means that patients are no longer treated in only one department or only in hospitals. A patient with diabetes, for example, is now treated in a unit for diabetic patients where all needed specialists are available instead of being referred to dieticians, ophthalmologists, and laboratories.

Another meaning of the expression "process-oriented health care" is that a patient should be treated in the unit where he or she can be treated at the lowest cost. This decision is made by the political administration and represents an "outsourcing" of patients from the hospitals to primary care and from there to home-care service and to "self-care." This means that information about the patient must be available at all these units at the same time and be instantly updated. There is also a need to include images, analogue information, and sound recordings in the CPR.

Patients are also changing, and the most important change is in their attitude, from passive receivers to active, knowledgeable, and demanding patients, aware of the quality of care. They want to have their own patient record at their own disposal and will demand only one record regardless of unit or provider and that the record should be presented in a way that is as understandable as possible for the patient. In Sweden these thoughts have resulted in a decision to find out what changes are necessary in legislation; this process is well under way.

The Future

Interoperability

Interoperability of all applications in a hospital, groups of hospitals, and primary care centers that work together, or in a region, should be the ultimate target for health data management. However, a single integration strategy to achieve this does not exist. The two most popular strategies that have been tried many times, without success, are the following.

- The single supplier solution whereby a solution is bought from one vendor who provides an integrated solution. This enables the entire organization to share a common database with no duplication of data elements, but it also means that no user will get exactly what he or she needs. Everybody within the organization must live with a compromise. These types of systems have proved unsuitable for groups and regions because of high cost and long lead times.
- The multivendor solution has the advantage of using "best of breed" systems, the investment can be spread over a longer period, and these systems are easier to adapt and grow. The disadvantages are that they present data integration problems; they are architecturally complicated and need meticulous planning and integration. The traditional method of linking systems was through point-to-point proprietary interfaces, which can be very costly. Interfaces might need to be amended if changes are made in the connected systems and could threaten to cost more than the individual applications. In attempts to avoid the limitations of point-to-point proprietary interfaces, generic interfacing tools, so-called interface engines, have been used with limited success.
- Open solutions based on standards. In 1997, OECD recommended solving the problems of interoperability by means of "open" modular solutions [13]. Such open infor-

mation systems for health and health care are being built on common architectures. Specific applications, or software products, should fit such architectures, which are "public" standards, and should therefore be available for both users and vendors. The applications are interconnected through interfaces that are also "public" standards. It is important to clearly distinguish between "quasi-openness" claimed by vendors for their proprietary systems and "real openness" of systems based on public standards.

The Future CPR

The next generation of the CPR must be independent from all organizational changes. Today many organizations produce one patient record for every unit where the patient has been and every patient has a number of records. These records are found by using a Master Index where all records are stored. It must be possible to create one CPR for each patient. This solution partly avoids requiring the patient to repeat his or her history. It needs to be possible to present only the amount of information that is needed at one particular time. Therefore, it needs to be possible to present the information as "views," where the healthcare provider has stated in advance the information needed for that patient. All healthcare providers can have a number of "views" for different occasions.

A format for long-time archiving of the CPR must be agreed on. Promising tests are being made using XML for that purpose [10].

Success Factors

The following success factors are the most crucial if a user-oriented CPR is to be developed:

- Cooperation.
- Clinical guidelines and/or treatment programs.
- Education.
- Standards.

The Vision

The goal is to describe how the future multiprofessional, multimedia, organization-independent electronic patient record, in which only new information is added instead of repeating the already-known data, should look like. Important prerequisites for the future CPR include:

- Being problem oriented and containing structured information as much as possible.
- Being capable of adding information instead of repeating already-known data.
- Making the different categories of staff responsible for collecting their part of the information.
- Making the CPR available in real time regardless of geographic location.
- The Health Care system has one CPR per individual, and each group of users is responsible for the design, content, and extent according to their needs.

References

1. Åhlfeldt H, Wigertz O. Study programs in medical informatics at Linköping University. In: van Bemmel JH, McCray A, editors. Yearbook of medical informatics 95. Stuttgart: Schattauer; 1995. pp. 115–120.

2. Abrahamsson S, Bergström S, Larsson K, et al. Information system for public health, medical care and social welfare in a county (in Swedish). Läkartidningen 1968;65:3196–3203.
3. Abrahamsson S, Bergström S, Larsson K, et al. The Danderyd Hospital Computer System. A total regional system for medical care. Computers Biomed Res 1970;3:30–46.
4. Fenna D, Peterson H, Abrahamsson S, Lööw SO. The Stockholm County Medical Information System. Berlin: Springer-Verlag; 1978.
5. Sjukhusrationalisering med databehandling (in Swedish). Stockholm: National Office of Organization and Management, 1970.
6. Hall P, Danielsson T, Mellner C, Selander H. Automation of data flow. Ann NY Acad Sci 1969;161:730–739.
7. Mellner C. The self-administered medical history (dissertation). Acta Chir Scand 1970; Suppl 406.
8. Hall P, Mellner C, Danielsson T. J5—A data processing system for medical information. In: van Bemmel, et al, editors. Data information and knowledge in medicine. Methods Inform Med 1998; [Special issue].
9. Hallén B. Computerized anesthetic record-keeping (dissertation). Acta Anaesthesiol Scand 1973; Suppl 52.
10. Peterson H. Introducing computer-based patient records. Prerequisites and requirements. Stockholm: Spri; 1998.
11. Sandström SÅ. RAM-X. A reference architecture supporting process-oriented health care. Stockholm: Spri; 1998.
12. Peterson H, Olhede T. Long-term storage of electronic health care information in XML format. Stockholm: Spri; 1999.
13. Electronic commerce, opportunities and challenges for governments. Paris: OECD, 1997.

Section 2
Preparing for Organizational Change

Section Introduction

Once the strategic plan is outlined (one cannot say "completed" because a strategic plan is always a work in progress), it is time to begin turning IT plans into reality by readying the organization for change. This section follows a systems analysis and design approach, integrating theoretical foundations with practical applications. To be considered are feasible alternatives, decision factors, consensus, organizational politics, and ethics. Three chapters in this section present "how to" approaches. Two domestic cases consider a design-driven strategy and a more focused approach to clinical documentation. A third international project used a leapfrog approach and created the Total Hospital Information System at Selayang Hospital in Malaysia. Here, the clinical, financial, operational, and administrative functions are paperless and wireless, and positive outcomes are being realized.

The key to getting the most out of this section is to understand that readers are being transported sequentially through a series of points and issues to consider and then apply to their own situations. The change process works, as is demonstrated by the numerous examples in this section.

7
Informatics in Health Care: Managing Organizational Change

Nancy M. Lorenzi and Robert T. Riley

As information systems proliferate throughout the healthcare organization, managing change is of paramount need.

Change is Constant

It is exciting to think about a new vision particularly when you are the creator/driver of it. You see the need clearly. You feel the urgency in your stomach. You are motivated to change. You see the fire with your own eyes. You smell the smoke in your own nostrils. The tent is on fire. Why are others in the organization so lackadaisical? Don't they smell the smoke? Don't they see the fire? Don't they feel the urgency to change? [1].

The healthcare profession as a whole is undergoing rapid changes with technology, politics, economics, and demographics all either forcing or enabling these changes. Change is a constant reality in both our personal and private lives. Our children grow up today taking for granted such things as powerful personal computers that we could not even envision at their ages. Our societies, our professions, and our daily work lives are changing. Moreover, this pace of change appears to be accelerating, not slowing down.

It is impossible to introduce a health informatics system into an organization without the people in that organization feeling the impact of change. Informatics is about change—the change of data into information with a possible evolution into knowledge. Data become information only after the data are processed (i.e., *changed*) in ways that make the data useful for decision making; those enhanced decision-making capabilities are inevitably going to affect the organization. The organization and its people influence, shape, and alter the nature and use of the informatics systems that, in turn, influence, shape, and alter the nature, operation, and culture of the organization that, in turn, etc.

Remember the saying, "Sometimes you get the bear; sometimes the bear gets you." The analogy in change processes is that if we do not manage our change processes, they

Nancy M. Lorenzi, PhD, is a Professor of Biomedical Informatics and Assistant Vice Chancellor for Health Affairs at Vanderbilt University Medical Center in Nashville, TN. Robert T. Riley was on the faculty of the University of Cincinnati and President of Riley Associates in Cincinnati and then Nashville, TN.

will manage us—an undesirable alternative at best. The lower our feelings of control during the change process, the lower our "resiliency" will be, and our ability to bounce back from the stresses of the change and to prepare for the inevitable next change in today's environment will be diminished [2]. When change processes are not managed well, the price is potentially high in terms of organizational stress. A Kepner Tregoe study conducted in a number of large U.S. companies found many of them suffering from "initiative overload" with high levels of cynicism among the employees. An article in *Management Review*, "Change for Change's Sake," described executives as seizing on one change after another, desperately seeking a quick fix [3]. These are the realistic outcomes of poorly managed change processes. This has become known as "change fatigue" in some organizations [4].

Change and Health Informatics: A Modern-Day Scenario

The following scenario presents an example of what happens when the introduction of a new system challenges perceptions about accepted practices. In this example, the perceived role of nurses as the integrators of patient data/information was challenged when physicians began doing direct order entry [5].

When using a *manual system* on an inpatient unit, the nurse usually serves as an integrator and reviewer. The physician scribbles something down on a piece of paper, which is given to a nurse, unit clerk, or paraprofessional to do something with. A nurse typically "cleans it up" and transmits the information or order to pharmacy, radiology, laboratory, dietary, etc. Occasionally the lab or pharmacy will call the physician back. However, the nurse in general serves as the conduit for the transfer of information. When nurses fill this role, they learn a lot. Moreover, they have a total view of what is happening with the patient as they filter and organize information from various sources. This is a classic workflow design. What happens when a system is implemented that calls for the physician to enter orders directly into the system?

In one hospital, the nurses did not like this type of new system. The nurses believed that the system reduced their role in the overall care process. It took them out of the reviewer, case manager, and integrator roles that they were trained to do and that they had always done. The nurses said their two most important roles are (1) the nurse as integrator and (2) the nurse as reviewer, and this new system usurped both roles.

The nurses were very concerned. In the old system, the physicians were used to issuing vague or approximate orders. For example, the physicians would scribble "d.c." or "d/c" for discontinue. They would order "X-rays" and the nurses would figure out that a P.A. and lateral chest were wanted. If the physicians tried to enter their orders as they traditionally did, they would either get nothing back or something they didn't want. The physicians did not know how to order because they had not actually placed orders before. When the physician scribbled an order, the nurse knew the physician, knew exactly what was wanted, and would make it happen. With the new system, this was not possible.

There was a significant decrease of the role of the nurse as an integrator and reviewer of care. Physicians began to make mistakes that nurses had previously caught, such as ordering incorrect drugs or incorrect dosages. There was less coordination between the nursing plans and the medical care plans. In their new role, nurses tended to show less initiative in making treatment suggestions. In summary, what was lost was the second overview review and analysis by a trained professional. The "second" person had lost the overview perspective. On the other hand, some positive things did occur. Relieved of the paperwork of ordering, nurses had 2 to 3 more hours per day to spend on hands-on patient care.

Using This Scenario

The remainder of this chapter presents practical techniques for dealing with informatics change processes. We suggest that you try to relate each of the concepts or techniques back to this scenario, especially in terms of your current or potential role(s) in the areas of health informatics and management. What change forces were at work? What might have been done to prevent the friction that developed?

Types of Change

Changes within an organization can often be identified as one of four types with the definite possibility of overlap between two or more:

- Operational—changes in the way that the ongoing operations of the business are conducted, such as the automation of a particular area.
- Strategic—changes in the strategic business direction (e.g., moving from an inpatient to an outpatient focus).
- Cultural—changes in the basic organizational philosophies by which the business is conducted, for example, implementing a Continuous Quality Improvement (CQI) system.
- Political—changes in staffing occurring primarily for political reasons of various types, such as occur at top patronage job levels in government agencies.

These four different types of change typically have their greatest impacts at different levels of the organization. For example, operational changes tend to have their greatest impacts at the lower levels of the organization, right on the firing line. Those at the upper levels may never notice changes that cause significant stress and turmoil to those attempting to implement the changes. On the other hand, the impact of political changes is typically felt most at the higher organizational levels. As the name implies, these changes are typically not made for results-oriented reasons but for reasons such as partisan politics or internal power struggles. When these changes occur in a relatively bureaucratic organization—as they often do—the bottom often hardly notices the changes at the top. Patients are seen and the floors are cleaned exactly the same as before. The key point is that performance was not the basis of the change; therefore, the performers are not affected that much.

Resistance to Change

It has been said that the only person who welcomes change is a wet baby! It seems to be part of the human makeup to be most comfortable with the status quo unless it is actually inflicting discomfort. Even then, people will often resist a *specific* change. This is probably the phenomenon of "the devil you know is better than the devil you don't know." It is a shock for inexperienced managers the first time they see subordinates resist even a change that they requested.

Resistance Against What?

There can be countless reasons for resistance to change in a given situation, and the term *resistance to change* is often used very broadly [6]. One of the first aspects that must be analyzed in a given situation is the difference between

- Resistance to a particular *change*, and
- Resistance to the perceived *changer(s)*.

In the first case, the resistance is actually directed against the changes in the system. In the second case the resistance occurs because of negative feelings toward specific units, specific managers, or the organization in general. In this latter case, virtually any change would be resisted just because of who is advocating or requiring it. Both forces have to be dealt with, but it is critical that we identify the primary one.

When a new health informatics system is introduced, three factors are very important:

- What is the general organizational climate; for example, is it positive or negative, cooperative or adversarial, etc.?
- What has been the quality of the *process* used to implement previous informatics systems?
- Was the process successful?
- What has been the technical quality of the informatics systems previously implemented?
- How did the users like the system?

Even if we may be new to an organization, we inevitably inherit, to some degree, the organizational climate and history. Negative "baggage" of this type can be a frustrating burden that adds significantly to the challenge of successfully implementing a new system. On the other hand, the ability to meet this type of challenge is a differentiating factor for truly skilled implementers.

Intensity of Resistance

Resistance can vary from the trivial to the ferocious. Also, the very perception of resistance can vary widely from one observer to another. One might perceive an end user who asks many questions as being very interested and aggressively seeking knowledge. Another might see the same person as a troublemaker who should just "shut up and listen!"

What causes resistance? First, there may be active resistance—users/people working with the system may flatly refuse to adopt it, resisting change through outright denial. Alternatively, problems embedded within the system may lead to resistance [7,8]. For example, poor communication inherent in a healthcare organization, failure to understand the office or clinical workflow, underestimation of the complexity of change, lack of ownership for change/technological implementation, and false assumptions about transferability of technology can contribute to systematic resistance to change [9].

We can safely assume that every significant health informatics implementation is going to encounter some resistance; however, the intensity can vary widely. In an organization with decent morale and a history of managing changes reasonably well, significant numbers of the people may be initially neutral toward a particular proposed systems change. However, there will still be a negative component to be managed. At the very least, this negative component must be prevented from growing. In other situations, the proportions of positive, negative, and neutral people may vary widely. Finally, for information technology (IT) to work, the system itself must be able to adapt to change.

The Cast of Characters

For any given change, people can occupy a wide range of roles that will strongly influence their perceptions of the change and their reaction to it. As on the stage, some people may occasionally play more than one role. In other cases, the roles are unique. Unless we clearly identify both the players and their roles in any change situation, we risk making decisions and taking action based upon generalizations that are not true for some of the key players. The following categories provide one way of looking at the various roles involved in an overall change process.

- The *initiator* or instigator perceives the problem situation or opportunity and conceptualizes the change to be made in response.
- The *approver* or funder is the power figure who blesses and financially supports the proposed change.
- The *champion* or cheerleader is the visible, enthusiastic advocate for the change. The champion constantly tries to rally support for the change and maintain that support during periods of adversity. In the case of successful clinical implementation, champions tend to be super-users; they are fast and reliable, and they really understand the inner workings of the institution and change process.
- The *facilitator* attempts to assist in smoothing the organizational change process. The facilitator is sometimes involved from the beginning, and sometimes is only called in for disaster relief once the change process has gone awry.
- The *developer* or builder is responsible for the technical aspects of the change (e.g., developing the new informatics system). These aspects can range from the broad technical conceptualization to the narrowest of technical details.
- The *installer* is responsible for implementing the change, including the necessary training and support activities.
- The *doer* is the "changee"—the person who has to perform his or her work in the changed environment. (Sometimes we refer to these people as end users.)
- The *obstructionist* is a guardian of the status quo and typically conducts guerrilla warfare against the change. If the obstructionist is also a doer, the reason may arise from a personal fear of the change. However, the obstructionism may also arise from forces such as political infighting (e.g., who gets the credit) or institutional conflicts (e.g., union resistance to a labor-saving system).
- The *customer* is the end beneficiary or victim of the change in terms of altered levels of service, cost, etc.
- The *observer* does not perceive that he or she will be immediately affected by this change but observes with interest. These observations often affect strongly how the observer will react if placed in the doer role in the future.
- The *ignorer* perceives that this change has no personal implications and is indifferent to it. In the broadest sense, this category also includes all those who are unaware of the change.

An overview term often applied to all these roles is *stakeholders*. With the exception of the ignorers, all the categories have some stake or interest in the quality of the change and the change implementation process. The roles are subject to change, especially during a change process that extends over some time. For example, an initial ignorer might hear rumblings of discontent within the system and change to an observer, at least until the feelings of angst subside. It is key for the implementation team to assess the people they will work with to determine which of these roles they occupy.

For those implementing change, the following steps are critical:

1. Identify what roles they themselves are occupying in the process.
2. Identify what roles the others involved in the process are playing, being careful to recognize multiple roles.
3. Identify carefully which role is speaking whenever communicating with those playing multiple roles.
4. Involve everyone in the change process from the start of the project.
5. Monitor throughout the process whether any roles are changing.

In addition to the preceding steps for successful change implementation, other critical success factors include visionary and supportive leadership; incentives and clear expectations; good support from technology vendors; sustainability of the information technology itself; energy and momentum for change (right personalities, work ethics, etc.); standardization and identification of customizable technological features; and an increasing effort to change organizational culture. Often, dedicated personalities and leaders can inspire change in places where successful IT implementation would be otherwise impossible.

Magnitudes of Change

Change—like beauty—is in the eye of the beholder. A proposed change that virtually terrorizes one person may be a welcome alleviation of boredom to another person. Also, the types and magnitudes of reaction are often difficult for an "outsider" to predict. When working with change and change management, it often helps to have a simple way of classifying the types and sizes of change.

Microchanges and Megachanges

A practical model that we frequently use divides changes into *microchanges* and *megachanges*, with no great attempt at elaborate definitions. As a first approximation, the following scheme can be used to differentiate between the two:

* *Microchanges*—differences in degree.
* *Megachanges*—differences in kind.

Using an information system as an example, modifications, enhancements, improvements, and upgrades would typically be *microchanges*, whereas a new system or a very major revision of an existing one would be a *megachange*. This scheme works surprisingly well in communicating within organizations so long as we remember that one person's microchange can well be another person's megachange.

Change Principles for Today's Organizations

Change may not be a strong enough word to fully express the challenge that organizations and the people in them face today. Writers such as Nicholas Imparato and Oren Harari [10] and Paul David [11] argue strongly that we are in the midst of a megachange from one social, economic, and cultural paradigm to another. Organizational strategies that worked under the old paradigm are no longer valid. Imparato and Harari describe this as "jumping the curve"—moving from an old growth curve to a new one rather than moving along the old curve as we have done for ages.

Imparato and Harari advocate four organizing principles for organizations wishing to jump the curve successfully [10]:

1. Look a customer ahead.
2. Build the organization around the software and build the software around the customer.
3. Ensure that those who live the values and ideals of the organization are the most rewarded and the most satisfied.
4. Make customers the final arbiters by offering an unconditional guarantee of complete satisfaction.

On the surface, the fourth principle may seem ridiculous for the area of clinical health care; however, given some thoughtful analysis and interpretation, it applies as much in health care as in any other organization. The crucial principle for health informatics professionals is the second one. New technologies must be organized around customer needs, not traditional bureaucratic boundaries. For progressive healthcare organizations, their largest assets will be the quality of their people, their software, and their databases, not their bricks and mortar or their equipment. Notice also a key implication of organizing around software: as the software continuously changes, so will the organizations. This flexibility will be a characteristic of successful organizations in the new paradigm.

A Practical Change Management Strategy

Change management is the process of assisting individuals and organizations in passing from the old paradigm to new ways of doing things. Therefore, a change process should both begin and end with a visible acknowledgment or celebration of the impending or just completed change. According to James Belasco [11], our culture is filled with empowering transitions. New Year's Eve parties symbolize the ending of one year and the hope to be found in the one just beginning. Funerals are times to remember the good points of the loved one and the hope for new beginnings elsewhere. Parties given to retiring or leaving employees are celebrations of the ending of the employee's past status and the hope for the new opportunities to be found in the new status.

Thach and Woodman define the three major informatics organizational change methods as follows [12]:

- *Technical Installation Model:* This traditional model focuses on the technical challenges, largely ignoring organizational and human issues. This model has often been sarcastically referred to as the techies "drop shipping" the technology or throwing it "over the wall" into the applications area. This model has often led to understandably high levels of organizational conflict.
- *Systems Approach:* This more recent model is the balancing of the technical with the organizational considerations in achieving an implementation. In this model, user inputs are often solicited and integrated into the project plan. Issues such as training are not left as afterthoughts, but a systems support team manages the project with a user-focused plan. The systems support staff are available for user "handholding" and train according to user expectations and needs.
- *Gap Analysis:* This model integrates informatics into the overall organization strategic planning process. This model, derived from Lewin's conceptual work, starts with an envisioning of the organizational future. Then, the steps necessary to reach that future are defined. The scope of the envisioning ensures that the informatics effort is well integrated into the necessary organizational changes.

Based upon our research, there is no single change management strategy that is effective in every situation. It is essential for the change management leader to take the time to know the desired state (vision–goal) and the particular organization and then to develop the appropriate strategies and plans to help facilitate the desired state. Over the years we have evolved a core model that is a combination of the systems and gap approaches described above. There are many options within this model, but we believe that it is helpful for change leaders to have an overview map in mind as they begin to implement new information technology systems. The five-stage model has proven effective for reducing barriers to technology change [13].

Assessment

The assessment phase of this model is the foundation for determining the organizational and user knowledge and ownership of the health informatics system that is under consideration. Ideally, this phase of the model begins even before the planning for the technological implementation of the new system. The longer the delay, the harder it will be to successfully manage the change and gain ultimate user ownership.

There are two parts to the assessment phase. The first is to *inform* all potentially affected people, in writing, of the impending change. This written information need not be lengthy or elaborate, but it will alert everyone to the changes in process.

The second part involves *collecting information* from those involved in the change. Information may be collected through surveys and interviews. There are a number of types of survey instruments; two include a general survey and a readiness assessment. The general survey instrument should be sent to randomly selected members of the affected group. One person in 10 might be appropriate if the affected group is large. Five to 10 open-ended questions could assess the individuals' current perceptions of the potential changes, their issues of greatest concern about these changes, and their suggestions to reduce those concerns. Recording and analyzing the responders' demographics will allow more in-depth analysis of the concerns raised by these potentially affected people.

The personal interview with randomly selected people at all levels throughout the affected portions of the organization is another data collection method. A sample interview survey is presented in the following Box 7.1.

Box 7.1   Sample Interview Instrument

Begin with a brief overview of what your organization is planning. Also ask important demographic questions, e.g., department/clinic/floor, and role, e.g., M.D., R.N. (Generally more accurate and useful information is received if the survey is anonymous.)

What have you heard about this information system from your colleagues?

- What is the most positive comment you have heard about this system?
- How do you think this system will affect your work/responsibilities?
- What are your concerns about the new system on your using this system?
- What are one or two ways that we can help to reduce your concerns?

Another type of survey is the readiness for change assessment. Readiness assessments are created based on the product, change required, and people/area involved. In a typical readiness assessment you would write the questions to capture the information needed to determine where strong support or resistance might be expected. The following is only a sample of a readiness assessment form that is based on the original ©Lorenzi-Riley Readiness Assessment Survey (unpublished) (see Box 7.2).

Box 7.2   Sample Readiness Assessment Process/Instrument

In an effort to prepare the _____ for the implementation of _____, our team has prepared a readiness assessment to identify questions that need to be answered as we develop strategies for implementation appropriate to your area. The objective of this survey is to collect data to determine the needs of your department. These questions are not a reflection on you, but rather an assessment tool used to gather data that the implementation team will use throughout the implementation process to ensure the successful rollout of _____.

Definition: *"The project"* is synonymous with "_____." This is followed by a more complete definition of the informatics tool.

Date: __/__/__ **Area/Division:** _____

Circle One:

MD   AA   Nurse   Technician   Management   Secretarial

If you have any questions regarding the project, you may contact _____ at _____.

Thank you for your participation.

	Fully agree 5	Somewhat agree 4	Neutral 3	Somewhat disagree 2	Fully disagree 1	Do not know 0	No answer
I believe the goal of the project to develop an electronic clinical information system for patient support is appropriate.							
I believe that an electronic clinical information system for — is critical to our future success.							
A great deal of change in — is required for the project to be effective.							
A great deal of change *in work processes and jobs* is required for the project to be effective.							

	Fully agree 5	Somewhat agree 4	Neutral 3	Somewhat disagree 2	Fully disagree 1	Do not know 0	No answer
A great deal of change *in working relationships with managers and administrators* is required for the project to be effective and achieve its objectives.							
A great deal of change *in working relationships with physicians* is required for the project to be effective.							
A great deal of support exists to make an electronic clinical information system succeed.							
Physicians in my organization will use an automated system to retrieve patient information.							
Physicians in my organization will use an electronic clinical information system to enter patient encounters.							

	Yes	No
The people who will be using the new computer information system must know and comprehend what the system will be realistically capable of doing. Do you believe this is true here?		
The people who will be using the new computer information system must be included in the communications and information regarding changes that are being considered and/or developed. Do you believe this is true here?		
The formal and informal leaders must support the system and push or pull through various times of success or failure. Do you believe this is true here?		
The people using the new computer information system must "see and know" the results of their comments about the system as rapidly as possible. Do you believe this is true here?		

Another type of interview is the focus group. If you do not have time for one-on-one interviews, you might gather five to seven people and ask your questions. One problem with the focus group arises if only the most opinionated person speaks. To control for the possibility, you might distribute the questions and ask each person to briefly write their responses, then ask each person to individually respond in addition to general group discussion.

It is important to listen to the stories the people are telling and to assess their positive and negative feelings about the proposed health informatics system. These interviews should help in ascertaining the current levels of positive and negative feelings; what each person envisions the future will be, both with and without the new system; what each interviewee could contribute to making that vision a reality; and how the interviewee could contribute to the future success of the new system. These interviews provide critical insights for the actual implementation plan. Often those people interviewed become advocates—and sometimes even champions—of the new system, thus easing the change process considerably.

Feedback and Options

The information obtained above must now be analyzed, integrated, and packaged for presentation to both top management and to those directly responsible for the technical implementation. This is a key stage for understanding the strengths and weaknesses of the current plans, identifying the major organizational areas of both excitement and resistance (positive and negative forces), identifying the potential stumbling blocks, understanding the vision the staff holds for the future, and reviewing the options suggested by the staff for making the vision come true. If this stage occurs early enough in the process, data from the assessment stage can be given to the new system developers for review.

When designing your model, this phase is important to establish that the organization *learns* from the inputs of its staff and begins to act strategically in the decision and implementation processes.

Strategy Development

This phase of the model allows those responsible for the change to use the information collected to develop *effective change strategies* from an organizational perspective. These strategies must focus on a visible, effective process to "bring on board" the affected people within the organization. This could include newsletters, focus groups, discussions, one-on-one training, and confidential "hand-holding." This latter can be especially important for professionals such as physicians, who may not wish to admit ignorance and/or apprehension about the new system. The manner in which the system is presented and represented will have an impact on its acceptance.

Implementation

This phase of our model refers to the implementation of the change management strategies determined to be needed for the organization. The implementation of the change strategies developed above must begin before the actual implementation of the new system. These behaviorally focused efforts consist of a series of steps, including informing and working with the people involved in a systematic and timely manner. This step-by-step progression toward the behavioral change desired and the future goals is important to each individual's acceptance of the new system. This is an effective mechanism for tying together the new technology implementation action plan with the behavioral strategies.

Reassessment

Three to 6 months after the new system is installed, a behavioral effects data-gathering process should be conducted. This stage resembles the initial assessment stage—written surveys and one-on-one and/or focus-group interviews. Data gathered at this stage allow measurement of the acceptance of the new system, which provides the basis for fine-tuning future efforts. This process also serves as input to the evaluation of the implementation process. It assures all the participants that their inputs and concerns are still valued and sought, even though the particular implementation has already occurred.

Conclusion

It is not always easy to know exactly why a particular person or group resists change. However, experience shows that an intelligent application of the basic five-step change model—coupled with a sound technological implementation plan—leads to more rapid and more productive introductions of technology into organizations. The process can be expensive in terms of time and energy but nowhere near the cost of an expensive technical system that never gains user acceptance.

Perhaps most importantly, overall success requires an emotional commitment to success on the part of all involved. People must believe the project is being done for the right reasons—namely, to further the delivery of higher-quality, more cost-effective health care. Projects generally perceived to be aimed at just saving money or boosting someone's ego/status are doomed to fail. Everyone needs to be involved in the change process from its inception, and the organization itself must be committed to the change. Furthermore, one must recognize that each organizational environment is unique—technology cannot be transplanted without first considering the needs of individual organizations. Adaptability on the part of users, administrators, and the technology itself is crucial to success.

A television commercial depicts a book editor, faced with adapting to major information system changes, commenting that "Art is constant; tools change." In the same vein, the ideals of all our professions are a constant; the tools change. The challenge facing health informatics is to successfully implement those new tools in organizations that often do not welcome them.

References

1. Belasco JA. Teaching the elephant to dance: empowering change in your organization. New York: Crown Publishers; 1990.
2. Conner DR. Bouncing back. Sky Sept. 1994;30–34.
3. Change for change's sake. Management Review Sept. 1994;9.
4. Morgan N. How to overcome "change fatigue." Harvard Management Update July 2001;1–4.
5. Horak BJ, Turner MDH. Case 9.1: Williams Memorial Hospital—nursing unit computerization. In: Lorenzi NM, Riley RT, Ball MJ, Douglas JV, editors. Transforming healthcare through information: case studies. New York: Springer-Verlag; 1995.

6. de Jager P. Resistance to change: a new view of an old problem. Futurist May–June 2001;24.
7. Argyris C. Overcoming organizational defenses: facilitating organizational learning. Boston: Allyn & Bacon; 1990, p. 169.
8. Argyris C. Overcoming organizational defenses (total quality management). Journal for Quality and Participation March 1992;15:2; 26+.
9. Vanderbilt University Conference on Clinical Provider Order Entry (CPOE), June 2002.
10. Imparato N, Harari O. When new worlds stir. Management Review Oct. 1994;22–28.
11. David PA. Computer and dynamo: the modern productivity paradox in a not-too-distant mirror. CEPR Pub. #172. Stanford, CA: Stanford Center for Economic Policy Research; 1989.
12. Thach L, Woodman RW. Organizational change and information technology: managing on the edge of cyberspace. Organizational Dynamics Summer 1994;31–33.
13. Lorenzi NM, Mantel MI, Riley RT. Preparing your organizations for technological change. Healthcare Informatics Dec. 1990;33–34.

8
The Role of Ethics in IT Decisions

James G. Anderson

As the role of information technology in health care changes clinical practice, existing values are being challenged.

This chapter addresses the ethical decision-making process in health care within the context of information technology (IT). Issues covered include the most prevalent ethical dilemmas encountered by healthcare decision makers, frameworks and guidelines that can be used to arrive at ethical decision making, and the best way to handle situations where questions of ethics arises. Specific cases are used as examples, and new dilemmas that are specifically posed by the emergence of e-health care are discussed.

The Changing Landscape of Health Care

Information technology pervades healthcare organizations. Surveys by the Healthcare Information and Management Systems Society (HIMSS) [1] and the Medical Record Institute [2] have found that healthcare organizations are implementing IT to meet information security requirements established by the Health Insurance Portability and Accountability Act (HIPAA) legislation, to improve patient safety by reducing medical errors, and to improve efficiency. IT applications are now viewed as essential in providing management information, containing costs, improving the quality of care, and ensuring patient safety.

At the same time, the rapid growth of IT in health care is transforming the delivery of health care. IT simultaneously changes clinical practice and challenges existing values. While many physicians still express skepticism, more healthcare providers are beginning to use online tools for patient care such as electronic medical records, electronic prescribing, online communication with patients, and remote disease monitoring. Developments such as the Internet and the World Wide Web that permit consumers to participate more actively in decisions regarding their care and to assume greater responsibility for managing their own health care represent a cultural change in health care that is far reaching. The traditional roles of physicians and patients are changing [3,4].

James G. Anderson, PhD, is Professor of Medical Sociology at Purdue University.

These new technologies raise a host of ethical and social issues. Some of these issues such as privacy and confidentiality of patient information are not new. However, electronic medical records and health information networks create the potential for far more serious violations and potential harm to larger numbers of patients than in the past. Other issues are new, such as the potential certification and regulation of online providers of healthcare services that cross state and national boundaries. While new developments in bioinformatics, the intersection of clinical informatics and genomics, show great promise, this new field also raises a host of ethical and social issues that need to be addressed [5,6].

Below we outline some of the major ethical issues raised by information technology. Specific cases will be provided to illustrate these issues and the questions they raise.

E-Healthcare

Increasingly, consumers are using the Internet to obtain health-related information, goods, and services [3]. A recent national survey found that more than three-fourths of respondents had used the Internet to obtain health information. A third had used it to locate providers, and more than 1 in 10 had looked for clinical trials, purchased medical supplies, and obtained support online [7] (Figure 8.1). Use of the Internet makes available to consumers a vast body of health-related information but at the same time potentially exposes them to out-of-date, inaccurate, and fraudulent information. It also changes the doctor–patient relationship and raises possibilities of conflict when the parties fail to agree on diagnosis and/or treatment decisions. While online communication with providers (26 percent), use of electronic medical records (22 percent), electronic prescribing (11 percent), and remote disease monitoring (5 percent) remain low in the United States relative to other countries [8–10], consumers express strong interest in using these tools (Figure 8.2). Almost 60 percent of respondents expressed

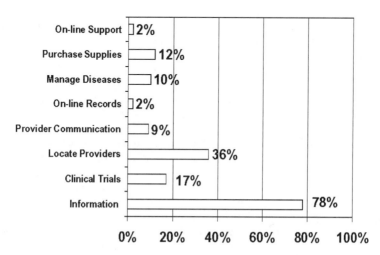

FIGURE 8.1. A national survey has shown that more than 75 percent of respondents have used the Internet to obtain various types of healthcare information. (From James G. Anderson, Business Briefings Ltd, with permission.)

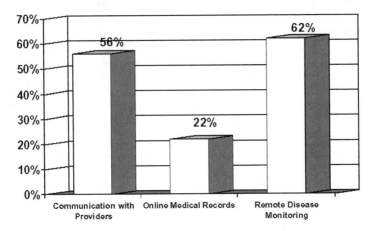

FIGURE 8.2. Consumers in the United States are showing growing interest in the use of online patient care tools. (From James G. Anderson, Business Briefings Ltd, with permission.)

interest in communicating online with providers, and 1 in 5 was interested in having their medical records online. Of those respondents who had a chronic disease, 62 percent were interested in remote disease monitoring [7].

Consumer use of the Internet is expected to increase dramatically, resulting in a $370 billion online healthcare industry by the year 2004 [11]. Online patient tools have the potential to dramatically affect clinical practice. Electronic medical records (EMRs) make comprehensive patient information more accessible to healthcare providers. Also, there is evidence that they reduce medical errors. Almost 90 percent of EMR users indicated that their use in practice improved efficiency and the quality of care provided. Providers who have not adopted EMRs in practice point to costs and concerns about how this technology will affect the doctor–patient relationship as major barriers to implementation [9].

A second IT application, electronic prescribing, improves efficiency by directly transmitting prescriptions to pharmacies. This tool helps to eliminate errors and delays caused by illegible handwriting and incomplete information. In addition, a Harris survey found that 45 percent of respondents indicated that the use of e-prescribing improved compliance with managed care formularies [9]. As e-prescribing becomes more common, it has the potential to increase the importance of managed care organizations in influencing the drugs that physicians prescribe. At the same time, the influence of pharmaceutical companies on physicians may be reduced.

Consumers overwhelmingly express interest in online communication with their healthcare providers. Over 70 percent of persons surveyed indicated that, if available, they would use the Internet to ask questions of their provider, arrange appointments, obtain prescriptions to refill medications they are currently taking, and to receive test results [7]. One survey found that 37 percent of respondents would be willing to pay for the ability to communicate with their provider via the Internet. In contrast, physicians express reluctance to initiate e-mail communication with their patients. They cite concerns about reimbursement, potential violation of the privacy of patient information, and potential malpractice liability [12].

Remote disease monitoring allows patients with chronic diseases to assume greater responsibility for managing their own health. In the survey cited earlier, more than

60 percent of respondents with chronic diseases expressed interest in remote monitoring [7]. IT is available that permits patients with diabetes, heart disease, and lung disease to collect and automatically transmit data on their condition via the Internet to a healthcare provider. The provider can monitor these data daily or weekly to decide when to see the patient or to intervene. One company, Health Hero, provides the Health Buddy monitoring and communication system. The system keeps track of patient data and automatically alerts the physician when the patient's condition changes and may require attention [13]. According to a recent survey, only 5 percent of physicians are currently using remote disease monitoring [8]. Reasons given for not adopting remote monitoring systems are costs and concern about how these systems will affect the relationship between doctors and patients. Although this patient care tool is currently not used extensively, it is likely that the number of physicians who use it to provide care to their patients will increase significantly.

While there is increasing evidence that IT applications can improve efficiency and the quality of care, their implementation in practice raises a host of social and ethical issues that need to be resolved. Some of the major issues are outlined below and illustrated by cases.

Consumer Health Information

Inaccurate Health Information

Surveys indicate that consumers are increasingly using the Internet to obtain health-related information. This tool helps them to make informed decisions about their own health care and to assume greater responsibility in managing their health. At the same time, information obtained from Web sites may be inaccurate, out of date, or fraudulent [14].

For example, an analysis of 371 Web sites that contain information on Ewing's sarcoma, a bone cancer that afflicts children and young adults, found that 1 of 3 sites contained information that did not come from peer-reviewed sources [5]. Some of the sites proposed treatment using alternative medicine. Estimated survival rates varied from 5 percent to 85 percent. This situation raises important ethical questions such as these: How can consumers effectively interpret and act upon contradictory Web-based information such as this? Are consumers able to effectively distinguish between peer-reviewed information and less reliable sources? What is the likelihood that parents who use the Web to obtain treatment information will delay or fail to consult their physician if they perceive a low survival rate for their child's medical condition?

Unverified Health Claims

Web sites that promote unproven or fraudulent claims are proliferating. The FTC in one study identified hundreds of Web sites that promoted unproven cures for ailments including AIDS, multiple sclerosis, liver disease, arthritis, and cancer [5]. Cures included the use of fatty acids to cure arthritis, laetrile for cancer, shark cartilage for cancer and AIDS, and magnets as a cure for various ailments. Although warnings were sent to many of these sites, more than 70 percent of the sites had failed to modify their claims a year later. Again this raises a number of important issues. How can consumers be assisted in distinguishing between good and bad health information that is available on the Web? Should federal and state governments assume responsibility to protect consumers from unverified and fraudulent health claims made by Web sites? What resources would be necessary for a government agency to investigate and initiate legal action against Web sites that fail to heed warnings about the information that they provide?

Conflicts of Interest

An additional problem that arises with Web sites that provide health-related information is potential conflicts of interest. The blurring of commercial content and professional information on these sites is a major problem for consumers. For example, the former dr.koop.com Web site provided advice on healthcare products and services. During its existence, the company that sponsored the Web site had stated that their goal was to "... establish the dr.koop brand so that consumers associate the trustworthiness and credibility of Dr. Koop [the former U.S. Surgeon General] with our company." In return, Dr. Koop was originally entitled to 2 percent of the revenue derived from sales of products. This financial arrangement was not made explicit on the Web site and was modified after the Web site received criticism for the potential conflict of interest [5]. As of this writing, dr.koop.com is currently in federal bankruptcy liquidation in Los Angeles.

Another feature of the Web site was its Community Partners Program, a list of hospitals described as "... the most innovative and advanced health care institutions across the country." The Web site did not mention that the healthcare institutions listed had paid $40,000 to be placed on the list. Questions that need to be addressed include: Did Dr. Koop and the corporation that sponsored the Web site have a responsibility at the onset to disclose the financial ties to medical services and products promoted on the Web site? Since the Web site also accepted advertising for healthcare products and services, did it have a responsibility to make the distinction clear between advertising and health education? In what ways, if any, is a Web site like or unlike newspapers, radio, and television in terms of the differences between news and advertising? How could a respected Web site make the fundamental mistake of selling endorsements for healthcare institutions and failing to disclose this practice to the public?

Physician–Patient Relations

As more and more people use the Internet to gather health information, they are assuming more responsibility for their own healthcare decisions. A number of consumer health services such as MedCetera and Health Responsibility Systems perform searches of the medical literature for patients. Fees range from $80 to $250. Customers receive bound notebooks containing abstracts of articles contained in Medline, the National Library of Medicine's database, and other sources. One company, HealthGate Data Corporation, offers a Web site where, for a fee, consumers can search and view summaries of articles related to their medical problems [5].

Some worry that patients who use the Internet to obtain specific disease-related information might not consult their doctors about serious health problems. Also, some physicians feel threatened when patients come to them with information gathered from the Internet about alternative diagnoses and treatments. In one instance, using the Internet, a woman with ovarian cancer found more than 200 reports of experimental treatments. She concluded that one experimental therapy using a combination of drugs would be more appropriate than the treatment that her doctors ordered. On the other hand, her doctors felt that the current treatment was more appropriate and that the woman was too weak to undergo the more intensive treatment regimen [5].

Cases such as this one raise a number of difficult questions. While patients are encouraged to learn more about their diseases and their treatment and to assume greater responsibility for their care and treatment, how should physicians respond to "clinical trial fishing" when this information is used to second-guess the professional's treatment plan? Should patients and family members be encouraged to question and even challenge decisions made by their healthcare providers? Or is shopping for additional opinions and protocols on the Internet counterproductive? Would patients be better off to find a physician they trust and accept their recommendations regarding the best treatment for their medical condition? Are there any safeguards for patients against faulty, misleading, or erroneous information about alternative therapies?

Online Health Services

Along with all the other goods and services available online, health services have become abundantly available. All manner of health services are available from virtual health calls to the sale of pharmaceutical products to mental health services. The money-making potential of these services has attracted the financial backing of a number of major corporations [5]. Below we review some of these online services and the ethical issues that they raise.

Virtual House Calls

A number of Web sites provide patient-specific health information. Mediconsult.com charges a fee of $195 to provide personal information on alternative therapies. Consumers submit online a detailed health history and receive a report suggesting the best treatment option.

Consumers can also shop online for surgery. Medicine Online, Inc. offers 36 procedures including breast augmentation, liposuction, dental surgery, and laser vision correction eye surgery. On some sites the consumer enters, on a Web site, his or her medical profile and the surgical procedure he or she wants performed. Physicians and dentists can bid on the procedure and patient and physician can negotiate the fee [5].

The proliferation of these online services raises a host of new issues. Is it appropriate to treat medical care as a commodity like other goods and services? Could advice and diagnosis really be effective and safe without any physical contact between online physicians and patients? What are the risks to consumers who shop on the Internet for the cheapest provider of services? Should the consumer be permitted to take these risks if they choose? What guarantees should providers of online medical services be required to supply that the healthcare providers are qualified to perform the services that they advertise online? Should physicians who advertise services online be required to state their qualifications? Is it unethical for physicians to bid on medical services before they see the patient in person?

Online Pharmaceutical Products

A survey by Forrester Research estimated that by the year 2004 consumers will use the Internet to purchase $15 billion worth of prescription drugs, almost $2 billion in over-the-counter nonprescription drugs, $3.3 billion in alternative health cures, and $1 billion in other health and beauty aids [11].

Web sites that provide prescription medications to patients who have not first seen a physician in person raise important issues. For example, Direct Response Marketing, a British-based Web site, sold $2.5 million worth of drugs in the first 18 months of operation. (See www.directresponsemarketing.co.uk.) The operator of the Web site is neither a physician nor a pharmacist. When consumers log on to the site, they are asked to complete an online questionnaire. A physician under contract with the Web site reviews the questionnaire, writes a prescription, and sends it to a pharmacy located near the offices of Direct Response Marketing. An employee of the Web site picks up the prescription and mails it to the consumer [5]. Questions raised by this practice include: Does the sale of prescription drugs over the Internet undermine licensing and regulation of the sale of drugs by the FDA? Are consumers who purchase drugs over the Internet without first seeing a physician placing themselves at risk? Should they be allowed to assume such risk? Is it necessary that a physician actually see a patient in person before prescribing a drug over the Internet? Should physicians who prescribe medications over the Internet without seeing the patient in person and/or the Web site providing the drug be held liable if the patient is harmed by the medication? Should drug companies be prohibited from providing drugs to Web sites that sell drugs without a doctor's examination and prescription?

Behavioral Health Services

Behavioral health services are beginning to move onto the Web. The National Mental Health Association sponsors a Web site to screen for depression. Patients can log onto the site and answer a set of questions on a diagnostic instrument developed by Harvard University and the National Mental Institute Screening Project. A score is printed out for the patient indicating whether or not the patient is clinically depressed. Concerned Counseling is a network of therapists who use the Internet to provide counseling to individuals and families. Some of the topics include marital conflict, eating disorders, and drug and alcohol addiction. When a patient sends an e-mail message they receive an answer within 12 hours; e-mail consultation costs $30 for each response. The cost of a chat room session is $45 for 30 minutes, $80 for up to 50 minutes [5].

One certified sex therapist operates a Web site that treats people online for sexual dysfunction. There is no personal contact between the doctor and many of his patients. In March 1999 the sexual and medical histories of 90 men and women who had consulted the doctor were inadvertently posted on a public Web site. The information included names, addresses, telephone numbers, and intimate details about their sex lives. This personal information from patient records may have been available to the public for months before the security breach was discovered [5]. Questions raised by the use of the Internet to provide behavioral health services include: Is there a danger that online screening and counseling may aggravate a sense of isolation and depression in some patients? Can patients receive adequate evaluations and treatments online? Will some patients who use the online service avoid seeing a therapist in person? Is information collected and stored online concerning a patient's psychiatric conditions or sexual dysfunctions adequately protected from privacy violations?

Electronic Medical Records

Almost half of all hospitals in the U.S. have implemented or are implementing EMRs [1]. Also, a recent survey indicated that 22 percent of U.S. physicians are using some type of EMR system in practice [8]. Physicians who have adopted EMRs report improvements in overall efficiency and quality of care. They also report reduced costs of transcribing, filing, storing, and accessing patient information. Hospitals and physicians who have not implemented EMRs point to cost and to concerns about the privacy and confidentiality of patient data as barriers to implementation.

Accidental breaches of security have occurred at a number of healthcare organizations that have implemented EMRs [15,16]. For example, an error on a Web server at a university health system made thousands of patient records open to public scrutiny. A hospital in Michigan where physicians use a voice mail service to record and access notes concerning patient examinations, consultation, admission, and discharge data could be accessed from outside the hospital without a user identification or password. The ready access to patient data raises a number of questions. How can currently available security measures be used to prevent errors like these from occurring? Is the healthcare organization obligated to inform all their patients whose records may have been affected by the breach in security? Will breaches of security like these result in patients withholding sensitive information from their healthcare provider? Who should be held responsible for any harm to a patient that occurs because of violations of confidentiality?

Privacy violations also occur when confidential patient data are used for inappropriate purposes. For example, medical students sold health records to malpractice attorneys. State employees in Maryland sold patient information from the state's medical database to HMOs. The *London Sunday Times* reported that anyone's medical records could be obtained by private investigators for about £200 [5]. These violations of patient confidentiality raise issues such as these: What should be the penalty for sale of patient information? Is it practical to make certain patient records or portions of the record that contain sensitive information such as substance abuse or mental illness off limits to employees? At the present time there are few restrictions on what states can do with medical information that they collect. Is it appropriate for states to use these data to identify potential criminals, to monitor family members suspected of child abuse, to detect drug users, etc.?

Moreover, secondary use of health information is growing [5]. Third-party payers use patient-specific data to process claims and to manage pharmacy benefit programs. Self-insured employers have legal access to employees' medical records. Data mining companies acquire medical information and link it with other sources of patient-specific information. The sale of personal information from these databanks for marketing purposes is widespread. One company, Acxiom, claims to have detailed information on 95 percent of U.S. households. Several large chain pharmacies have been sued for selling patient-specific information on prescriptions to a number of drug companies including GlaxoWellcome, Warner-Lambert, Merck, Biogen, and Hoffman-LaRoche. Some of the issues that these practices raise are: Should the consent of the individual patient be necessary before his/her medical data are included in shared databases? Who should be held accountable if patient data contained in these shared databases are used inappropriately?

Patient Safety

The Institute of Medicine has estimated that between 44,000 and 98,000 Americans die each year due to medial errors [17]. IT, when implemented appropriately, has the potential to significantly reduce medical errors and the resulting harm to patients [18–21]. At the same time, information systems when not properly implemented or integrated in a healthcare system have the potential to harm patients. This suggests that there is an ethical imperative to utilize IT to reduce risks to patients wherever possible and to thoroughly evaluate these systems [22–25].

In one instance, a young woman was admitted to the emergency department of a hospital with a high fever. When her blood pressure dropped she was admitted to the ICU with a presumed diagnosis of sepsis. The clinical information systems in the emergency department and ICU were separate. The physician ordered an antibacterial medication but the pharmacy filled the prescription with an antiviral medication. By the time the error was discovered the woman had experienced irreversible brain damage [26]. This case raises issues such as whether medical errors like this could be prevented if the hospital had implemented an integrated clinical information system. Are hospitals and other healthcare systems ethically obligated to implement available IT such as EMRs and e-prescribing to provide improved patient safety?

Another hospital hired consultants to design and implement a computer-based pharmacy system [5]. The system that was implemented included data handling and a user interface from a warehouse inventory system. Within months of implementation the system had to be discontinued due to risk to patients resulting form the large number of medication errors. The problem was traced to the fact that the new system eliminated much of the oversight provided by staff in using the old paper-based system. Questions raised from this case include: Did the hospital technical staff, which was responsible for testing and evaluating the new system against specifications, do enough testing? Could many of these problems have been foreseen and avoided by testing the new system? How can the hospital regain the confidence and support of its professional staff and employees when they implement a new system?

Bioinformatics

Bioinformatics involves the use of IT to acquire, analyze, store, manage, and transmit genetic data [27]. In the future, gene chips will be used to acquire genetic data; data mining will be used to extract data from large databases and warehouses; and decision support systems will be used to analyze data and to make clinical decisions.

The rapid growth of bioinformatics presents additional social and ethical issues. Acquiring and using genetic data for clinical purposes will raise issues concerning consent and appropriate use of these data. Questions that need to be raised include whether patients have given their consent to the collection of genetic data that will be used for clinical purposes. When there is no treatment or cure for diseases that have a genetic origin, would most patients prefer not to be told about the results of genetic testing? Who can appropriately access and use patient-specific genetic data? Should certain uses of these data be prohibited? For example, insurance companies may use this information to determine eligibility for coverage. Employers may use genetic information to hire and assign employees to specific jobs.

Ethics in Health Informatics

Cases discussed here raise issues that occur in the use of IT in health care. They reflect day-to-day situations that arise in health settings that require decisions. Issues such as privacy and confidentiality, conflicts of interest, harm to patients, and the nature of the physician–patient relationship are fundamental and pervade the U.S. healthcare system [28].

Biomedical ethics provides a common frame of reference to address these issues [5]. First, ethics helps us to identify issues that involve questions of right or wrong, appropriate or inappropriate actions on the part of individuals and organizations. For example, when, if ever, is it ethical to sell or use private patient medical information for commercial purposes such as marketing pharmaceutical products? Additional questions include: How can we distinguish between legitimate and illegitimate access to patients' medical information? How can we safeguard the confidentiality of patient data? When should patient consent be required before medical data are used for secondary purposes such as management, research, marketing, etc.? Who should be held accountable for breaches of confidentiality?

Actual cases are ideal for identifying and analyzing ethical issues that arise in practice as a result of IT. Cases can be selected and used to identify, discuss, and debate controversies and challenges raised by informatics applications such as decision support systems. The discussion of cases permits participants to share opinions based on their experiences and values. It also allows principles to be tested for comprehensiveness and for whether they can be generalized to other situations that may arise from the use of IT. In this sense, case studies provide reference points when participants experience analogous situations in their professional work.

Bioethics also provides a framework and tools to address controversies involving ethical issues and resolve conflicts that arise in practice. An effective approach involves the following steps [29]: collecting information on the controversy or challenge that arises from using IT; identifying the nature of the problem; analyzing the problem using ethics approaches; outlining practical alternatives and actions that can be taken by individuals and/or organizations; and, finally, evaluating the outcome.

Also, discussion of challenges, problems, and issues can lead to the development of institutional policies and procedures. Often there needs to be balance between potential harm and benefits of uses of IT. One way to assess these issues and resolve conflicts is to establish institutional ethics committees. Members of these committees can also serve as consultants when issues arise. In fact, the Joint Commission on Accreditation of Healthcare Organizations (JCAHO) requires accredited organizations to establish a mechanism for addressing ethical issues [30].

Another way that bioethics can contribute to medical informatics is by contributing to the development of professional standards. A number of codes of ethics have been proposed for health information professionals [31]. These codes help to ground the profession in a body of values and standards. Courses, seminars, workshops, and other educational activities can be used to raise the awareness of professionals concerning ethical issues in informatics.

Acknowledgments. Portions of this chapter are taken from reference 5, with permission. I wish to acknowledge the assistance of Marilyn M. Anderson in the preparation of this chapter.

References

1. Healthcare Information Management Systems Society. 13th annual HIMSS leadership survey, 2002. Available: *http://www.himss.org/2002survey/final_report_01.htm*. Accessed 4/22/2002.
2. Medical Record Institute. Fourth annual survey of electronic medical records trends and usage, 2002. Available: *http://www.medrecinst.com/resources/survey2002/overview.shtml*. Accessed: 9/13/2002.
3. Anderson JG. The business of cyberhealthcare. MD Comput 1999;16:23–25.
4. Anderson JG. CyberHealthcare: reshaping the physician-patient relationship. MD Comput 2001;18:21–22.
5. Anderson JG, Goodman KW. Ethics and information technology: a case-based approach to a health care system in transition. New York: Springer; 2002.
6. Goodman KW, editor. Ethics, computing and medicine. New York: Cambridge University Press; 1998.
7. Anderson JG. CyberHealthcare: patterns of consumer use and barriers to Internet use in the United States. In: Business briefing: global health care 2002, vol. 2, 53rd World Medical Association General Assembly.
8. The increasing impact of e-health on physician behavior. Harris Interactive, Health Care News 2001;1(31):1–14.
9. U.S. trails other English speaking countries in use of electronic medical records and electronic prescribing. Harris Interactive, Health Care News 2001;1(28):1–3.
10. European physicians especially in Sweden, Netherlands and Denmark lead U.S. in use of electronic medical records. Harris Interactive, Health Care News 2002;2(16):1–3.
11. Dembeck C. Online healthcare expected to reach $370 billion by 2004. EcommerceTime.com, January 4, 2000. Available at *http://www.ecommercetimes.com/perl/printer/2128*. Accessed October 4, 2001.
12. Patient/physician online communication: many patients want it, would pay for it, and it would influence their choice of doctors and health plans. Harris Interactive, Health Care News 2002; 2(8):1–4.
13. Available: *www.healthhero.com*. Accessed: November 22, 2002.
14. Anderson JG. Health information on the Internet: let the viewer beware (caveat viewor). MD Comput 2000;17:19–21.
15. Anderson JG, Brann M. Security of medical information: the threat from within. MD Comput 2000;17:15–17.
16. Anderson JG. Security of the distributed electronic patient record: a case-based approach to identifying policy issues. Int J Med Inf 2000;60:111–118.
17. Kohn LT, Corrigan JM, Donaldson MS, editors. To err is human: building a safer health system. Washington, DC: National Academy Press; 2000.
18. Hunt DL, Haynes RB, Hanna SE, Smith K. Effects of computer-based clinical decision support systems on physician performance and patient outcomes: a systematic review. JAMA 1998; 280:1339–1346.
19. Raschke RA, Gollihare B, Wunderlich TA, et al. A computer alert system to prevent injury from adverse drug events. JAMA 1998;280:1317–1320.
20. Bates DW, Teich JM, Lee J, et al. The impact of computerized physician order entry on medication error prevention. JAMA 1999;6:313–321.
21. Anderson JG, Jay SJ, Anderson MM, Hunt TJ. Evaluating the capability of information technology to prevent adverse drug events: a computer simulation approach. J Am Inf Assoc 2002;9:479–490.
22. Anderson JG. Evaluating clinical information systems: a step toward reducing medical errors. MD Comput 2000;17:21–23.
23. Anderson JG, Aydin CE, Jay SJ, editors. Evaluating health care information systems: methods and applications. Thousand Oaks, CA: Sage Publishing; 1994.
24. Anderson JG, Aydin CE. Evaluating the impact of health care information systems. Int J Technol Assess Health Care 1997;13:380–393.

25. Anderson JG, Aydin CE. Evaluating medical information systems: social contexts and ethical challenges. In: Goodman KW, editor. Ethics, computing and medicine: informatics and the transformation of health care. New York: Cambridge University Press; 1998. p. 57–74.
26. Ash JS, Anderson JG, Gorman PN, et al. Managing change: analysis of a hypothetical case. J Am Med Inf Assoc 2000:7:125–134.
27. Goodman KW. Bioinformatics: challenges revisited. MD Comput 1999;16:17–20.
28. Anderson JG. Information technology in health care: social and ethical challenges. In: Witten M, editor. Building a man in the machine: computational medicine, public health and biotechnology, part III. New Jersey: World Scientific Publishing, 1995. p. 1533–1544.
29. Purtilo R. Ethical dimensions in the health professions, 3rd ed. Philadelphia: Saunders; 1999.
30. Joint Commission on Accreditation of Health Care Organizations. Ethical issues and patient rights across the continuum of care. Oakbrook Terrace, IL: JCAHO; 1998.
31. Kluge EHW. Fostering a security culture: a model code of ethics for health information professionals. Int J Med Inf 1998;49:105–110.

9
CASES IN REDESIGN, I
Memorial Hermann Healthcare System: Redesign and Implementation of a Multifacility Clinical Information System

DAVID BRADSHAW and BEVERLY BELL

This narrative chronicles the development of a standardized, multidisciplinary clinical information system from the perspective of design and implementation, rather than of technology.

Enterprise Background

Located in southeastern Texas, the Memorial Hermann Healthcare System (MHHS) encompasses nine facilities whose services span specialty care, community, and academic settings. The facilities range in size from 50 to 870 beds. Specialty clinics affiliated with MHHS are in excess of 80. MHHS identified the need to develop a systemwide, consistent approach to patient care, providing healthcare professionals with information, resources, and processes that facilitate optimal, efficient clinical decision making. The phases of project initiation, design, build, test, and implementation at the first two facilities were accomplished over a 10-month period. The deployment throughout the MHHS enterprise was accomplished in 15 months.

As MHHS looked for vehicles to support their goals, they turned to their Information Systems Division (ISD). Throughout the enterprise, ISD faced several challenges, including:

1. The existence of multiple databases and associated hardware platforms across the enterprise.
2. Disparate/standalone applications across the enterprise.
3. Patient information replicated in multiple applications.

These challenges led to several concerns that MHHS identified:

David Bradshaw is Vice President and CIO of Memorial Hermann Healthcare System. Beverly Bell, RN, BS, HMA, CPHIMS, is Vice President at Healthlink Incorporated.

1. The difficulty of obtaining aggregate data.
2. Concerns about data integrity being compromised.
3. Requirements that ISD have expertise in multiple applications, operating systems, networking technologies, and hardware platforms.

Meeting Business and Quality Care Needs

An enterprisewide Clinical Information System Coordinating Council (CISCC) was established to work with ISD to define the direction for a clinical application system. These two groups compared the functionality, integration, and vendors of the three clinical information systems that were currently installed throughout the enterprise. Once they defined the future direction of clinical information systems for their enterprise, CISCC was able to articulate a vision that would provide the enterprise with a standardized, multidisciplinary clinical information system. They named the project Care[4], Care to the fourth power, because the new system would assist them in delivering the Right *care*, at the Right *time and place*, with the Right *resources*, and with the Right *information*. More specifically, the new system would be designed to support the following objectives:

1. Improve patient safety by the use of automated rules and clinically approved and standardized protocols.
2. Increase patient and staff satisfaction by improving communication between clinical staff and physicians and providing timely access to information.
3. Increase staff productivity by optimizing departmental workflows supported by the new systems design.
4. Improve gross revenue by developing standardized charge processes for clinical events.
5. Reduce average length of stay (ALOS) by automating the support of the clinical decision-making process.

CISCC made the decision to install the Cerner Millennium suite of products for their clinical information system needs. They opted for a single vendor solution, rather than a "best-of-breed" solution, to minimize integration issues. This decision supported MHHS's need to have an integrated system that encompassed order entry, documentation, and results viewing within a single application.

While MHHS already had Cerner Millennium installed at the academic facility, it was evident to the Coordinating Council that the clinical information system solution had to be designed for use by every facility within the enterprise. They realized they would need to undergo a design phase that would include representation from all their facilities.

Due to a project of this magnitude, ISD decided to select an implementation partner whose responsibility would be to:

- Facilitate project approach, scope, design, methodology, and project plan.
- Monitor scope and issues to ensure the project schedule was met.
- Coordinate among the multiple entities and projects.
- Ensure that training enhances user acceptance.
- Recognize and address roadblocks.
- Prepare the facility to accept change associated with the new system.
- Provide Cerner Millennium application expertise.

Rather than sending out Requests for Information (RFI), MHHS decided to hold a bidder's conference and invited several consulting firms that were widely known throughout the industry. MHHS presented a history of MHHS, their enterprisewide mission and goals as well as the goals and objectives of their Care[4] project, and identified their information systems functional needs. Each attendee was to draft a proposal that included a project organization chart, the number of full-time equivalents, project phases and related activities, length of phases, and deployment strategy. The Coordinating Council and ISD reviewed the proposals and listened to the presentations before selecting their implementation partner. It was very apparent to ISD that they needed the implementation partner to work closely with their vendor as well as themselves.

In addition to the implementation partner, MHHS also partnered with their clinical data repository vendor, Cerner, to provide Cerner Millennium application expertise. Cerner's responsibilities included:

- Management of Cerner points that were logged.
- Information of Cerner Offline Code Distribution (OCD) and product knowledge.
- Obtain fixes and provide education associated with the new functionality.
- Act as liaison to other Cerner sites that may be experiencing similar challenges.
- Act as liaison between corporate Cerner and client site.
- Participate in design decisions to optimize value and functionality.
- Provide Cerner Millennium application expertise.

Operational Methodologies

At the conception of the project, MHHS identified the techniques for meeting management, decision making, and issue tracking that would carry them throughout the project. Brainstorming and nominal ranking were among the techniques regularly used during planning sessions. Additionally, it proved very useful to hang 3-foot by 5-foot sheets of paper on the wall to capture points expressed in the sessions. A standardized meeting plan and minutes format was identified and adhered to by all project participants. For permanent electronic storage of project documents, the project folders were organized in a standardized fashion to coincide with the overall project.

When possible, a laptop with PC viewer was used to project the Cerner application screens to meeting attendees. This allowed for visual and audio learning techniques to be used by meeting participants. It was quite common to have "handouts" at each meeting so that attendees could use them to take information back to their coworkers as well as to have visual aids during the meeting.

Project Initiation

Project Governance Structure

Now that the project was being initiated, it quickly became apparent that ISD needed to identify the project governance structure. This activity was a priority because it set the foundation for the project participants and project direction. The project governance structure established the roles and responsibilities of each position.

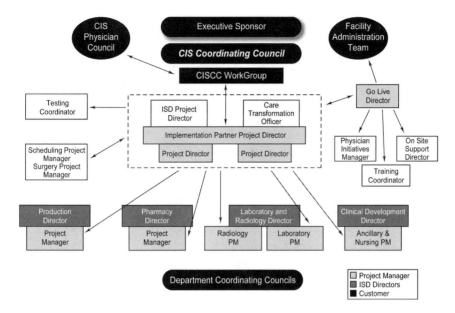

FIGURE 9.1. Chart of Project Governance structure for Care[4].

The Clinical Information System Coordinating Council (CISCC) had overall project responsibility (Figure 9.1). The CISCC was composed of MHHS administrative leaders representing all disciplines and was chaired by the project sponsor. In this case, the project sponsor was the enterprisewide COO. The sponsor and council members established project goals, objectives and approach, ensured quality output, guided enterprise-wide standardization process, held project team and business/operational owners accountable for achieving predefined results, and assisted ISD with decision making for clinical application development. This council met monthly while a subset of its membership called the CISCC Workgroup met weekly to make decisions on issues that required immediate attention. One example is the approval of system change requests that affected project scope.

The Clinical Information System Practice Committee (CISPC) was established in an effort to meet the enterprisewide clinical information system needs of the medical staff. The membership was diverse across numerous medical and surgical specialties. Each facility within the enterprise had at least one member on the council. The council did not solely consist of information system champions, as there were many novice technology users as well. The representatives sat on their respective Medical Informatics Committee at the facility in which they primarily practiced. The CISPC met monthly and made high-level decisions that affected physician, physician employee, and resident use of MHHS computer systems. The CISPC steering committee met every other week to determine design decisions and discuss system change requests that were relevant to physicians, physician employees, and residents.

The Care Transformation Officer and Go-Live Director worked very closely to prepare each facility for the workflow process changes as a result of an enterprise-wide system design. The ISD Project Director managed the overall project plan that was fed by other plans such as Testing, Training, Pharmacy, Radiology, Ancillary, Nursing, and

Production (code shared by all applications). All these areas had their own Project Manager to oversee their particular project. The Project Executive and Practice Director provided information, guidance, and expertise relevant to Cerner products. The Implementation Partner Project Director provided project guidance to the clinical information systems leadership team. The Physician Initiatives manager was responsible for project plans that instilled physician acceptance of the new system.

Project Goals

Although MHHS knew they wanted to have a single data repository for patient information, the goals specific to the project needed to be defined. The CISCC decided the project goals were to:

1. Establish a standardized product and operational procedures to be utilized by all facilities.
2. Gain confidence of facilities with the use of a standardized product.
3. Manage current and future functionality.
4. Collect and analyze metrics to document critical project success factors.
5. Minimize deployment time.

Project Scope

It was now time to solidify the project scope. Multiple planning sessions of the CISCC were held to reach consensus. It was decided that nursing would enter all orders, except medications. With regard to Pharmacy orders, the Pharmacy department would enter all medication orders into the system. The following departments would use the system for documentation, resulting and charging as appropriate: the cardiac catheterization lab, cardiology, neurophysiology, food and nutrition service, care management, physical medicine (speech, occupational, and physical therapy), radiology, radiation therapy, rehabilitation services, respiratory therapy, sleep lab, antepartum testing, chaplaincy, and social work. The pharmacy would use the system to dispense and charge medications and intravenous fluids, print and distribute Medication Administration Records (MAR), and monitor staff productivity. Surgery would schedule all cases and enter all physician preference cards, charges, and limited intraoperative documentation, while scheduling would use it to schedule all inpatient and outpatient procedures for every ancillary department. Additionally, electronic signature of dictated physician reports was mandated with the project.

After having documented the scope, it was necessary for the CISCC to identify the functionality that was outside the scope of the project. Using the same meeting management and decision-making techniques, they decided that the following functions would not be included in the project: nursing documentation, electronic documentation of medication administration and bar coding for positive patient identification, Emergency Room documentation, and computer-based physician order entry (CPOE).

Rapid Deployment Strategy

With an open mind, MHHS pursued how it could deploy the new system to as many facilities as possible and as quickly as possible. They wanted to minimize the length of time each of its facilities was on different clinical information systems. There were several additional benefits to a rapid deployment strategy:

1. Rapid deployment of operational model to all facilities.
2. Benefits of process standardization would be realized sooner.
3. Completion approximately 6 months sooner than consecutive model.
4. Reduce the time that facilities are on different applications.
5. ISD would be available to deploy additional functionality sooner.

Several models were considered: each had to be evaluated with relation to staffing resources, cost, time spent before and after deployment, prerequisite activities, and postdeployment activities. The CISCC decided upon a deployment strategy that included two facilities going live on the same day followed by two more facilities coming up on the same day 4 months later. Eight weeks after the second set of facilities went live, a single large facility was scheduled to go live. The three largest facilities went live between January and September 2003.

Enterprise Design Solution Methodology

There were several reasons to justify a standardized enterprisewide design:

1. To lay the groundwork for a rapid deployment across the enterprise.
2. To minimize change during the deployment process.
3. To expedite the return on investment across the enterprise.
4. To achieve faster delivery of functions by advanced information technology utilization.

Project Phases and Timeline

While this is a description of the phases of the project, it is important to realize that the steps did not necessarily occur consecutively. The success of the project rested in the ability of MHHS to have tasks in different phases of the project happening concurrently.

I. Project Initiation Phase

During the project initiation phase, the project governance structure, project goals, scope, charter, and project work plan were documented and kickoff held. This phase lasted 4 months.

II. Enterprise Design and Build Phase

The enterprise design and build phase lasted for 6 months and consisted of the activities that follow.

First, a clinical systems functionality questionnaire was completed by ISD. Second, an in-depth, facility questionnaire was circulated to all department directors. Third, an analyst interviewed department directors, validating their understanding of the responses on the questionnaire. Fourth, 37 multidisciplinary Joint Application Design (JAD) sessions were held to identify how specific functions would be built in the new system. Fifth, current and future states were flowcharted. The future states were based on the JAD sessions. Sixth, after ISD completed building 10 percent of the system, ISD held build validation sessions with the JAD participants. Seventh, the CISCC, Chief Nursing Executives, and Chief Financial officers went through a review session and accepted the design. Each of these steps was critical in designing a model that could be used across the enterprise.

1. *Clinical Systems Functionality Questionnaire.* This step required that the analyst complete a detailed comparison of all functionality across the current systems. This provided the analyst with a basic understanding of the functionality needs of the enterprise in place at that time. The 61-page document included items such as work lists, schedules, security, authentication, authorization, audit trails, assessment documentation, problem lists, care plans, medication documentation, vital sign documentation, result entry, charge capture, etc. This document was resurrected and referred to during the system design phase of the project.

2. *Facility Questionnaire.* The questionnaire was circulated across all ancillary and nursing departments that were to use the new system. The questionnaires were quite long and covered department operations as well as functions that they performed on their current computer system. The department directors were given 2 weeks to complete the questionnaire.

3. *Interview of Department Directors.* After having familiarized themselves with the responses on the facility questionnaire, the ISD analyst scheduled interviews with each department director and reviewed the questions with the director. The purpose of this exercise was to validate that the ISD analyst accurately understood the responses and to obtain a better understanding of the current state. Obtaining the current state information was important to help understand the operational processes and the potential for change necessary for the individual hospitals.

4. *Joint Application Design (JAD) Sessions.* For this enterprisewide design, the purpose of the JAD session was to assess the operational needs and end user expectations for the new system. Each JAD session was tasked with creating a standardized design that could be implemented in every facility. The outcome was a detailed design document that would be used by the analyst to build the appropriate system functionality.

Joint Application Design (JAD) sessions had been used by the organization during previous enterprisewide projects such as replacement of registration and patient billing applications. Having experienced success in the past with this methodology, the ISD and CISCC members decided to use this methodology again.

The benefits they had experienced with previously held JAD sessions included:

1. The ability to consolidate multiple design meetings into one meeting.
2. Identifying and organizing items that required decisions.
3. Quantifying for system builders what was needed to build the system.
4. Validating customer requirements agreed upon in the JAD session.
5. Alignment of workflow process redesign with system functionality design.
6. A means to satisfy clinician needs.

An overview of the planned JAD sessions was given to the members of the CISCC. Following approval of the design methodology, a letter describing the JAD process and calendar of JAD sessions was sent electronically to the administrators at each of the enterprise's facilities. The CISCC representative from each facility was to reinforce support of the initiative at their respective facility.

MHHS conducted 37 sessions covering departments such as pharmacy, radiology, nursing, surgery, and all other ancillary departments except Laboratory. Several multidisciplinary JAD sessions were held following the completion of the individual department JAD sessions. For example, frequency or schedules (i.e., BID was 0900 and 1700) of exams were streamlined to an enterprise-wide common list. Representatives from all the hospitals were invited to attend each session. Hospital administrators identified the attendees they wanted to participate in the JAD sessions. Despite staffing constraints that are prevalent throughout the healthcare industry, for the most part each facility was represented at each session.

To lend equality and ownership to the JAD participants and to have continuity to the JAD sessions, the same JAD guidelines were used for every JAD session:

- The voices of all participants are equal.
- Pagers and cell phones should be set to silent mode.
- Avoid using technical jargon.
- Everyone is responsible for adhering to the agenda and to associated timeframes.
- The timekeeper will signify the midpoint and 1-minute point.
- Items where decisions are not finalized will be placed on open list.
- Unrelated topics will be noted on the parking lot list.
- Discussion will be centered on normal business operations.

Each JAD session had a facilitator, recorder, and timekeeper to keep the session productive. Tools such as 3-foot by 5-foot sheets of paper hung on walls and personal computers connected to overhead displays were used in addition to the JAD booklets during the JAD session to enable all participants to see examples of what was being presented and to see design decisions.

For each JAD session, the analyst generated a booklet that was used to facilitate attendees through the decision-making process. The JAD booklets were specific to the individual JAD sessions. Each decision that needed to be made had a chapter divider and its corresponding supporting information behind the chapter divider. It took approximately 40 to 50 hours of work for each 8-hour JAD session. The analyst also distributed questionnaires to the JAD participants for completion.

It was imperative to have the vendor participate in the development of the JAD session booklet and to participate in the JAD sessions. This allowed design decisions to be realistic rather than establishing design requirements that were not supported by the software vendor. If the vendor representative did not know if a feature could be accommodated, the vendor performed the research and provided accurate expectations to the person documenting the outcome of the JAD session.

Because the JAD participants were not familiar with the vendor software, when applicable, they were shown actual screens in the software application. It was also very important to explain how the decision they were making affected them during normal operations of their department. For example, if the decision was to have BID as 0900 and 1700, they needed to be given examples of when they would be using this decision.

In the JAD sessions, the future state processes were discussed with a focus on the major process changes from the current state. The analysts constructed future state workflow process maps using Microsoft's Visio based on the responses during the JAD sessions.

Corporate policies and procedures were documented to accommodate JAD decisions as appropriate. However, some procedures were left for each facility to decide upon given their uniqueness, for example, the decision to have a nurse collect blood samples or have a phlebotomist collect blood samples. Also, regulatory requirements such as HIPAA requirements, JCAHO standards, and state laws were taken into consideration during the JAD sessions.

At the conclusion of JAD sessions, the analysts documented the decisions in the same format as the JAD booklets. The Design Review/Approval process was the final step in the JAD process. It was essential in providing a final validation for JAD participants, facility management, and administrators. This step gave participants the opportunity to review their decisions and provide approval that the design will meet their expected needs and produce the stated project objectives.

The nursing and ancillary departments used three levels of review and approval. The responsible analyst assigned to that department facilitated the first level of review in a series of design approval meetings. The purpose of these sessions was to present design decisions made by the JAD participants to the ISD clinical development team to better coordinate the build process of the project. The ISD clinical development team was the team responsible for building the application. They would use the information obtained in the JAD sessions to facilitate the build process.

The purpose of the following two levels of review and approval was to present future state design and the associated process impacts resulting from the JAD process. The second level was obtained from the original JAD participants in the JAD validation sessions. The third level was the Chief Nurse Executives, Chief Financial Officers, and the CISCC Workgroup.

The departments of Pharmacy and Radiology obtained approval from their respective councils (permanently established enterprise-wide departmental coordinating councils). The councils reviewed the design decisions made in the JAD sessions and approved or revised the decisions as needed.

Laboratory departments at all the facilities had achieved standardization of both work process and computer system in previous years; therefore, JAD sessions were not necessary.

The analysts on the surgery team established a design methodology that varied slightly from the other departments included in this project. They too evaluated current state processes to help with the identification of process changes and changes to the current system and its related workflow processes. The surgery team did not conduct JAD sessions; however, a Task Force of the Operating Room Council composed of 30 individuals was assembled to make the necessary design decisions. Ten task force group meetings were held. In these meetings the attendees standardized procedures, delay codes, cancellation codes, item file, anesthesia types, acuity codes, and service types. The Operating Room Council reviewed and approved the standardization decisions made by their task force and authorized the analyst to start building their system.

5. *Gap Analysis*. After documenting the current and future states, it was necessary to identify the delta between the two states. The current and future states were documented by department, as was the gap analysis. Using Microsoft's Visio, the new functions and steps were boldfaced and in another color. This documentation allowed MHHS to quickly visualize the impact on adapting new system functionality, workflow, and processes once the facility was using the new system.

6. *Ten Percent Build and Validation Sessions.* ISD came to the facilities training room where they reviewed the decisions from the JAD in conjunction with screens that had been built. A demonstration of the actual build work was shown to the customer. The session lasted 8 hours and covered items such as staff positions, charge screens, and orders screens.

During this phase, over a 2-week period, MHHS received, loaded, and tested multiple new OCDs to gain new functionality offered by their application vendor.

7. *CISCC and CFO Review.* During this session, the CISCC members saw a demonstration of the 10 percent build and reviewed how the JAD sessions supported an enterprisewide design. As a committee, they approved the enterprisewide design and

build. The CFO's designee reviewed charge descriptions and numbers appropriate to their facility.

8. *Build Finalized.* The ISD team completed the remaining 90 percent of the build after approval by the CISCC. This effort required 2.5 months of build time.

III. Testing Phase

The duration of the testing phase was 7 months. Several types of testing took place and required numerous individuals. The testing coordinator had managed the effort to draft a testing project plan, test plan, test scripts, and issue tracking database. All testers were brought together in a testing room set up for the purpose of testing. The types of testing included:

1. *Functional.* The purpose was for each analyst to ensure each selection on the screen worked as intended.

2. *Integration Testing.* The objective was to test the interfaces and data flow between multiple applications such as financial and clinical applications.

3. *Usability Testing.* The objective was to confirm the usability of the system by emulating daily transactions and ensuring the user interface was acceptable with respect to functional, operational, and technical adequacy of the system. This included testing of policies and procedures and reporting outputs.

4. *Regression Testing.* This confirmed that the build did not adversely affect any software that had been previously tested and incorporated into production.

5. *Security and Controls Testing.* This verified that security and control mechanisms provided in the integrated system are effective in preventing unauthorized use and invalid business scenarios that have the potential to corrupt business data.

6. *Device and Routing Testing.* This determined that the devices (workstations and printers) were configured correctly to operate.

7. *Performance Testing (Data Volume).* This confirmed that the system met all specified performance criteria when executed under stated full-load conditions (data volume). Specifically, it determined the ability of the system—hardware, operating system, network, and software—to operate under heavy data entry workloads, and determined processing time of interface routines under peak workloads.

IV. Implementation Phase

The implementation phase required 4 months and included conversion planning, training of employees, and conversion support.

The first step in preparing for conversion was to communicate with the facility. A facility-based communication plan was developed that targeted five different audiences within a facility: administration, management, super users, end users, and physicians and their employees. The communication plan stated, week by week, what topics needed to be addressed and what meetings needed to occur.

1. *Administration.* Information was disseminated to the administrative team before distribution to other bodies. This allowed the administrators to understand what their team was doing before they did it. It also allowed the administrative team to provide direction to ISD. The following is a sampling of topics that were discussed on a regular basis: training requirements, distribution of sign-on codes and passwords, activities on the night of conversion, conversion support schedule, charging mechanisms, new procedures and policies, and physician initiatives.

2. *Management.* The items that were discussed with the administration team were discussed with the management; however, more depth was given to the topics. Department-specific meetings were held with regard to ancillary departments such as Pharmacy, Laboratory, Radiology, and Health Information Management so department directors could learn and understand the new system and its impact on their individual department operations.

In addition to the departmental meetings, several multidisciplinary process meetings were held. In these meetings, ISD showed real screens and described the purpose of functionality. Simultaneously, ISD reviewed the future state workflow. This allowed department management to see the new system their employees would be using and see how the new system would be incorporated into their employees' workflow. Because there are different styles of learning, ISD also documented, in textual format, the old and new procedures and whether there was a need for education, a new policy, or a new procedure. This document served as a plan for those items needing follow-up activity. For example, each facility drafted any policies or procedures that were new for them. The document was also used to train employees on the new procedures that would accompany their new workflow processes.

The charge capture meeting was across departments in that it included the business office director as well as department directors. A flowchart was used to demonstrate how charges flowed between the business and clinical systems. A table was created to demonstrate into which application employees entered charges and how each department charged (on completion of order, retrospective) and credited items. Actual charge and credit screens were shown to the department directors. Reports from both the business and clinical systems were reviewed and discussed. Department directors were also asked to validate that all their charges were in the new system, charge master, downtime charge form, and where applicable on the tick sheet. Even though the process was not changing, we reviewed the process in which to obtain new charge numbers and delete numbers that were no longer needed.

Several planning sessions were held to discuss activities on the night of conversion. Discussion centered on when and who would review and document current orders, when and who would enter the current orders into the new system, when and who would validate census in the new system, when and who would generate patient labels and stuff charts with enough paper documents to last through night, when and who should ensure reports would come off the printer as planned, etc. The ancillary department and nursing activities were documented according to date and time in a conversion manual.

Downtime procedures were reviewed and in some cases were revised. For example, Respiratory Therapy was moving to "chart charging." Therefore, they needed to adjust their downtime forms to reflect actions to be taken if Care[4] were unavailable.

3. *Super users.* The super users were trained the first week of training, and they were asked to participate in at least one training session. Two meetings specific to super users were held prior to conversion. Agenda items included a review of the activities that were going to happen the night of conversion, review of new process changes to accompany the new system, review of their ISD resources, and practice time on the new system.

4. *End users.* "News You Can Use" e-mail messages were distributed to all the facilities' employees on a daily basis for a matter of 3 weeks prior to conversion. It included a countdown of the days to conversion and "tips and tricks" that would help them when using the new system.

5. *Physicians.* ISD worked with the administrative team to identify physicians that would both challenge and support the project. Quite naturally, this group of physicians

became the project champions as they learned more about the new system and felt comfortable using it. This was accomplished via small group demonstrations and training sessions that were performed by a physician and ISD personnel.

To communicate the functionality for physicians, demonstrations were conducted at various medical staff meetings such as general staff and section meetings. A letter from the CEO of the facility was sent to each physician office, and educational posters were placed in designated areas within the facility.

ISD offered a variety of training methodologies to meet the needs of the physician. Computer-based training was available via the Web and on disk. One-on-one instructor-led sessions were available in the physician dining room, Health Information Management department, or physician office. Physicians were also accommodated with regard to training times. Because electronic signature of dictated reports was included in the project, physicians were required to demonstrate competency in this function.

The facility sponsored luncheons for the physician office personnel. The purpose of the luncheon was to provide a PowerPoint presentation of the new functionality the physician and office personnel would have. The sessions were usually scheduled a few weeks prior to the conversion and one or two following the conversion.

An instructor using a Web-based learning management tool trained the office staff personnel in a classroom setting. The class provided 60 minutes of training on the new system. Separate classes were held for business office personnel and for those who were patient care providers.

6. *Conversion activities.* In an effort for the facility administration to discern whether or not their facility was indeed ready for the conversion, a Readiness Checklist was drafted. This document addressed such items as super users scheduled, hardware placement, testing of printing, training completion, policies and procedures documented, downtime procedures revised, and attitude of employees and physicians.

After the facility decided they were ready, they met with the project sponsor (enterprise COO) and a subgroup of the CISCC to enable all involved parties to state their readiness and reach consensus to convert systems as planned.

The project sponsor and CISCC meeting was followed by a conversion kickoff meeting with the facility management team and anyone who was working the night of conversion. A conversion manual was distributed to every department and nursing unit during this meeting.

7. *Usability lab.* At the conclusion of training, super users practiced system functionality and processes that had been previously identified. Scenarios were established to guide the super uses through the exercise. This enabled the super users to practice on the system as well as become familiar with the new processes. One example of how a process was affected was that while orders could be entered on pre-admitted patients they were not encounter specific. Therefore, it was necessary to review the preadmit process to know who was entering and retrieving those orders.

8. *Metrics.* The CISCC wanted to be able to monitor the overall success of the project at each facility. A subgroup of the CISCC met to identify the metrics to be collected. An example included the daily charge posting for Pharmacy, Laboratory, Cardiopulmonary, and Respiratory Therapy. Also for pharmacy, the volume of orders entered into the system and the volume of actions taken against the orders were collected. Regarding Radiology, the Turn-Around-Time (TAT) was tracked.

The facility management and administrative teams were educated on the metrics before and during the conversion period. All the metrics were submitted to a single person who would compile the values in a spreadsheet. Values were displayed numerically and in a run chart. At the conclusion of each week, the spreadsheet was shared with the facility and ISD administration. Any concerns were addressed as appropriate.

V. Postconversion

The support team structure for conversion support encompassed four tiers. First tier were the super users, second tier was the conversion team, third tier was the ISD production and development team, and the fourth tier was the vendor and implementation partner. There was 24/7 support for the first 2 full weeks of postconversion. The second week postconversion had fewer people supporting than the first week; however, it was still 24/7 coverage. For week three following the conversion, the conversion team provided on-site support from 6 A.M. to 8 P.M. The last week of on-site support was week four. The hours of support were 8 A.M.–5 P.M.

Once the conversion period was completed, the super users continued to provide first-tier support while the ISD Support Center provided a second tier of support. The third tier was the ISD production and development teams.

Because two separate facilities went live on the same night, there were three command centers, one primary and two satellites. The primary housed personnel from the vendor, the implementation partner, and the corporate production support personnel. The satellite command centers were staffed with clinical development analysts (who built the system) and conversion support staff (ISD employees who supported facilities). The conversion support staff answered "how to" questions and supported the facility super users.

The primary command center recorded all problems, system change requests, and facility process issues into three separate categories in the Support Center's database. The questions related to "how to" do a task were not tracked. At the primary command center, the team worked to resolve open problems. The conversion team worked with the facility to resolve open process issues.

During the week of conversion, three daily conference calls were held between the three conference centers. At 12 noon (High Noon) each day, an open forum meeting was held. Any employee, management staff, or administrator could stop by to voice concern or get an update on a particular problem. An open forum meeting was not held during the night shift because the conversion support team was able to keep them informed.

The fourth week postconversion was considered to be a week of transition. It was during this week that the conversion team prepared the facility management team to assume responsibility for collecting ongoing metrics, finalizing any open process issues, understanding how future enhancements were to be communicated, ensuring they knew how to request a change to the system, understanding how training for new employees would occur, understanding how they would be notified of downtimes, etc. A Transition Checklist was created and reviewed with administration before exiting the facility.

All the tasks stated above were instrumental in the healthcare organization's efforts to successfully implement multiple modules of an application simultaneously at multiple facilities. Above all, the teams' steadfast commitment to quality as well as to on time and on scope completion was of utmost importance in achieving success. Job Well Done!

10
CASES IN REDESIGN, II
UPMC Health System: Transforming Care Through Clinical Documentation

DARINDA E. SUTTON

Automated clinical documentation represents a major milestone for UPMC in its drive to improve the quality of care and achieve an integrated electronic health record.

Challenges for Health Care

The healthcare industry currently faces the serious challenge of needing to transform the delivery of care to be able to continue providing quality care. One of the key issues confronting the major players in today's healthcare environment is the increasing shortage not only of nursing staff but also in radiology, pharmacy, and other direct patient care providers. Several solutions come to mind to cope with this dilemma: one is to increase the supply of patient care providers, another is to decrease the demand for those services. The latter is not the most advantageous option as it implies that we would be decreasing the quality of care (or access to health care). If we cannot effectively increase the supply of care providers, or decrease the demand of services by patients, then we need to look for solutions in the process of the work that we do and in the way in which we provide care.

How can we transform the delivery of care to make it more efficient? How can we take advantage of technologies that promise to support more efficient and effective healthcare delivery, while maintaining quality care characterized by high patient safety and no adverse reactions or adverse outcomes? No single silver bullet exists that can solve these problems from either the technology or the process redesign perspective. In lieu of looking to the elusive silver bullet, we may need to attack the current crisis from many different angles. This case study chronicles one approach—the process that one large Integrated Delivery Network (IDN) in western Pennsylvania has undertaken to transform care from the clinical documentation perspective in preparation for the implementation of an integrated electronic health record.

Darinda E. Sutton, RNC, MSN, is Director of Clinical Systems for the UPMC Health System in Pittsburgh, PA.

The UPMC Health System Mission and Vision

The University of Pittsburgh Medical Center (UPMC) Health System (UPMCHS), a large integrated delivery network affiliated with the University of Pittsburgh, is a premier healthcare system in western Pennsylvania and one of the largest nonprofit healthcare systems in the United States. UPMC's primary service area is Western Pennsylvania's nearly 4 million residents, as well as regions in West Virginia and Ohio. The UPMCHS includes 20 hospitals and more than 400 physician offices in 29 counties in the region. Annual patient activity for the UPMC Health System includes approximately 4300 licensed beds, more than 150,000 inpatient admissions, and nearly 2 million outpatient visits. Our emergency medicine specialties oversee more than 350,000 visits each year, and surgical services participate in more than 115,000 surgeries annually. Our home care arena is involved in excess of 1 million visits a year. In addition, the health system supports the education and training of approximately 1100 medical residents in 70 specialty areas, as well as 1200 nursing students and hundreds of other allied health students in pharmacy, radiology, respiratory therapy, and social work. UPMC is the largest employer in the region with 35,000 employees and contributes more than $15 million annually in community services, charity, and other uncompensated care.

In 1997, the health system embarked on the journey of automating and transforming care across the continuum through the development and implementation of an integrated electronic health record (EHR). Mission and vision statements were adopted for the EHR that not only underscored the importance of the initiative but also established a framework for the project.

The EHR Mission was "To improve patient care and organizational effectiveness through clinical and consumer interaction with computer based technology. This will occur at the point of care everywhere in the Health System." The EHR Vision was to "Create a singe Electronic Health Record (EHR) that crosses the continuum of care and spans the UPMCHS enterprise and that will:

• Improve the quality of patient care.
• Increase the efficiency within the organization as a whole.

The EHR will be immediately accessible to physicians and clinicians and will allow consumers the opportunity to be informed and participate in their care."

Examining Current Data

To inform our process, a review of literature was conducted to examine current data related to redundancy and duplication of nursing documentation and the impact on workflow efficiency when documentation is standardized, streamlined, and ultimately automated. Filho identifies the problem of duplication and redundancy of documentation for nursing as a global phenomenon that is demonstrated in Brazil as well as in England [1]. Paperwork continues to frustrate nurses in most healthcare settings. Bowles estimates that nurses spend up to 50 percent of their work time documenting patient information [2]. It is not known how much of this time is spent on documenting duplicate information found in the paper chart. Pabst et al. studied the impact of computerized bedside documentation on the time that nurses spent documenting. Preimplementation baseline studies revealed that nurses spent 13.7 percent of their time in documentation. Three months postimplementation revealed a decrease to 9.1

percent, or a 20-minute savings per nurse per shift. Although this was not enough gain in efficiency to increase the nurse-to-patient ratio, a decrease in overtime to finish documentation and a shift to more direct patient care activities was reported [3]. There were many other examples and studies reported in the literature that demonstrated a correlation between time savings, cost savings, and the implementation of automated documentation systems. Few studies existed that demonstrated clear time efficiencies directly related to the elimination of duplicate documentation or to the benefits of standardizing documentation across a large IDN.

A project that was undertaken in Norway in 1996 describes the process that five regional hospitals took to develop an interdisciplinary electronic patient record. Part of this project focused on the development of a standard framework for nursing documentation as well as determining the main components that need to be implemented in an EHR [4]. The project identified issues, obstacles, and challenges that were similar and paralleled what we encountered with our own documentation standardization project for nursing.

The three objectives of the Norway project included the primary objective of developing electronic nursing documentation that would improve the quality and continuity of patient care. In the second objective, the team set out to define the main components of nursing documentation in the electronic patient record. The third and final objective focused on the development of a specification of user requirements for a nursing documentation system on which all the hospitals agreed. The outcome of this project was the development of a standardized organizational model and working methodology for nursing practice and documentation on which five regional teaching hospitals in Norway agreed. Although the author identifies many struggles and further work that needs to be done, all project participants understand the great benefits that will be reaped from the nursing documentation as they move forward. The ability for regional facilities to have standardized nursing documentation that is based on standard language will allow nursing managers to receive richer data about what providers do as well as information on nursing service in general. Researchers will gain a database that will provide them with valuable information about the impact of the computer on nursing documentation [4].

The UPMCHS Time Study

At UPMC, a time study project was conducted across 13 of the hospitals to determine the amount of time that RNs were spending on specific activities. A total of 25 nursing units were enrolled in the study. The study revealed that charting accounted for 20 percent of the time spent by RNs, medication administration took 17 percent, and direct patient care came in third at 15 percent of the time. Twelve other categories of nursing activities accounted for the remainder of nursing time. As UPMC moves through the process of realizing the EHR across our facilities, we will use these data as a starting point for measuring improvements in documentation efficiencies.

The UPMCHS Franchise Model

Similar to the work undertaken in Norway, our global objective was to develop a standard "Franchise Model" of clinical documentation and order entry that would support the most efficient and effective delivery of patient care. The Franchise Model would also be implemented across all our facilities. The term Franchise Model was coined to emphasize the principle that the EHR was being developed for the Health System, and the design was not being customized to meet nonstandardized processes at each facility. The example of national restaurant chains was used to help illustrate the franchise model concept. For example, even though each McDonalds® is independently owned and operated, it is part of a larger network of franchises. Whether in the United States or abroad, you can still get the same food items and generally the same process of service if you are at the base of a Japanese shrine on the main street in Kyoto, Japan, or under the golden arches in suburban America. We were striving for this same effect in the development of the Franchise Model of the EHR. It should not matter to the consumer at which hospital he or she is visiting; the same process and methodologies of care delivery and documentation should be visible at all facilities.

To make it more manageable and reasonable to deliver outcomes along the way, this huge initiative was organized into three phases. The first phase focused on the standardization of the clinical data and content that was needed for the interdisciplinary team of caregivers. Once a baseline for repository of content was established, the second phase looked at the content in conjunction with the process of workflow of the patient as well as the workflow for each discipline. How did the patient flow through the system? How were data gathered and recorded? How were data and information retrieved and reviewed? How were intershift and interdepartmental communications about the patient handled? The final phase consisted of the development of manual forms that supported the standardized content and processes designed in the first two phases. It took about 19 months to complete all three phases.

Phase I: Clinical Documentation Standardization

The overall goal for the Clinical Documentation Standardization project was to provide a foundation to support UPMC's strategy of enabling systemwide practices and standards that support the academic and clinical missions of the organization. The specific goals outlined for this initiative focused on five main areas:

1. To facilitate improved clinical standards and enterprise-wide documentation practices by standardizing inpatient clinical documentation across UPMC's 17 hospitals. (Since the kickoff of this project, the health system has expanded to 20 hospitals.)
2. To eliminate redundancies and duplication in documentation.
3. To enhance the quality and reporting of clinical care from a multidisciplinary perspective through standardization.
4. To define and standardize common clinical documentation data elements needs for all patients.
5. To develop an approach for standardizing clinical documentation practices for both automated and manual (paper) settings.

As mentioned previously, the literature search did not reveal any detailed information that quantified how much redundancy or duplication of documentation actually occurs in practice today. The UPMC Health System is probably not unlike most healthcare delivery counterparts across the country, or even in the world, in terms of the amount of duplication of charting that occurs. As part of the initial work of the team, an inventory was conducted of all the existing paper forms used in acute care from all the facilities. This resulted in more than 2700 forms from 35 clinical departments in the 17 hospitals. The survey showed that allergy documentation redundancy ranged from

18 to 60 different forms per hospital across the enterprise. Twenty-five forms asked for family history and 36 different forms include past medical history. For the most part, the data in these three examples are static and do not change dramatically from hospital encounter to encounter, let alone within one encounter. One can easily see how the redundant nature of charting also affects patient perception and satisfaction. Even if the number of times that questions about allergies were reduced by 50 percent, it would still be between 9 and 30 times per admission in some cases and unacceptable as a standard of practice. This analysis provided more support for the goals and objectives of this project as a method of transforming care.

Phase I, which became known as the Clinical Documentation Infrastructure project, spanned a period of about 4 months, from May 2001 through the beginning of September 2001. An interdisciplinary clinical group was organized, representing all the facilities in the health system. Each facility collected the manual documentation forms and submitted them to catalog data elements and content in a database. The database would then be used to query data elements and would help quantify the frequency of use and, in turn, redundancy of information. This phase of the project focused more on determining the common nomenclature and content of data rather than on the process that surrounds how the data are gathered, charted, used, and or retrieved. This occurred in the second phase of work when we married content and process.

An original deliverable output of the Clinical Documentation Infrastructure team was to focus on the documentation content for two patient service lines, diabetes and cardiovascular. This involved developing the in-depth and detailed multidisciplinary charting required for these two patient populations. The plan was to then conduct a pilot evaluation of the development on several demonstration units. Four nursing units in three facilities were identified as the demonstration units; two units were selected as the cardiovascular demonstration units, one for a manual or paper process evaluation at one of the community hospitals, then one unit at one of the tertiary academic hospitals that was to go live with the automated EHR first. The same occurred for diabetes. One unit at a community hospital was selected as the paper demonstration unit, and another unit at the tertiary academic hospital as the demonstration unit for the automated process. When the final common data elements and nomenclature were determined, manual charting forms were to be developed to reflect the content that was on the electronic screens. The automated and the manual processes would be piloted and evaluated on the demonstration units in preparation for the full house implementation of the automated EHR at the tertiary site.

Unfortunately, this methodology could not be implemented as planned. The EHR project embarked on an organizational restructuring about this time, which altered the implementation strategy and assumptions upon which the plan had been based. As a result, the final output of the clinical documentation infrastructure team was a set of common multidisciplinary data elements and content and served as the basis for the electronic forms design for the EHR. This in effect was the end of this phase of the project and did provide a firm foundation that was used as the starting point for the next phase, where process and content were brought together.

Phase II: Content → Process Workflow

The second phase involved work across all disciplines, but for the purpose of this case study, nursing will serve as the basis for illustrating how we worked through the operational details of putting content and workflow process together. While the work of the Documentation Infrastructure team did provide us with a strong foundation of content and a defined list of automated documentation forms for nursing, there were gaps when we tried to apply all the charting forms to the "day in the life of a nurse." This became one of the biggest lessons learned from this project, and it is strongly recommended that anyone considering such an undertaking always consider the process of how the data will be collected, documented, stored, retrieved, and communicated, hand in hand with whatever data or content are needed. Although it may take longer to accomplish this, in the end it will be more efficient.

When process reengineering began, more of the clinical systems analysts who were on the project team were pulled in because they would ultimately have to build, test, and eventually support the EHR clinical documentation. All the clinicians who were part of the first phase were not included as this would have created a Phase II project team that was too large to make any decisions and would have become paralyzed in the process. The "dream team" organized consisted of eight clinical nurses who represented five of our facilities. They were empowered by the Vice Presidents of Patient Care Services and the Chief Nursing Officer of the health system to make the final process and design decisions for nursing documentation. The author served as the tiebreaker during this process, in the event the clinicians were split on how they wanted to proceed. The other key role that the Director of Nursing Informatics played was to challenge the group to think creatively and out of the box. This included asking hard questions to help the clinicians determine "Why do we need these data or information?" and shifting the paradigms away from "That's just the way we have always done it."

The dream team became known as the EHR Nursing Focus Group (NFG). Three of the members had participated in Phase I and in the Clinical Documentation Infrastructure group. The three provided some continuity between the first two phases and were able to provide background on why some decisions on content had been made in Phase I. This is the main reason why combining content and process within one group should be encouraged. There was a lag time of about 6 months between the two phases. The lag time, combined with the limited knowledge transfer and crossover between the two phases, paved the way for in-depth and redundant discussion on certain topics that had been thoroughly discussed in the first phase. When the majority of people were not part of the initial decision making, those decisions were constantly being challenged as part of the Phase II project. This was one area of frustration for people who participated in both phases of the project, and at times was paralyzing for the group. A guiding principle was adopted early on with this group because of this problem. If a decision had already been made in Phase I of the project, the only way it would be opened for discussion and be revisited would be *if* there were any issues directly related to it from a process and operational workflow perspective.

Before the Nursing Focus Group began to meet regularly, a gap analysis was performed that looked at the nursing documentation forms that had been developed to date and were applied to the nursing process for several key workflow areas. These workflow processes included:

1. Admission/Transfer/Discharge throughput.
2. Shift Report and intradepartmental communications.
3. Daily Ongoing Patient Care charting.
4. Multidisciplinary patient education.
5. Physical Assessment based on CBE (Charting by Exception).

The team walked through the future state of care delivery for each process and applied the nursing charting forms that were developed in Phase I. This clearly outlined the gaps in nursing documentation for each of the workflows and provided the basis for the work of the Nursing Focus Group. This preliminary work was essential for identifying the scope of work of the Nursing Focus Group.

The Nursing Focus Group met every Wednesday for 8 hours, over a 2-month period. Each session was focused on one area or segment of the nursing workflow processes and the specific documentation that was required to support the future process in the EHR. If there was more than one reasonable option for a process, the clinical analysts developed and built the options in one of the development environments for the EHR. At the meeting, the EHR development domain was available and the options were presented to the focus group online, so the group could readily see the different options in the system and make educated decisions. All discussions and decisions were documented in real time during the meeting so that everyone on the team could reference this as needed in the future. This is another key item that the group viewed as essential to the success of this project. Phase I showed that incomplete documentation of decisions and discussion can lead to unnecessary rework and analysis paralysis. A second guiding principle that emerged from Phase II was that although the perfect decision on the design might not be made, it is important to stick with the decisions that the group has made to date, begin to use the new process (whether in manual or automated form), then evaluate and make changes as needed. A strong facilitator is essential to making this a successful process. A credible facilitator can enforce the guiding principles and not allow the group to stray from the task at hand and be able to effectively move the group forward.

The 8 weeks of work by the nursing group culminated in an all-day session in the computer training room to which the NFG, EHR clinical systems analysts, and members of the Corporate Nursing Standards of Care (SOC) team were invited. All the final decisions that were made by the NFG were built in the EHR development domain. A detailed scenario was developed that resembled a test script. The scenario covered each of the detailed processes and charting and documentation decisions that were finalized as the Nursing Franchise Model for the EHR. Each person who attended the session was able to sit at a computer terminal and go through the entire patient scenario with assistance from EHR project analysts. This allowed each nurse to step through each process in relation to the future state automated workflow. This served as the final sign-off on the design for nursing. Once sign-off occurred, the overall clinical documentation standardization project moved into the third and final phase.

Phase III: Standardized Manual Documentation Forms Project

In preparation for the implementation of automated clinical documentation in the EHR, manual charting forms needed to be developed for use by nurses during periods of computer system downtime. Because the electronic forms developed were based on the franchise model concept for the Health System, paper forms did not exist that mirrored the future state process for nursing documentation that could be adopted for downtime charting. Given that we had to develop the paper forms for downtime that reflected the EHR design, we decided to take advantage of this opportunity to develop a systemwide standardization project for nursing at UPMC.

An existing working group within the Health System undertook the task of developing the standard manual documentation forms. The Corporate Nursing Standards of Care (SOC) team was a group that had a strong and established working relationship and had been in existence for about 4 years. As mentioned earlier, this was the one group of individuals who was invited to the all-day review session at the end of Phase

II. They were also part of the final review and sign-off in the hands-on session to begin to expose them to the electronic forms. The session also helped the SOC team understand the future state processes that the manual forms would need to support. The SOC team was charged with the development of manual charting forms based on the EHR Franchise Model for charting. The team would also develop the associated policies and procedures. The forms would be used for the manual downtime charting for those facilities that are live on automated EHR. In addition, the standard forms would be implemented across all UPMCHS facilities to standardize nursing documentation and some nursing processes.

The goals and objectives for Phase III were:

1. To standardize nursing documentation across the inpatient nursing facilities.
2. To allow non-EHR facilities to implement and use the Franchise documentation.
3. To decrease the learning curve when EHR is implemented at a facility.
4. To allow for more efficient changes to all forms if regulatory, or if standards are changed across the Health System.

This work began in May 2002 by the SOC team after the project proposal was approved by the Vice Presidents of Patient Care Services and the HIM Directors for the Health System.

Screen prints of each of the electronic forms for nursing were made with copies for the SOC team. These screen prints served as the basis for the documentation content. The first task was to decide how many paper forms would need to be developed. Would there be a one-to-one relationship, or could some of the electronic forms be consolidated onto one paper form? It was decided to develop 4 paper forms from the approximately 12 electronic forms for nursing. The SOC team was divided into four smaller working groups, and each group was responsible for developing the draft of their assigned form. The Interdisciplinary Patient Education form was the easiest to develop. It was drafted and then presented to the Corporate Patient Education committee for review with few issues or problems encountered. The admission assessment was straightforward from a content perspective, but we encountered a lot of discussion and process issues that influenced the final formatting and layout of that form. The future state process would be to have the inpatient admission assessment initiated at the point of entry or at the point in time when it is known that the patient is to be admitted; this would include initiation of this form in the Emergency Department (ED) and/or in any other preadmission area. This process was not one that was standardized in the current state across the facilities of the Health System. As the paper design was finalized, the data elements that should be collected in the ED for an inpatient who would be admitted were identified and placed at the beginning of the assessment. Analysis of the process revealed that additional work would need to be done with the ED nursing managers to begin looking at all their specific charting within that area to include triage forms and ED treatment records. This entire process of an ED patient coming into triage through the ED to an inpatient bed had to be taken into account along with the data and forms. This was a clear example of one of the lessons learned from Phase I, namely, one always needs to look at content and process together.

Originally, we began to develop a separate form for the physical assessment and a separate form that would combine several miscellaneous items such as vital signs, intake and output, activities of daily living (ADLs), and IV site assessments. The final draft combined all these items onto one bifold form that would serve for 3 days of charting and serve as the Patient Care Record.

At the time of this publication, we are just beginning the pilot evaluation of the manual nursing forms at four of our facilities. Each of the early adopter hospitals has selected one to two of their med-surg units to serve as the initial evaluators. Each facility will come with its own challenges from a process reengineering perspective. We will begin to use the forms and conduct an aggressive evaluation of content as well as workflow and make modifications to forms and or process as needed. After an evaluation period, a Health System implementation plan will be developed for the manual forms.

References

1. Filho JR. The complexity of developing a nursing information system: a Brazilian experience. Comput Nurs 2001;19:98–104.
2. Bowles KH. The barriers and benefits of nursing information systems. Comput Nurs 1997;15:191–196.
3. Pabst MK, Scherubel JC, Minnich AF. The impact of computerized documentation on nurses' use of time. Comput Nurs 1996;14:25–30.
4. Helleso R, Ruland CM. Developing a module for nursing documentation integrated in the electronic patient record. J Clin Nurs 2001;10:799–805.

11
INTERNATIONAL PERSPECTIVE
Selayang Hospital: A Paperless and Filmless Environment in Malaysia

HADIS ROSNAH, MOHAMAD AZRIN ZUBIR, and Y. NOR AKMA

Successfully operational for 3 years, Selayang Hospital in Malaysia integrates clinical, administrative, and financial functions in a totally paperless environment.

A Thousand-Mile Journey

Selayang Hospital has set a milestone in Malaysian history for being the first hospital in the country to create a "paperless and filmless" environment for its outpatient and inpatient services. The fully integrated information system in Selayang Hospital is known as the Total Hospital Information System (THIS), which encapsulates integration between clinical (including imaging and critical care), financial, and administration systems.

As of time of publication, the system is up and running. Having all care providers, that is, physicians, nurses, paramedics, billing clerks, and others, use computers in their daily work is no longer just a concept. It is a reality. Physician's notes, nurse charting, radiology reports, requests for laboratory investigation, ordering of patient meals—are all done online at point of care. Furthermore, the filmless setting—where physicians retrieve digital images in the wards, consultation rooms, and operating theater—is also a hospitalwide reality that distinguishes Selayang Hospital from others.

Looking back at how we did it, and what we went through, is a thousand-mile story. To have the entire integrated system working, as prescribed, within 36 months is a distinctive accomplishment. No doubt the journey of creating Selayang Hospital was "painful"; however, it was also an ever-enriching and courageous endeavor. The payoff of information technology (IT) investment is of utmost importance, but the lessons learned and the value created is the culmination of benefits realization. Selayang Hospital is an epitome of the perseverance and sheer determination of the people involved who made it a reality.

Hadis Rosnah, MD, MHP, is Director of Telehealth. Mohamad Azrin Zubir, MD, MSc IT, is CIO of the Selayang Hospital. Y. Nor Akma, MD, MHA, is Deputy Director of the Selayang Hospital.

Setting Strategic Objectives Through IT

Selayang Hospital is a 960-bed government hospital, owned by the Ministry of Health (MOH), and located about 15 kilometers from the city of Kuala Lumpur. It provides 20 secondary and 6 tertiary clinical care disciplines. This state-of-the-art hospital is the Malaysian showcase for the use of IT in all aspects of operation.

One of the major causes of fragmentation in healthcare delivery is the existence of inadequate information systems that do not allow for sharing of information to facilitate better patient care. This covers a wide spectrum, from patients' records to information related to quality and health outcomes [1]. In addition, the lack of coordination and integration of activities within or between hospitals has resulted in little or no continuity of care; this not only caused redundancies in patient management, which has cost implications, but also inefficiencies in delivering patient care services with resulting poor patient management and outcomes.

Thus, the strategic objective of improving hospital operations through IT was the driving force behind the MOH effort to pursue implementation of THIS in Selayang Hospital. The emergence of THIS is also in line with the Malaysian Multimedia Super Corridor (MSC) flagship application initiatives. It is the vision of the Government of Malaysia to connect all hospitals and health clinics and to create a lifetime health record (LHR) and lifetime health plan (LHP) for every member of its society.

The Total Hospital Information System

Even at the onset of planning stages, the objective of IT implementation in Selayang Hospital was not to have systems that focused on specific areas like order entry, emergency system, results reporting, and so forth. This ultimately creates an incomplete electronic medical record (EMR). It is also believed that such business strategies will create systems that are fragmented in terms of clinical practice compatibility and information sharing. Thus the Total Hospital Information System (THIS) was conceived as a hospitalwide information system that allows for sharing and exchange of information among all the functional units in a hospital.

From the technology viewpoint, THIS is made up of a highly integrated suite of applications encompassing clinical systems, which includes digital imaging, critical care, and financial and administrative systems (Figure 11.1).

For the clinical systems, a nearly full suite of Cerner Millennium clinical applications is deployed across the facility. The Picture Archiving and Communication System (PACS), Sienet, is provided by Siemens. The patient accounting, human resources, and payroll software is from Peoplesoft, while the financial and materials management software is from Oracle. Critical care and operating theater applications are from Spacelab, and the Central Sterile Central Supply Department (CSSD) application (SteriSys 2000) is from Team Vantage. Microsoft Office is being used for office automation and intranet operations. THIS runs on networked Compaq computers and Sun Microsystems servers linked by 3Com Fast Ethernet switches. In terms of hardware, the whole system encompasses 1200 personal computers, 150 bar-code readers, 30 wireless laptops, and 300 printers including label printers located throughout the hospital. All integration of clinical and financial data is based on HL7 standard. The DICOM 3.0 standard is used for image integration.

In essence, THIS was envisioned to meet the following objectives:

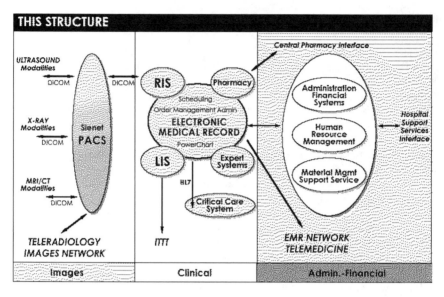

FIGURE 11.1. Selayang Hospital's Total Hospital Information System (THIS) is made up of a highly integrated suite of applications covering clinical and administrative functions and includes digital imaging, critical care, and financial and administrative systems.

- To embark on an Electronic Medical Record project where all patient records will be archived into a single clinical data repository.
- To create an enabled hospital that operates efficiently by leveraging new technologies.
- To create a paperless and filmless environment in the delivery of patient care.

Having stated these objectives, THIS was designed and developed around functions that focus on patient workflow and work processes rather than locations or administrative divisions of services. The applications are designed to support physicians and other healthcare providers in delivering patient care across different episodes and settings in a seamless and continuous manner. Capabilities include order entry, retrieval of laboratory results, radiology reports, radiology images, generation of patient lists, and others. Patients' progress notes, nursing assessment, intake and output, and vital signs are entered online into the system at point of care. Indeed, THIS provides an enterprise wide solution for real-time, online, accurate, and cost-effective electronic access to patient information across the hospital.

Going Live in Just 36 Months

Planning for THIS was done as part and parcel of the overall physical project planning dating back to early 1995. Rollout of THIS implementation began in September 1996 when a core team was appointed to look into the overall structure of the system; set the implementation methodology; and put in place policies, functional requirements, the work process, operating procedures, the decision-making process, and so on. Inevitably, various committees and workgroups were formed consisting of key players with a mix of skills and backgrounds in hospital management, IT management, and clinical fields. They were responsible for managing various issues during the course of the project.

Taking into account that Malaysian experience in IT was still lacking, especially in the healthcare industry, the strategy adopted was to implement proven solutions that had been functioning at successful sites that could support current and future MOH clinical and business requirements. A core team was sent on a fact-finding mission to explore sites with suitable applications that met the THIS requirements. At the time, however, no site existed that had a system as complex and as highly integrated as required. The team, therefore, had to draw up specifications for the activities that would need to be performed over the period of implementation. At the initial phase, the focus was on business process reengineering. The overall project timeline is illustrated in Figure 11.2.

The project tasks were carried out in seven major steps:

1. *Project Preparation/Initiation.* The scope of this phase included initial project meetings; defining the project organization; identifying resources, especially staffing; and performing implementation planning.

2. *System Planning.* This included a detailed requirements study and process review, analysis of process improvement opportunities, business process reengineering, developing policies and procedures, and knowledge transfer.

3. *System Design.* This entailed identifying data elements, process design, architectural and database design, system and structure design, and hardware and interface design. It also involved other requirements, such as design and specifications of furniture and workstations, power supply and uninterrupted power supply (UPS), air conditioning, and fire protection.

4. *System Building.* This phase included construction of database, contents creation, data entry forms, templates and reports, build and customization of applications, and production of the database.

5. *System Validation.* This included development of the testing and simulation script, acceptance test plan, functional and integration testing, simulation and dry run, and downtime procedure testing.

6. *System Training.* This included development of the training program and the schedule covering various aspects of the systems, training manuals, basic and applications training, training of key users and end users, and mass training.

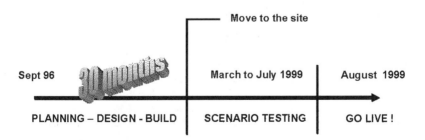

FIGURE 11.2. It took 36 months to plan, design, build, test, and commission THIS. To ensure smooth migration and acceptance, testing was done for a period of 6 months. The system went live in August 1999 when the hospital opened its doors to the public.

7. *Convert and Operate.* This included defining the conversion requirements, creation of the build and production domain, data conversion program, steps for "Go Live," postconversion review, revision, and change control.

The project was explicitly clinically driven, and the involvement of the clinicians in the project was given prominence from the planning stages to all the stages of implementation up to going live.

The team involved was divided into four groups and recruited at various stages of the project:

• *The Core Team.* This group consisted of 20 members of management executives and senior physicians. They were in charge with overseeing the whole project, providing guidance and decision making. They were also responsible for high-level reengineering of work processes and for setting the operational policies and standards.
• *Application Analysts (AAs).* This group consisted of senior nursing managers, paramedics, and clerical staff taken from their positions in existing hospitals. They were involved in the initial training, requirement study, process design, and system building. As the project moved toward completion, they were involved in the acceptance testing and simulation of the various systems. There were about 30 AAs actively involved in the project.
• *Key Users.* The key users were recruited from the respective departments, representing specific areas and disciplines. They included doctors, nurses, and other care providers. Their primary role was to be the champions of the system. They had to prepare function-based training materials and finalize the detailed workflow and work processes. Along with the AAs, they were also performing the simulation testing. A total of about 300 key users were identified, representing various disciplines and business units.
• *End users.* These were ultimately the main system users who carry out their day-to-day activities.

It took 36 months to plan, design, build, test, and commission the system. To ensure smooth passage to going live, aggressive acceptance testing, as well as workload simulation, was done for a period of 6 months. The system went live in August 1999 when the hospital opened its doors to the public.

A New Scenario with New Relationships

Despite teething problems in the initial operation, all started out well. The system is currently being deployed throughout the whole hospital and is used by all physicians and other healthcare providers. As illustrated in Figure 11.3, an average of 1000 users are concurrently accessing the system during peak hours.

The working environment at Selayang is totally different from that of a conventional hospital. Physicians in the clinics no longer use pens to take down notes. "Since I have worked at Selayang Hospital, I can't remember the last time that I bought a pen," claimed a doctor. With electronic rounds, a team of doctors and nurses can discuss their cases before making ward rounds. Physical rounds are conducted efficiently because decision making is based on the information acquired before the rounds are made.

The system has improved the quality of service as it reduces paper and duplication of work and enables easy access to patient data and records. No request forms are required when doctors are entering orders. Once the physician places an order for

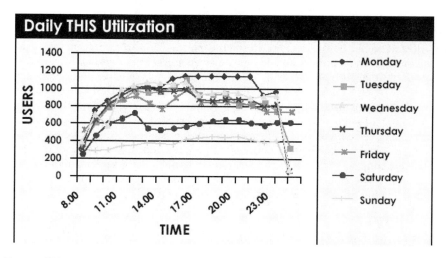

FIGURE 11.3. Analysis of usage shows that an average of 1000 users are concurrently accessing the system during peak hours.

drugs, X-rays, or laboratory tests, the information is collected in a work list, which is then routed to the respective service department and staff. A nurse will know exactly her workload for the day through the work list assigned to her. The system provides fast and accurate information and streamlines the method of data entry, storage, and retrieval, thus freeing the staff from laborious time-consuming tasks. The robust clinical information system also supports clinical decision making with reminders and alerts in real time. Searching for paper records has become a myth.

Using the Critical Care System, a patient's vital signs can be accessed remotely via computer monitors. With PACS, the delivery of patient care has also been definitely revolutionized. This can be seen through instant access to image and radiological reports including previous images, simplified workflow of radiological examinations, shorter turnaround time, better quality control, and so forth. Doctors can view digital images through special monitors placed in all the clinic rooms and also in various parts of the hospital. This removes the need for X-ray films and transfer of films from one section of the hospital to another. It is a very common scenario to see a clinician already viewing an image and making a decision before the patient returns from the imaging department after taking the X-ray!

Because both clinical and financial data are integrated, any chargeable procedures, examinations, and laboratory investigations carried out for patients automatically trigger charges to the patient bill. This enables the hospital to generate bills and collect payment as soon as the patient is discharged. In the long term, the hospital will benefit in terms of revenue collection.

The greatest visible impact is not just in the use of computers but also in the work behavior among the staff. At Selayang Hospital, THIS has definitely changed the way information is being managed. New information and telecommunication technologies encourage healthcare providers to adopt a more virtual, more integrated, and more distributed approach to the delivery of health services [1]. As described by Berg, the technology will affect the distribution and content of work tasks and change information flows [2]. This creates a model of information delivery that will change relationships among healthcare professionals.

All staff employed by Selayang Hospital from the CEO to physicians, nurses, and even the attendants, porters, and drivers are given access to the system. Thus, communication throughout the hospital is mainly through e-mail. Notices and circulars are issued online electronically, meaning less paper but more messages. Various requests from the staff are made online using a user-defined structured template. Thus, the traditional way of sending paper memos around is very remote. In the wards, laboratory, and radiology departments, the environment is quiet and more organized with fewer phone calls and less talking. All information required, including laboratory results, is available at any desktop. This allows Selayang Hospital to have a minimum number of porters. The common phenomena of calling, checking, and seeing people buzzing around hunting for laboratory results is very much reduced.

Challenges and Opportunities

Being the pioneer in a paperless and filmless environment presented a daunting challenge. Venturing into the type of project where no one has gone before also posed difficulty in adopting the right model. Implementing a very complex system in one stroke, rather than gradually, and on a fast track was also a very ambitious undertaking, particularly when it is known that numerous IT projects have crashed and burned along the way. As it is, it is common knowledge that the more comprehensive the technology, the more difficult the implementation [2]. As Gerber has pointed out in his book *The E-Myth Manager*, it is an act of courage to stumble from one phase to the next, against all odds [3]. One plays Russian Roulette at every step of implementation, realizing that at times one is not sure of the breadth of the project's perspective. In terms of team building, it is like building a ship while sailing on a turbulent sea. However, the uncertainty and unpredictability of the IT implementation process should be accepted and even nurtured, rather than considering it a threat. It should be taken as an opportunity to learn [2].

Being a green site, it was much easier to lay out the functional requirements for THIS, since they could be incorporated as part of the overall hospital planning and design. However, given that IT implementation in health care is still lacking, embarking on a complex IT project from scratch was indeed a difficult task, albeit a testimonial to emotional tolerance. It goes without saying that "Wisdom is knowing what to do, virtue is doing it!" One thing is certain: facing an existing set of circumstances presents an obstacle to your goals. Vision, leadership, determination, teamwork, and support from all involved are needed.

The major challenge faced in the early phases of implementation was defining process reengineering in the absence of policy. Having sound operational policies and detailed standard operating procedures (SOPs) is tremendously vital for achieving a well-designed system that meets the functional requirements. In reviewing the fundamental conventional process, enormous efforts were made to translate the traditional bricks-and-mortar process into electronic protocols. It is an unavoidable fact that the IT landscape is littered with landmines. We had to look for practical insights and pay close attention to pick lists that would work [4].

Perhaps the lack of uniform standards for medical terminology, vocabulary, and even basic naming conventions is one of the most challenging tasks in enabling interoperability among various entities. Associated with this, the unavailability of standards pertaining to data sets, data elements, and data content is another obstacle in setting up centralized patient records. Being the first electronic hospital, the creation of data elements and the database structure had to be done from scratch, that is, in transforming paper-based data into electronic form. For example, data for the following needed to be structured and developed electronically from the paper-based document for physician order entry: a total of 2349 surgical procedures, 1024 prescriptions, 642 laboratory investigations, and 433 radiology examinations. Another 1300 user-defined structured forms and templates were created, which are used by doctors, nurses, and all healthcare providers for clerking, charting progress notes, and documentation. Inevitably, a system of approval process also had to be put in place to ensure acceptance from users and create a sense of ownership about what had been built.

Physician involvement in the approval process facilitated project buy-in and generated leadership among physicians in adopting the various innovations and new working methods. One challenge, however, was ensuring that customization of the system also met the requirements of user interface design for hospitalwide use. When every discipline pushes for an individual request, there can be an explosion of variables that results in numerous individual screens. The balance between the "needs, wants, and nice to have" of different user groups has to be handled effectively, weighing the impact of changes in one application upon other applications as well as on the interfaces between them. This ensures that changes have been thoroughly considered and agreed upon by all affected parties. Thus, a stringent change control mechanism has to be in place. To navigate this enduring task requires strong leadership.

Along with concern about the lack of IT knowledge, issues that users are skeptical about include security of patient medical records and systems integrity. Security features, which include access, approval, and an audit trail, are inherent in the system and need to be addressed to fulfill the requirements of EMR and the electronic process. A delicate decision needs to be made that weighs the trade-off between easy access to a patient's record and confidentiality and privacy. A well-defined delineation of privilege across the enterprise needs to be established where access to medical records is based on a "need-to-know" basis and in which any access can be tracked through the audit trail, including access to read-only files.

Another key issue facing IT implementation is people. A long delay in user participation, especially that of hard-to-find senior clinicians, can allow vendors to design systems based on what they think is right, ignoring clinical needs. Consequently major changes and rework may need to be done if a significant number of clinical configuration settings are not addressed. Needless to say, absence of experienced staff can cause relentless pressure on the team scrambling to keep the project on schedule. In THIS, acquiring staff in a timely manner for the right migration track was fundamentally crucial in ensuring that they received adequate training and understanding of the system right from the beginning. However, it is also essential to get people with the right attitude. Managing change with a project team that is skeptical, apprehensive, inflexible, and, worse still, does not believe in what it is doing, is a heart-burning experience.

Leapfrog implementation using vendor's solutions is another ballgame altogether. The question is, Are there reference sites with similar systems that can share their experiences? Even if there are, the premise that "If it works for you, it'll work for me" should not be taken for granted. There is no way a clinical information system designed for use in one country can match the realities of another country [5]. Although there may be proven solutions, the degree of integration adopted at another reference site may not be as comprehensive as that required at Selayang Hospital, for example. Thus, making THIS work is definitely not easy.

The risk of acquiring "off-the-shelf" software also has to be addressed. In an attempt to understand the systems acquired, the debate is not on whether to use them or not, but how to align the systems with specific clinical needs. It is always claimed that any vendor can deliver a good system. However, a commitment in terms of providing continued support and backup is also required. Other than introducing new solutions, is the vendor committed to providing support on required changes and upgrading, as well as involvement in research and development? Thus, along the course of the project, immense effort should be made to work in partnership with the vendor to achieve excellent outcomes.

Leadership as a Critical Success Factor

Central to the successful implementation of THIS is leadership and the unwavering commitment by the topmost level of management as well as by the project team. The requirements to balance the numerous trade-offs between the various parties involved, and to perform the arduous task of sifting through a bewildering array of uncertainties puts the leadership in a vital, but unenviable, position [6]. It is, indeed, very fortunate that the centralized health system in Malaysia provides a direction for what the Hospital of the Future in the country should be [7]. The creation of Selayang Hospital is not only a short-term agenda, but envelops the country's vision to move forward in shaping the health system of the future. Furthermore, leadership capability at every level of the decision-making process is a key factor in inspiring the core team and mandating change.

The question of whether the implementation is seen as a success or a failure is ultimately not merely a technical matter. Patient Care Information Systems (PCIS) need to be conceived as organizational development as well as organizational change [2]. With the emphasis on the improvement of the work process as a result of business process reengineering, applied in tandem with project implementation, it is no surprise that THIS has brought efficiency to the hospital operation. This can be shown from the findings of the user survey after 2 years of operation in which 94 percent of the respondents agreed that THIS improves their work efficiency.

To get a full-blown clinical information system off the ground at one stroke requires sheer determination as well as a solid foundation. It took 6 months to perform system testing and simulation to ensure that there would not be a potential disaster when the system was moving from a build to a live environment. Intensive user acceptance tests and simulation testing were done to every application as well as to the whole system, focusing on functionality and interface issues between various applications as well as applications to equipment. In addition, load testing was performed before the conversion by using numerous scenarios based on a patient walkthrough for both outpatient and inpatient settings. Besides looking into system integrity and security, system performance, system architecture, and other critical areas, the testing and simulation were also done to evaluate whether the system fulfilled work process and policy requirements.

The implementation of patient care information systems has to be managed by a project group, not limited just to the IT department. The involvement of representatives from future users and the institution's top-level management was crucial [2]. It is imperative for the project team to be represented by cross-disciplinary expertise. The commitment of the people in setting up committees and workgroups at various levels of implementation, with specific roles and responsibilities, has also driven the project team to the right perspective.

A key issue in any IT project is the organizational buy-in, especially by physicians. Adequate user involvement is vital to fostering ownership of the system [2]. In Selayang Hospital, the project team succeeded in bringing users onboard, even from the onset of the project. In view of such commitment from the physicians, the acceptance of THIS for their daily work is very compelling. The user acceptance survey reveals that 80 percent of Selayang Hospital employees are comfortable with THIS and prefer using a computerized system compared to traditional paper-based records.

Achieving Strategic Payoffs

The far-reaching vision that has been set for the country drove the Ministry of Health to take a bold step toward implementing a leapfrog conversion. By making Selayang Hospital a test bed for future IT rollout, the MOH has created a sound foundation and has definitely achieved strategic payoffs in reshaping the health system of the future. Being a centralized system, once THIS is successfully implemented in Selayang Hospital, the planning for the rest of the country will be in place. One year after Selayang Hospital went live, Putrajaya Hospital, the second hospital with a paperless and filmless environment went into operation. Next in the pipeline is the development of 14 new hospitals, currently under different phases of construction, to be equipped with IT. Seven of them will be Total Hospital Information Systems. Ultimately this group of IT-enabled hospitals will be the main catalyst for the creation of a Lifetime Health Record and a Lifetime Health Plan. This goal will make the country a showcase for nationwide, networked, paperless, and filmless hospitals.

The strategy of having a fully integrated hospital system and going live at once, rather than gradually, was achieved through the implementation of this paperless and filmless environment. This accomplishment has definitely brought profound benefits to the MOH, not only in terms of having achieved its goals, but because this implementation is much easier in an environment where users have never used a computer. The approach has also eliminated dual overlapping operations, both paper and electronic, as in a more traditionally phased-in IT implementation. This means that developing the best process for all aspects of patient flow is done at once. This approach also prevents prolonging the implementation schedule, which, in the long run, achieves significant overall cost savings.

Another valuable achievement was the creation of solid partnerships with vendors. Realizing that MOH is still lacking in IT experience, and that support staff was very scarce, one of the most effective ways to develop a robust integrated system, in a comparatively short period of time, was to appoint a systems integrator. Through this integrator, issues were solved in a coordinated manner, and the MOH was able to increase its odds of achieving interoperability and interfacing.

The MOH is also using this as an opportunity for knowledge transfer. With the extensive technology transfer that occurred during the course of the project, a significant number of IT champions were created, including senior clinicians. New career moves were also accomplished. A number of nurses and paramedics, as well as radiographers and laboratory technicians, have been given positions as application analysts (AAs). With the skill and competency they have gained in using the application software tools, they can further enhance and improve the system without depending on the vendors.

They are also responsible for troubleshooting and IT training. This will result in overall cost savings brought about by system improvements that will also be reflected in the future nationwide rollout.

Another area of interest is how the practice of medicine in an electronic environment has benefited care providers as well as patients. What does IT mean for healthcare workers? Like any revolution, we will see winners and losers, those who adapt successfully and those who do not [8]. There are also early and late adopters. Although initially the benefits of THIS were yet to be seen, for care providers, the easy access to integrated and comprehensive information at point of care and the reduction of paperwork have led to improvements in productivity and quality. The use of user-defined data entry forms with discrete data provides standardization and improves clinical documentation. Order entry eliminates illegible handwriting, reduces medical errors, and improves patient care. Mobile workstations provide doctors and nurses with vital information about patients during ward rounds. The system has taken nurses away from writing records repeatedly so they can spend much more time on the comfort and education of the patient. The ritual process of gathering records before the clinic day is totally eliminated.

Since it lags far behind in the development of knowledge-based systems, the health sector is considered one of the most inefficiently run, compared to other industry sectors. The argument has also been made that healthcare costs have soared because of the absence of knowledge-based systems [9]. By virtue of the wide use of information sharing, Selayang Hospital has explicitly ventured into knowledge management. Furthermore, the networked environment has brought high-quality knowledge to physicians and patients through the availability of online guidelines and protocols, the integration of library resources via clinical workstations, system-generated leaflets, and so forth. This has enhanced staff motivation because they feel empowered and more confident of their work. The network environment will also populate databases, creating and expanding a pool of shared knowledge and producing more accurate outcomes-driven protocols. Evidence for clinical and management decision is available to all staff instantly through databases at the right time and place. For example, the creation of a centralized public folder and a hospital intranet act as an effective platform for sharing information among all staff.

With the enormous investment in THIS, it is important to note its payoffs. Many agree that return on investment (ROI) should be used to justify the business case for IT projects. However, this may not always be the right way to measure payoffs because not all returns are financial. Similar to e-business, THIS demands significant change management and the focus should be on the value created, especially to the customers [10]. A firm, economic analysis of THIS has yet to be carried out. Suffice it to say that savings in terms of time, resources, and money are definitely on the agenda. Looking at the business case, the realization of benefits of the IT investment for Selayang Hospital is evident from its intangible impact, which is primarily focused on nonfinancial outcomes, that is, improving hospital operations such as business process reengineering, quality improvement, reduction of medical errors, and service efficiency.

The initial findings of a comparison study between Selayang Hospital and similar-sized non-THIS hospitals have shown that THIS has brought significant benefits. There is a 36.7 percent time reduction during admission, an 8.3 percent time reduction during a patient's stay, a 71.1 percent time reduction at the time of patient discharge, a 73 percent reduction in reporting following a portable X-ray, and an 80 percent reduction in time to view a patient's record. In terms of resource utilization, there is an 11.32

percent reduction in staff for registration and scheduling functions and a 51.6 percent efficiency gain in scheduling patients.

It is evident that by having PACS, the move to teleradiology is much easier. Because Selayang Hospital does not have a neurosurgeon, head injury patients are being referred to the nearest neurosurgeon in Kuala Lumpur Hospital. However, since teleradiology is being practiced routinely in real time between the two institutions, a study over a period of 1 year showed that 72 of 110 head injury patients are managed at Selayang Hospital. The study also shows that Selayang Hospital is able to reduce referrals of head injury patients by 30 percent. This signifies cutting costs in transporting patients, reducing congestion at the neurosurgical unit in Kuala Lumpur Hospital, and, obviously, providing more comfort and convenience to patients.

Conclusion

It is indeed an achievement for Selayang Hospital to have implemented THIS, thus enabling the sharing of information to facilitate better patient care. The leapfrog approach taken needed sound planning and commitment, not only from the team members who were directly involved but also from the vendors involved and from the top management at the Ministry of Health. Getting clinicians involved from the start of the project was another key factor contributing to its success.

The experience described by all involved in implementation has shed some light on the challenges, namely, the lack of experience in healthcare IT among the team members involved, the lack of a reference site, and the deadlines to be met. The message is clear, however. Successful implementation has resulted in unmatched payoffs. The IT environment has demonstrated value to the organization in leveraging the quality of healthcare delivery. It has changed work behavior among staff. Easy access to integrated and comprehensive information at point of care, online clinical guidelines and protocols, and reduction of paperwork has resulted in improved care and outcomes for patients. Even more significant, the networked environment has created a knowledge-based organization.

Selayang Hospital has been tenaciously laying the groundwork for growth of information communications technology in the Malaysian healthcare industry. No doubt the journey to implement a system that is extremely complex as THIS is not just one line in the sand. Nevertheless, it has provided abundant learning opportunities. The extensive transfer of knowledge has created IT intellectual capital whose expertise will be very valuable for future undertakings. The Selayang Hospital experience will propel future hospital IT development in the country. In a true sense, Selayang Hospital shall lead the way in reshaping the healthcare system of the future in Malaysia.

References

1. Suleiman AB. Health system of the future: patient centered services through integration and teamwork [keynote address]. Directors Conference. Ministry of Health, Malaysia, September 2000.
2. Berg M. Implementing information systems in health care organizations: myths and challenges. Int J Med Inf 2001;64:143–156.
3. Gerber ME. The e-myth manager. Harper Business 1998;97–136.
4. Cronin MJ. Unchained value: the new logic of digital business. Boston: Harvard Business School Press; 2000. p. 1–21.

5. Heeks R, Mundy D, Salazar A. Why health care information systems succeed or fail. Information Systems for Public Sector Management Working Paper Series. Institute for Development Policy and Management, University of Manchester; 1999 June; No. 9.
6. Sittig FD. The importance of leadership in the clinical information system implementation process. Inf Rev November; 2001.
7. Brouwer S. Malaysian revolution wins hearts and minds. IHACJ 2000;5(5):46–47.
8. Masys DR. Effects of current and future information technologies on the health care force. Health Affairs Sept/Oct 2002;5:33–41.
9. Laudon KC, Traver CG, Laudon JP. Information technology and society. Belmont, CA: Wadsworth; 1994. p. 474–479.
10. Sawhney M. Damn the ROI, full speed ahead. Net Gains. CIO Magazine July 15, 2002. Retrieved from http://www.cio.com/archive/071502/netgains.html.

Section 3
Transformation: Making IT Happen

Section Introduction

Section 3 continues the journey of implementation. The emphasis on transformation in this section, and, indeed, in the whole book is hard to miss. The message is not only the transformation of individual institutions, but of the industry as a whole. Transformation takes place through culture shifts, acceptance of information technology, the positive outcomes achieved by the new technologies, and by the Chief Information Officer.

Health care and information technology are two of the most evolving fields today, and the role of the chief information officer (CIO) follows suit. A chapter on the evolution of the role of the CIO brings to light how the role of the CIO has been perceived over time and explores what that role needs to bring to ensure organizational success. To supplant the theoretical perspectives, a variety of chief information officers share their stories of technology transformation. Written from the eyes of "worker bees," these stories show how the impetus of transformation survives hurdles, politics, and cultural issues.

Two chapters round out this section. One provides insights into the successful governance of a highly celebrated Integrated Delivery Systems in the United States, and the other transports readers "down under" for a firsthand look at IT implementation at a private facility.

12
IT: Transition Fundamentals in Care Transformation

JEFFREY S. ROSE

Success with clinical computing requires the simultaneous navigation of important sociocultural pathways, all aimed at the transformation of the ways in which we function.

It must be considered that there is nothing more difficult to carry out, nor more doubtful of success, nor more dangerous to handle, than to initiate a new order of things.
—Niccolo Machiavelli, *The Prince* [1]

The potential of information technology (IT) to safeguard patients, communicate medical information, accrue and organize health data, facilitate knowledge discovery, enhance process efficiency, and weave best "evidence" into the fabric of medical practice has been demonstrated in a variety of settings [2–14]. Widespread success in actually transforming care practices through clinical computing, however, remains unusual. A recent survey of health system chief information officers (CIOs) revealed that only about 2 percent had ever successfully implemented a comprehensive clinical system [15], and the health industry trails other endeavors in their adaptation to the information age [16–19].

Success with clinical computing depends on far more than automation and attention to hardware, software, and networks. It requires the simultaneous navigation of important sociocultural pathways, each dependent on the other and all aimed at the "transformation" of the ways in which we function as a team-based profession [20,21]. The purpose of this chapter is to provide an overview of what "care transformation" means as it relates to information in medicine and to relate some organizational approaches to the transitions necessary to improve the way we think and act as an industry.

Transformation

Transformation, for the purposes of this discussion, is defined as *a state of profound, lasting, individual and organizational behavior, enabled by the strategic acceptance of information systems, resulting in health practices of optimum value, safety, and appropriateness.*

Jeffrey S. Rose, MD, is Vice President and Chief Medical Officer for the Cerner Corporation.

This definition emphasizes several important concepts:

1. Transformation is profound and lasting—a *fundamental and persistent* new way of acting that is *perpetuated culturally*.
2. Transformation is enabled by information and computing tools that are *strategically introduced, accepted, and used* by practitioners.
3. Transformation is focused on bringing maximal *value, safety, and appropriateness* to the health of both individuals and populations.

A *transformed* health system would consistently and pervasively:

- Have knowledge of and perform *all* interventions that have a demonstrable positive impact on the health status of individuals and populations (*value*).
- Have knowledge of and perform *no* interventions that have a demonstrably negative impact on the health of individuals or populations (*safety*).
- Have knowledge of and perform no interventions that have *no* demonstrably positive impact on health status of individuals and populations (*appropriateness*).

There are many societal and cultural elements that come into play in achieving this transformation, of course, but at their core, value, safety, and appropriateness depend upon information availability to caregivers—about patients, communities, and health disorders. The use of information to maintain health and cure disease is the essence of medical practice, and the goal of IT, therefore, is to make relevant personal, population, and disease-specific knowledge available to practitioners at any time or place so that best possible judgment (wisdom) can be exercised. To be more concrete, transformation means that we function in an information environment where the computing tools assure that there are no adverse events resulting from our interventions, no delays in streamlined diagnosis and treatment, no errors or inefficiency in our care delivery processes, and no *unnecessary* variance or waste in our actions.

Today, we practice with *incomplete information* about the people and disorders we are treating almost all the time [22–25]. We have alarming error and iatrogenic injury rates, most of which involve system errors involving drug knowledge dissemination, drug dosing, patient identity checking, and *patient information availability* [26,27]. We spend 30 percent to 50 percent of our precious resources on activities that produce little or no demonstrable benefit to patients [28–30]. We base less than 30 percent of our decisions on firm scientific evidence of intervention efficacy [31,32]. We cannot possibly be cognizant of, let alone assess the quality of, newly discovered information in our profession [33]. We practice in very complex systems involving handoffs of information and activity dependencies among a host of individuals with nonstandardized, poorly measured processes in which errors are virtually assured [34–38].

Our capacity to change this state will be necessarily gradual, and imperfect, but Figure 12.1 represents the idealized transformation we hope to achieve through improved IT use in health care.

Focus on Transition

The most important step toward success with IT in health care is the recognition that all the five spheres of the transformation process depicted in Figure 12.1 must be addressed together as a firm part of a health enterprise strategy. Each requires attention and resources, and none may be shortchanged or omitted without significant risk of failure. The troublesome effects of neglecting one or more spheres have been noted

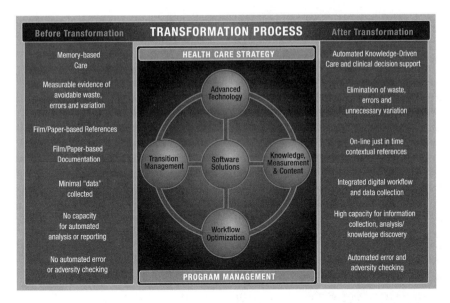

FIGURE 12.1. Core elements that need to be present to achieve transformation in health care through the application of information technologies.

in other industries: among general IT projects—where more than 50 percent of all capital expenditures are directed—31.1 percent are canceled before completion; more than 50 percent overrun cost estimates by upward of 200 percent; and few implementations yield anticipated gains or savings [39–41]. In health care, the complexity of our thought processes and systems makes methodical attention to each area even more critical.

The utility of advanced technology and software in these transformation issues is more completely addressed in this and other texts on medical informatics [42]. The concepts of optimizing clinical workflow in light of "digital" processes (doing things the way we always have with new tools simply does not work), of measuring and demonstrating the efficacy of IT efforts, including selecting clinical content and business knowledge to strategically and responsibly affect those measurements, are equally important and also addressed elsewhere. The primary focus of the remainder of this chapter is on the transition process, which is the most commonly mishandled of the spheres (see Figure 12.1).

In my experience, successful transition efforts in health care through IT contain common elements:

1. There are simple clear goals and well-conceived strategies for accomplishing each transformation goal, formulated by a balanced team of clinical, operational, and IT leaders together.
2. There is a fundamental shift in focus within the enterprise placing the patient (person) at the center of a cultural move toward care safety and quality rather than profit or pure provider benefit in the model. Understanding and managing clinical culture becomes a primary activity.

3. There is an early and consistent focus on clinician teamwork and workflow and recognition that transforming health care through IT is not an information systems project, but a clinical and operational one.

Successful technical "installation" remains critical, that is, the software and technology must "work," but the other important activities that must be undertaken by enterprises to gain system acceptance and yield higher-quality professional behavior are key. The myth that "perfect" software with high technology pervasive computing will yield transformation (if you build it RIGHT, they will come) has been perhaps the greatest obstacle to badly needed change in our profession.

The overriding problem with failed IT projects in general, and particularly in clinical culture, is lack of attention to the human elements of changing behavior among professionals—the initiation of a "new order of things" as Machiavelli pointed out. Nearly 65 percent of major organizational change efforts of all kinds, IT related or not, fail in the United States [43]. Conversely, suboptimal software and technology, which are realities of the evolving digital age, have been used to advantage when attention has been paid to the other spheres [44,45] and of those spheres *transition leadership is the key* [46–49].

Understanding and Managing Clinical Culture

Clinicians faced with the presence of *information tools* in their sacrosanct medical environment have often rejected computing initiatives, despite the fact that the use of IT in health care is perhaps the most pressing matter for their profession today. In general our culture has key common elements:

- A stern belief in professional autonomy and opinion-based methods rather than in validated knowledge.
- A view of guidelines as constraints, implying restriction of independent judgment.
- Emphasis on recollection, intuition, and uniqueness.
- The belief that repetition establishes validity.
- The idea that relationships are authoritarian, not cooperative.

The major sectors of healthcare practice (broadly divided into academic and community practice settings) provide variations on these cultural themes, based on the values and goals of the providers in the particular setting—teaching, research, and tenure in academia versus efficiency, service, and autonomy in the private sector. Experience has taught that these common elements create unique challenges to the progress we need, and this will become clearer as our discussion proceeds.

Managing the transition depends upon cooperation, cultural understanding of fears that impede adoption (resistance), understanding of cross-domain clinical workflow, ability to create the impetus for change and to harvest the gains from transition, and the ability to balance policy with technology. These factors are addressed in turn.

Cooperation

Successful transition requires "countercultural" actions, not least of which is cooperation (Figure 12.2). Three dependent but remarkably different communities exist in most healthcare enterprises (clinical, IT, and operations/administrative subcultures), which can be visualized as clusters at each of the three corners of the triangle. These groups think in entirely dissimilar ways, use disparate language, and approach problems with

Barriers to Progress

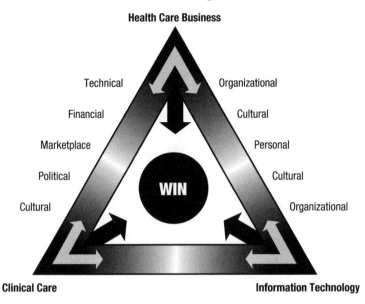

FIGURE 12.2. As this triangle indicates, successful transition requires "countercultural" actions among the three communities that exist in most healthcare enterprises.

completely different methodologies. Migration together is key to reaching the winner's circle and actually transforming care processes in the enterprise as a whole [50]. This coalescence depends upon each faction understanding, empathizing, and working closely with each other. Most failures with healthcare IT initiatives can be traced directly back to the exclusion of one or more of these communities from the information system selection or implementation process. (Actually, the shape should be pyramidal, with a fourth base corner representing patients/consumers, but in the interest of simplicity, we will pursue the triangle.)

The obstacles listed along the sides of the triangle exist along the bottom as well (they simply are not represented on the diagram). Organizational, cultural, and personal barriers are formidable as the corner dwellers attempt to work collaboratively. When the subcultures naturally clash, many organizations re-isolate the groups to avoid conflict. Some organizations have tried appointing liaisons to move between the cohorts, thinking that this subverts the need to actually "work together," but the liaison is usually destroyed or worn out before success is anywhere close. *The only way to get to the winner's circle is to eliminate the organizational barriers first, by forming balanced committees, work groups, or task forces.* The instinctive thing for enterprises to do is to skip this step of cultural melding altogether, or to give it short shrift in the effort to move quickly.

Despite the discomfort of conflict and the time and talent required for successful negotiation, this unification is critical to reaching goals and solving operational problems for staff and care providers without breaking the bank or creating unrealistic expectations. Establishing ground rules for group conduct from the beginning seems tedious as well, but encouraging each subgroup to understand the capabilities, needs, and resources of the others is *the* most important key to the win. Subcultural differences can be mitigated by having meetings, sessions, and project governance that fully involve members of all three domains. The *technologists* should spend time with clinicians in their medical settings to observe workflow and information flow and to understand the ways in which teams function in the care environment. The *clinicians* likewise (at least those who are leading the clinical system efforts) should participate fully in discussions of technological applications to their problems. They should come to understand the limits of technology and the methods by which the technologists will contribute to useful solutions. The *operations and administrative* leaders should spend time in the clinical environment (if they don't already) and participate in all sessions with the clinicians and the technologists regarding system acquisition or creation.

In this cooperative manner, the clinicians become familiar with project concepts and methodology, software production, testing, implementation, training, and operational processes. The technologists better understand what happens in a clinical day and the nature of the interactions among doctors, patients, and staff. The operations/administrative contributors come to understand all these things and can contribute their requirements for reporting, solvency, and process efficiency to the creative work. The operations leaders in their role are ultimately accountable for funding, implementing, and reaping gains from the automation.

Transformation using information technology is not solely, or even primarily, the purview of the information systems department as has traditionally been the case.

Managing Resistance

Distilled for simplicity, the core behavioral barrier to success with IT in the clinical subculture is a powerful apprehension—infobia—which is a combination of two dominant fears: *fear of appearing incompetent using information systems technology and fear of the potential harmful effects information might have on practice, position, prestige, or job security* [51].

Infobia keeps us doing things in ways that are familiar—working on our overwhelming responsibilities (increasingly large numbers of patients seen in detrimentally brief appointments, overloading of professional support staff with clerical duties, inordinate bureaucratic burdens mandated for remuneration, litigation-phobic decision making in a void of patient information, and error commissions of every conceivable kind despite our best intentions)—in traditional, or instinctive, ways.

It is important to bear in mind that the process of medical training and the tradition of clinical autonomy render physicians unusually susceptible to the fear of appearing incompetent in front of patients or colleagues. Although clinicians may be quick to accept new technology that enhances professional esteem (laparoscopic surgery, MRI, etc.), there is far more squeamishness about approaching a machine that most pediatric patients can use with greater facility. It is important in the merging of cultures for all parties to understand the psychological basis for this unique apprehension [52,53].

The second element of infobia has to do with the way information has been used, as a weapon, in futile attempts to control clinical decisions and the costs they engender.

Clinicians instinctively fear that incomplete or misleading information will compromise their clinical autonomy and adversely affect the quality of care.

The cultural resistance to clinical computing can be represented as a hill leaders must scale *with their troops* to get to a transformed state, and the largest part of this resistance, with respect to information technology, is infobia. Figures 12.3 to 12.5 illustrate the resistance challenge hill and the instinctive and counterinstinctive methods of dealing with it.

The details of dealing with resistance in this model are available elsewhere [54], but recognize that the most traditional response to resistance is to ignore it. At the time of project Go Live when the resistance can no longer be disregarded, which is inevitable, traditional managers commonly start manipulating the opposition, using force of reason, rather than reason itself, extracting deals and favors, and eventually threatening and intimidating "nonbelievers." These tactics set up winners and losers and create the fear, suspicion, and polarization that we have seen repeatedly in unenlightened change efforts.

Countercultural responses to resistance are difficult to exercise, particularly under pressure. These include giving serious attention to the anxiety and reality involved in the change, respectful listening to and communicating with resistors, and promoting reasons for implementing the solution for the benefit of the organization as a whole as

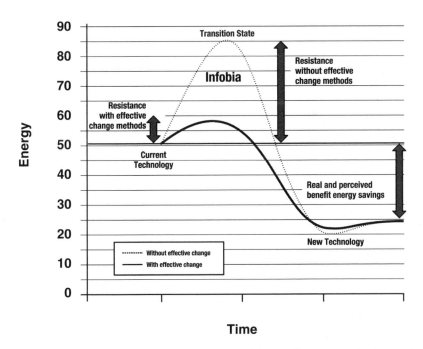

FIGURE 12.3. The transition hill to be scaled is lowered by excellent communication, copious training and support, clear vision and direction, and ongoing steadfast commitment to success by leaders from each subculture. All three must manage their own versions of infobia to get to the winner's circle.

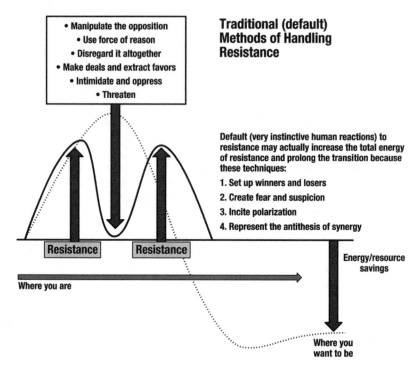

FIGURE 12.4. There are traditional and very instinctive ways of handling resistance that do not work very well. These include manipulating the opposition; using "force of reason," rather than promoting true big-picture sincerity; disregarding resistance altogether, which is really easy; making deals with individuals, which inevitably backfire; or simply using intimidation, oppression, or threatening behavior, which approach some Machiavellian tactics. Notice that this is really application of pressure from the outside, which does not do anything to diminish resistance and actually prolongs the transition process and which ultimately does not get to a preferable energy state. The default reactions set up winners and losers, create fear and suspicion, incite polarization, and are the antithesis of synergistic cooperation [43].

well as for each individual in the organization. It is extremely important *to train adequately, to support users after implementation, and to reward and broadcast success.* Using these techniques, synergy and trust can be built and cohesiveness established. It is remarkable how many times the entire system budget is spent on technology and nothing is left for adequate training and support; it is counterinstinctive to limit expenditures on the systems to preserve funds for user education and support.

Workflow and Well-Defined Pathways

To paraphrase a leading expert on the logic of failure, we have been loosed upon the information age with prehistoric brains [55]. We tend to think in an immediate cause-and-effect manner. It is in our innate (instinctive) wiring, and such thinking may lead to short-term gains but subsequently to long-term losses; more often it leads to impressive and expensive disasters. There has been recent overemphasis on the process labeled CPOE (Computer Physician Order Entry) with claims of markedly enhanced safety and efficiency that could result from addressing this subelement of a subsystem. While this is a critical component of a clinical transformation strategy, it is also a prime example of rushing to a solution without understanding the comprehensive nature of the problem or the potential for more comprehensive progress that such an immediate effort might cause.

Many healthcare enterprises prefer to skip the crucial process of "enterprise modeling" and workflow assessment. They do not take the time to define and integrate work pathways, and they fail to see that making one process more automatic creates chaos elsewhere or prevents problem solutions further downstream. If we lose sight of the grand design, we risk stopping prematurely at a critical juncture because it fails to yield tangible benefits, not recognizing that the next step, for which we readied ourselves, is the one with the enormous payback. Fortunately, there is increasing acknowledgment of the importance and complexity of understanding and building and implementing solutions, rather than fixes [56–58].

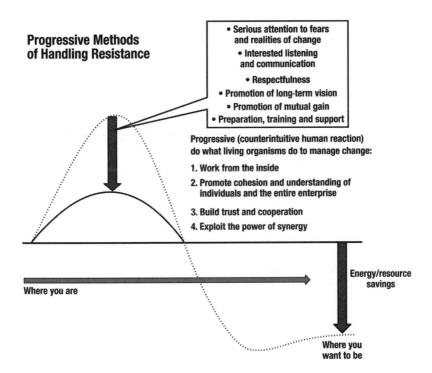

FIGURE 12.5. The counterinstinctive, but much more effective ways of dealing with resistance (infobia), are exercised from the inside. Note the pulling down of the curve from within rather than more oppressive pressure from outside as in Figure 12.4. By paying serious attention to the fears and realities of the change, by careful listening and extensive communication, by ongoing respect, by promotion of vision and evangelism about organizational gains, and by appropriate training and support, the changes can be more easily obtained. Effective techniques promote cohesion and teamwork, build trust and cooperation, and build synergy [43].

The determination of how healthcare processes occur is complex and intimidating. Great emphasis placed on understanding workflow has shown that medication prescribing and dispensing seem simple on first glance and might be easily automated. More careful analysis reveals the medication ordering administration process to be among the most convoluted, multifarious, and constantly changing in health care, and designing systems that meet the needs of the clinicians, the patients, the pharmacists, and the health plans is a monumental task. As much as we know about the hazards of medication-ordering errors for patients, it is becoming increasingly apparent that the variability, unnecessary complexity, indeed, immeasurability of errors in many other areas of service and care delivery are problems of even more intimidating immensity [59,60].

Our instincts also lead us to idiosyncratic, proprietary, but relatively "easy" solutions, rather than to systems founded on IT standards and knowledge commonality. We have often used the "best of breed" approach to system selection in particular niches, which presents a nearly insurmountable obstacle when the desired endpoint is actually comprehensive information integration.

A very important concept for traditional short-term "nonpathway thinkers" to grasp is that not every step in a pathway must produce resources, that is, return on investment (ROI). Sometimes no gains can be harvested from a step, and at other times resources need to be donated to a step simply to prepare the organization for the next cascade of changes. These resource-consuming steps are sometimes called "infrastructure plays" or "preparatory expenditures."

The IT world is a prime example of where money must often be spent without immediate gain but with anticipation of return on the investment *by the end of the pathway*. It is important to understand that subsequent pathway steps will restore energy balance and ultimately yield a net gain. *The individual transition steps involve one-time expenses, but the pathway as a whole (transformation), if well executed, yields enduring riches, a base for evolution, and perpetual market advantage.* If we do not create the infrastructure for long-term success, we cannot expect to transform.

Effective pathway analysis requires the input of user communities from the very beginning of the effort, because *successful transition begins with system requirement definition, design, or selection.* In the case of IT design or acquisition, frontline workers' evaluation of current procedures and analyses of where and how workflow can be improved with information systems is critical to success. Lack of user involvement from the earliest developmental stages has been found to be a major reason for failure with change and with IT adoption [61].

The early investment of those who will be affected by the new system results in a sense of responsibility and ownership. It also inspires trusted coworkers to help each other with transition. Involvement of middle managers in the same way is crucial too, because they are often the most influential people working with employees—and they may also be the operations people most susceptible to infobia, with potential for inordinately high resistance to change.

Impetus and Benefits

It is instinctive for humans to keep things as they are unless there is some pressing reason to change. To stimulate transition, leaders must convince their followers that there is enough pain in staying with the status quo or enough pleasure inherent in a new way of doing things. The impetus for transition is what John Kotter refers to as *decreasing complacency*, or *establishing urgency* (Figure 12.6) [62]. Others call this cre-

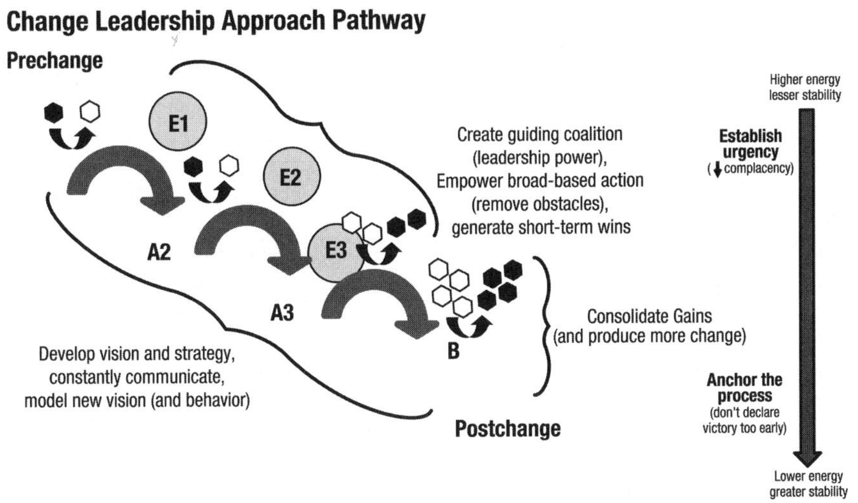

Change Leadership Approach Pathway

Figure 12.6. Notice that establishing urgency is represented by the energy diminution from the pathway that is to be achieved, and that once the pathway is traversed and the end state achieved, anchoring the process with good user support is important to keep things at the desired stability. Thinking through the pathway and integrating business and IT objectives is represented as vision, strategy, communication through appropriate means, and managing infobia at each step by creating coalitions and empowering change agents, removing obstacles (diminishing energy of activation), and generating a string of short-term wins that lead to overall success [62].

ation of a "burning platform." Patient safety issues, declining reimbursements, or publicity around horrific medical errors may constitute such motivational events, but so far they have not ignited platforms to the degree that transformative efforts have become dominant. The use of counterinstinctive resistance management techniques suggests active listening, understanding, and perhaps posing a question to the resistant clinician such as, what if our positions were reversed and I came to you protesting use of our *paper record system*, promising that I could remember everything about my patients and needn't record anything at all, how would you respond? (see Figure 12.5).

Harvesting Gains

The phenomenon of "successful" IT *installation* in health care (and in other industries), without a yield of expected gains, is startlingly common. Management discipline is crucial to realizing benefits from the new systems pathways in tangible ways for the enterprise: measurable performance, quality and service enhancements, as well as demonstrable cost reductions or avoidance. The main difference between successful *implementation* of an information system and *transformation* of an enterprise is that *only* transformation yields a truly beneficial return on investment. This is where detailed work in the sphere of measurement and knowledge is required (see Figure 12.1).

More often than not, a new information system is purchased, predicated on a return on investment involving reduced personnel over some time period. The new information system does improve efficiency and operations, but the "potential" recovered resources escape. Even when the ostensible goal of a system is "safety" rather than ROI per se, much sociocultural change is required to maintain positive impact.

When successful change processes have been completed, and if benefits are actually realized, it is instinctive for the community that underwent the change to feel exclusively entitled to those benefits. One of the most difficult concepts for traditional corporations to comprehend and promulgate as their structures shift to more integrated (matrix) and less hierarchical (organization chart) models is the notion that recovered resources are *not* necessarily the property of the department that generated them. Rather, they are riches that accrue to the organization as a living whole. Kotter refers to this as "consolidating gains" to produce more change (see Figure 12.6).

Disciplined accountable managers must assure that resources saved via IT are captured, authentic, and demonstrable. They must also determine where those resources should be best used for enterprise stability. The expectation must be clear, from executives through frontline workers, that benefits recovered from information systems are guaranteed (budgeted as concrete savings—money or FTEs, going forward), and become the property of the enterprise as a whole. It takes foresight, planning, and courage for managers at all levels to extract gains in efficiency and improved processes from the enterprise; this must be done with fairness and diplomacy, or the infobia around potential savings will prevent the change from ever occurring. Budgeting personnel reductions ahead of time and working toward them through attrition rather than layoffs, communicating enhanced workplace skills, and increased job satisfaction are important in this process.

Balancing Technocracy with Policy

Once the power of information systems is recognized and leveraged for success, there is a tendency for institutions to view it as a panacea. Not every problem is soluble through technology. Months and months of time and effort can be wasted trying to automate something that humans do with great efficiency. Simple policies and good auditing can circumvent problems that are beyond the capabilities of information systems today.

It is natural for enterprises to either attempt to replicate the paper world in software or to solve all human problems with computational methods and machines. The desire to use computers to enforce policies, restrict information access, regulate workflow, and provide detailed security needs to be resisted. Although the electronic world renders many of our current processes obsolete, humans still handle some complexities better than computers. A familiar example is the use of technology to strictly govern information access—complex rules for trying to determine who can see what information depending on personal characteristics and fleeting relationships—which introduces inconsistency and complexity into systems that destroy usability.

In the frenzy of automation design it is counterinstinctive to simply agree that people do a task better than the computers could and allow them to continue those tasks. A straightforward illustration is that of "delegation," which becomes an issue with in-baskets and desktop medicine processing. To find a reliable set of rules about who takes over for whom when an individual is gone, and what the fallback is when the delegated person is absent for some unforeseen reason, and then to depend on machines to follow these shifting, convoluted rules, becomes impossible. On the other hand, nurses on a ward or in an office are quite good at distributing work: they know who is there, who is not, who is double-booked, and even who is in a lousy mood, and they can distribute the work accordingly. The automation solution is simple, not complex: let the nurses keep distributing the work as they see fit, but via electronic means.

Similarly, a security-confidentiality policy that clearly sets forth regulations about suitable information use and enforces them, combined with proper auditing of information access in a system, is much more effective than automated software (with indeterminate variables) to preemptively determine proper access. Trying to discern who is a VIP, who is a "family member," or who is an "employee," and then revealing information based on shifting role definitions becomes unfeasible and only succeeds in preventing needed access to information for treatment because of the limitations of the software.

The Road Map

The principles outlined above for focusing on the five spheres involved in transformation, and the overview of the challenges of transition specifically in the healthcare environment, suggest that a great deal of organizational planning and activity must surround any IT project that is to support the operational, clinical, and financial goals of a particular enterprise. Given the complexity of the transformation, and the multiple areas of work that assure success, we have found a transformation road map, which can be reviewed with various levels of detail and is helpful in ensuring that all bases are covered. A high-level example of such a road map for purposes of illustration is provided in Figure 12.7. Recognize that for each of the high-level activities indicated

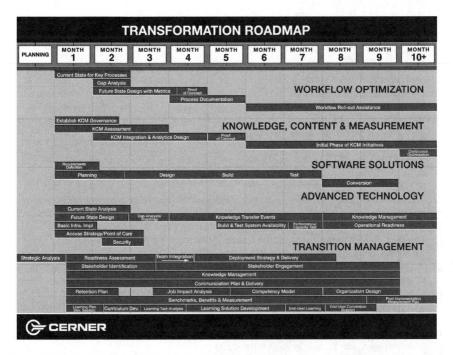

FIGURE 12.7. For each of the high-level activities indicated along the timeline in the five threads in the road map, there are specific roles, responsibilities, deliverables, risks of incompletion, and alternatives that must be delineated.

along the timeline in the five threads, there are specific roles, responsibilities, deliverables, risks of incompletion, and alternatives that must be delineated (and are at deeper levels of the road map tool).

The transformation of healthcare practices using IT is a complex process that requires clear goals, thorough strategy, multidimensional organization thinking, attention to detail, and a great deal of discipline. In addressing some of the core elements of transition management and the challenges of dealing with change in clinical culture, my hope is that as each enterprise determines specific transformation goals, it will return to the key ideas here, and determine their own road map to success, bearing in mind that having a map is essential to getting to the destination, but success is equally dependent on the ability of leaders to persuade, understand and support their teams during the process, and particularly to realize the value of making the trip . . .

References

1. Machiavelli N. The prince. 1537. ch. 6.
2. Overhage MA, Middleton B, et al. Does national mandate of provider order entry portend greater benefit than risk for health care delivery: the 2001 ACMI Debate. JAMIA 2002 May–June; 9(3):199–208.
3. Hunt DL, et al. Effects of computer-based clinical decision support systems on physician performance and patient outcomes: a systemic review. JAMA 1998;280(15):1339–1346.
4. Shiffman RN, et al. Computer-based guideline implementation systems: a systemic review of functionality and effectiveness. JAMA 1999;6:104–114.
5. Patrino K, et al. EMR reduces costs and protects revenues. In: Kiel JM, editor. Information technology for the practicing physician. New York: Springer; 2000.
6. Teich JM, Merchia PR, Schmiz JL, Kuperman GJ, Spurr CD, Bates DW. Effects of computerized physician order entry on prescribing practices. Arch Intern Med 2000;160: 2741–2747.
7. William LG, Robert JD, Audrius P. Preventing exacerbation of an ADE with automated decision support. Journal of Healthcare Information Management 2002;(16)4.
8. Raschke R. A computer alert system to prevent injury from adverse drug events: development and evaluation in a community teaching hospital. JAMA 1998;280(15):1317–1320.
9. Bates DW, Leape LL, Cullen DJ, Laird N, et al. Effect of computerized physician order entry and a team intervention on prevention of serious medication errors. JAMA 1998;280: 1311–1316.
10. Bates DW, Teich JM, Lee J, Seger D, Kuperman GJ, Ma'Luf N, Boyle D, Leape L. The impact of computerized physician order entry on medication error prevention. JAMA 1999;6: 313–321.
11. Tierney WM, Miller ME, Overhage JM, McDonald CJ. Physician inpatient order writing on microcomputer workstations: effects on resource utilization. JAMA 1993;269:379–383.
12. Mekhjian HS, Kumar RR, Kuehn L, et al. Immediate benefits realized following implementation of physician order entry at an academic medical center. JAMA 2002;9:529–539.
13. Miller AS. Hosp Pharm 2002;37(6):644–646, 695.
14. Taylor R, Manzo J, Sinnett M. Quantifying value for physician order-entry systems: a balance of cost and quality. Healthcare Financial Management 2002; July.
15. Geerlofs JP. Clinical software for strengthening the physician-patient relationship. In: Kiel JM, editor. Information technology for the practicing physician. New York: Springer-Verlag; 2000.
16. Coddington D. Beyond managed care: how consumers and technology are changing the future of health care. San Francisco: Jossey-Bass; 2000.
17. 13th Annual HIMSS Leadership Survey 2002. Superior Consulting.
18. Drazen E, et al. A primer on physician order entry. First Consulting Group, California Health-Care Foundation Publications; September 2000.

19. Strassmann P. The squandered computer: evaluating the business alignment of information technologies. New Canaan CT: The Information Economics Press; 1997.
20. Edmondson B, Edmonson P. Speeding up team learning. Harvard Business Review 2001; Oct. 1.
21. Lawrence D. From chaos to care: the promise of team-based medicine. Boulder, CO: Perseus; 2002.
22. Wood GC. Serving the information needs of physicians. N Engl J Med 1972;286(11):603–604.
23. Covell DG. Information needs in office practice: are they being met? Ann Intern Med 1985;103(4):596–599.
24. Gorman P. Information needs in primary care. Med Info 2001;10(pt 1):338–342.
25. Tang PC. Traditional medical records as a source of clinical data in the outpatient setting. Proc Annu Symp Comput Appl Med Care 1994;575–579.
26. Kohn LT, Corrigan JM, Donaldson MS, editors. To err is human: building a safer health system. Committee on Quality Health Care, Institute of Medicine. Washington, DC: National Academy Press; 2000.
27. Sharpe VA, Faden I. Medical harm: historical, conceptual and ethical dimensions of iatrogenic illness. Cambridge: Cambridge University Press; 1998.
28. Eddy D, Billings S. The quality of medical evidence: implications for quality of care. Health Affairs 1988;7(1):19–32.
29. Halvorson G. Strong medicine. New York: Random House; 1993.
30. Berwick D, Fineberg H, Weinstein M. When doctors meet numbers. Am J Med 1981;71: 991–998.
31. Weinstein M. Checking medicine's vital signs. The New York Times 1998; April.
32. Berwick D, Nolan T. Physicians as leaders in improving health care. Ann Intern Med 1998;28(4):289–292.
33. Chassin M. Is health care ready for Six Sigma Quality? Millbank Quarterly 1998 Oct; 76(4).
34. Millenson M. Demanding medical excellence. Chicago: University of Chicago Press; 1997.
35. Leape L. Controversies Institute of Medicine medical errors are not exaggerated. JAMA 2000;284:95–97.
36. Wilson RM, et al. The quality in Australian health care study. Med J Aust 1995;163(9):458–471.
37. Gopher D, et al. Human Factors Society, 1999.
38. Steel K, et al. Latrogenic illness on a general medical service at a university hospital. NEJM 1981;304(11):638–42.
39. Davenport TH. Information ecology. New York: Oxford University Press; 1997.
40. Sheehy B. Train wrecks: why information technology investments derail. San Diego, CA: The Governance Institute; Fall 2001.
41. Johnson J. Chaos: the dollar drain of IT project failures. Appl Den Trends 1995;2(1):41–47.
42. Shortliffe EH, et al, editors. Medical informatics: computer applications in health care and biomedicine, 2nd ed. New York: Springer-Verlag; 2001.
43. Maurer R. Beyond the wall of resistance. Austin, Texas: Bard Books; 1996.
44. Lorenzi N. Antecedents of the people and organizational aspects of medical informatics: review of the literature. JAMA 1997;4(2):79–93.
45. Worthley JA. Managing information in healthcare: concepts and cases. Chicago: Health Administration Press; 2000.
46. Senge P. The dance of change. New York: Doubleday; 1999.
47. Dickout R. Designing change programs that won't cost you your job. McKinsey Quarterly 1995; No. 4.
48. Liebowitz J. Failure and lessons learned in information technology management. An International Journal, Cognizant Communication Corporation.
49. Robbins H, Finley M. Why change doesn't work. Princeton, NJ: Peterson's Press; 1996.
50. Rose J, Ippolito L, Garver S. Run toward the roar: six counter-instinctive actions for organization success with health information technology. Connexions MGMA; Jan. 2001.
51. Rose J. Medicine and the information age. Ivvins, TX: ACPE Press; 1998.
52. Clinicians for the restoration of autonomous practice (CRAP), EBM: unmasking the ugly truth. Br Med J 2002;325:1496 [satire].

53. Robinson AR, et al. Physician and public opinion on quality of health care and the problem of medical errors. Arch Intern Med 2002;162:19.

54. Rose JS. Lessons from life: the biology of business transformation. The Physician Executive 2001; Sept.–Oct.

55. Dorner D. The logic of failure. Reading, MA: Addison-Wesley; 1996.

56. Gartner 24 January 2002.

57. Birkmeyer JD, et al. Leapfrog patient safety standards. Eff Clin Pract 2002;66(8).

58. Anderson, et al. JAMA 2002.

59. Goodman T. Utah's medical error toll:18 deaths in one year [based on Report of the Utah Department of Heatlh]. Salt Lake Tribune 2002; Dec. 21.

60. Boodman J. No end to errors. The Washington Post 2002; Nov. 30.

61. Ives B, Olson M. User involvement and MIS success: a review of research. Manag Sci 1984;30:586–603.

62. Kotter JP. Leading change. Boston: Harvard University Press; 1996.

63. ••

13
The Role of the CIO:
The Evolution Continues

BETSY S. HERSHER

> *In today's complex healthcare environment, we are relying more and more on the CIO as a comprehensive leader who touches almost every aspect of the business.*

A Role in Transition

History is history, and it is usually considered old. In exploring the history of the chief information officer (CIO) role, however, one of the issues and challenges we have had is that it is not old. We are all familiar with the definitions of CEO, COO, CNO, CFO, etc. The definition of these roles has been known for many years, and they are well understood. Even though those roles have changed significantly throughout the years, they have always been seen as very senior leadership roles on the executive management team. When the CIO role was instituted, however, no one really knew what it meant or who the right kind of person was to fill that role. Enough thought was also not given to what the job responsibilities and accountabilities would be. The title of CIO was bestowed with the hope that the title would make the job, or it was bestowed as a reward for years of service. Isn't the designation of CIO enough? Perhaps it was thought that a fairy godmother would create an executive with her magic wand. Some of that illogical reasoning is still present today. There has also been much confusion as to the type of professionals the CIO needs to have as part of his or her information technology (IT) team to do work that was sometimes undefined.

Creating a successful CIO role has involved many processes. There have been births and rebirths, course corrections midstream, and CIOs, themselves, have changed their own vision of what they think the role should entail. With that, questions have also been raised to determine the need for the position, its place in the reporting structure, its overall function, and its impact on cost benefits to the organization. In organizations that have outsourced IT operations, the role has taken on a much broader scope—to be more strategic and focused on managing relationships.

In the past, IT has been seen as an expense, rather than as a service. It has been hard to measure the success of a new program managed by a CIO in dollars and cents. However, very strong imperatives now indicate that this type of data is necessary to

---

Betsy S. Hersher, BA, is President of Hersher Associates, Ltd.

face the future. Not only is IT now recognized as a service, it is also a major factor in customer satisfaction and a driver in successful clinical redesign. In fact, patients, particularly those who are becoming more IT savvy, want to see information online. IT is a very valuable asset in providing and directing care delivery and more and more a part of strategic initiatives for the healthcare enterprise. There are multiple complex issues today facing executive management healthcare teams across the country. There is much reliance on data as a resource and on the CIO as a comprehensive leader who touches almost every aspect of the business.

Complex Issues

In general, health care has always been an unusually operated business. For a service that is one of the largest contributors to the Gross National Product in this country, interestingly enough, few policy leaders have helped or provided guidance on the road passed, as well as on the very complex road to be traveled in the future. Some CEOs are expecting the CIO to fill the critical role of key advisor and confidant on new initiatives. They want to be able to turn to the CIO for sage advice and council, understanding almost every endeavor related to IT. Forecasts for the future are entirely positive, challenging, and exciting. What an outstanding time to become or to be a CIO—at this very important junction of change and growth.

There has been so little policy agreement on how to provide services that it appears to many that the cost of healthcare delivery is way out of line and, in many cases, uneven. For years, it was believed that care delivered in an academic medical center was far more costly than care delivered in a community setting. Is it the cost of insurance? Is it the cost of malpractice insurance? Is it unions, insurance, or the pharmaceutical firms charging astronomical amounts of money for prescription drugs? What is it that has driven up costs? Whatever the reason, a great deal of time has been spent focusing on the cost instead of concentrating on the delivery of care. This is why managed care entered the picture in the first place and exercised a stranglehold on the industry for a period of time. Fortunately, drastic change has occurred in this particular arena, and reason appears to be prevailing. Still, one must question why a visit to check up on a minor problem, involving a 5-minute examination, no tests, and a bill for $96, can occur in a small internal medicine practice that insists on payment in cash because the group no longer accepts insurance.

Where have we gone wrong? Until recently, how have we, as an industry, supported our key consumers? Who are they? Patients? Physicians? The insurance industry? What about help for older adults who come in for care and have to document their entire medical history on a scrap of paper folded in their wallets? Sometimes, these patients even have to remember the results of previous blood pressure and other tests to remind their doctors. Interestingly enough, there are many nonautomated offices that function well and are capable of keeping excellent paper records. However, they are the exception, not the rule. There are currently few electronic medical records vehicles in place in hospitals, clinics, or physician offices.

Why is a national pharmacy chain capable of keeping, online, nationally and internationally, a patient's ailments, drugs to which they are allergic, the date of their last purchase, their prescription records, and, more than anything else, maintain the security and privacy of their records? Why can't our healthcare providers function in this way? Because of their automated system, a pharmacist at one of these chains may be a better resource for drug-related questions than our own physicians.

Clearly, security, privacy, and full access to those data on a national basis are mission critical to pharmacy chains. Now that it is becoming a mandate to healthcare providers, a move is occurring as quickly as possible into an environment that will support and secure the records of patients in hospitals and clinics and in physicians' offices. Hopefully, those records will soon be available anywhere, anytime.

The Evolution of the CIO

The role of the CIO in the healthcare enterprise evolved as a result of the 1982 TEFRA (Tax Equity and Responsibility Act) regulations, reporting requirements, and other historical developments. As hospitals fought to remain viable and competitive, they began to view information as a key corporate resource—a drastic change from their previously rather laissez faire attitude toward data and the departmental folks in the basement cranking out checks and bills.

We must remember that we are a product of whence we came. So, when TEFRA hit in 1982, and CEOs were hoping it would be a fad, everyone probably failed to notice the need for a senior IS executive, let alone one that would report to the CEO or COO and sit at the senior executive table.

The role of the CIO in health care and his or her associated required skill set have evolved rapidly in response to the acceptance and requirement for information as a key corporate resource. The relevance of past history, however, has very little to do with today's IT leadership success factors, although many of the skills we looked at 10 years ago are still critical. While expectations for the CIO have changed, many new accountabilities have also been added. There are many supporting factors that are allowing senior IS executives to share their workload so that an increasing portion of their time can be spent providing creative, strategic direction. Outsourcing has had an effect on this issue in a major way. We will be discussing the viability of many new positions with emphasis on succession planning and critical clinical implementation leaders.

Cause and Effect

Managed care, mergers, and advanced technology were the buzzwords of the 1990s as well as of government regulations. These elements catalyzed the growth of multiple integrated delivery systems and recognition of the importance of the continuum of care. Mergers and demergers have strongly affected healthcare enterprises, along with deep financial stress. For the majority of our organizations, serious financial stress occurred even before Y2K, with the Balanced Budget Act, and it has continued in a more disastrous vein thereafter. Along with that, three other factors affected CIO and IT initiatives.

The first was that a great deal of money was spent on IT during Y2K efforts, leaving other major capital needs on hold. Second, because Y2K was a technical issue, some CEOs thought they needed strong technicians in the CIO role. Since CEO and other executives on the management team thought that technology leadership was what got them through Y2K, there was a very brief change in the skill sets that CEOs were looking for in their CIOs. For a period of about 6 months to a year, they wanted to make sure that their CIO and CIO executive team was very technical, and the need for strategic executive skills diminished. Fortunately, that trend was short-lived, as the industry evolved to focus more on clinical systems, concern over delivery of services, and issues of patient longevity. CEOs suddenly got the message that they needed a CIO who was both skilled in business as well as a healthcare strategist. The position became much more strategic and executive. Third, outsourcing became a major factor with its promise to solve recruitment issues and ease the need for upfront cash to financially challenged organizations.

After approximately 1 year of upheaval following Y2K, the profile of the new CIO emerged as someone who was extremely well regarded, considered a key player on the executive management team, and a creative leader and influencer who can support the direction of health care. In many cases, new hires were candidates who fit the new parameters. Information technology's mission became critical to CEOs, given the combination of changes in health care, potential longevity of the baby boomer generation, pressure from government regulations, the Leapfrog Group, and JCAHO requirements.

Health care is chaotic, showing strong indicators of response to changes being mandated by the federal government, as well as by business groups. An immediate planning effort is also essential to address the demands of baby boomers (approaching 65 years of age), who will soon comprise 25 percent of the population. It is estimated that by 2010 we will have 74 to 76 million individuals who will be age 65 and older. Health care will be advancing so that people are getting better medical treatment. Therefore, we will be treating older, healthier adults in an outpatient setting that will require significant data. In addition, if people are living longer, they will end up with the same chronic illnesses and the same 2 years of expenses at the end of their lives, no matter their age when they pass away. To support these people, an electronic patient record will be vital, along with many other computerized systems.

Fortunately, advances in technology in general will support the exploding need for and creative utilization of technology. The decreasing cost of technology and the increasing availability of powerful departmental tools dictate that someone must orchestrate the flow of information, foster the integration of systems, ensure the integrity of data, and monitor for redundancy. The CIO must have the vision to view these issues from a senior executive perspective and to match business and organizational needs to the appropriate information and technology platforms.

There are few crystal balls needed now. Many of the valuable uses of technology are becoming obvious. The need for computerized records is not only being mandated by outside sources, but consumers need their information stored in one place. Not only has IT advanced, but medical advances also portend that the next generation may live longer. Couple that with the fact that much of nonacute health care will be delivered in an outpatient setting or at home. Compelling arguments exist for connectivity from the home to physician offices or to help lines.

Current and Future Skills and Issues

During the past 18 months, a new era for the CIO has emerged due to changes in care delivery systems, internal and external challenges, and future predictions. There is a yin–yang aspect to these challenges representing threats that must be dealt with quickly. Since health care as an industry has done very little to pay attention to healthcare future policy, we are suddenly seeing consumers, patients, doctors, and insurers pressing the industry for change, and there is a great deal of impatience. Some organizations are choosing to outsource IT because they think that by outsourcing, these problems are handled more efficiently. That is yet to be proven.

Until recently as an industry, we have paid little attention to succession planning or coaching our next group of leaders. Therefore, as our CIOs begin to consider retirement, there are not enough potential CIO candidates coming up through the ranks. In addition to all these issues, CIOs are working diligently with executive teams on issues of patient safety, clinical redesign, security, and the Health Insurance Portability and Accountability Act (HIPAA).

Physician order entry (POE) is a major issue that also must be handled. The business coalitions have more formally organized groups, such as the Leapfrog Group that is demanding POE, and JCAHO, which has its own set of demands. It would, however, be wonderful if we had electronic patient records that were usable in all areas of the enterprise to support physician order entry.

There is a lot on everyone's plate. Additionally, as healthcare costs continue to rise, coupled with insurance costs, it is becoming very difficult to provide the money to support all these critical areas. As the dust clears, it appears that questioning the need for CIOs with strong supporting IS executive teams has subsided, but new landmines have surfaced at all levels of the IS organization.

As noted earlier, the basic skills needed for a CIO have not changed in at least 10 years. However, there are additional skills and attributes critical for success. These skills are imperative to meeting goals, as the CIO can bridge the gap between the business side and delivery side of health care. We need to have the right people in the right positions. CIOs need to be innovative in these dynamic times of change. It is finally time for their creativity and leadership to be utilized. At the same time, CIOs need to keep the big picture in mind. It takes a great deal of professional commitment to face today's challenges. These leaders must have the appropriate skill set.

Hard Skills

Skills fall into two equally important categories that are referred to as "hard" and "soft" skills. Hard skills are learned, innate, or associated to experiences. They include:

- Leadership.
- Business orientation.
- Excellent communication skills.
- Results/action orientation.
- Team player.
- Partnering.
- Change agent.
- Architect.
- Facilitator.
- Negotiator.
- Coalition builder.
- Politically savvy.
- Risk taker.
- Educator.
- Entrepreneurial.
- Ability to deal with formal/informal relationships while building consensus.
- Managing relationship priorities.
- Ability to develop a strategy.

The CIO needs to have the strategic vision to set the overall architectural platform for the organization and to function as a change agent and risk taker. Leadership, communication, and political skills are paramount. The CIO must be able to ensure the continuity and integration of systems, thereby supporting the future growth of the enterprise without controlling all resources. Flexibility is a key success factor in all these initiatives.

The CIO also needs to be a great negotiator, building long-term business relationships. Business sense and the ability to communicate ideas and priorities are important for success. The CIO has to be a survivor and viewed as absolutely credible to set standards and procedures for the organization. The successful CIO is viewed as a leader and resource for technology. A CIO must be comfortable dealing in ambiguity and dramatic change and be capable of responding quickly to initiatives and challenges that face the organization. A CIO must possess a global view of managing relationships and systems. Because there are often several CIOs involved in an integrated health network (IHN), a mature, credible leader is "comfortable" and manages by influence and facilitation rather than by control. Partnering, using influencing skills without formal power, and creating comfortable formal and informal relationships in a variety of venues are not simple talents. It is a real asset to be able to balance the need for immediate action and decision making within a service and enabling environment. The CIO in an IHN serves many masters with complex problems. Developing a broad vision and network strategy, while at the same time juggling the needs of cooperation, specific entities, and departmental priorities, requires the skills of an excellent leader.

Soft Skills

Experience has shown that senior leadership positions will be filled successfully only if there is a match to the corporate culture. Soft skills, in reality, are those skills that hiring executives seek. If you are a potential CIO and have prepared yourself with the proper experience, then review this list carefully. Your ability to match the corporate culture will be evaluated based on instinct, style, and the following soft skills as they apply to various cultures:

- Image/presence.
- Global view.
- Vulnerability.
- Decisiveness.
- Comfortable with self/mature (not judged by age).
- Comfortable taking charge.
- Comfortable following.
- Confident.
- Credible leader.
- Honest/high integrity.
- Courageous/risk taker when appropriate.
- Sense of humor.
- Flexible.
- Energetic.
- Creative.
- Resourceful.
- Perceptive/intuitive.
- Tenacious.
- Achiever.
- Balanced.

Each organization has its own unique culture, values, and way of life. For a CIO to be most effective, he or she will need to be compatible with that culture and demonstrate a strong understanding of those corporate values. Essentially, the CIO should match the corporate culture and be flexible enough to grow and change with it.

Current Issues

Issues facing current CIO and CEO leadership include:

- Demergers.
- Lack of succession planning.
- CIO retirement.
- Embracing new roles.
- Reporting structures.
- CEO and senior executives retiring and/or forced to leave.

Mergers and Demergers

So much energy goes into a merger that IT is often neglected in the planning process. Suddenly, senior leadership realizes that they have two separate computer systems and have not spent any time talking to two CIOs about a planning process. Most often in merger situations, the information systems (IS) teams manage to work well together. However, IS is also the group that tends to be overstressed as demands start flooding in with no one available to help set priorities. If everyone is fortunate enough to make it through the early merger time period, things begin to settle down.

Recently, it has become apparent that many mergers are not working, resulting in demerger situations. When a demerger occurs, the IT organization that has been blended faces the trauma of splitting up the resources, personnel, and contracts. Morale issues will be just as severe as they were during a merger situation, with employees concerned about whether and where they will be retained and how their position will be affected.

A demerger requires very careful planning and execution and may result in the IT organization continuing to provide services for all the entities for a period of time. Frequently, CIOs who have taken positions as the heads of large IT organizations that resulted from mergers, may find that the diminished scope that a demerger creates may eliminate the need for their positions.

Planning for Succession

In the past, health care in general has not been very proactive in the area of succession planning. You need only to look at the number of COOs that have not been elevated to the CEO position, or the Controller or Assistant CFO who has not been elevated to the top job. For some reason, it seems that part of the healthcare culture is to avoid internal development. Due to financial constraints, however, a trend is developing to look internally for leaders of new initiatives, and with proper coaching, it is working, both in IT and within the entire organization.

In the IT world, we are now backed into a corner as it relates to succession planning. Only recently have CIOs begun preparing the next generation of IT leaders to take over. It takes time to train successors and strategically align them with the executive team so that they will be accepted as leaders when they are ready to take over a higher role. Accordingly, CIOs must prepare for the future of their organizations and the industry by identifying and developing the second or third generation of IT leadership. Succession planning is imperative at all levels of the IT organization. Many of the key directors are the same age as the CIO. Although few of us want to face the issues surrounding CIO retirement, numbers do not lie.

As we look at the history of the CIO, the position really did not take life until around 1985. Generally, it was a midcareer move up. It took several years for CIOs to iron out specific areas of needed growth and the kind of support they needed from their management teams. So if the individuals who were identified as CIOs stayed in their jobs 3 to 5 years or longer, and then moved into one or two other positions, without having to do very complicated algebra we find that most of our current CIOs are within 0 to 10 years of retirement. Hopefully, the CIO has been a good mentor and coach to the members of the senior IS team and has been smart enough to have two or three individuals prepared and ready to move into the CIO role when they retire or leave for a better position.

A succession plan requires a great deal of support from senior leadership, as well as excellent coaching and mentoring skills from not only IS leadership, but also leadership throughout the organization. To be most effective, succession planning requires two components:

1. An overall organizational program that not only prepares for problems and changes, but also develops leadership for the organization.
2. One-on-one planning for mentoring and developing successors.

The CIO must make a personal commitment of time and effort in sharing responsibilities and giving successors exposure at meetings and conferences. Mentoring a successor should be treated as a professional responsibility. It is also important to work with a successor to develop a documented plan that provides a time-and-events calendar with specific accountabilities and deliverables.

As with many other aspects of an executive-level position, becoming adept at coaching and mentoring is a learned art. To dedicate the time and commitment required, one must have an agreement with the person that one wants to develop that he or she truly wants to be coached and grow into a more demanding role. Without bidirectional commitment, both parties may become frustrated.

Once the succession plan has been completed, delegating specific tasks and projects leads to a good start. Examples include spending time talking about approaches to certain situations; giving freely of ideas that might be valuable and spending time reviewing the results periodically with specific feedback that will help ensure success; establishing an open-door policy whereby a successor feels free to approach the mentor with questions and ideas; and helping them avoid future landmines. Someone tapped as a successor must exhibit the potential to move into key leadership positions based on their skills, education, communication style, attitude, and motivation. Keep in mind that recognizing talent and developing that talent can benefit the entire organization.

If information systems organizations have such a narrow talent pool, when a critical person leaves, the organization falls into chaos. It is important not to let that happen; plan for the future by hiring and developing the right people.

No matter how much effort one devotes to succession planning and developing talent internally, situations occur in which it will be necessary to recruit from outside the organization. This could include a successor leaving for another opportunity, lack of talent internally, time pressures requiring immediate action, or new initiatives requiring new skill sets, just to name a few.

In considering the executive responsibility involved in providing succession planning, developing capable new leaders is essential to the future success of healthcare information system organizations. The more senior a position on the executive team, the more critical a successor becomes to the health and well-being of the organization—especially when the unexpected or expected change occurs. In coaching a successor, it is also useful to draw on one's previous experience with a personal mentor or coach who was instrumental in helping one to prepare for management and leadership responsibilities.

Now more than ever, it is important to plan for the future. We need "farm team" players ready to move to the major leagues. Developing talent, creating career paths, and promoting from within does a great deal for morale, retention, and organizational stability. Having senior leadership aging or retiring and no clear successors in sight could easily create a situation where a whole generation of growth is wiped out. This would be a shame as the years ahead should be fun and strategic, creating opportunities to utilize information as a key resource in patient care delivery.

New Roles

Other key positions that will work with or report to the CIO are being established. These include security and privacy roles, as well e-health and a significant number of Chief Technical Officer positions. There is an explosion in the need for clinical IS leadership, which is opening up substantial opportunities for medical information candidates. None of these new roles need to be technical, but the candidates need to be able to work well across the organization since they affect the future and business aspects of the healthcare enterprise. There is a major effort taking place around clinical planning, redesign, and systems installation. As a matter of fact, the effort to bring in seasoned physicians who have been involved in implementation of clinical systems is absolutely an immense change that has taken place over the past 5 years. Many of these physicians have the opportunity to lead large implementation projects. First of all, it gives them a wonderful opportunity for management and, more importantly, there is a possibility that some of them will obtain enough executive experience to move into the CIO ranks when, as mentioned previously, CIO turnover occurs.

There is also an interesting competition taking place surrounding new positions in security, privacy, and clinical systems as to where these positions report. It is most appropriate to have IT physicians reporting to the CIO with a potential dotted line to the Chief Medical Officer. This relationship will allow the CIO to benefit from the physician's clinical knowledge and credibility and will give the physician adequate training and exposure required to lead an IT organization.

Outsourcing

Outsourcing became very appealing to CEOs who were tired of managing expensive resources during a time when finances were tight and recruitment was a major problem. Selective outsourcing proved to be very valuable. However, when the outsourcing firm came in, one ran the risk of losing key members of the IT management team to the firm. Therefore, in many cases, outsourcing became very problematic, particularly if the CIO role can be outsourced as part of the agreement.

Managing a complex outsourcing agreement requires a CIO who is an employee of the health system with some additional skills than those found in traditional CIOs. The CIO's job has become one of relationship building and change management. The success of a CIO is partially dependent on a strong IS management team, although the CIO must manage the technologists and lead the executive team through technology-based business decisions.

Very early on in the development of the CIO position, there was unfounded concern that these multitalented executives did not exist in health care. That being the case, it was assumed that a respected executive could be trained to be a CIO, except, in some very rare instances, CIOs have IT somewhere in their backgrounds, and are not administrators who learn on the job.

Reporting Structure

To have optimal effect on the organization, the CIO should be reporting to the highest level possible. As time goes on, the position is gathering more and more influence. As a matter of fact, there are new labels being given to these individuals. Many CIOs now carry the title of Senior Vice President/CIO. There is very little disagreement on the fact that the CIO must have an office in close proximity to his or her peers.

For a brief time, actually, right after Y2K, some CIOs were reporting to CFOs. That trend is continuing somewhat, but slowly returning back to a reporting structure to the COO or the CEO. Individual managers reporting to the CIO have also taken a jump in influence, strategy, and operational responsibility. The key executives in IT generally reporting to the CIO can include a Chief Medical Information Officer, a designated successor, a contract manager (if they are in an outsourcing mode), and a CTO. This is generally considered to be the CIO's cabinet. These individuals are strong supporters of the CIO, allowing him or her the freedom to work very strategically with peers.

The Future

Well, it has finally come: an opportunity for the IS leadership to be embraced by the executive leadership because a competent, creative CIO is suddenly being thrust into the forefront of many major decisions occurring within the organization. There are a few new skills that need to be added, because these are very, very challenging times. Success will only come by staying flexible and creative and by understanding the changing market's need to provide additional IS service as it applies to the industry as well as to the consumer. It is critical to keep up with the changing environment, including skills that need to be kept up to date, or perhaps even one step ahead of the status quo.

To provide a new perspective, Arthur Gross, a leading CIO, shares his views on the future role of the CIO. He notes that:

One somewhat different facet of the emerging environment that may be useful for consideration is the confluence of:

1. The role of academic health science centers in spawning the prototype CIO of the future (i.e., "If you can do it there, you can do it anywhere").

2. The emergence of the medical technologies that have embedded within them information technology infrastructure and, in turn, the blurring of the distinctions between the medical technologies and the information systems technologies, the latter which historically have been the province of the CIO, while the former has been owned by hospital physicians and administrators.

3. The emergence of the physician CIO.
4. The increasing focus on informatics in medical school education.

This confluence has raised interesting issues of:

1. Governance (who owns what technologies).
2. Who is best qualified to lead the technology strategic planning that, going forward, needs to integrate future medical technology planning initiatives with conventional information technology initiatives.
3. How to parse responsibility within provider environments in which the medical technologies are often considered competitive differentiators in the market place occupied by high-end providers.
4. What strategies need to be invented by the nonphysician CIO who is responsible for managing risk for all IT in the provider environment but may not be the "acknowledged expert" in some quarters due to the absence of formal medical training.

Now, perhaps these issues are relevant only in academic health science centers but, even if that is the case, it appears that trends in health care are often detected early in these high-end academic provider environments and subsequently migrate to the larger community.

One way of viewing this "trend" is to compare it to the trend in CEO searches in which, increasingly, physicians are being tapped for these leadership positions. Actually, from my perspective, the physician CIO "trend," if it exists (and I have no data), is a potentially good thing insofar as healthcare IT is the intersection of two arcane disciplines—medicine and technology. Theoretically, the best minds to move the industry forward should be armed with in-depth knowledge of both.

Factors for success include carefully aligning your IS strategies to the business strategy and giving absolute support to any and all corporate directional changes that need to occur. However, the CIO role has changed to such an extent that CIOs are being looked at as confidants and visionaries in terms of solidly assisting and predicting where the organization should go and, most importantly, how technology can be used to provide better patient care, clinical redesign, patient safety, and any number of things that 5 years ago may have seemed unreal.

A successful CIO will be able to manage the vendors, the consultants, the technicians, and in some cases, an outsourcing organization. If a CIO manages outsourcing, however, he or she needs to do it through a contract manager so that all the time is not spent managing outsourcing, but in being creative and strategic for the rest of the organization.

Continued success will be measured by knowing who your customers are and managing those relationships. It will continue to be important to have the skills to manage expectations and priorities, manage major change efforts, and deal extensively with outside resources. Additional skills that will be highly valuable, in addition to those we have already highlighted, are related to CIOs being strategists, people who know how to form alliances and can facilitate access to data. We, of course, are looking for the Holy Grail in a CIO, asking him or her to manage strategy, bring in the appropriate operations and technology expertise, and be leaders by example. They will need to manage it all and should be the key strategist responsible for selecting, motivating, and growing the operational leaders of tomorrow.

They should be heavily invested in looking at e-health for the organization and be able to draw out those innovations that are valuable for the growth and planning of their enterprise. Soon, there will be an imperative that will have the CIO leadership interface with medical devices internally and externally throughout the organization. They should be concerned with the Intranet and Extranet, making sure that it is usable and that the information architecture is appropriate for all contingencies.

In several recent surveys, the answer to what CIOs want was fairly uniform. They are looking for the opportunity to improve delivery of care, challenge, growth, creativity, resources, and support. What about the CIOs who have been there, done that, and are now looking for new challenge? Many organizations that already have an excellent operational CIO are looking to hire a super CIO, a true strategist and a leader on the executive team. There are a variety of these positions opening up all over the country. Another position that very experienced CIOs may want to consider is interim CIO management, although it most likely requires significant travel.

The majority of IT changes will be connected to clinical redesign to support healthcare delivery. This will certainly change the CIO role, which must continually change in response to new challenges. The CIO position is becoming more and more exciting every day.

The future for all of us in the healthcare industry is exciting. We are growing in the services we offer. We are growing in the need for access to data. And the day has finally come where information as a resource is a valued and required commodity. The leaders of that commodity are ready to go, but to succeed fully, these leaders need to make sure that there is a team behind them that can succeed when they are ready to move on and a flexible technology structure to support sudden changes.

Acknowledgments. Betsy S. Hersher would like to thank Arthur Gross for his contributions to this chapter. Mr. Gross is the Executive Vice President and Chief Information Officer of the Henry Ford Health System in Detroit, Michigan. Ms. Hersher would also like to thank *ADVANCE For Health Information Executives* magazine for allowing portions of a previously published article, "Succession Planning," to appear in this chapter. Special thanks also to Damon Popovich for his contributions as editor.

14
CIO STORIES, I
Northwestern Memorial Hospital, Chicago: Patients First, from the Ground Up

TIMOTHY R. ZOPH

> *The decision to invest in a new facility and in technological advancements that support state-of-the-art treatment has been a critical factor in the success of this much-lauded center.*

Imagine . . . You enter a healthcare facility from any entrance, and you are welcomed as a valued guest. The traditional registration process is replaced by "smart desks" where attendants review your information, already in the computer, and then send you on your way. *Imagine . . .* You take a seat, and when it is time for your appointment, a patient escort, wearing a headset, appears at your side and greets you quietly and confidentially before accompanying you to and from your procedure. In constant electronic communication with your caregivers, your escort has kept you informed of any delays. *Imagine . . .* While at the facility, you and members of your family have access to a Health Learning Center where you can electronically explore the most advanced information available on your health concerns.

We have accomplished all this and much more at Northwestern Memorial Hospital, one of the country's premier academic medical centers in Chicago, Illinois, by making information technology (IT) an integral part of the planning process as we built for the future. Three years ago, in 1999, we opened a new $580 million hospital facility that was built from the patient's perspective. The hospital is acknowledged to be one of the most technologically advanced healthcare facilities in the world.

The new facility was more than 10 years in the making, and it challenged the organization to make careful and strategic decisions about how technology could best advance our *Patients First* mission over the long term, and, in doing so, address some of the functional and operational issues affecting health care. The timetable was such that our 5-year, $50 million IT Strategic Plan had to be fully tested, executed, and operational in 4 years if we were to meet organizational goals.

At Northwestern Memorial, we worked to create the ideal experience for our patients in a high-touch, high-tech environment. Since the grand opening of this new facility, we have experienced double-digit volume growth, patient satisfaction scores among the highest in the country, and external recognition for contributions as a leader in health care.

Timothy R. Zoph, BS, MS, MBA, is Vice President of Information Services and Chief Information Officer for Northwestern Memorial Hospital.

The decision to invest both in a new facility and in the technological advancements to support state-of-the-art treatment is a critical success factor in positioning for the present and future demands of health care. It requires a strong vision, solid management, careful planning, clearly articulated goals, and an uncompromising execution strategy that includes a willingness to test and rethink and make tough choices along the way.

By sharing this experience, my goal is to provide a useful framework for other organizations with an opportunity to invest in a new facility with new IT systems to achieve a vision of patient care.

Advancing a Patients First Mission

Northwestern Memorial Hospital is located in downtown Chicago, an organization with a history of more than 137 years of service to the community. It is the primary teaching hospital for Northwestern University's Feinberg School of Medicine and an organization known for its commitment to excellence in clinical care, education, and research. The hospital itself was created in 1972, the result of a merger of two of the oldest and most distinguished patient-focused medical facilities in Chicago. Three years later, the Prentice Women's Hospital and Maternity Center and the Norman and Ida Stone Institute of Psychiatry became part of the hospital organization as well.

By the mid-1980s, however, it was clear that facilities had become a major issue in planning for the future. The aging buildings throughout the 18-acre campus shared with Northwestern University were expensive to maintain and could not support the technological advances rapidly changing the delivery of health care. A study commissioned by the Northwestern Memorial Board of Directors in 1989 cemented our direction when it concluded that "Our current physical facilities are the single greatest obstacle to achieving greatness."

The *Patients First* mission required focus on what it would take to create the ideal experience for patients in all aspects of facility function. From this came the clear vision to plan, design, and build a world-class facility that would provide the community with integrated and advanced care in a healing, patient-focused environment. It was to be much more than a replacement hospital for the existing campus buildings and the more than 20 disparate outpatient facility sites in the primary service area. It would be a facility designed and built by all members of the Northwestern Memorial family, with input from patients, physicians, employees, caregivers, and community leaders—with the patient foremost in mind.

The new hospital presented an opportunity to redesign patient processes and enhance patient care through an investment in new IT capabilities that would help set the standard for health care in the 21st century. This vision of patient care could not be realized without a substantial investment in IT.

The Planning Philosophy

Northwestern Memorial has been aptly described as a planning-driven organization, and this was clearly the case in setting sights for a new facility. The planning process for the new hospital began in earnest by early 1993, when senior management developed a set of guiding principles intended to move the entire organization forward in a new vision of patient care. More than 400 principles were created, covering some 60 different operating categories that affected the process of delivering health care in areas such as "point of service care management" and "common communications architecture," for example. This principle-centered framework served as the common reference for all user groups and drove strategic planning efforts organizationwide.

Already in place, the Northwestern Memorial Corporate Strategic Plan focused the organization for the years 1995–2000. However, as we prepared for and planned for the new facility, six new strategic plans were created, each directly supporting and advancing the organization's mission and strategic goals. These new plans, addressing areas such as Long-Range Finance, Fundraising, and Campus-Wide Facilities, focused on strategically moving the organization forward and into a new hospital building by 1999.

The guiding principles for technology served as a model for the 5-year, $50 million Information Technology Strategic Plan, which was developed in 1995. The primary goal was to implement IT solutions to enhance clinical decision making, patient outcomes, and effective operations. The IT plan was specifically designed to make the necessary investments in technology to achieve the organizational vision. However, because a most important guiding principle was "no first use" in the new facility, there was a requirement to execute the plan fully in 4 years instead of 5.

The objective, then, was to implement new IT solutions in existing buildings before moving these advancements into the new hospital. This strategy provided an opportunity to validate technology, introduce new patient care and administrative processes, and reduce the overall risk if new technology and patient care commenced at the same time. Uncompromising adherence to "no first use" drove accelerated project timeframes and mandated pragmatic decision making along the way.

Contingency planning is crucial when pursuing high-risk technology projects tied to a new facility. In this case, for example, even though plans included filmless radiology and paperless medical records, square footage was still maintained in the new facility for film file rooms and medical record storage. Operational contingencies were also developed in the event that plans for the new technology could not be fully realized.

What We Set Out to Achieve

The construction of the new Northwestern Memorial Hospital was the largest privately funded construction project in the state of Illinois and one of the largest of its kind in health care. The connecting two-tower structure, which opened on time and on budget, was built over one city block with 2 million square feet of space. Hospital inpatient facilities were located in one tower and outpatient ambulatory care in the other. The driving goal throughout the project was to exceed patient expectations with the most technologically advanced and patient-friendly hospital we could create.

We focused on leveraging information technology to the greatest extent with new patient encounter models, filmless radiology systems, an exploration of paperless medical records, a Health Learning Center, and an advanced communications infrastructure. Importantly, the vision represented a bringing together of the Northwestern Memorial medical family with on-site location for 600 of more than 1200 affiliated physicians, a number that included our entire academic clinical group of 400.

The vision for on-site clinical practice extended beyond location. Information technology would be the foundation for the orchestrated flow of patients and information throughout the new facility. The patient would receive a coordinated care experience even when many points of service and multiple providers were involved. Patient information would be captured only once, and then would become available to all caregivers providing a service in the facility. The building would be designed to optimize this coordination, and, at the same time, provide for future flexibility. Although remaining organizationally separate from the physicians, the hospital looked toward a unified commitment to this patient-focused approach.

Moreover, a new facility presented a significant opportunity to provide the "ideal patient encounter" with seamless administrative processing and a dramatically improved patient process flow that would be respectful of the patient's time and expectations for care. The goal was to remove all unnecessary administrative steps and guide patients to the point of service in a friendly and expeditious manner. In advancing our guiding principle of integrated information systems, the hospital agreed to develop a common process for patient identification, scheduling, and registration for all services. There was recognition that these systems are vital to the operational flow of the facility and to provide the cornerstone of the clinical information systems strategy.

All steps involved in patient movement through the facility were analyzed carefully. As a result, centralized admitting and registration areas were removed from architectural plans. In doing so, our core admissions process would be trimmed by 15 to 30 minutes through the use of automated preregistration and 45 electronic check-in areas. The concept of "smart desks" also provided a centralized view of consolidated patient information from all systems conveniently located at all points of entry. These "meet and greet" locations were designed to personally attend to patients, then guide them to a scheduled service.

More than 45 ancillary services were targeted for automated scheduling. New call centers for preregistration would be created. Admitting and registration processes would be merged into one. All new systems and new process flows would be substantially implemented in existing structures throughout the Northwestern Memorial campus before the grand opening, a tough challenge in buildings more than 50 years old and designed for centralized patient flow.

Significant technological enhancements would come with implementation of filmless radiology systems. The arrival of a visionary Chairman of Radiology, an industry-leading vendor partnership, and a solid team of radiology and IT professionals all contributed to our commitment to a filmless facility. The prospect of a new data communication network with 80 times the capacity of our existing systems linked by fiber connections to every clinical location, including physician offices, also propelled our vision.

This new technology enabled a new means of using digital information from all radiological exams including MRI, CT, mammography, and X-ray to speed the turnaround of diagnosis, to allow for simultaneous consultation among physicians and other healthcare professionals, and to assure that images would be permanently archived and instantly available for future use. Institutional and vendor commitments were solidified in the spring of 1998, with archiving technology and the initial pilot accomplished in our existing Emergency Department later that year continuing through early 1999. The new hospital opened with filmless flows in the Emergency Department and image inquiry in intensive care units. Radiologists changed to filmless readings for all images within the first operational year.

The outcome was evidenced by improvements in radiology service delivery to patients such as a reduction in diagnosis and treatment delays and reduced exposure and test time. In addition, departmental productivity increased due to improved workflow and immediate and simultaneous access to current and historical studies. Operating costs in the areas of staffing and film cost decreased, and lost studies approached zero, with retakes reduced from 10 percent to 1 percent. As a result, a real transformation occurred for physicians and radiology that, at the same time, offered major benefits for patients.

The *Patients First* tradition also was evidenced in the design of the new 5000-square-foot Health Learning Center, which would become the largest hospital-based learning center of its kind. The vision here was to create a comfortable place where patients, families, and the broader Chicago community could actively engage in learning about health care through traditional methods such as books, periodicals, visual models, and lectures as well as through advanced features of electronic learning. The center, which offers 25 private workstations and private learning rooms, provides the nucleus for our electronic and Web-based education efforts. Visitors can access the latest medical information in a confidential manner, with any questions facilitated by care professionals on the center's staff. Materials also can be accessed through computer workstations located in a remote location in the facility, designed so that patients waiting for diagnostic tests or family and friends waiting during a surgery can take advantage of electronic access to research health concerns.

As a concluding design element, a communications architecture was implemented with the capacity, flexibility, and standardization to meet healthcare needs in the 21st century. Standards demanded the capability to move information quickly anywhere in the facility, and recognizing that health care is at the early stage of automation, this anticipated the facility's digital future. All areas of the new facility—common areas, patient care, diagnostic services, and physician offices—share a common architecture. The vertical fiberoptic core and a horizontal distribution to all areas of care marked the path for movement of high-density information unique to our industry such as imaging, video, and, in the very near future, a fully electronic medical record. The wiring infrastructure alone accounted for more than 25,000 connection points and 600 miles of cable. The facility houses 110 communication closets, each a generous 150 square feet and vertically aligned to provide for convergence of all systems needing access to the common network.

The Hard Choices/Scaling Back

One of the lessons learned during this process was that while we tend to view technology as a means to bridge organizational boundaries, in reality it is only a tool—the difficult work is in aligning the people and changing the culture. Technology, we learned, can move no faster than organizational change. The vision of the ideal patient encounter demanded new technology solutions, but, most importantly, it required that the hospital and the physicians work as a single operational entity. Although common information systems were the vehicle, the challenge was to agree on a new operating framework that would join the hospital, the physicians, and ambulatory care services in a commitment to standardized information and seamless patient flow.

A representative task force was formed and aggressively explored the standards that would create the ideal encounter through information captured at one single point and then shared throughout the facility. However, although the technology strategy moved forward, we could not reach consensus on an organizational structure and a new operating framework. The fallback position for the hospital, then, was to develop the ideal encounter for all hospital-based services in the new facility and gain cooperation from all entities so that scheduling information for patients would be shared and the smart desks would be operational. The shared communications framework provides the pathway for future integration, which remains the goal.

Another lesson learned was that available technology did not always meet our standards. Early in the planning process, in 1993, Northwestern Memorial was awarded a 3-year, $3 million research contract from The National Library of Medicine to develop electronic patient record systems beginning in the physician setting. Working with a team of physicians who enthusiastically piloted the system, we acquired firsthand knowledge of the promises, complexity, costs, and the state-of-development of vendor-based paperless solutions.

At the end of the contract, however, it was clear that the move into the new facility would be done with paper medical records. Available technology was simply not reliable, and a decision was made to put this project on a longer timeline so that vendor-based solutions would have further time to develop. There are encouraging signs that this will become a reality in the future. The infrastructure exists in the new hospital to support future development, and Northwestern Memorial's academic clinical physician practice, the Northwestern Medical Faculty Foundation, signed an agreement to fully automate their clinical practice based on the results of the pilot project.

How We Did It: Execution Strategy

Identify Threshold Changes in Information Technology

Early in the process, during the reviews of the schematic design and in the beginning stages of the detailed design, we sought to identify technologies that would drive threshold changes in patient care processes and, as a result, influence the facility design. Although technology continues to change rapidly, facility design is often set 5 years in advance of the opening of a major healthcare facility. The objective is to design for the future and execute in the present. There are few threshold choices to choose from, but these choices can have a significant impact on success. As such, questions such as "What can be done to enable our vision?" and "What can actually be achieved?" became very important. As technology leaders, our role is to see that these questions get asked and answered, early and often, by the collective management team.

When undertaking a project of this magnitude, healthcare institutions are affected by factors including available resources, time constraints, level of risk, and, perhaps most importantly, by the ability to manage simultaneous change within the organization. At Northwestern Memorial, the entire senior management team was actively engaged in the planning and review process and in making choices about project commitments, sequencing, and achievability. The process of arriving at a "team consensus" was a key predictor of success. For example, implementing filmless radiology systems was a late-stage commitment in 1998, after achieving alignment of clinical leadership, vendor partnership, and a clear articulation of benefits to patient care and hospital operations. In contrast, electronic implementing medical records was an early-stage commitment in 1993, but ultimately deferred to postmove to allow for further product maturity.

Anticipate Construction Deadlines in Execution Timeframe

The IT execution strategies embraced the Northwestern Memorial commitment to an "on time, on budget" process and a passionate attention to detail. The discipline of planning narrowed the choices based on resources, achievability, and time, with construction deadlines being a major factor. We were challenged with less than a 4-year window to redesign hospital processes, implement new systems, and prepare hospital staff for major technology change while working from a 5-year strategic plan. Accomplishing this required the coordination of the execution strategies for major initiatives along with other commitments to automate all ancillary service functions in some 30 new departmental systems. At the same time, it was important to stay current with system maintenance, upgrade schedules, and fully prepare and test all systems for year 2000 compliance. Mindful of the internal resource capacity required to undertake so many simultaneous technology projects, the tactical strategy was revisited each year of the process and necessary adjustments were made. Progress of technology deployment was carefully assessed, and the value, risk, and resource capacity necessary to be successful were calibrated.

Actively Manage Change Through Visible Leadership

Northwestern Memorial worked to invest all its more than 5000 employees in the success of this project, reinforcing throughout the process that building a new hospital was the work of the entire organization. Senior management articulated a clear vision and demonstrated a strong commitment throughout the planning, development, and construction, constant reminders of the hospital's investment in the future as leaders in health care.

More than 125 functional user groups participated in evaluating the patient-focused design of all aspects of the new facility, which in turn created excitement about the project and drove the development of full-scale visual representations of the future with mockups of patient rooms, recovery bays, emergency department treatment areas, and surgical suites. Our information technology plan used full-scale pilots to prove in advance the concepts of all the technology strategies.

Managing technological change of this magnitude requires visible leadership. For an IT leader, there can be no substitute for personal and active commitment to technology, making sure that systems are fully integrated in the new facility. At the same time, the IT leader must be a part of the senior management team responsible for the project's overall success. Approximately 1 day a week of my time was devoted to the new hospital project during the 5 years of construction; this included senior project leadership meetings and weekly project leadership meetings to ensure synchronization and technology alignment with decision making related to construction. Budgets, timetables, technology acquisition, and transition planning all were essential components.

Finally, it is important to establish a physical presence on-site. Take the time to tour the construction site and the buildings where your technology is being tested, because you never know what you might learn when you experience it firsthand. Visible leadership is essential in communicating commitment to the project and support for members of the IT team working to make the vision come true.

Manage Transition Risk

Some of the biggest challenges came with managing the overall transition process during the final year of construction. As moving into the new facility was anticipated, our IT team became a part of the hospital's comprehensive transition effort, which focused on all aspects of a successful move. All technological systems were configured and validated for the parameters of the new facility and final year 2000 compliance testing. New communication networks were fully installed in the new facility and tested.

The design allowed for the prestaging of new technology components necessary for the opening of the hospital such as PCs, diagnostic equipment, and filmless radiology workstations. The transition plan called for sufficient technology staging on the common communications network to provide for initial operation without physical transfer and setup of equipment from older facilities. The ability to do this required careful management of life cycle technology decisions throughout construction so that new equipment for prestaging the new hospital could be purchased.

On May 1, 1999, the CEO of Northwestern Memorial, Gary Mecklenburg, escorted the first patient transported into our new 492-bed medical/surgery facility. That day, a total of 250 patients were moved, and ancillary services, surgical suites, and a Level One Trauma Center were up and running. Within 1 week, nearly 500 physicians had moved their clinical practices into the designated facility space.

We created an Information Technology Command Center that operated 24/7 in the weeks leading up to opening day and for several weeks following. Management and IT staff were assigned to rotating 12-hour shifts that allowed for tracking of, and immediate response to, all reported issues. This plan also provided a supporting structure for the revalidation of all technology components postmove. Our entire Information Services organization became a singular transition team in support of the move.

The discipline, the commitment, and the team spirit that developed during the transition would serve us well for the year 2000 event, incident response management, and major system conversions that were in store.

Realizing the Benefits

It is no accident that patients often remark that the new Northwestern Memorial doesn't "feel" like a hospital. Uniformed attendants at "smart desks" anticipate the needs of patients and visitors and retrieve the necessary information quickly through the computer network. Our Health Learning Center services generate 3000 visits every month. A magnificent collection of healing art is displayed throughout the facility. Every room is private with a pullout bed for visitors and a window with a view. Our hospital cafeteria attracts a lunchtime crowd from throughout the downtown area. Other amenities directed at convenience include a coffee shop, a local bookstore, a florist, a bank, two gift shops, and a specialty café.

The benefits of the new facility were evident in patient satisfaction ratings. The impact was immediate, with patient satisfaction related to the new building itself soaring significantly with the move. During the first 6 months of operation, overall patient satisfaction indicated that patients were more likely to recommend our facility, as evidenced in improvements in the "likelihood to recommend" section of the patient satisfaction survey [1]. In addition, improvements were also realized in the room and staff and visitors and family areas.

Volume increased as well. In the first year of operation in the new facility, our admissions went up 16 per cent with an increase of nearly 12 per cent in Emergency Department visits and nearly 15 per cent in Outpatient registrations. Today, the facility hovers at full occupancy with a 35 per cent increase in volume growth since the grand opening. Enhanced clinical effectiveness and productivity improvements have also been witnessed. Most significantly, throughout the process, Northwestern Memorial has maintained a solid financial position, and today it is one of only three hospitals in the United States with the highest AA+ bond rating issued by Standard & Poor's.

The Northwestern Memorial organization has received widespread external recognition since the move into the new facility. This includes:

- From the patient and service perspective, HCIA-Mercer honored Northwestern Memorial in 1999 as the "Best Overall Hospital in Chicago for Clinical Excellence." In 2001, we received "Best Patient Service" in the *Sodexho-Modern Healthcare* magazine Excellence Awards. *U.S. News & World Report* magazine's "America's Best Hospitals" report ranked Northwestern Memorial in the top 50 hospitals in 11 of 17 specialty categories in 1992.
- From the consumer's perspective, in 2002, Northwestern Memorial received the "Consumer's Choice Award" from the National Research Corporation and was ranked the No. 1 hospital by consumers in Chicago and the surrounding nine-county area. The hospital has been ranked the "most preferred" in this survey since 1992. The Consumer's Checkbook 2002 national survey published in the *AARP Modern Maturity* magazine listed Northwestern Memorial as one of "America's Top Hospitals," ranked No. 5 nationwide.
- From a technology perspective, since 1999, Northwestern Memorial has been recognized yearly as one of the "100 Most Wired Hospitals" by *Hospital and Health Networks Magazine*. Our Internet technologies also have been recognized. In 2001, the hospital was awarded the "Platinum Award, Best Overall Internet Site," in the 400+ bed category, by *eHealthcare Strategy and Trends*, an industry publication, for best Web site design, usability, portrayal of the organization's information, quality of health content, interactivity, ability of the information to drive business, and general impressions of the Web site.

Looking to Our Future

Vision is both a destination and journey. Although everything we set out to achieve was not fully realized when the hospital opened, we remain committed to the full promise of this new facility in the coming years. If anything, the accomplishments and lessons learned offer us confidence to take additional steps into the future. While it is indeed a great challenge to undertake technology and process changes contemporaneous with the development of a new facility, this is the most opportune time to align enabling technology with the future of an organization.

Technology is once again an integral part of the process as we plan for the future of women's health care. Our Prentice Women's Hospital and Maternity Center has become the largest birthing center in Illinois, with 9000 births last year. But an aging facility and population projections that our births will increase substantially over the next several years have created the need for a new facility. And with that comes the opportunity for a new vision and a new approach to women's health.

We are working to create the new Prentice Women's Hospital, a state-of-the-art facility designed to provide comprehensive health care for women at all stages of life. It will house one of the largest maternity care facilities in the world with the capacity for up to 13,600 births a year. The lessons learned during the planning and development of the new hospital will serve as useful markers as we move forward with this new project.

We look forward to this challenge, as it is yet another opportunity to invest in the future of health care. Technology enhancements bring a decided value to our educational outreach efforts as we work to lure students to our workforce of the future, and our state-of-the-art facility enriches our ability to attract the best workers and leaders to our organization. At Northwestern Memorial, our vision is to provide the best experience for our patients—a vision that is fully realized through investments in information technology.

Reference

1. Briggs P, Barnard C. The New Northwestern Memorial Hospital: planned, constructed and operated through the patients first philosophy. J Qual Improvement 2000;26(5):287–298.

15
CIO STORIES, II
The Jewish Home and Hospital Lifecare System, NYC: Paving the Way for Long-Term Care

KRISTINE M. CERCHIARA and NANCY STODDARD

> *Knowing that the current marketplace did not support its needs, this organization sought out a proven system that could be adapted to the long-term care environment.*

The long-term healthcare industry has been slow to recognize clinical systems as a strategic tool and information as a corporate asset. As a leader in the long-term care environment, the Jewish Home & Hospital (JHH) Lifecare System pursued an information systems strategy unlike that of most other long-term care organizations.

JHH Lifecare System has long held a vision of a computerized patient record as an effective and economical method to support clinical processes, one of the factors that drew both authors to the organization in 1990. In turn, this strategy supports the mission of the organization to provide the highest quality care in the most cost-effective way.

As a long-term care organization, the JHH Lifecare System serves the needs of older adults by providing a wide spectrum of care at whatever level their needs demand. We serve more than 5000 older adults each day through comprehensive inpatient services, home care, community services, and housing programs. Our inpatient services comprise 1600 beds on three campuses, providing skilled nursing care, rehabilitation services, subacute care, Alzheimer's specialized care, respite care, and hospice.

The U.S. Department of Health and Human Services projects that in the next 30 years the number of individuals over 65 will more than double, from 33 million to 72 million, and will represent more than 20 percent of the population in the United States. Our industry is evolving in reaction to this complex changing environment, and as reimbursement revenues decline, it is forcing us to balance often-opposing goals of improving quality of care while reducing the cost of managing and delivering that care. As with successful organizations in other industries, long-term care organizations will succeed when cost-effectiveness and quality are exhibited.

To assist in achieving that goal, the JHH Lifecare System looked to information technology early on to gain a competitive edge and focus on operational process improvement. As one of the largest not-for-profit long-term care organizations in the country,

---

Kristine M. Cerchiara is Vice President and CIO of the Jewish Home and Hospital Lifecare System. Nancy Stoddard, RN, BSN, MBA, is Director of Clinical Information Systems for the Jewish Home and Hospital Lifecare System.

our demographics do not fit the typical nursing home model (100 beds or less), and systems available in the marketplace do not support our needs. The systems that do exist are little more than tools to track census and walk clinicians through standardized assessments and care plans. They are deficient in that the actual care processes are not supported, resulting in duplication of effort to maintain a patient's clinical record and document regulatory requirements. To support our organization's vision, we went looking for a proven clinical system that we could adapt for long-term care.

Selection Process

The selection of a clinical information system is a decision that will live on in the organization for years to come. Therefore, it is important that the selection be done in a thorough and comprehensive manner, designed to educate the users and the organization as to the magnitude of the undertaking. To quote Sy Syms, "An educated consumer is our best customer." We followed a very structured approach, developing objectives, functional requirements, and expectations, and allocating adequate resources while including representation from administrative, financial, and clinical operations. Although this represented a significant investment on the part of the organization, it was time and money wisely spent. Our evaluation and selection strategy was guided by several key principles:

- *Patient-Centric.* The system would support clinician workflow and the operations of delivering patient care. Historically, our organization, like many others, has employed systems selection strategies that were either financial, regulatory, or hardware driven and not driven by the business we are in, the delivery of patient care [1].
- *Flexibility.* We would spend more time evaluating the design and flexibility of the system rather than specific features and functions. Since we anticipate care requirements and technology to change, we did not want to narrow our scope by focusing on specific reports and data presentations.
- *Criteria/Rules Driven.* The system would provide decision support links to clinical knowledge and alerts/reminders with data review at point of decision. It would also support real-time warnings and alerts at all points of care with automatic routing of abnormal or critical results or "need-to-know" information.
- *Long-Term Care "Hooks."* Although we were not focusing exclusively on long-term care systems, the systems had to enable compliance with federal and state regulations. Necessary components include the Resident Assessment Instrument (RAI), which incorporates the Minimum Data Set (MDS) and Resident Assessment Protocols (RAPs), and, in New York State, the Patient Review Instrument (PRI). We sought a tool that would allow these assessments to be done as a by-product of completion of "routine" clinical activities (for example, admission assessment) and *not* as an additional process.

Overall, we wanted the system to allow us to immediately realize enhanced efficiency by improving processes, streamlining workflow, and sharing knowledge between every "touch point" in the delivery chain. The system selected at the end of the process was a highly sophisticated system with a price tag unknown to the long-term care industry, 4 to 15 times more than any of the others we evaluated—quite a sticker shock. Nevertheless, an analysis of processes demonstrated the value we could obtain from the system. We constructed a study to test the features and functionality of the system fully in relation to specific processes, identifying intangible benefits and projecting tangible ones.

TABLE 15.1. Model of return on investment (ROI) calculations for Nurses Order Accountability Record.

Nursing orders		Facility #1	Facility #2	Facility #3	SUM
Staff type	RN				
Benchmark (b)	1 hr/patient /month	1	1	1	
Efficiency factor (e)	100%	1.00	1.00	1.00	
Salary factor (s)	$32	32	32	32	
Volume factor (v)	Patient census and admissions/month*12	6,816	10,788	3,672	21,276
Savings/year	(b)(e)(s)(v) =	218,112	345,216	117,504	680,832

Source: From Ref. [2].

Working with members from the vendor's product development division, and by comparing the system capabilities to our organization's known documentation and business operations, the team identified eight key processes to improve, which would yield a high level of return on investment (ROI). These processes were:

- Order transcription.
- Results reporting (Laboratory, Radiology, Rehabilitation).
- Medication order entry and administration.
- Appointment Scheduling (Clinic and Rehabilitation).
- MDS assessment.
- MDS scheduling.
- Care Planning.
- Medical Records Management.

The study demonstrated significant savings in order entry and transcription, mostly due to physician direct order entry and direct routing of requests for service to ancillary service departments. The preparation of the Nurses Order Accountability Record each month requires significant manual effort. Table 15.1 provides an illustration of how the ROI calculations were performed. For each staff type and activity, a benchmark was derived, that is, how long it takes to complete a task given the current process. The efficiency factor was assigned based on the level of transformation expected by automating (in this case, 100%, because the activity was to be eliminated). Finally, salary and volume factors were applied to the final calculation [2].

Opportunities with regard to medical record management were also significant. They included savings in purchase and maintaining inventory of paper forms and a marked reduction in efforts devoted to filing of results. Savings were also projected in processes supporting MDS assessment and care plan, primarily in the reduction of duplicative efforts.

Workflow Transformation: A Process unto Itself

These target processes formed the framework by which our vision of a transformed nursing home was conceived. Workflow analysis was directed by a team of analysts provided by the vendor and supported by the JHH project team. Extensive data collection, interviews, and observation of clinical activities were conducted. The existing workflow was analyzed, and then the vendor team proposed a system workflow. We now realize that the opportunities for transforming our paper-based workflow were limited by this vendor-driven approach. Some of the vendor team, and the JHH project team, had limited expertise with the full scope of database functionality and tools to reap the full benefit it could offer.

Complicating the workflow analysis and database build was the fact that this sophisticated product, with all the clinical information it offered, was still designed for the acute care setting and was virtually untested in the long-term care environment. The vendor made some critical assumptions about our requirements, which fell far short of the actual needs. The vendor's implementation team did not include an experienced analyst with long-term care expertise, so we did not have "best practices" to draw on and struggled to translate the clinical excellence we practiced into procedures and workflow that were efficient. We had contracted for implementation support to customize 40 percent of the "off-the-shelf " program. Once we were deeply embedded in the system design and database configuration, the vendor's calculation showed that the difference between Jewish Home's desired design and the system's existing modeled capabilities was about 20 percent. This gap was significantly underestimated. As a result, target dates were not met and budget estimates were exceeded.

Although the vendor agreed to absorb some of the overruns, our stakeholders lost a considerable amount of confidence in the vendor's ability to produce, and negative perceptions of the product overshadowed our successes. In an apparent attempt to minimize losses, the vendor was reluctant to further develop the product utilizing the enhanced functionality that attracted us to the software in the first place. The combination of these and other factors caused JHH to revise the plan and defer implementing the PRI, MDS, and Care Plan modules to the following year. Unfortunately, these modules supported key processes that were identified early on as having the most opportunity for return on investment. We put ourselves in the difficult position of rolling out a product that did not capitalize on the unique strengths of the expensive tool we purchased and, in our haste, lost sight of the vision.

Impact on Clinicians

Nursing

One of the most clearly stated and often quoted goals of system implementation was to decrease administrative tasks so as to increase clinician time spent with patients. This was particularly important with nurses, because at the onset of the project we were beginning to feel the pain of the nursing shortage. The profession of nursing is in crisis. Nurses enter the field to make a difference interacting with patients and families, but a large percentage of nursing time is spent in nondirect care activities such as scheduling, documenting, and communicating with other disciplines and support departments [1]. In fact, in our organization, and most likely typical to most long-term care organizations, nurses provide the hub whereby all patient-centered communication passes. Doctors write orders for referrals to ancillary departments that must be processed and scheduled by nurses before patients can get the services they need. Many processes depend on the nurse to duplicate clinical and demographic information found in the clinical record, transcribe it to request forms, and then track the completion of the requested service via labor-intensive lists and ticklers.

Nevertheless, in redesigning these inefficient processes, it was often difficult for nursing management to "let go" of the traditional role of the nurse as the center of communication. "But the nurse has to know what is going on with the patients!" In response, we went overboard in ensuring that the nursing "review queue" contained an item for every order, assessment, and result documented for all the patients. Not long after we implemented the pilot units, it was evident that we had to narrow the scope and focus of notifying the nurse on an exception basis. For example, we modified the queue routing by sending only orders that required a nurse's direct participation and assessment/results in the abnormal or critical range. This demonstrates why pilot units are so valuable; integration testing in a simulated environment had not revealed the "information overload" we were to inflict on our nurses.

The promise of computerized process is appealing, but PCs have not yet become integrated into the workflow of the typical clinician's day. Nursing knowledge and expertise is hard to define, measure, and communicate. There is a vast body of knowledge that expert nurses use to provide high-quality care to their patients, but extracting and representing this knowledge and structuring it for a computer system in an efficient real-world way remains difficult. Our nursing leadership was inclined to highly structure nursing assessments and treatment documentation, responding in a detailed way to every policy, regulation, and professional standard. The overall intent was to prompt the nurse to include all pertinent information and ensure compliance and excellence, with particular attention to deficiencies that had been experienced with the paper system. The novice nurse found the sheer volume overwhelming, and the expert nurse was prevented from zeroing in on the most important clinical observations and overlooking those that were insignificant or irrelevant. The nurses felt that the computer had added to their documentation burden, rather than reduced it. There was acknowledgment that nursing time usually spent in transcription was saved, and system modifications made shortly after Go Live were well received. But, coupled with the reality of the increasing nursing vacancies due to the shortage and the difficulty surrounding "floating" nurses unfamiliar with the system to the pilot units, the net effect on many nurses was not positive. Considerable resources were consumed in our attempt to meet the nursing leadership's requirements, so the failure was particularly disappointing and frustrating for the project team. The solution will be found somewhere in between the two extremes, and it remains a challenge for future development at JHH.

Certified Nursing Assistants

On a brighter note, we experienced great success with regard to system acceptance with our Certified Nursing Assistants (C.N.A.). In the early days of implementation planning, this group was identified as being at great risk due to their limited exposure to computers either in higher education or in the workplace. They had responded to a "self-assessment" conducted by our Staff Development Department as having a high degree of perceived discomfort with technology. In response, a targeted education program was delivered in partnership with the Local 1199 union that represents a significant portion of our nonprofessional staff. The program included open access 24 hours per day to "kiosk" computers loaded with games and basic PC training programs, manned at intervals by intern volunteers from a local commercial computer school, along with structured classroom training with 1199 instructors. The trainees were rated by the instructors and invited back for more training when it was indicated, but, more importantly, they were able to rate their own level of comfort and could opt to attend again. The program preceded actual system training, and we have no doubt it was integral to the ease with which the transition from paper-based documentation to computer-based charting was accomplished in the C.N.A. group.

Physicians

A similar feat, of no smaller proportion, was achieved with our physician staff. The literature is filled with examples of physician resistance and aborted computerized physician order entry (CPOE) implementations in hospitals. Armed with a healthy fear of what could happen, we strategized to nurture the support of physician leadership at the highest level. Biweekly sessions were held with the VP and Directors of Medicine to design typical order sets and protocols, keep them current with the activities of the steering committee and the project team, dispel misconceptions about the project, and build trust. At their request, the basic PC training included all levels of staff, including physicians. The sessions continued long after the initial Go-Live and incorporated hands-on training and support, and as a result, champions emerged. The groups of physicians on the pilot units were initially overwhelmed by the requirements of entering orders and completing all their documentation online. To ease management's concern over the risk of serious medication error, we instituted 100 percent audit of all new pharmacy orders. As their requests for enhancements were fulfilled, and with the support of leadership, the physicians were able to overcome the initial pain and realize the benefit of improved workflow and ease of access to patient data. When we implement beyond the pilot units, we will delay the implementation of medication order entry until competence is demonstrated with simpler orders. Until a high level of proficiency is achieved, the potential risk of harming a patient secondary to a data entry error outweighs the benefit that direct physician order entry can provide.

Rehabilitation Services

Significant efficiencies were realized in our rehabilitation therapy areas, not only with automated patient and resource scheduling (which was one of our target processes) but also with ease of access to patient information. It was easier for management to ensure that staff was compliant with documentation standards and automated routing of periodic progress notes to work queues for completion enhanced compliance. Because rehabilitation therapy contributes significantly to case mix and reimbursement revenue in long-term care, the system was employed to provide a real-time monitor on the process. The difference between achieving the highest possible payment category may only be a matter of minutes of therapy not provided or not documented. The system prompts the therapist to comply with the "plan" for his or her individual patient and, if the patient is not able, to document the reason. With the assistance of exception reports, all attempts are made to "make up" missed therapy appointments, and in doing so, patient care and revenue are optimized.

Lessons Learned

Cultural Issues

Unwillingness to dramatically change current process, methods, systems, responsibilities, and documentation limit progress and impede the transitions to automation [3]. When you change processes, it affects people. Getting people to let go of their old ways and embrace new ones is a difficult challenge. All change represents a loss [4]. Even when change is for the better, there is still loss. Change management involves helping people cope with this loss and cannot be implemented overnight.

Immediate Return

Focus on the areas where there is the greatest potential to show some marked improvements quickly. This will demonstrate system effectiveness and help gain buy-in and commitment to the overall IT strategy. Our experience taught us that the "big-bang" approach to implementation is not a viable option at JHH. After initial stumbles, our stakeholders did not trust the IT team or the vendor. Once we demonstrated successes in a pilot unit, there was a breakthrough. But, pilot testing can have its downfalls also; the objectives need to be limited and clearly defined, and, if possible, key staff involved needs to "volunteer" to participate. Having the involvement of people who have a sincere desire to see computerization succeed is probably more than half the battle. Implement gradually. Bringing up everything, everywhere, at once can be overwhelming—to users, resources, and the entire organization. We ultimately opted instead to implement the system in pieces, creating a staged process that is easier for us to manage and easier for users to absorb.

Training

Training should not be limited to the system being implemented, but include changes in processes, job contents, and impact to the workplace. Organizations need to budget for and invest in training and education—both short term and long term. As the pain of the nursing shortage grew, so did our ability to replace nurses taken away from patient care for training. This factor should not be overlooked in the planning stages.

Roles, Responsibilities, and Accountabilities

These factors must be clearly defined and redefined throughout the implementation process. User involvement in all appropriate aspects of the implementation must be budgeted and nonnegotiable. Development of super users is key. Stakeholder participation can be promised sincerely, but it is hard to "wrap one's mind around" a project of this scope in the abstract, and once budget realities are known in relation to required resources, promises become economically untenable and plans change. Employment of "pilot" implementations in targeted areas prior to full-house implementation is one way for the stakeholders to get an understanding of their role. For our group, it was absolutely necessary because the product was being customized to long-term care and, for some users, the "big picture" was not clear until it was "live."

Fight Battles Early

We eventually regretted some concessions that were made early on, specifically with regard to the staffing of the project team. In an attempt to cooperate with local management, we did not insist that only middle management and line staff be selected. In retrospect, department head-level staff could not be freed of their primary job responsibilities, even on a part-time basis, and the result interfered with the morale and effectiveness of the team. In addition, we inappropriately assigned one promising member to an area for which this person had little clinical experience and set the stage for stress and discontent. Project team members should possess clinical skills across the key clinical/operational areas that the system will be deployed in and be qualified for the roles they are filling.

Set Realistic Goals and Expectations

Users obviously become impatient if it takes them more time to do a task, such as filling out a patient record or using a new computer application, than doing the job manually. However, even well-designed computer applications always require a learning period before users begin to see productivity gains. Emphasis should be placed on the long-term gains of suffering through temporary productivity setbacks. Ability to derive return on investment is contingent upon achieving a critical mass of users at an advanced level of sophistication, which may not occur for 6 to 18 months after the full deployment effort. In our case, this fact was exemplified by staff that was initially resistant and vocal in their criticism of the system being transformed into active defenders.

Scope Management

It needs to be well understood, throughout the organization, that any changes to scope for any reason at any time adds cost, uses resources, and affects the timeline. Similar to designing and constructing a building, each time the architect's blueprint is altered after it has been finalized, rework occurs, and the costs of rework should not be underestimated.

Contractual Issues

The contract should support expectations. In other words, get it in writing. This relates not only to the functional requirements of the software, but expectations of the implementation team, system development, and senior executive support. For example, if the expectation is that the vendor will guide the implementation against best practice standards, this should be supported by contractual language that specifies the terms and conditions of delivery.

Looking Forward

The JHH Lifecare System has high hopes for this system. We believe its long-term care functionality will improve the overall process of delivering quality patient care across the combined 1630-bed, three-campus site. This CPR tool will streamline paper documentation and care planning to increase patient safety, reduce medication-related errors, and improve outcomes and decrease rising administrative costs. Ultimately, the improved clinical care process might even aid in recruiting and retaining clinical staff by reducing arduous paperwork and freeing caregivers' time to devote to patient care.

References

1. Healthmedx 2002. Productivity loss is greatest in non-patient care activities. http://www.healthmedx.com/about/challenges.asp. Accessed November 20, 2002.
2. Stoddard N. Benchmarking for long term care clinical system investment. HIMSS Long Term Care Conference; 2002 March 9 [abstracted from presentation].
3. Toepper M, Cerchiara K. Integrating long term care into a delivery system. Presentation and Proceedings of the HIMSS Annual Conference; 2000 April 9–13; Dallas, TX [CD].
4. Hammer M, Stanton S. The re-engineering revolution: a handbook. New York: HarperBusiness; 1995.

16
CIO STORIES, III
Methodist Healthcare System, San Antonio: Redesign of Clinical Documentation

JENNIFER ALLAN BROWNE

It was back to the drawing board when design problems surfaced in the clinical documentation module of an already installed system.

In 1994 the Meditech[1] hospital information system was installed in four hospitals within the Methodist Healthcare System (MHS) in San Antonio, Texas. Most modules, such as Lab, Radiology, Pharmacy, and Order Entry, stabilized rapidly and well. The Clinical Documentation module, however, stalled with design problems. Two years after installation, unresolved clinical issues remained:

- Documentation time had increased.
- Complex care plans did not effectively communicate patient problems.
- Excessive interventions were needed to support daily documentation.
- The patient care plan did not connect with the daily documentation record.
- Accuracy of the medical record decreased.
- Fragmented data were produced.
- Medical records accumulated duplicate and conflicting information.
- Extracting concurrent and retrospective data proved difficult.
- Physician dissatisfaction with nursing and the medical record had increased.

By 1996, mounting nurse and physician dissatisfaction demanded redesign of the clinical documentation module [1].

The goals of redesign included:

- Improved patient care.
- Meeting legal, regulatory, and clinical requirements.
- Decreasing documentation time and eliminating repetitive documentation.
- Reducing costs (associated with overtime, resources, and support).
- Streamlining the medical record.

Jennifer Allan Browne, RN, BC, is Clinical Informatics Coordinator for the Methodist Healthcare System in San Antonio, Texas.
[1] Medical Information Technology, Inc., MEDITECH Circle, Westwood, MA 02090 (platform: MAGIC).

- Improving data retrieval in the form of audits and reports.
- Producing a multidisciplinary/interdisciplinary documentation record.
- Providing a foundation for quality assessment, clinical benchmarking, and outcomes measurement.
- Increasing nurse satisfaction and decreasing physician complaints [1].

Redesign Model

Approach: Standards of Care/Standards of Practice

An aggressive literature review began to find a clinical language that would support all clinicians in a computerized environment. No computerized documentation approaches supported the streamlined, interdisciplinary vision sought. Some nursing nomenclatures seemed to work well on paper, but fell short when used in the computer environment. As a result, in 1996 Patient Centered Documentation© (Standards Based Documentation) was drafted [2].

Trial implementation began with a small nursing group, working closely with a medical malpractice attorney [3]. Patient Centered Documentation (PCD) unites the foundational plan of care and documentation via the Standards of Care for the hospital, the Standards of Practice for the unit, and age-appropriate care guidelines for the patient.

- Primary Objective: To ensure that every patient entering the healthcare system at any level will receive the same standard of care. Launching of this foundational plan of care starts upon admission and results in (a) a complete patient record, (b) no delay in documentation, and (c) reduced intervention duplication.
- Secondary Objective: To separate core standards of practice from patient problems and physician orders. This way, any clinician can review the record and immediately identify specific patient needs/problems.

Abbreviated Documentation

Documentation time was decreased in two ways. Nursing interventions were split into those that required documentation and those that only required acknowledgment. Interventions requiring acknowledgment only were grouped to allow complete documentation with just one keystroke. This approach shortens documentation yet provides a complete record.

Assessment documentation works in a similar manner. A normal assessment requires only one response for verification, but the clinician is prompted to chart, in detail, variances if the assessment is abnormal. PCD highlights abnormal assessment information. Data entry is minimized while still producing a complete documentation record that emphasizes abnormal findings.

Patient-Centered Plan of Care

During PCD development, it became clear that a single clinical language was needed to seamlessly integrate all phases of the patient's care. Thus, the care plan problem list shows only actual patient problems. No duplicative or ambiguous problems exist, and only potential problems that require intervention are addressed.

- Goal of the problem-based, patient-centered terminology revision: To create a language that all care providers could easily understand and use. For example, the nursing terminology "Altered Cardiac Output" was replaced with the terminology "Problem: Cardiac." Goals and interventions associated with each problem were designed as unit/specialty specific and allow patient-specific response. When problems are unique to a discipline (i.e., respiratory therapy, pastoral care), data entry remains exclusive to that specialty, but information is universally communicated. The simplified, universal, clinical language enables the bedside RN, as primary care coordinator, to assess, integrate, evaluate, and prioritize patient and family care needs.

Pilot Study

In 1997, PCD was piloted in two intensive care units at Metropolitan Methodist Hospital. Parallel trials were conducted for 2 weeks, followed by a 1-month structured implementation. During the 6-week period, rigorous chart review was conducted, assisted in great part by the attorney working on our team. It was imperative that the pilot produce not only a comprehensive clinical record but also a record defensible in court. The pilot succeeded, and the model was installed in all inpatient units of the 200-bed Metropolitan Methodist Hospital.

Evaluation of PCD performance on four medical surgical units used a survey of users, analysis of incremental overtime, and content analysis of records 3 months after implementation. *Nurses from these four units reported a 55 percent decrease in charting time per patient.* The average daily census and patient acuity remained constant during this evaluation period. *Incremental overtime decreased 45.1 percent during this same 3-month period.* This translated to an actual 8.2 percent decrease in salary per patient day and an annual savings of $107,923 for the four nursing units involved in the study. *Nursing satisfaction related to documentation improved from a mean score of 3.43 to 4.47 on a five-point scale.*

Implementing PCD Throughout the Methodist System

Systemwide installation became a strategic objective for 1997–1998. PCD would be installed at three more hospitals in 1997 and our largest facilities, Southwest Texas Methodist Hospital (SWTMH) and Methodist Children's Hospital of South Texas, still charting on paper, by 1998.

Two projects remained that would prove essential to the success of PCD. Carried on simultaneously, the implementation team created a system structure that would provide ongoing synchronization at all hospitals and redesigned charting screens to maximize automation of reports.

Organizational Framework

Redesigning clinical documentation at hospitals already documenting on the computer required dedicated executive support. The key to this support was development of a unified charting approach that made the computer a productive system tool, rather than just a warehouse of information. Our original goals could only be realized by maintaining synchronization of documentation screens at all hospitals.

The primary obstacle to this universal redesign was that information specialists, educators, and end users at each hospital had invested years of work into the hospital-specific documentation currently in place. To overcome this problem, information specialists were appointed (one person per facility) as a core redesign team. An unbiased facilitator was appointed to coordinate this group. Although the specialists still reported to their parent hospital, work roles were assigned by area of specialty rather than by hospital. This diffused team member allegiance to any one site.

The Nurse Executive appointed a Steering Committee to oversee all computer documentation, policies, and related material. The steering committee maintains the system vision established at the executive level. Steering acts as the buffer and the referral source for solutions whenever disagreements occur.

Forms Framework

With a system redesign commitment firmly in place, form standardization came next. Past experience told us end reports and the appearance of the Clinical Patient Repository (CPR) would only be as good as the data entered. In earlier implementations, paper forms had been replicated in the computer, with no plan for output data. Redesign reversed the strategy: *Data output became the key focus rather than data input.*

The team met with all disciplines, assessed needs, and coordinated documentation to meet the requests of end-user groups. For example, risk management, admitting, dieticians, case management, infection control, physicians, and nursing are just some of the groups that reviewed and assisted with the editing of assessment forms. These groups revised documentation within their area of expertise with the primary goal of incorporating precise questions and screening tools into the admission and daily documentation that would allow automated generation of necessary reports. These reports would meet all legal and regulatory requirements as well as improve the efficiency of tracking data. The secondary goal was clean organization of information in the CPR.

Once draft forms were complete, approval was required from the clinical specialty, legal, and the regulatory committee. With approval at this level, original forms went to the steering committee for final approval. With rare exception, once a process has been approved at the steering level, it becomes a system standard and must be utilized in all forms. For example, advance directive information is standardized across admitting and nursing area to produce a seamless flow of information. One audit reviews the timeliness of placement of the advance directive document on the chart, while presenting the information in the CPR in identical format across the entire spectrum of care at all facilities.

Results and Realized Benefits

Final Installations

The redesigned system was installed and implemented at the four "Live" sites by early 1998. Informal evaluation 3 months after installation confirmed the results obtained in the original pilot. The PCD methodology was then installed at our fifth site. The 750-bed Southwest Texas Methodist Hospital and the Methodist Children's Hospital campus was a new installation, with caregivers moving from paper to computer (both order entry and documentation) for the first time. In previous initial installations, where caregivers charted on the computer for the first time, MHS experienced significant increases in overtime during the first 6 months. The new system was installed in our largest facilities in September 1998 using a "Big Bang" approach. No increase in

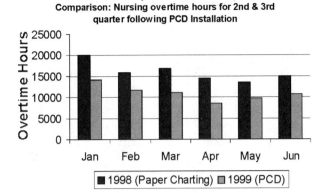

**Methodist Hospital & Children's Hospital
Comparison: Nursing overtime hours for 2nd & 3rd
quarter following PCD Installation**

FIGURE 16.1. Following installation of Patient Centered Documentation, overtime declined from 0.84 hours per adjusted patient day in the quarter preceding implementation to 0.47 hours per adjusted patient day in the quarter following implementation. (From 2000 HIMSS Annual Conference Proceedings [1].)

overtime occurred; in fact, overtime declined from 0.84 hours per adjusted patient day in the quarter preceding implementation to 0.47 hours per adjusted patient day in the quarter following implementation. The following two quarters maintained decreased nursing overtime while the volume of patient days remained constant (Figure 16.1).

Evaluation of Care

By standardizing problems, interventions, and queries, detailed audit and variance reports are now available. RN accountability, high nutritional risk, suspected domestic violence, falls, restraint, isolation, advance directives, and pain assessment are just a few of the produced reports. In the past, this type of chart review had been labor intensive. For example, prior to PCD, it required one part-time RN to manually audit 100 records per quarter related to pressure ulcer documentation and patient medication education. Currently, with PCD, more than 600 records can be reviewed in 1 day (Figure 16.2).

Regulatory/Clinical Compliance

The PCD-driven computer has now become a tool for MHS, which allows for problem identification, solution implementation, and immediate evaluation of the revisions. For example, in 2000, all MHS facilities were delinquent in documentation of the essence of a patient's advance directive. Initial audits revealed an 87 percent error rate systemwide. By redesigning documentation, staff was prompted by the information system to enter correct data. As a result, no in-services were required and the error rate dropped to 4 percent in less than 8 weeks (approximately 2400 records were screened weekly with a 2-hour compilation time).

Another advantage is the immediacy of reports. Identification of patients in restraint for any given year can be produced in less than 1 hour. Behavioral restraint is now reviewed on a daily basis. When a behavioral restraint is identified, the reviewer goes to the patient unit and reviews the chart for completeness of record. Medical/surgical

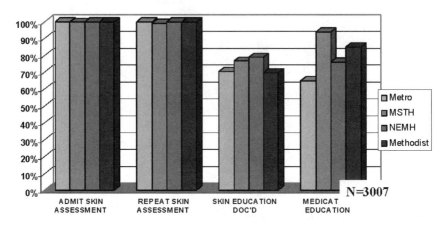

FIGURE 16.2. Prior to PCD, chart review had been labor intensive. For example, it required one part-time RN to manually audit 100 records per quarter related to pressure ulcer documentation and patient medication education. In this example, more than 3000 records for a single quarter were reviewed in 4.5 days. (From 2000 HIMSS Annual Conference Proceedings [1].)

restraint is also evaluated in the same manner, resulting in complete records being delivered to medical records at the time of patient discharge.

Process Improvement/Productivity

High-Risk Nutritional Screening

An automated process was designed utilizing weighted criteria embedded transparently into nursing documentation. Stratified degrees of risk identification and automated communication to the dietary department ensure that dietician referrals and assessments are prioritized accurately. Key indicators are individualized for the adult, obstetric, and pediatric populations. The enhanced computerized process resulted in a 22 percent improvement in appropriate identification (specificity) of patients at nutritional risk and a 20 percent improvement in overall timeliness of assessment (Figure 16.3).

Respiratory Therapy

The Respiratory Therapy Department (RT) has redesigned both documentation and charge processes. This enables the department to evaluate both quality service indicators and productivity. Completeness of documentation improved from 72 percent in 1997 to 97 percent in 2000. Delay in treatment initiation time greater than 60 minutes decreased from 48 percent to 13 percent. During the same time period, on-time treatments increased from 84 percent to 97 percent.

From 1998 to 1999, total Respiratory Therapy FTEs at our largest facility decreased from 124.38 to 100.41. This translated to a decrease in expense per patient day from $32.02 to $24.71. During the same time period, patient days increased 3.6 percent. Total expenses from year-end 1998 to year-end 1999 dropped $783,897.00 (−19.73 percent. This can be attributed directly to increased productivity. Prior to the computer, work assignments generally ran 345 minutes in a 480-minute shift (72 percent). By reassigning work units, and evaluating using the computer, current assignments target 425 minutes (88 percent), resulting in an average departmental personnel productivity at our three largest facilities of 109 percent [4].

In both clinical examples, the specialty departments participate fully in the interdisciplinary care process using the established documentation framework. They are, however, able to individualize the approach to meet unique, specialty specific needs.

Revenue Support /Financial Savings

Prior to the computer, all bedside blood glucose charting/charging was done on paper, with forms being hand-delivered to Lab for review and charging. Lost/delayed paperwork resulted in College of American Pathologists (CAP) citations and an unknown amount of lost charges. After automation of charges, revenue increased $2,230,330 for the same 8-month period in 1999 over 1998. The volume of glucose reagents ordered and utilized remained the same both years, demonstrating that testing volume had not increased, but the actual data captured were more efficient. This approach also brought

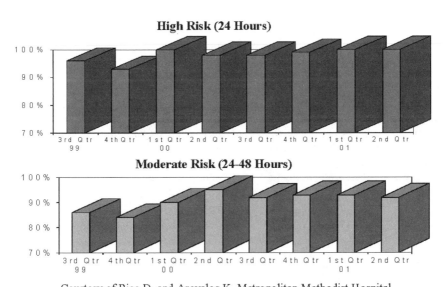

Courtesy of Rice D. and Arevalos K. Metropolitan Methodist Hospital

FIGURE 16.3. An enhanced computerized process facilitates identification for stratified degrees of risk and communication to the appropriate department. In this example, this process has resulted in a 22 percent improvement in appropriate identification (specificity) of patients at nutritional risk and a 20 percent improvement in overall timeliness of assessment. (From 2000 HIMSS Annual Conference Proceedings [1].)

the Lab into immediate CAP, JCAHO, and Medicare compliance. The accuracy of charge entry from nursing units is also monitored, with error rates approximating 0.7 percent.

Because documentation is standardized, practice polices are identical at all MHS facilities. As a result, staff is educated identically and a seamless continuity of care can be demonstrated. Standardization has produced immediate resource savings in the following areas: (a) consolidated training and orientation classes, (b) ease of shared staffing citywide, and (c) resolution of float nurse/agency nurse/student nurse issues. MHS has been able to reduce the number of instructors and resource materials.

Patient Safety

Computerized documentation has enabled clinicians to immediately identify patients at safety risk in multiple categories. Examples include fall, skin breakdown, suicide, and latex allergy alerts. The computer tabulates a score and adds suggested interventions to the plan of care as triggers to clinicians in the prevention of injury. The computer can also identify patients at risk for communicable diseases, providing staff an early opportunity to initiate protection for themselves and other patients.

Most recently, MHS has implemented an electronic medication administration record at three facilities. This bar-coded approach to medication delivery cross-checks the medication, dosage, route, patient, and allergies. Numerous medication errors have been identified and averted. Systemwide installation is targeted for year-end 2003.

Clinical Communication

PCD has automated computation and distribution of information. Nursing risk assessments now autocalculate, based on previous assessment indicators to produce 100 percent compliance in risk screening and continuity of care between outpatient and inpatient services.

Data are collected once and distributed multiple ways. For example, assessment of the patient's neurological status calculates scores into the fall risk, high-risk skin breakdown, initial and ongoing nutritional risk assessments, as well as the hospice/palliative care referral report. Six required data elements are satisfied with the entry of one query.

Similarly, data entered once can populate other forms. Clinical data flow to physician forms, multidisciplinary care conferences, the collaborative education record, change of shift reports, and chart audits. The goal is to maximize the efficiency of data entry while facilitating interdisciplinary communication. Equally important is the ability to present information identically at all facilities.

Conclusion

Redesign of clinical documentation using PCD has resolved the majority of clinical documentation issues. Documentation time has decreased, the plan of care and documentation of care are consistent, and the medical record is smaller. Nurse satisfaction has improved and physician complaints have declined.

The monitoring of records for legal and regulatory purposes has been automated. We can address immediate needs and monitor effectiveness of interventions with ease. Revenue support and quality monitoring have improved significantly, and clinical communication is being optimized.

Patient Centered Documentation has provided a powerful framework that has proved highly versatile and adaptable. We are confident this approach will support any future healthcare challenges the Methodist Healthcare System may encounter.

References

1. Allan J, Englebright J. Organizing clinical information systems to manage and improve care. Proceedings of the 2000 Annual HIMSS Conference and Exhibition; 2000 April 9–13; Dallas, TX. Session 80. p. 269–284 [CD].
2. Allan J, Englebright J. Patient-centered documentation. J Nursing Admin 2000;30(2):90–95.
3. Comerio A. Partner, Adams, Comerio, and Vowell Law Firm. San Antonio, TX.
4. Information, courtesy of Michael G. Freiling, Director of Pulmonary Services, Methodist Specialty and Transplant Hospital, Southwest Texas Methodist Hospital and Methodist Children's Hospital of South Texas.

17
CIO STORIES, IV
ThedaCare, Wisconsin: Successful Integration Through Leadership

KEITH J. LIVINGSTON

ThedaCare's transformation into a nationally recognized integrated health system is as much a technological achievement as it is a model in leadership commitment.

ThedaCare is an integrated delivery network in northeast Wisconsin with three hospitals, more than 100 employed physicians, over 350 affiliated physicians, behavioral health services, a laboratory, home health services, and a full spectrum of retirement, assisted living, and skilled nursing facilities. ThedaCare also has controlling ownership of Touchpoint Health Plan, a leading provider of managed health care in the United States.

ThedaCare ranks among the nation's 25 best integrated delivery systems, according to *Modern Healthcare* and Verispan (2002). It is also among the American Hospital Association's (AHA) 100 "Most Wired" health systems.

Each of ThedaCare's three hospitals is a three-time designee on *Modern Healthcare*'s annual "Top 100 Hospitals" list, as rated by HCIA-Sachs. ThedaCare hospitals were also named 2002 "Consumer Choice Award" winners, based on consumer perception surveys conducted by the National Research Corporation.

Overcoming the Challenges of Fragmentation

In 1997, ThedaCare's vision was not unique:

". . . to provide the best health care to our customers at the lowest cost."

Neither were ThedaCare's challenges unique. The organization was facing increased competitive pressure, higher costs, lower reimbursements, and a nationwide nursing shortage. Through consolidation and acquisition, it had also grown quickly beyond its ability to operate as a cohesive unit. What seemed like a health system uniquely positioned to achieve its vision—encompassing hospitals, physicians' offices, and a health plan among a broad spectrum of other services—was in actuality a conglomeration of independent units. ThedaCare found itself with disparate computer systems, discon-

---

Keith J. Livingston, BBA, is Chief Information Officer of ThedaCare.

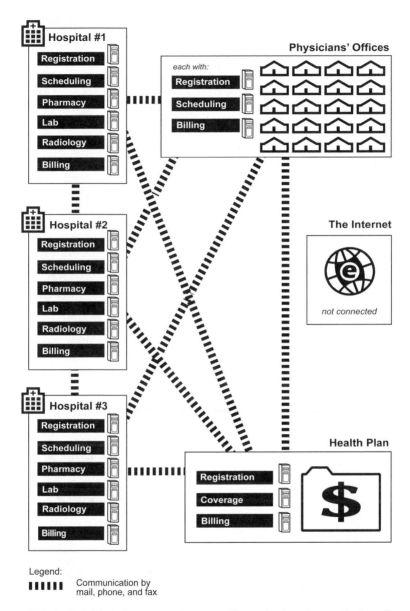

Legend:

▌▐▌▐▌ Communication by
       mail, phone, and fax

FIGURE 17.1. In 1997, ThedaCare was a "fragmented" organization, characterized by disparate systems and platforms within facilities, between facilities, and among individual business entities.

nected care processes, and, often, conflicting goals (Figure 17.1). Ironically, the name of the organization back then was "United Health."

ThedaCare acknowledged the challenges it faced and went to work on a plan to overcome them. While many provider organizations at the time were divesting themselves from the payer business, ThedaCare set out to prove that a partnership between payer and provider could exist under one roof, that hospitals and clinics could work together, and that the results would be higher-quality care, reduced costs, and improved organizational viability.

ThedaCare leadership had already redefined the term "patient" to "customer" in all internal discussions, as an acknowledgment of the emerging consumerism in health care. This change of mindset would be necessary to frame the drastic organizational changes that ThedaCare was planning to pursue. A central strategy for differentiating ThedaCare in the eyes of customers would also be to redefine the role of the primary care provider (PCP), adding value through improved continuity, better communication, and more active health management. Integrated information technology (IT) systems would play a critical role in achieving this goal.

Several years into the project, ThedaCare has encouraging results to support its theory regarding the benefits of a unified health system. In 2002 Touchpoint Health Plan was named the "highest performing plan in the nation overall" by the National Committee for Quality Assurance (NCQA), based on results of the HEDIS survey. (HEDIS is NCQA's Health Plan Employer and Data Information Set, an objective set of performance measures of clinical care and member satisfaction used to compare health plans nationwide.) The organization has also set national benchmarks for breast cancer screening, beta-blocker treatment after heart attack, diabetic care, and cholesterol control. Along the way, ThedaCare's strategic hypothesis was also confirmed— that improvements in care quality and service quality do indeed make a difference to customers when selecting a health provider. This case study will tell the story of how ThedaCare built its customer-centric IT foundation, highlight the results achieved, and look forward to new customer-focused transformations on the horizon.

Leadership

On January 1, 2002, ThedaCare became the first health system in the nation to unify its hospitals, physician practices, and health plan with a single enterprise database and integrated applications for clinical care, registration, scheduling, billing, and managed care functions. The hospital systems "go-live" on New Year's Day was the culmination of the organization's integration plan begun in 1997. Despite this unique technological accomplishment, ThedaCare's integration story does not start with technology. It starts with leadership.

Early on, ThedaCare realized that breaking away from its fragmented past would require a commitment from company leadership on every level to new processes, new methods of communication, and new technology. The targeted change would be swift and massive—a fundamental rethinking and rebuilding of core processes—an operational "do over." The timeframe was years, not decades.

Working in Uncharted Territory

ThedaCare's IT approach has traditionally been conservative and practical, but with the destination so clearly defined, the organization was looking to the IT department for something special. It was the job of ThedaCare's technical team to construct a strategy that would do more than "approach" the ultimate vision. The team needed a plan to make it all the way there. To guide its decisions, ThedaCare identified three strategic ground rules that would enable it to realize the vision of a truly unified health system.

Translating the Vision: Strategic Ground Rules

Rule No. 1. Full Information Everywhere

ThedaCare determined that when a customer comes to any facility or interacts with anyone in the organization, that customer's entire health record should be right there, instantly available. No longer would physicians and nurses (especially nurses) be focused on gathering information. Select pieces of the record would not suffice. The entire clinical, demographic, and financial record would need to be available on demand, with "no assembly required" by the end user.

Rule No. 2. Ambulatory First

It was decided that when doctors started to use systems heavily (for ordering and documentation), they should not have to learn an ambulatory system and a separate inpatient system. From the beginning, ThedaCare's clinical leadership knew that if physicians could learn how to use the system in their clinics first—essentially their "home"—the organization would achieve more consistent computerized physician order entry (CPOE) usage in the hospital. In addition to the training advantage, the "ambulatory first" approach would provide a useful, richly populated inpatient/ambulatory record—instead of a blank slate—for hospital caregivers. With a high proportion of physician users not employed by ThedaCare, it would be important to implement a system that physicians would voluntarily embrace.

Rule No. 3. Engage the Customer

Back before the explosion of the Internet, nobody knew for sure what the mechanism would be, but ThedaCare correctly anticipated that its customers would want access to this wealth of personal health information once it was recorded. It was recognized early on that great potential existed for differentiating ThedaCare in the eyes of customers and for extending care continuity beyond the scope of the admission or office visit.

The IT team knew intuitively that the only way to live up to these ground rules in real life was with integrated applications—a single code for core systems, sharing a single, customer-centric enterprise database. Going down that path would put ThedaCare in uncharted territory and in a position of considerable organizational risk. A measure of comfort was found in the shared belief that it would be far riskier trying to approach the challenge any other way.

Choosing Integration over Fragmentation

In these early days, ThedaCare's computer systems were not a rallying point for organizational change. They were, in fact, pretty unpopular. The health system needed a quick and solid IT "win" to build momentum for the organizational redesign that was soon to follow. With this in mind, and after a rigorous selection process, ThedaCare chose Epic Systems Corporation of Madison, Wisconsin, as the vendor that would help fulfill the bulk of the integrated vision. Epic had two decades of experience with the patient-centric database approach and a solid track record of hitting implementation dates. The needed momentum was provided with a fast-track implementation of Epic's enterprise master person index (EMPI), clinical data repository (CDR), and Web-based CDR viewer in August 1998.

Timeline of Transition

The CDR project was a smooth implementation and an overwhelming success in practice, giving users in clinics and hospitals a central, Web-accessible source for historical lab, pharmacy, radiology, and transcription data. The CDR implementation was an important precursor to the "ambulatory first" strategy for advanced clinical systems. Successful rollouts followed of Epic's ambulatory electronic medical record (EMR), registration, scheduling, and billing systems, which went live at initial sites in the year 2000. Later, patient Web access, affiliate Web access, provider home access, and health plan systems were added. With the January 1, 2002, go live of Epic's inpatient suite—including the enterprise EMR, order entry, registration, ADT, patient lists, and billing—ThedaCare completed its integrated IT foundation (Figure 17.2).

While building continues upon the integrated platform, ThedaCare has already seen significant success, especially in the clinics, where the EMR is now a way of life. Integrated registration, scheduling, and billing have worked hand in hand with the EMR to streamline workflows in some areas and to eliminate old, time-consuming workflows in many more. In the hospitals, only a few months postlive at this writing, ThedaCare is already seeing the expected benefits of inpatient/ambulatory integration.

Adding Value to the Ambulatory Encounter

With the implementation of the EpicCare Ambulatory EMR, Ground Rules 1 and 2 were quickly satisfied. ThedaCare had a central, comprehensive source of patient information that physicians were comfortable using in their daily workflow. Financial benefits followed, including:

- Decreased transcription costs.
- Reduced paper costs through elimination of route tickets and encounter forms.
- More patients seen per week per physician.
- Fewer lost charges per visit.

In addition to these welcome financial gains, the health system was positioned to achieve the larger goal of transforming care in its market.

Better Health Through Proactive Disease Management

As mentioned before, a major strategic driver behind ThedaCare's decision to pursue integrated IT was the desire to redefine the primary care provider (PCP) value proposition. The goal was for the PCP to be viewed as an ongoing healthcare advisor, rather than a provider of reactive, episodic services. This perceptual shift would set ThedaCare apart in the market and significantly influence customer decisions. Continuity of care would be central to the change, so it was critical to have information systems that would support the PCP proactively, with comprehensive patient information at every point of care and the ability to communicate outside the scope of a traditional visit.

Customers with chronic health problems are the primary beneficiaries of continuity. Proactive management of diseases like diabetes, asthma, and hypertension not only keeps people out of the hospital, it also builds a stronger relationship between the PCP and the customer. Results to date are excellent. En route to its recognition by the NCQA, Touchpoint scored in the top 5 percent nationally in 17 of 28 Effectiveness of

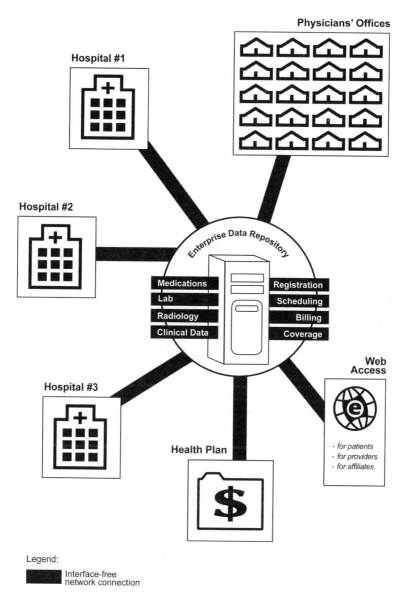

FIGURE 17.2. With its hospital go-live on January 1, 2002, ThedaCare's integrated IT foundation, based on Epic's enterprise repository, connected inpatient, ambulatory, payer, and Web environments to a single data source.

TABLE 17.1. Comparison of improvements for Touchpoint health plan.

Effectiveness measure	1996 (%)	2001 (%)
Pediatric immunizations	77.9	85.2
Adolescent immunizations	53.0	82.7
Mammography	76.9	90.4[a]
Cervical cancer screening	76.4	90.8
Prenatal visits	78.1	94.4
Postnatal checks	78.1	87.4
Beta blocker	72.2	100[a]
Diabetic eye exams	58.4	94.7[a]
Cholesterol control	64.0	75.9[a]

[a] Leads the nation.

Care measures, and led the nation in the four categories. Some notable improvements are illustrated in Table 17.1.

Orchestrating Care

Successful disease management requires more coordination of effort outside the scope of the physician visit than it calls for actual intervention during the office encounter. Success requires a true orchestration of multiple information resources.

- *Step 1: Build a system that knows your customers.* Before you can tackle diabetes, you need an easy way to identify the people with diabetes in your care. Leveraging the single repository, ThedaCare has a single registration, whether customers enter the system through the health plan, a hospital, or a clinic. How does this help manage diabetes? Just as you give your address only once at ThedaCare, you only have to be recognized as having diabetes once, and all the core information systems—the EMR, the payer system, scheduling, and billing—will instantly share this knowledge. This single entry in the record will automatically put a customer in the appropriate management program, triggering added attention from systems and staff. The system also automatically identifies healthy people who fit health maintenance criteria, such as women over 50 who should receive regular mammograms.

  What's the alternative to a single registration database? Before switching to Epic, ThedaCare sent its data away to a data specialist to be cleaned for duplicates. The number of duplicates crashed their system. Trying again with Epic's EMPI, 1.5 million duplicate records were eliminated that had grown out of the previous tangled web of systems.
- *Step 2: Push alerts to the point of care.* During an office visit, ThedaCare's clinical system automatically checks the customer's record for membership in disease registries and for other health maintenance criteria. If an intervention is appropriate, the system will notify the physician with an alert from within the standard visit workflow screen. ThedaCare's Physician Users' Group prioritizes which alerts are active based on identified deficiencies and the potential for a significant health impact. Currently, ThedaCare has active alerts for diabetes, coronary artery disease, pediatric immunization, adolescent immunization, Pap tests, and mammograms.
- *Step 3: Involve everybody.* Disease management works best when relevant information is in the hands of more people. At ThedaCare, alerts are not limited to the exam

room. Schedulers making unrelated appointments receive health maintenance alerts from within the scheduling application, so they can allocate time for necessary procedures and properly sequence appointments requiring multiple steps.

- *Step 4: Measure your progress and make adjustments.* Because all ThedaCare's clinical data are stored in one place, it is easy to create reports that pinpoint opportunities for improvement. The system creates lists of noncompliant patients who will receive a personal phone call or letter. It also reports disease management outcomes by provider to help physicians compare their individual results with standards and peers—stimulating consistent levels of care for all customers.

The Next Step: MyThedaCare.org

It is tempting to call this the final step, but that would be selling the future short. ThedaCare's most recent initiative toward expanding continuity is bringing the electronic record into the customer's home. This is Ground Rule No. 3 in its purest form. The organization is now in the early stages of rolling out MyThedaCare.org, a secure Web site that lets customers view large portions of the same medical record ThedaCare providers use, allows them to schedule an appointment online, enables them to refill prescriptions over the Web, and lets them securely e-mail physicians. It is also yet another vehicle for delivering automatic health alerts, based on membership in disease registries, preventative health criteria, and other alerts chosen by physicians to address individual health needs. Customers benefit from Web access because they do not have to wait on hold for results or appointments, and ThedaCare users benefit because it makes for fewer interruptions to their care workflows.

Physician and customer feedback has been strongly positive. The expectation is that Web applications will become major strategic differentiators for ThedaCare in the near future. One doctor reported that one of his patients—an older woman—had moved an hour north and switched to a new provider outside of ThedaCare. When she learned that her new doctor did not have her record available online, she decided to switch back to her ThedaCare doctor and simply drive the hour for appointments.

ThedaCare is also enabling better customer–physician relationships by making the system accessible in the provider's home over the Web. One physician reported recently how home access to the EMR led to better care. A young patient of hers had an asthma attack after hours, and the answering service had paged the physician for advice. She reviewed the child's record from home and placed a medication order, which the system autofaxed to a 24-hour pharmacy. Because of this technology, the child was spared a trip to the Emergency Department, the physician was able to deliver effective care without driving into the office, and the mother was given peace of mind.

Sustaining Better Care with Integrated Revenue Systems

Customer billing and managed care round out the integrated picture at ThedaCare. Redesign efforts here fulfill the "lowest cost" part of the organizational vision. The ability of ThedaCare's IT infrastructure to capture charges more accurately, decrease lag time for reimbursement, and eliminate unnecessary human intervention imparts an operational edge as well as an edge with customers. It supports continued efforts in the clinical realm while allowing ThedaCare to price its health services more attractively to employers.

Crossing Clinical and Financial Boundaries

Charges captured by clinicians in the EMR are billed automatically, without a paper form and without the need for a data interface. Co-pay and coverage information are easily accessible from within the registration workflow, scheduling, and even in clinical settings. Some of the results:

- *Increased percent of co-pays collected at the time of service.* This measure has gone from 53 percent to 82 percent, contributing to a decrease in AR days and leading to a 15% drop in mailing costs alone.
- *Decreased days to posting.* Epic sites currently average 4 days. Sites on the old system are at 8 days.
- *Decreased Accounts Receivable days outstanding.* Epic sites average 50; sites on the old system average 55.

Electronic Claim Transmission Cuts Costs and Billing Lag

ThedaCare's integrated billing system electronically transmits claims and posts reimbursements, leading to increased efficiency and lower third-party costs. Some examples:

- *Reduction of electronic claims submission costs.* Prior to implementation, ThedaCare paid separate transaction fees to submit and retrieve claims from a clearinghouse. Now, claims go directly to Touchpoint without clearinghouse involvement, saving 59 cents per claim roundtrip.
- *FTE savings from electronic posting of Touchpoint and Medicare payments.* With the reduced need for staff intervention, the billing department realized a 15 percent FTE reduction.

Hospitals Capture Return from Integrated Investment

Here is a vision of the future in ThedaCare hospitals: It's 9 A.M. on a Tuesday. Responding to a trauma en route via helicopter, a physician quickly gathers whatever patient information he can that will help treat the case. Instead of picking up the phone to medical records or asking someone to track down a fax copy of the history from the PCP's paper chart, he logs on to a workstation, searches the database easily by name, and brings up a full inpatient and ambulatory medical record. By the time the helicopter touches down, the physician has reviewed a full history, current medications, problem list, and recent lab results. The ensuing treatment is more informed, more confidently delivered, and actively monitored by electronic decision support.

That is the vision. It is also the reality. It happened not long ago at ThedaCare. What makes the story remarkable is that it happened on a holiday. Had that electronic record not been there, there would have been no information to support the treatment of this incoming trauma. With physicians' offices closed, nobody would have been on the other end of that phone call. Nobody would have been around to fax a history. What makes this story even more remarkable is that the holiday was New Year's Day 2002 and the physician, Dr. Raymond Georgen, was using a clinical system that had gone live only 9 hours earlier.

The story is a great example of how technology can really affect care, but it is all the more encouraging when you consider that the results realized so far in the hospitals are just a small sample of what is to come. ThedaCare is still at the "foundation" stage with its inpatient redesign, but has already seen measurable benefits. Hospital staff has documented over 350 service improvements, better charge capture, lower hospital AR days, and an improved Medicare Secondary Provider (MSP) questionnaire completion rate, currently 99.9 percent by time of discharge.

At this writing, ThedaCare has just gone live with CPOE in two hospital units. In preparation, the messy catalog of orthopedic order sets was trimmed from 28 paper forms to three standardized electronic templates. ThedaCare hospitals are truly poised for a clinical redesign much like its physicians' offices have experienced.

Looking Back

ThedaCare has enjoyed uncommon success with the implementation and user acceptance of its integrated systems. The senior leadership, IT team, clinical leaders, and vendor team all played important roles in developing this positive track record. Of course, there were inevitable challenges and plenty of lessons learned. The following are, based on ThedaCare's history, some of the most important things you can do to improve your odds of success with an integrated implementation.

- *Pick the right vendor for your organization.* While a vendor cannot single-handedly "make" an implementation, it can "break" it. ThedaCare has been very happy with the selection of Epic for the core of its integrated system.

  Prior to partnering with Epic, ThedaCare was unsuccessful in implementing enterprise systems from another vendor whose software, in retrospect, simply was not ready for live use. It was a short but painful relationship, one that could have derailed many broader strategic initiatives had it not ended quickly in favor of a better fit.
- *Start with the CDR to gain momentum.* Ask anyone involved with ThedaCare IT, and that person will tell you the decision to implement the Web-based, view-only CDR prior to any advanced clinical systems was the best tactical decision of the entire project. It gave users in the clinics and hospitals an early view of what was to come and gave the IT department a strong foothold for future implementations.

  Starting with the CDR contributes to two major drivers of clinician acceptance:

  1. Make it indispensable.
  2. Make it easy.

  The CDR combined information previously found in multiple systems (labs, radiology, medications, allergies, patient history, etc.) with multiple log-ins and multiple passwords. This was one easy place to find it all. After a brief adjustment period, the organization had an overwhelmingly positive experience to build on, as more difficult projects were unveiled in the future.
- *Be honest with end users for better system acceptance.* ThedaCare has developed a strong culture of user acceptance surrounding its technology initiatives. Part of that comes from the fact that its IT goals are in line with the goals of the end users. The other element is that ThedaCare leadership is extremely honest and committed to communicating, prior to go-live, the inevitable challenges that are soon to follow.

ThedaCare's clinical leaders have significant experience with this. They equate the change management process with the steps of mourning—denial, anger, etc. ThedaCare Medical Director for IT, John Barkmeier, MD, once said, "You can tell what week of rollout a clinic is in the moment you walk through the door." The process is predictable—as if scripted. But the clinical leaders do not just sit and watch it happen.

They communicate. They counsel. Invariably, users get through the rough times and, invariably, life is better on the other side.

Looking Ahead

Looking back, there is no question that ThedaCare took a successful approach to unifying a fragmented system. Looking ahead, the organization is better equipped than ever to effect real change due to its flexible IT foundation. The plan for the future is to continue to build on the integrated foundation and to continue to create stories of better care and improved service that were not possible just a few years ago. The now-integrated ThedaCare will leverage the flexibility of its technology to achieve differentiation in the market. It will turn a wealth of data into new forms of usable knowledge. It will challenge the remaining boundaries that separate customers from caregivers. Finally, ThedaCare will continue to push the percentages toward the ultimate goal of delivering the best possible care.

18
CIO Stories, V
University of Illinois Medical Center at Chicago: Best of Breed, Single Vendor, or Hybrid

Anne LeMaistre and Bernadette Biskup

> *After weighing the pros and cons of best of breed versus integration, UIMCC opted for a hybrid approach in its journey toward a multidisciplinary electronic health record.*

A Backdrop of Challenges

The changing requirements of health care in a highly competitive marketplace have given rise to many new challenges that encouraged the University of Illinois Medical Center at Chicago (UIMCC) to embark on a journey of transformation that fully utilizes health information technology. These challenges include national nursing and pharmacist shortages, increased complexity of ensuring safe care delivery, and changing care delivery models in the midst of an environment of increased costs and reduced revenues. All these challenges have augmented the long-standing desire of clinicians to improve the communication of clinical information within the healthcare organization.

UIMCC's journey is ongoing, striving to deliver to patients and community safe and efficient care that is of the highest quality. As you follow this journey, understand that it was a partnership forged with these goals in mind and could only be accomplished with the investment and commitment of the board, medical center administration, physicians, nurses, and clinicians. The current results of this journey have yielded an integrated and multidisciplinary electronic health record that is used and depended on by all clinicians to document and obtain patient information. The foundation for the electronic health record is in place, and UIMCC is now well positioned to coordinate patient care across the continuum of care as well as begin to use information to reengineer the care process.

Anne LeMaistre, MD, is Medical Director of Information Services for the Seton Healthcare Network in Austin, TX. Bernadette Biskup, RN, MSN, is interim CIO for the University of Illinois at Chicago Medical Center.

A Journey of Transformation

Founded in 1882, the University of Illinois Medical Center Chicago (UIMCC) is today the largest publicly owned hospital in Illinois and among the busiest teaching institutions in the nation. UIMCC includes a 507-bed hospital, an outpatient surgery center, a new, $100 million, 245,000-square-foot Outpatient Care Center, and 8 satellite facilities located within a 20-mile radius of the primary campus. The Outpatient Care Center houses 12 primary care and specialty centers. Approximately 800 primary care physicians and specialists are affiliated with the medical center. The medical center generates revenues of about $400 million annually and employs 3200 people, including 1200 nurses. UIMCC handles approximately 20,000 inpatient admissions and about 420,000 outpatient visits annually.

Located on Chicago's west side, the medical center is a comprehensive health sciences center that includes colleges of medicine, nursing, pharmacy, dentistry, applied health sciences, and a school of public health. The medical center serves an ethnically diverse community composed of many nationalities and languages along with professionals who are migrating back to the inner city. The diversity, language, and cultural variety of the community present numerous challenges to providing high-quality health care.

A recent *U.S. News & World Report* survey ranked the medical center in the top 4 percent of America's hospitals in the specialties of AIDS, cancer, cardiology, endocrinology, gastroenterology, geriatrics, gynecology, neurology, otolaryngology, ophthalmology, rheumatology, and urology. As a tertiary site for many complex medical procedures, UIMCC supports major programs in neurosurgery, ophthalmology, oncology, cardiology, neonatology, and obstetrics.

In the mid-1990s, implementation of an electronic health record (EHR) was proposed to the medical staff by senior administration as part of a strategic plan aimed at integrating ambulatory and inpatient care delivery. The plan described an EHR that would provide a longitudinal patient record and knowledge tools to support education and clinical care objectives. The clinical care emphasis was to maintain and improve quality and patient safety as well as transform the care delivery process.

The vendor selection was conducted in a standard manner by forming a committee composed of diverse clinical and technical members. The committee was charged with finding a vendor suited to be a long-term partner. The first decision by the committee was one of establishing a philosophy and approach on how to build the future. Should the solution be "best of breed" or one that favored an "integrated" approach?

Best of Breed Versus Integration

Similar to many healthcare systems in the 1990s, UIMCC purchased information systems with a best-of-breed mentality. One of the first cultural changes was to begin to consider the organization's information system as a single entity, even though it was made up of a number of discrete and dissimilar subsystems that supported various departments or user disciplines. A prerequisite for achieving the goals set and long-term success was to develop an effective plan to integrate the data from these subsystems. The complexity of this integration is not unique—and has long been discussed in the industry. Many technology solutions have been proposed. The discussion of this topic at UIMCC revolved around the following:

- Continue to choose best-of-breed systems with the consequent complexity of managing a variety of hardware platforms, operating systems, programming languages, and databases. This path would be the most challenging because the systems with their different architectures would need to be connected to communicate with each other to support the integrated care process workflow.
- Acquire an integrated system from a vendor that would replace many of the current systems. The trick would be to provide sufficient capabilities to meet the needs of the various disciplines.

There are, obviously, pros and cons for both best-of-breed systems and single-vendor integrated systems. Best-of-breed systems provide for departmental control, optimization of the application for user requirements, and the ability for an institution to replace any system without replacing the entire information system structure. However with a best-of-breed philosophy, the complexity of dealing with numerous vendors and architectures increases the risk that data failure will occur. Maintaining disparate databases increases the total cost of ownership, and the organization is faced with how to manage the training for viewing the same information in different formats and presentation. Segregated data within individual systems also limit the ability to use the data in clinical alerts, aggregated analysis, reporting, and clinical summaries. Integrated systems, on the other hand, are a "mirror image" with respect to the pros and cons of a best-of-breed solution.

The complexity of supporting an integrated system is lessened through the elimination of duplicate interfaces, databases, and maintenance. The shared database, similar to the sharing of clinical information in the medical record, enhances the software's ability to optimize the clinical workflow process. However, the negatives are the cost of acquisition, and concerns that the application may not be ideal for single department functionality and that integration requires dependency on a single vendor. After weighing these two strategies, a hybrid solution seemed appropriate.

A Hybrid Clinical System Solution

A hybrid solution, combining a partially integrated system with interfaced systems, can be a cost-effective and clinically effective alternative. In this approach, departments that are supportive but *not directly* integrated in patient care activities are allowed to continue their system selections with a best-of-breed philosophy. This approach affords the freedom to apply a single department solution, but does not prohibit selection of an integrated vendor's application. Adverse consequences of choosing a nonintegrated vendor are generally limited to reduced functionality for that department and do not affect the broader care process or providers. To support the care process, data (optimally in the form of discrete results) do need to be interfaced back to the integrated system and a vendor must provide high-quality interfaces meeting national standards. Departments that generally consider use of a best-of-breed-strategy are laboratory, radiology, and dietary.

Clinicians and departments that *directly* participate in the care process are optimally supported by integrated systems. The rationale behind this approach is that the workflow and the data utilized in the workflow are patient centered and shared between clinicians. An integration of these support processes to one common database provides high-quality data in an efficient manner. The integrated approach allows for consistency in data presentation, clinical alerts, and provides less data risk since there are reduced technical reasons for failure (data not able to be interfaced, data loss during interface transmission, etc.).

Although the committee felt that full integration was the best long-term goal, the group recognized that a hybrid strategy of integration was the most cost-effective place to start. The selection committee chose a vendor to integrate the clinical processes for direct care providers that included physician order entry and clinical documentation for both the hospital and ambulatory environment. Clinical results and demographic data from existing legacy systems were interfaced for registration, laboratory, radiology, and transcription.

Managing the Project

Goals of the Project

To be successful, the project required a close partnership among administration, clinical department leaders, physicians and clinicians, the Information Technology department, and the vendor. A multidisciplinary steering committee was formed to execute the vision, develop a tactical plan, and provide project oversight. Throughout the project, physicians were actively engaged and provided the leadership for committees and work groups. Where possible, existing committee structures were utilized for communication to stakeholders and review of key design elements. Objectives for the project included:

1. To combine the inpatient and outpatient medical record into one longitudinal record with improved clinical access and availability.
2. To support educational and teaching objectives.
3. To integrate clinical information available from various legacy systems.
4. To support enterprisewide data integrity and process efficiencies.

Project Planning and Leadership

A project implementation team was recruited from within the organization and was composed of primarily clinicians. A senior nurse was appointed as liaison between the project staff and the Chief Nursing Officer to facilitate communication. An ambitious timetable was outlined due to the lack of Y2K compliance of various existing systems. The project team immediately assumed high visibility in the organization, and the project was given priority status and support.

The vice chancellor for health affairs, chief executive officer, chief operations officer, chief medical officer, and chief nursing officer, as well as other key administration officials, were tireless in their support and endorsement of the system and never ceased to encourage the skeptics. The chief medical officer kept the focus on patient safety and insisted on system features to support both efficiency and enhanced decision support for quality of care. The advocacy of the chief medical officer and nursing officer with their respective clinicians ensured the engagement of clinicians in system design and helped to sustain the project.

Implementation

Looking back, the planning phase was the most underrated yet pivotal phase of the project. During this phase, functional and interface requirements were defined, business processes were reviewed, and changes to policy and procedures were identified. In addition, the anticipated benefits of the system were understood, quantified, and assigned to appropriate phases of the project. Realization of these benefits became critical to success as the clinicians were rewarded for their transformation and the information technology staff recognized the value of their efforts and hard work. Other very practical parts of the transformation were solidified during the planning process, such as these:

- Design and renovate space for information technology staff.
- Design and build a training facility.
- Create a project team for implementation and support.
- Develop user support procedures and train personnel.
- Design and build network infrastructure; plan and install hardware.
- Redesign clinical workflow and data analysis processes.
- Develop a transformation implementation plan.
- Define historical data requirements and determine legacy data integrity.

System configuration began after building a detailed project plan with defined resources. During this phase, the reference database was created and shown to clinicians to ascertain usability issues and level of acceptance. These sessions were important not only to validate and perfect the design but to reinforce the key goals and objectives of the project and sustain interest. The most important lesson learned during the design and build phase was a very simple one: Listen to the clinicians; they know what they need for patient care. Eliminate processes that waste time and are redundant, and explore all options to support those that are critical to the provision of safe patient care. For UIMCC, having system analysts who were also clinicians was immensely helpful in understanding how to incorporate user wishes into system design. Other important items accomplished in this phase were the institution of stringent change control practices, a risk management plan, and constant communication to the organization regarding project progress. As this phase closed, simulated real-life scripts of key patient care processes were executed by untrained clinical users who assisted in uncovering any remaining errors that had not previously been identified during controlled testing.

Because a legacy patient care system existed for the inpatient setting and the ambulatory setting was dependent solely on paper medical records, the decision was made to introduce the new electronic health record to the ambulatory clinics. This decision had the immediate benefit of eliminating issues with the delivery of the paper medical record. The rollout began with a pilot clinic in October 1997 by populating the EHR with patient demographic data, laboratory, surgical pathology, and radiology results. Shortly after a successful pilot, the EHR was introduced to the remaining clinics. During the rollout, additional functionality was added to the system to bring more benefits such as clinical documentation and electronic signature.

The introduction of the EHR to the inpatient setting was approached differently as the legacy patient care system was not Y2K compliant and a gradual phased-in approach was not possible. Use of dual systems was not an acceptable option from the clinician's perspective, particularly in light of the fact that the implementation included physician order entry, physician documentation, and nursing medication documentation. A modified "big bang" approach was chosen to convert from one system to another. Although a big bang approach was chosen, a very short "dress rehearsal" was conducted on a pilot inpatient unit for 1 week. Doing a dress rehearsal provides the opportunity to flush out unforeseen issues that are easily corrected in a controlled environment but can result in chaos when released to the entire user community, such as print routing, user access, and build corrections. After a successful pilot, all inpatient nursing units, services, and departments were brought online over 3 days. Physicians reentered all orders, and the nurses assisted the physicians in a quality assurance role. The Chief Medical Officer played a key role facilitating communication between the clinical staff and the information technology (IT) department.

In addition to the order entry functions introduced in 1999, other functions such as charge services, components of nursing documentation, rules, and patient care tasks were also included. In July 2001 the medication process was fully integrated with the introduction of the pharmacy system, resulting in a fully automated medication process starting with physician order entry and ending with electronic medication scheduling and charting. All the components were now in place to assure knowledge-driven care and decision making could be enhanced through an event-driven decision support application that employs a graphical user-interface-based editor that allows for the easy creation of the rules.

In 2002, patient registration was integrated into the EHR. Reporting quality outcome measures for cardiology has also been introduced. Future plans include completing the clinical documentation process for all disciplines, enterprise scheduling, and automating the supporting functions of the intensive care unit, surgery suite, and the emergency department.

User Training and Support

Clinician acceptance of an EHR is less about software and technology and more about change management. It is critically important for trainers to have an understanding of adult learning and change principles. People generally have a fear of the unknown, and often prefer the known because it is understood and comfortable. Users have varying degrees of tolerance for change, learn at different rates, and need the time to adapt. In most cases those who are recalcitrant and against the change will convert to the new practices. Generally the trainers are the first to identify change management issues with clinicians and need to help them through at a pace that is tolerable to them.

Because of the vast numbers of users to be trained and a constrained timeframe, a computer-based training (CBT) program that guided the user through the system's features was developed and used to provide training on demand for all levels of staff. This CBT program could be accessed from anywhere on the network and also in open learning laboratories for those who felt the need for additional support by trainers. One of the features of the training program appreciated by the clinicians was its ability to track their progress through the modules so that upon their return they could start at the point where they left off. At the end of training, passing a competency test is required before a user is given access to the system.

Only employees who require patient information receive training, and the level of training varies depending on the individual's role and responsibilities. For example, clerical staff, physicians, and nurses all have different security levels and access to information that is tailored to the role they play in the provision of patient care. Establishing consensus on access for each role requires extensive discussion since it is a process unique to the EHR. Users must sign a confidentiality agreement before receiving system access. Access to a patient's data is automatically recorded along with a declared relationship of the care provider to the patient. Over time there continues to be a need to train physicians and clinicians because:

1. Physicians float between hospitals, requiring refresher training upon return.
2. Continuous system design improvements are constantly implemented.
3. New functionality is continually released by the vendor, tested, and implemented.
4. There is an ongoing need to optimize a clinician's use of the technology for improved efficiency and safety. At UIMCC today, a skilled clinician can no longer function successfully in clinical practice without EHR training.

Technology

Patient information can be entered into or retrieved from UIMCC's electronic health record from any one of 2500 personal computers located throughout the institution. These personal computers are hardwired to the network in both the inpatient and outpatient settings at every nurse station, in each exam room, in clinician workrooms, and in ancillary departments. For protection of the network, the use of local modems on individual personal computers is discouraged. As technology has progressed, additional wireless devices have been added for clinical care in the inpatient setting. These wireless devices are the favorites of the clinicians because they follow the clinician as he or she moves from patient to patient through the care delivery process.

In addition to access to the EHR, all personal computers and wireless devices provide access to reference applications including drug databases, patient education material, medical literature, and reference texts. These knowledge databases are integral to support the clinical care and teaching mission and many are also intelligently linked inside the EHR as well. Currently, document imaging, radiology picture archive images, ultrasound clips, EKGs, and endoscopic images must be accessed through the personal computer desktop. Future plans include integrating these images within the EHR.

The network has grown significantly since 1997, and today 185 Intel servers support the organization's business functions including clinical applications, e-mail, business desktop applications, printing, Intranet, and security services. The network is a shared physical infrastructure, and no separate network(s) exists for ancillary systems such as radiology. The network structure has evolved with technology over time and varies among the different buildings in the medical center. The newest building, the Outpatient Care Center, has a 10/100 Mbit switched Ethernet, and all the digital radiography equipment is connected to this infrastructure. Image traffic is segregated with the use of a Virtual LAN (VLAN). A gigabit Ethernet backbone network connects all switches in the Outpatient Care Center to the hospital. The hospital building runs at lower speed connections supported by 10/100 Mbit Ethernet switches. As remodeling or construction occurs, the wiring plant is improved and data jacks are upgraded to the 100 Mbit speed. Two physical gigabit paths connect the hospital switches to Outpatient Care Center. Local data centers in each building are maintained for application servers, ancillary databases, and e-mail servers. Minimal communication services (network access, e-mail, and local database applications) can be delivered if the building is isolated from the campus network.

The Information Technology Data Center provides a high security environment, and all mission-critical clinical databases are housed in this center. Database servers and key computing hardware are connected on a 100-Mbit FDDI network within the data center. External access to the network is strictly limited to data center routers and communications equipment. Redundancy of each feature of the data center was incorporated, including power feeds from two different grids in the city and dual air conditioning systems.

System Description and Functionality

The EHR is based on a three-tiered Health Network Architecture (HNA) provided by Cerner Corporation, Kansas City, Missouri, which includes mainframe servers, application servers, and personal computers or thin clients. Along with dependency on the electronic medical record comes the need for high availability and disaster recovery, and these must be planned for in the project. Components of disaster recovery to be considered are strategies for drive shadowing or redundancy, backup and recovery, and an off-site recovery plan if an unexpected disaster occurs requiring restoration. All points of failure must be considered, both inside the system as well as critical systems connecting to the EHR, for instance, backing up transactions that flow through the interface engine.

An interface engine utilizing Health Level 7 (HL7) standards exclusively manages interfaces between application systems. The medical center's approach since inception has been to define in detail and document interface specifications to later ensure their supportability. Among the external interfaces is a link to a transcription services vendor. This capability supports transcribed dictation to flow into the EHR for review, editing, and signature. The system directs documents to the correct physician's work center and into the patient's EHR.

Information available in UIMCC's EHR includes patient demographics, insurance information, allergies, problems/diagnosis, patient history and physical exams, diagnostic test results, medication lists, progress notes, consult reports, procedure notes, operative reports, inpatient medication administration records, inpatient orders, transcribed reports, and discharge summaries, as well as numerous other documents and reports. All the data are stored in a patient-centric data repository. Prior to the activation of the EHR, the existing legacy master person index was scoured to eliminate duplicate entries and loaded into the system. The system today includes basic patient information from as far back as 1995 and laboratory and test results beginning in 1997.

Functionality within the system is designed to enhance communication and teamwork between and among caregivers. The physician work center was designed to support workflow, organize information, and enhance clinician-to-clinician communication. The work center utilizes a desktop metaphor and exception-based processes to support the presentation and execution of clinical tasks. Data content and vocabulary are standardized by the system, which provides for consistent presentation of terms and vocabulary and further enhances communication. An example is the patient problem list that presents problems in both standard textual and codified terms (either ICD-9 or Snomed).

Cultural Change

As UIMCC has progressed past the initial implementation of the electronic health record, clinical staff gradually adapted and became competent working with the technology. Their interaction with user support personnel has become much more sophisticated such that initial troubleshooting is often done before contacting the IT department. For instance, users often know when rebooting will solve a problem, and they can convey information about which network server they are logged onto when they place their call. These new skills have transformed the way that staff, at all levels, manage patient information and their access to it. Use of a common chart with a defined nomenclature and standardization of terms has resulted in an evolution in clinical practice as well. Integrated data presentation views provide consistent views of the information for all caregivers.

The organization has developed higher expectations regarding the availability and transfer of information. Reflective of care delivery in this new electronic world, a seemingly insatiable demand for data has developed, whether it is for additional data capture, enhanced presentation, displays, or data reporting. With each improvement in efficiency and performance, the bar is raised, and the seconds that it takes for information to appear on the computer screen seems like an eternity despite the fact that in the past it could take hours to get an old chart from medical records. Keeping it simple and quick is the key to satisfying clinicians and provides a compelling argument to transform. Understanding clinical needs for data assimilation up-front during design can aid in acceptance and making the system seem simple and quick. The clinicians at UIMCC have developed an acceptance of the EHR as a continuously developing system. However, it is important to set expectations correctly since users are forced to straddle two worlds, paper and electronic, during transition periods. The continuous introduction of new functionality requires equal waves of training to assist the learning curve and related commitment of time on the part of the clinicians. Despite these issues, the improvements clinicians find in access to information tend to outweigh the time and effort investments and lead to acceptance of the system.

Electronic Health Record Benefits

The system's greatest benefit is its provision of immediate access to patient-specific information and communication of that information to all caregivers who need it. Integrated displays present data in intelligent summaries regardless of the source, be it bedside testing, clinic instruments, or laboratory instruments. The system also presents customized views to ascertain data trends. Graphing capabilities enhances this trending, highlights the trend, and is often utilized as a patient education tool. Communication between caregivers also has been vastly improved, which has enhanced the quality of patient care. Before the system, the emergency room physician often treated the patient in the absence of past clinical information because the patient's medical record seldom reached them during the care event. With the EHR in place, the emergency room physician has all the medical record available, including the name of the primary physician to contact for further consultation.

Nurses have reported saving time during their discussions with insurance companies since the information they request is readily available. Patient's satisfaction has risen since the ubiquity of the desktop record means the patient is no longer asked the same questions numerous times by a variety of caregivers throughout the institution. Physicians particularly like the fact that communication with other caregivers is a by-product of their interaction with the system and does not require additional steps. For example, the physician work center includes folders that contain documents to sign, documents to review, phone messages, and consult orders. Documents post to folders through a variety of methods, including a transcription interface, from another caregiver, via a phone message taken regarding a specific patient, or from a new consult order. Prior to the system, these processes were performed on paper. The result was much slower turnaround time to complete these tasks, and charts were unavailable to others while awaiting review.

Online documentation by clinicians has paid big dividends in quality and completeness of clinical documentation. In addition, the legibility and prompts for required information makes the documentation easier to audit. While compliance has risen and adherence to strict standards has increased, the problems of overdocumentation and the consequent loss of time and efficiency from the effort have risen. Design efforts to provide the clinician with guidance on acceptable levels of documentation are necessary.

Integration of the EHR with knowledge tools and alerts provides a powerful tool for the clinician. Before the implementation of the EHR, departments (laboratories, radiology, cardiology, etc.) printed at least two paper copies of every patient result. The first was sent to medical records to be filed in the paper chart. The second was printed in batches by ordering location, and then either delivered or left in mailboxes to be picked up. These efforts caused delays that could be measured in days, not hours. Print-outs might be delivered to the wrong location and were not sorted by, or delivered to, the specific caregiver who ordered the test. In the electronic world, the physician work center displays results within seconds from their release to the clinician who ordered the diagnostic test. Certainly the medical center has benefited from eliminating some paper storage costs. However, to the clinician, the instantaneous availability of the record, which despite best efforts could never be accomplished in the paper world, provides the greater benefit.

Subsequent to implementation of the new physician order entry software in 1999, the additional benefits not previously available such as duplicate order entry checking, alerts, and other knowledge reference tools were recognized. Synchronization between the orders and the Medication Administration Record (MAR) improved accuracy and timeliness and provided a real-time view of the patient's current medication status.

Patient Safety and Quality Care

The level of quality and safety in our nation's healthcare delivery system has been called into question, with unprecedented national attention and with business groups taking a hard line that improvement is necessary. Our journey toward patient safety, led by our chief executive officer, began with a commitment for high-quality and safe care at all levels of the organization.

Through its centralized design and standardized data, the EHR has enhanced patient safety efforts by delivering reliable, more comprehensive, and readable information. Utilization of paper records with multiple clinical systems is fragmented and may result in each having different values from points in time and thus providing misleading views of the patient's current condition. For example, the nursing documentation system may show the patient is allergic to a drug while the pharmacy system indicates "no known allergies." An integrated patient-centric database minimizes discrepancies and ensures better data integrity by standardizing formats and requiring critical data to be recorded in one location and shared with all. With shared information, clinicians are more likely to read what others have documented. Also, the reduction and in some cases elimination of transcription in the process has led to a reduced opportunity for errors.

Errors from omission have also been eliminated. With paper medical records, there were frequently problems with misplaced reports and/or notes that delayed the clinician in decision making. Legible, complete documentation eliminates these frustrating delays and improves patient safety. Because availability of online patient information is assured at all times, fewer departments feel a need to hoard charts or maintain "shadow charts" locally. In the past, this practice interfered with the Health Information Management (HIM) department's ability to keep the record complete and provide it to all clinicians wishing to review it. Now, HIM resources formerly assigned to filing mountains of loose paper in patient's charts have been reassigned to other duties such as quality audits leading to improved compliance by clinicians.

Access, timeliness, and appropriateness of care have been improved with the implementation of the system. Nurses take calls from patients and document details of the encounter and advice given to the patient in the patient's electronic record. This documentation can be easily routed to the correct physician's work center for review and follow-up. The physician can add information to the documentation, leveraging the work already performed by the nurse.

In summary, our progress can be attributed to an effective partnership between leadership, clinical knowledge experts, and operational process improvement efforts all combined with supporting information technology. The supporting IT combines improved data integrity with interactive rules and knowledge databases to enhance care processes such as orders and documentation. As a result, we were better able to address myriad safety needs including medication safety, infection management, pressure ulcer prevention, restraint management, and fall prevention. This part of the journey is an ongoing cycle of review and assessment leading to future improvements. Establishing medical staff review and approval will be essential to the acceptance of these efforts.

Medical Decision Support

Since the medical center had limited experience with rules and alerts, it was decided to take a "walk before you run" approach. One of the first issues that arose was how to and who should provide clinical oversight and judgment. In previous years, the medical staff had always handled practice standard development between affected service chiefs informally. No medical staff process existed for building consensus on practice standards that were key to the development of rules and alerts at an enterprise level. The payoff can be large if the consensus-building initiative is characterized by diligence, perseverance, and compromise along with a bit of tenacity. From experience, the consensus-building efforts should begin well in advance of the need to design and develop a decision support process.

Recently, the chief medical officer has established a new medical staff committee to oversee the evolving practice standards automated by the system. The rules and alerts are presented to this committee after development and testing have been completed. Two clinicians, paired with content experts in the discipline that the rule will affect, are assigned to formulate the rule(s) logic. The rule is presented to this new committee for review and approval after it has been created, tested, and its impact on system performance validated through a background process. At present there are a number of successful rules running that include preventing the ordering of a medication in the absence of documented allergy status, guidelines to govern anticoagulant therapy, and alerts to clinicians regarding renal status when a renally cleared medication is ordered. While these rules and alerts have been effective in changing clinical practice, they have also shown great benefit in adjusting operational behaviors as well.

Reengineering processes to enhance access and operational processes have also been core features of the system design. An automatic search against a medication database for adverse drug interactions and allergies is done each time a physician orders a medication. If a potential adverse reaction is detected, the user is presented with a Drug Allergy/Interaction Summary window. This alert summarizes the ordered medication, the existing allergy, medication previously ordered for which there is a conflict, and the severity of the interaction. The caregiver then has the option to discontinue the ordered medication, discontinue the existing medication, or continue with the order.

Medical error reduction and the improvement of care quality are key benefits that automatically accrue through the use of the EHR. Now that foundational systems are in place, this is an area that strategically will grow and evolve within the system. For all that has been achieved, we know much more lies ahead. We have only just begun to scratch the surface of all that can be accomplished by incorporating rules, knowledge, alerts, and content into the equation. At this point, some paper remains as part of the paper chart and is waiting to be converted; this includes outpatient orders, nursing assessments, and consents for treatment.

The Destination

We hope you have enjoyed learning about our Transformation Journey. We are certain that because no two health systems are exactly alike, no two transformation journeys will mirror each other. Similarly, no two transformation journeys within UIMCC share exactly the same features. From physician order entry to meds integration, from going paperless to decision support, our experiences in achieving distinct milestones have all been decidedly unique. What's more, transformation is not an end state. Our ongoing transformation most certainly will continue to offer new lessons, new knowledge, and new improvements.

Acknowledgments. The efforts and accomplishments detailed here are the result of numerous individuals who have worked tirelessly to achieve a clinical information system for improved patient care. The heroes of this project are the administration, clinicians, and staff who have dedicated their lives toward aiding others, but, most of all, the men and women of the UIMCC Information Technology Department, physician champions (Drs. Sarne, Galanter, Hier, and Chamberlin), and Joyce Coundourides and Marikay Menard, who have each made a personal investment in building this dream.

19
CIO STORIES, VI
Maimonides Medical Center, Brooklyn, NY: A Technical and Cultural Transformation

ANN C. SULLIVAN

Maimonides' new information environment features the only known deployment of four integrated EMR systems plus 100 percent physician order entry.

Brooklyn, New York's Maimonides Medical Center is the third largest independent teaching hospital in the country and site of the nation's first human heart transplant. Maimonides is also an institution with deep roots in the community, particularly the nearby Orthodox Jewish neighborhood of Borough Park. Bound by tradition, the institution had resisted the transition to modern information systems that most U.S. hospitals had embraced for decades.

In the mid-1990s, the information environment at Maimonides was operating in a time warp—1950s vintage keypunch machines, ancient mainframes, no network, no desktop PCs. From my perspective as new chief information officer (CIO), it was quaint—but also deeply troubling. Forces such as healthcare deregulation and managed competition were bearing down on us like a steamroller.

We had a lot of catching up to do, and top management knew it. In 1996, Maimonides's CEO, Stanley Brezenoff, and COO, Pamela Brier, committed one third of the hospital's capital budget for the next 3 years to build a state-of-the-art information environment—buildings, staff, and technologies—all at once.

The project would mean altering the daily work activities of thousands of people and was a transformation as much cultural as technological. We had to address several challenges in parallel: building an MIS team capable of leading the transition, identifying and deploying new technology where virtually no foundation existed, and preparing the organization to embrace the new system. One key constituency would be particularly affected: the hospital's physicians, as the CEO took a strong stand requiring 100 percent adoption of Computer Physician Order Entry (CPOE).

Our efforts led to the emergence of Maimonides Access Clinical System (MACS), a new information environment that has transformed the delivery of health care at Maimonides and positioned the institution for long-term growth. MACS features a number of technical achievements, including the only known deployment of four inte-

---

Ann C. Sullivan, MBA, is Senior Vice President and CIO of the Maimonides Medical Center.

grated electronic medical record systems. But more to the point, we have achieved our goal of 100 percent physician order entry as well as dramatic improvements in patient safety and efficiency. In recognition of these accomplishments, Maimonides was awarded the 1998 Computerworld Smithsonian award and the 2002 CPRI Davies award.

Building the Team

The first challenge was to build an MIS staff with the talent and credibility to sustain a project of this magnitude. Above all, I was looking for people with clinical experience, since they were most knowledgeable in how a computer system can best meet caregiver needs. Whenever possible, our strategy was to hire people from within the hospital and teach them the necessary technology, particularly the clinical systems and electronic records. We discovered that it was almost always faster to teach internal people computer technology than for technology people to learn the inner workings of the medical center.

During this time, the hospital was undergoing a redesign through Ernst & Young. The threat of a reduction of hospitalwide personnel led many of the nurses, pharmacists, and lab and radiology technicians, several of whom who had been with the hospital for years and knew the organization intimately, to join the MIS Department. Since MIS was growing, I offered to hire interested clinicians and train them in our new Computer Patient Record. We hired 16 people this way, trained them well, and they became the backbone of our department.

As physicians were going to be prime users of the new system, it was clear that they had to be closely involved in the design for the project to succeed. However, most physicians cannot afford to take time away from their practice. The solution was simple: we put several physicians on the MIS payroll, representing different departments and medical specialties. Their ideas and knowledge were essential during construction of knowledge-driven order sets, screen design, and documentation.

The participating physicians brought enormous credibility to the project while serving as advocates for MIS with their colleagues. It was also important that they continue to practice during their MIS engagement, both for ongoing credibility and to experience the system from the same perspective as their peers.

Elements of MACS

MACS includes a core of four electronic medical record (EMR) systems, which integrate with over 30 ancillary, clinical, and administrative systems. While the original intent was to deploy a single EMR system hospitalwide, as the project unfolded, it became clear that some specialty areas had needs that were distinct enough to require their own dedicated solution. As a result, Maimonides selected discrete departmental EMR systems for Ambulatory Care, Obstetrics, and the Emergency Department, all integrating with an Inpatient EMR system. These core systems are:

- *Ambulatory Care:* NextGen EMR (NextGen Healthcare Information Systems, Horsham, PA).
- *Emergency Department:* HealthMatics ED (A4 Health Systems, Cary, NC).
- *Obstetrics:* Intelligent Patient Record for Obstetrics (IPRob) (E&C Medical Intelligence, Glen Rock, NJ).

- *Inpatient:* Eclipsys HCM 7000, to be replaced by Eclipsys Sunrise Clinical Manager in 2003 (Eclipsys Corporation, Boca Raton, FL).

Laying the groundwork for the EMRs meant creating a complete information technology (IT) infrastructure. The Maimonides MIS department started literally from the ground up, building a new headquarters with the facilities necessary to support a major urban medical center. We installed a SONET enterprise network, deployed 2058 PCs throughout the hospital, and built a new server farm and mainframe data center. Most hospitals would take years to complete these tasks, but we did not have the luxury of further delays. MIS successfully completed these projects in only 9 months, winning the credibility needed to lead the hospital in further technology initiatives.

Few ancillary systems were in place prior to 1995, which meant that MIS had to plan and implement a number of new systems including radiology, voice recognition, document imaging, transcription, and Picture Archive and Communication System (PACS). The few existing systems had to be upgraded, including the laboratory, blood bank, and anatomical pathology systems. New administrative systems were deployed simultaneously, including Peoplesoft Financial and Human Resources applications as well as new patient registration and accounting systems.

Building Vendor Relationships

Before the project got underway, technology vendors were fleeing because software purchased years before had not been installed. We needed to turn these relationships around: to make Maimonides an institution that vendors would want to do business with. We met with our major vendors and discussed how we could partner together for mutual benefit. Technology vendors place strong value on organizations that successfully implement their applications, but we were not in that position. We therefore had to define creative new relationships that vendors would find attractive.

The solution was "vendor partnerships": a win–win arrangement where the hospital and the vendor work together to create the best solution for the healthcare IT market. This could range from advising vendors in products and services for the healthcare market to serving as a Northeast center of excellence for vendors to showcase their latest products. It could also mean engaging in codevelopment efforts with vendors to provide the precise functionality required by individual departments within the medical center. In short, Maimonides and our vendor partners were willing to do whatever was necessary to ensure each other's success.

MIS also worked closely with vendors to develop systems with the precise functionality that individual departments require. For example, the Obstetrics EMR was built in Israel as a standalone departmental system, but at Maimonides it had to integrate with the Inpatient EMR. To achieve the needed functionality, the vendor worked with the medical center to develop interfaces to patient accounting, radiology, food and nutrition, and other systems.

Upon the project's success, the Obstetrics EMR vendor approached Maimonides to become its national application implementation partner. Future goals include joint development of a fully integrated comprehensive EMR for obstetrical patients from prenatal through postpartum. As a result of this and other strong relationships, Maimonides founded Technology4HealthCare, LLC, a for-profit enterprise dedicated to bringing advanced EMR solutions to hospitals across the United States.

Engaging the Physicians

The success of MACS depended on physician participation and ownership—not just grudging tolerance, but recognition that their input would have a significant impact on the care they provided to their patients. Maimonides developed several strategies to win physician engagement and obtain their input. We were also determined to be as flexible as possible to accommodate their needs. (For example, MIS conducted training in the middle of the night to meet the crammed schedules of some doctors.)

Recruiting Physician Leaders

We sought out physician leaders who were already advocates for physician systems and recruited them to help lead the project. For example, the chairman of orthopedics is also a degreed engineer who develops and sells his own software products. He was a natural choice to chair the MACS Physician Task Force, the body charged with setting policies and making decisions affecting physicians and other users. His peers looked to him as a technology mentor, which made him an ideal champion for the new project, and he also loved the challenge of spearheading the transition through the various factions within the physician community.

Two project sponsors, one representing the hospital's salaried attending physicians and one representing voluntary community-based physicians, were also chosen for their personal and professional attributes. The attending physician sponsor is the chair of the Emergency Department, an individual very interested in technology and widely known as a driving force behind the hospital's EMR efforts. The sponsor for the voluntary physicians was also highly respected as a former President of the Hospital's Medical Staff.

Finally, we benefited greatly from a "coach" (our Medical Director) who had an intimate knowledge of the institution, its politics, and informal organization. While he had no formal authority in the MACS project, he was invaluable in guiding us through the implementation process, frequently steering us away from landmines that people did not even know were there.

Physician Segments

The different physician groups each had their own needs and priorities, including community physicians, paid attending physicians, residents, medical students, nurse practitioners, and physician assistants. MIS made certain that these different groups were well represented on the task force and other governing bodies. We also learned that tailoring the implementation to fit the needs of each segment greatly increased the likelihood of acceptance and project success. For example, community physicians were very concerned about gaining access to the system from their home or office. To meet their needs, MIS developed a special version of the system called *OfficeMACS*, providing remote access to patient data and results.

Small Details That Go a Long Way

We also paid attention to small but important details where MIS could provide value to physicians and help them work more productively. For example, we made it much easier for doctors to find current pager numbers for their colleagues. A physician only had to enter his or her pager number once, and it would appear in every pathway where it was needed. These types of details, properly communicated, went a long way in securing physician buy-in.

Communicating the Results

As the project evolved, it was important to communicate the results and show that we were acting on physician input as much as possible. MIS obtained a standing invitation to attend monthly meetings of the various medical specialties. This participation greatly enhanced communication, allowing MIS staff to provide project updates as they affected different medical disciplines and hear physician concerns firsthand. To convince caregivers to buy into the new system, we also had to communicate how the new system would benefit each user community. For example, for obstetricians, the ability of the Obstetrical EMR to cut potential for lawsuits made a strong impression.

Training Strategy

The medical staff credits the MIS training approach as the single most important factor in the overall success of the project. Even in the mid-1990s, most of our hospital community had no basic computer skills. MIS launched a massive training program that would enable caregivers to meet the demands of a 21st century healthcare institution. We started literally from the ground up: creating a training center, building classrooms, hiring six nurse educators, developing courses, and training manuals. As of March 2002, 13,722 individuals had received over 61,000 hours of formal training.

We knew that getting physicians to use a CPR system in their daily work would determine whether the entire project would succeed or fail. Therefore, we created a training environment bringing together several crucial elements, including the right instructors, the right curriculum, the right manuals, the right schedule—even the right names for courses.

We learned that when it came to computer training, most physicians hated the "T-word" and the stigma of being seen as computer novices. So we didn't call it training—instead we used terms like "Navigating the Internet," and attendance was standing room only. The sight of a stack of pizzas being delivered to a classroom was another effective tactic!

Physicians, nurses, and ancillary staff all receive separate customized training. Not only do clinical pathways differ, but also each caregiver, although looking at a common patient, sees the information from a different perspective. Within the Inpatient EMR, physicians' classes are customized to each specialty. For example, a surgeon would be taught the screens for postoperative order entry, while an oncologist would be instructed in using chemotherapy order screens.

MIS recruited nurses that physicians knew and trusted, who became MIS employees as MACS instructors. "Just-in-time" training ensures the material is fresh in the user's mind. Training demand intensified during new application launches, and in the month of June, when new physicians start. During these periods, classes were scheduled in the morning, afternoon, and evenings, including weekends. If a physician's schedule conflicted with the training schedule, MIS would arrange a class to accommodate that physician, even in the middle of the night when necessary.

Careful attention was given to instruction materials. MIS created personalized manuals for each caregiver, explaining each screen used for their clinical specialty along with a quick reference guide. Physicians also received a customized pocket guide with directions to their clinical pathways, such as lab and medication order screens, along with phone numbers to call for assistance.

Support by Clinicians

The second most important success factor (besides comprehensive training) was providing support by trained clinicians. During go-live times, support staff was tripled.

Clinical Command Center

Support is coordinated from a dedicated facility, the Clinical Command Center. Available by dialing MACS, the Command Center is equipped with the latest help management software and staffed 24/7 by nurses, physicians, and other clinicians who are experts on the four EMR systems and ancillary applications. When a caregiver on the floor reports a problem, a clinically trained MACS expert can walk them through the screens on the phone, or in person on the unit. (To avoid distracting Command Center staff with nonclinical issues, MIS also maintains a conventional IT Help Desk, which can be reached by dialing *HELP*.)

"Super Users"

Complementing the Command Center staff, a cadre of expert nurses were designated as "Super Users" to provide clinical support on the floor and conduct on-the-job training, especially during fast-paced go-live periods. The program was initiated by seeking volunteers, but we discovered that it was possible to identify individuals who would make good super users and then recruit them. Successful super users were characterized by a commitment to transforming service delivery, a flair for working with physicians, and an upbeat attitude.

Continuous Improvement Processes

MACS is a work in progress that belongs to all Maimonides caregivers, and is as effective and valuable as its users are willing to make it. User feedback is vital, and various processes have been put in place to ensure ongoing improvement and consensus.

User Groups

Maimonides has a very active and vocal culture of user groups. Nobody holds back at user group meetings, which provide an ongoing forum to raise application issues, debate workflow changes, and prioritize upgrades and enhancements. There are user groups for specific types of caregivers as well as integrated groups representing a cross section of user types. For example, the OB integrated user group includes representatives from attending physicians, residents, nursing, medical records, and legal. Each user group submits its requests for improvements to the physician task force, which determines overall priorities.

Command Center Database

Calls to the Clinical Command Center are logged in a Microsoft Access database to identify potential areas for improvement. For example, if the software flags recurring questions about how to enter a particular IV, the correct procedure can be emphasized in training sessions and highlighted in the training manual. This process of tracking

Command Center calls also helps audit MACS itself, since numerous calls about a clinical pathway may indicate that a change to the pathway is required. MIS communicates these updates via regular bulletins to affected departments and also makes personal visits to demonstrate the changes.

Training Improvement Cycle

The MACS training program is specifically designed to enable continuous improvements. Caregiver training leads to feedback on the training process, which leads to enhancements to the curriculum. Questions from the floor come into the Clinical Command Center, where they are used to adjust either the curriculum or MACS screens. The information is posted to an expert system, which guides improvements to the training curriculum and MACS.

Assessing the Benefits

Results at Maimonides demonstrate that physician order entry with knowledge-based decision support leads to more accurate and efficient treatment. Since implementing the EMR systems, the medical center has shown remarkable improvements in patient outcomes, greater efficiency, and increased hospital revenues. Among the highlights:

- *Patient safety:* The hospital has seen a sharp reduction in medication errors and adverse reactions. In 2001, the decision support feature of the inpatient EMR identified 164,250 drug–drug, drug–allergy, drug–food, and drug–duplication alerts, resulting in 82,125 beneficial changes in treatment. In addition, problem medication orders decreased by 58 percent and medication discrepancies by 60 percent. Electronic medication management eliminated pharmacy transcription errors as well as errors such as incorrect date, time, quantity, route, or frequency.
- *Length of stay:* With improved efficiency and patient outcomes, the average length of stay at Maimonides decreased from 7.26 days to 5.05 days from 1995 to 2001. (This is 1 full day less than all other New York City voluntary hospitals.)
- *Efficiency:* The time required to deliver medications from an order to the patient's bedside was reduced from 276 minutes to 88 minutes—a 68 percent improvement. Duplicate medical tests (which are both costly and prolong the length of stay) were reduced by an average of 20 percent. In radiology, the introduction of PACS and voice recognition helped reduce the time to deliver a final radiology report from 180 hours to within the same day.
- *Patient access:* The reduced length of stay enabled an increase of 32,168 admissions since 1995, 8000 of which are directly attributable to MACS. With the additional admissions, the hospital realized a $19.8 million increase in revenue the first year alone. Patient access also improved significantly in the Emergency Department, where faster turnaround time resulted in an increase in visits from 57,795 in 1996 to 77,118 in 2001.

The Payback

Although traditional cost–benefit analysis is difficult for clinical systems, Maimonides outcome data show real and measurable benefits. MACS has shown a return of investment (ROI) for all investments of 9.4 percent in a payback period of 46 months, plus marked improvements in patient care and cost efficiency. Table 19.1 provides details of the ROI model, showing the payback for the $43.9 million investment.

TABLE 19.1. ROI worksheet for tangibles at Maimonides.

Option Description MACS Summary Factor (in thousands of $'s)*	Year 0*	9.4% ROI: Return on investment 46 PP: Payback Period (Months) Year 1	Year 2	Year 3	Year 4	3.84 PP: Payback Period (Years) Year 5	Year 6	Total
INITIAL INVESTMENT:								
Inpatient CPR	6,033	3,050	696	200	723	423	0	11,125
Laboratory	1,223	0	106	0	0	56	931	2,316
Blood Bank	101	1	0	0	0	0	0	102
Interface & Integration Engine	294	245	0	147	259	298	431	1,674
Enterprise Network	1,830	874	3,992	339	72	0	0	7,107
Decision Support	1,078	1,508	111	468	253	0	0	3,418
Radiology	426	138	0	0	0	0	0	564
PACS	2,159	1,344	420	544	0	0	0	4,467
Voice Recognition	186	0	0	0	0	0	0	186
ED CPR	677	34	0	1,046	829	864	0	3,450
Ambulatory CPR	1,654	1,632	1,813	1,017	1,077	0	0	7,193
Perinatal CPR	556	1,134	617	0	0	0	1,362	2,307
Total Initial Investment	16,217	9,960	7,755	3,761	3,213	1,641	1,362	43,909
Capital Reimbursement		649	1,047	1,357	1,508	1,636	1,053	7,250
Grant Revenue: Ambulatory CPR-CHCCDP	0	1,166	1,632	1,398	466	0	0	4,662
Grant Revenue: Perinatal CPR-FOJP	0	0	100	100	100	0	0	300
New Total Initial Investment	16,217	8,145	4,976	906	1,139	5	309	31,697
ONGOING EXPENSES:								
Inpatient CPR	0	0	2,046	2,122	2,211	2,301	0	8,680
Laboratory	0	239	246	254	262	270	279	1,550
Blood Bank	0	38	39	41	42	43	0	203
Interface & Integration Engine	0	0	160	164	169	174	180	847
Enterprise Network	0	414	828	1,741	1,744	1,748	0	6,475
Decision Support	0	0	0	254	363	367	0	984
Radiology	0	67	119	121	123	125	0	555
PACS	0	358	362	365	369	373	0	1,827
Voice Recognition	1	41	49	61	62	62	0	276

	Year 0	Year 1	Year 2	Year 3	Year 4	Year 5	Year 6	Total
ED CPR	0	0	0	0	0	0	543	543
Ambulatory CPR	0	0	0	0	0	855	881	1,736
Perinatal CPR	0	0	0	645	669	689	710	2,713
Total Ongoing Expenses	1	1,157	3,849	5,768	6,014	7,007	2,593	26,389
Total ALL Expenses Per Year	16,218	9,302	8,825	6,674	7,153	7,012	2,902	58,086
Total ALL Expenses Cumulative	16,218	25,520	34,345	41,019	48,172	55,184	58,086	58,086
SAVINGS & EFFICIENCIES:								
Inpatient CPR (Includes Revenue)	4,625	7,372	14,100	14,568	14,430	0	0	55,095
Laboratory	0	0	0	0	0	0	0	0
Blood Bank	0	0	0	0	0	0	0	0
Interface & Integration Engine	0	0	0	0	0	0	0	0
Enterprise Network	0	0	0	0	0	0	0	0
Decision Support	2,048	2,048	2,048	2,048	2,048	0	0	10,240
Radiology	186	278	282	282	282	0	0	1,321
PACS	908	2,724	1,593	1,604	1,616	0	0	8,445
Voice Recognition	155	155	155	155	155	0	0	775
ED CPR	Not Yet Available							
Ambulatory CPR	Not Yet Available							
Perinatal CPR	Not Yet Available							
Total GROSS Payoffs Per Year	7,922	12,577	18,178	18,657	18,531	0	—	75,876
Total GROSS Payoffs Cumulative	7,933	20,510	38,688	57,345	75,876	75,876	75,876	75,876
Total NET Payoffs Per Year	6,765	8,728	12,410	12,643	11,524	(2,593)	0	49,487
Total NET Payoffs Cumulative	6,775	15,503	27,913	40,556	52,080	49,487	49,487	49,487
NET CASH FLOW								
Net Cash Flow Annual	(16,207)	(1,380)	3,752	11,504	11,504	11,519	(2,902)	17,790
Net Cash Flow Cumulative	(16,207)	(17,587)	(13,835)	(2,331)	9,173	20,692	17,790	17,790

* Year 0 = First Year Of Project.

Ancillary systems have also provided measurable benefits. PACS is an example of an application that has clearly proven its worth, with a payback period of less than 20 months. Electronic access to images allows faster image interpretation and improved decision making, while allowing Maimonides to eliminate film processing and storage costs. In another example, a voice recognition system in radiology delivered a payback period of 18 months through elimination of transcription costs and faster turnaround of reports.

While MACS has demonstrated its worth from a strictly financial perspective, it is impossible to place a value on more rapid access to more complete and accurate patient information for clinical providers and staff. How is the value of reduced medical errors, or most important, of satisfied customers, measured? Clearly, clinical information systems are justified—and by more than strictly quantified financial benefits. Today, the vision for MACS has come to life: an information system environment that has brought dramatic improvements in the delivery of patient care while positioning Maimonides as a world-class medical institution for the years ahead.

20
CIO STORIES, VII
Children's Hospital, Columbus: Realizing CPOE Through an Effective CIO-CMO Partnership

ROBERT A. SCHWYN

In this implementation of computerized physician order entry, the CMO's role was instrumental in helping to achieve physician buy-in.

The current ongoing rollout of computerized physician order entry (CPOE) across the clinical areas of Children's Hospital in Columbus, Ohio, and the success achieved to date, would not have been possible without executive sponsorship by the Chief Medical Officer (CMO) and a close partnership between the CMO, the Chief Information Officer (CIO), and the entire Information Services (IS) Division. The components of this successful partnership are multifaceted and continue to evolve as the organization shifts to a more *centric focus* that recognizes information technology (IT) as a key enabler in improving clinical care. Even more important is the cultural transformation of the organization to one receptive to change as a result of new and evolving technologies. This chapter describes the approach and a framework that Children's Hospital used to build an effective partnership with the physician constituents.

Previous Attempts at Physician Order Entry

Children's Hospital began its first endeavor with computerized physician order entry back in the early 1990s and recognized fairly early that

1. While the concept of CPOE was acknowledged as a top priority for the organization, it lacked strong physician leadership to sponsor the initiative.
2. Commercially available software to meet physician needs was unavailable in the market.

These two factors led Children's to "table" the initiative until both aspects improved. In the late 1990s, Children's began another attempt at CPOE, this time with a half-time (0.5 FTE) appointed physician informatics representative and a newer, more functionally rich commercial software product. Children's was able to implement

---

Robert A. Schwyn, MBA, is Vice President for Information Services at Children's Hospital in Columbus, OH.

CPOE in November 1998 in a Neonatal Intensive Care Unit. While this effort was successful in garnering general awareness for the importance of the project, it continued to lack the necessary physician involvement and buy-in from the medical staff and other clinical disciplines to be effective in changing clinical practice and maintaining a focus on continuous improvement. Unfortunately, at this time, the vendor also announced that this product was scheduled to be "sunsetted," so all efforts to continue expansion were discontinued. Having made significant progress in implementing this one-unit pilot, however, Children's proceeded yet a third time, focusing on the lessons it had learned from the two previous attempts, and in early 2000, Children's began working with a new vendor and a new product.

Knowing that a limited number of hospitals across the country had achieved successful CPOE implementations, although *without* the robust clinical functionality that was desired, the CIO of Children's Information Services division recognized that the biggest hurdle to cross was physician acceptance and buy-in. An opportunity arose, allowing a new physician informatist to begin working with Information Services for 50 percent of his time. This physician was a recent graduate of the Children's Pediatric Residency program, was well accepted and known at Children's, and already had proven himself capable of leading IT initiatives that enabled improvements in clinical care. It was obvious that this physician could be instrumental in bridging the clinical–technical gap, but it was unrealistic to assume that he could address the long-standing cultural and political challenges involved in IT-enabled change.

For nearly a year, the CIO focused his efforts on educating the executive leadership on the pitfalls and lessons learned from the previous attempts, as well as on other relevant industry best practices. His goal was to engage the senior leadership in understanding this effort as a key strategic priority. As can be seen from the representation of organizational "readiness" in Figure 20.1, for an organization to be successful in

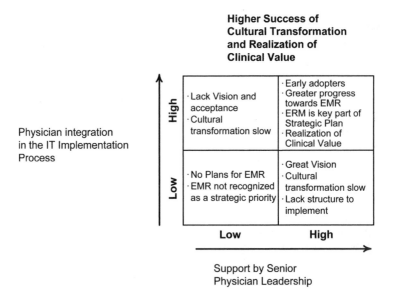

FIGURE 20.1. There is a clear relationship between strong physician leadership and involvement and an organization's state of readiness for it to be successful in implementing IT initiatives.

implementing IT initiatives, both strong physician leadership and strong involvement on the part of physicians are essential.

Establishing the Partnership

In late 2000, the Institute of Medicine and the Leapfrog Group began to exert a visible influence in patient safety initiatives on most healthcare organizations. Partially as a result, Children's CMO, who was relatively new in this role, began to actively recognize the value of IT as an enabler in achieving patient safety goals. The CIO and CMO began to collaborate on the CPOE initiative; it was clear from the onset that understanding each other's roles, agreeing on approach, and providing collaborative leadership was critical in making this venture successful.

The process began with numerous one-on-one sessions, whose goal was for them to grasp the complexity of the project they were contemplating before roles could be defined. Fortunately, since the scope of the project had not been finalized, an opportunity was available for the CMO to be involved from the "ground up." Because of his commitment to the project and willingness to invest his time personally, the CMO stated explicitly his expectation that other key leaders would participate in helping set the scope and in being involved in the design process for the project. This effort, to get other clinical leaders to participate as part of the process, would prove paramount in achieving buy-in later on. In the past, the CIO had attempted to involve clinical leaders, but, unfortunately, he lacked the authority and institutional commitment that the CMO was able to obtain by stating his vision and focus. On several occasions, the CMO stated, "I see this as part of my job" and commented that "spending over 50 percent" of his time each day working on IT issues was critical in changing the culture of the organization.

Crafting a Road Map

As the partnership started to evolve, it was clear that both the CMO and CIO needed to be "on the same page" in articulating a clear, consistent vision for how IT, and more specifically, the Electronic Medical Record (EMR) would evolve at Children's. Mounting industry pressure to improve patient safety, coupled with Children's goal of becoming a national leader in pediatrics, was useful in helping to establish a definition of quality and, more specifically, how it would be measured. Establishing a defined and documented description of quality as it related to the EMR was a pivotal process in driving all organizational quality and safety initiatives, particularly those practices and procedures that could be enabled with the use of technology. Having these goals in place is critical in strategically grounding an organization in the importance of quality as the driver. Physicians also clearly understand the need for quality initiatives and have a heartfelt passion for providing the best and safest care to their patients. Having a strategy driven on quality, rather than on a historical approach driven by utilization review and/or financial enhancement, is instrumental in achieving physician buy-in.

Creating the EMR Vision and Direction

Children's needed to have a clear, concise vision for how the EMR would evolve to support its strategic quality goals. The CMO and CIO collaborated on a strategy that was simple, yet effective, in communicating plans for the EMR. It included developing a template that identified the following:

- Major components (e.g., Inpatient, Emergency Department, Perioperative, Ambulatory).
- Timeline.
- Priorities.

Children's EMR Vision Template (Table 20.1) was not a comprehensive model that addressed every area and every constituent; it was more important to have a simple model that was easily understood by everyone and did not overwhelm the organization. This template, while very dynamic, has served as a tool for setting organizational priorities and is also a key element in the individual performance plans of the organization's leadership.

Defining Key Investment Principles

Despite having a clear vision within the organization about direction and priorities relating to the EMR, a disparity still existed within the leadership about how various clinical areas would utilize technology to support the EMR. Other organizations have struggled with disparate technical solutions that lack integration or are difficult to interface. Children's wanted to assure that every dollar invested not only helped move the organization closer to an EMR but also to ensure that the goals of a totally integrated EMR would be achieved. Therefore, it was important to establish key investment principles that would serve to govern all future investments related to the EMR. Historically, developing these principles at Children's was purely an IT initiative. However, as partnerships within the organization strengthened, the Chief Medical Officer recognized the value not only of collaborating on the creation of investment principles but also of supporting them. These key principles are defined as follows:

1. Every investment must address patient safety, improved quality, enhanced security, and greater availability of care.
2. All solutions must be capable of supporting full integration of the patients' data, whether through integration with existing solutions or through interfaces, supporting a goal of a single access to all components of the patients' information.

   a. Niche clinical systems would only be acquired if there were a compelling short-term return on investment (ROI).
   b. Scanning technology would only be used to provide access to those components that could not be computerized or enhanced to provide improvements in patient safety.

TABLE 20.1. Children's EMR Vision Template.

	Inpatient	Perioperative	Emergency Department	Outpatient
Documentation				
Lab				
Reports				
VS, I & O				
Notes				
Attending				
Residents				
Nursing/staff				
Consults				
Order entry				
Scheduling				

3. All investments would support a single sign-on process utilizing a two-factor authentication process using biometrics.
4. All solutions will be capable of supporting industry standards relating to data transmission (e.g., HL7), image transmission (Dicom), and a standard clinical vocabulary.

Garnering Financial Support

The process of creating a long-range IT plan with projections for financial investments was a traditional IT process, and, on many occasions, the CIO had proposed well-defined and well-thought-out plans for implementing technology to support clinical initiatives. These plans were historically met with reservation with regard to the accuracy of the projected financial investments as well as skepticism regarding the ability for the anticipated outcomes to be realized.

In this new model, both the CIO and the CMO teamed up in an effort to convey a level of confidence that the anticipated benefits could be achieved. Historically, the CIO had made many compelling arguments justifying the value of investing in technology, but they fell short of convincing the organization that the investments would truly have an impact on patient care. Thus, having the CMO articulate that needed improvements in patient care could be achieved using IT was critical in generating confidence. In addition, both the CMO and the CIO are accountable from an individual performance perspective; if the stated goals are not achieved, both individuals are held accountable.

Having achieved a moderate amount of success in the improvement of patient safety and quality from several other recent clinical technology projects, also helped make the compelling case that any investment would have a high probability of success. Traditionally, these projects had been seen as IT projects and lacked the senior-level commitment needed to address the cultural changes required. Interestingly enough, because of this collaborative model, and recognizing that Children's was clearly at the forefront of the "early adopter" stage of technology availability, the senior leadership and the board were willing to assume a higher level of risk in making an investment. This willingness by the senior leadership to take a more aggressive position with regard to investing in the EMR helped tremendously to support the organization's strategic transformation to one that uses technology to achieve patient safety and quality benefits because it values high-quality care.

Implementation/Minimizing Risk

Fortunately for Children's, the CMO's involvement in supporting IT initiatives did not stop at the senior level. The EMR experience brought about recognition that the CMO's role in the implementation of technology is paramount if processes are to be changed to truly bring about clinical enhancements. Consequently, the CMO took on an active role in three major areas involving implementation.

1. *Getting the medical leadership involved.* It was important to get the medical staff involved and committed to a change process that would enable technology to add value to the care process. The CMO recognized that his ability and personal investment in this change process were critical in communicating the vision and convincing the medical leadership that their involvement (and belief in technology as an enabler) were

critical to achieving improvements in patient care. At every medical staff meeting (Grand Rounds, Section meetings, etc.), the CMO made time to discuss the importance of striving for improvements and how the EMR would be instrumental in achieving these goals. When encountering resistance on several occasions, the CMO would often counter with "You aren't against patient safety are you?" This tenacity and resilience for championing a strategy for an EMR evolution was the first step in creating a cultural transformation that spawned broad clinical interest in using technology in the clinical setting.

2. *Facilitating multidisciplinary process/change issues.* Previous attempts at implementing technologies that involved change in clinical practice often faced serious conflict between different disciplines. For example, implementation of physician order entry has traditionally had an array of complex process issues that involve different practices in the way physicians place medication orders and the methodology in which pharmacists process those orders. As an organization moves to a computerized method of transmitting those orders, it is important to reconcile these variances in practice. The CMO is the most senior medical leader responsible for patient safety and quality; therefore, it is important that any change in practice be well thought out to ultimately provide benefit in clinical practice. To achieve the best and most optimal practice change, it is important to have both the CMO and CIO jointly at the table to address all conflicts. The CIO and the IT project team bring the appropriate facilitation skills to help manage all issues and to identify conflicts in practice change. Having the CMO as an integral part of the project team assures that changes in practice result in an optimal practice change for patient safety. On many occasions it was clear that an improvement in one area of practice could potentially result in a decrease in safety to another area. The CMO in these situations is critical in facilitating team efforts toward the most optimal clinical solution.

3. *Active collaboration with vendor(s) in the delivery of features/functions.* Management of vendor activity, both during the selection process and implementation, is traditionally challenging. Vendor solutions often lack the functionality desired in their base or "vanilla" products. It is important to present a strong united front with both senior IT and medical leadership to clearly communicate the desired features and functions necessary to optimally enable change. Having the CMO involved in communicating the need for desired functionality and the relevance to clinical quality is invaluable in escalating those needs to a very senior level within the vendor organization.

As of this publication, the components of this framework continue to evolve at Children's. Establishing a strong partnership with all levels of physician leadership is essential in building an organizational culture that is receptive and willing to undergo major changes to leverage IT as a key enabler in improving clinical care.

21
CIO STORIES, VIII
Sutter Health, California: IT Governance in an Integrated Healthcare Delivery System

JOHN HUMMEL, LEE MARLEY, and ED KOPETSKY

> *Creating and sustaining a successful IT governance structure requires commitment, leadership, and close attention to the political, economic, and fiscal environment.*

It is common knowledge that an organization's business strategy must be linked to its information technology (IT) plan. To achieve effective alignment, the IT management and governance structures are either integrated with, or a replication of, the overall organization structures. The challenges of creating and sustaining a successful IT governance structure in a complex business organization takes executive commitment, strong leadership, and close attention to the political, economic, and fiscal characteristics of the environment.

The remainder of this chapter presents the evolution and status of the IT management and governance structures at Sutter Health, a complex, multientity healthcare delivery system.

Sutter Health Background

Sutter Health is based in Sacramento, California, and is composed of more than 30 hospitals throughout Northern California. Sutter began in 1923, with the opening of Sutter General Hospital. A second sister hospital, Sutter Memorial, was added in 1937. By the 1980s the landscape of health care was changing dramatically, especially in Northern California where the presence of HMO Kaiser Permanente created the single largest provider in a highly capitated managed care market. Mounting fiscal pressures would threaten the survival of stand-alone hospitals without negotiating leverage to address this rapidly growing managed care environment.

In 1981 the governing organization of Sutter General and Memorial Hospitals formed Sutter Health. Pat Hays, appointed President and CEO, began a controlled and constant growth strategy through acquisition and affiliation of stand-alone acute care facilities and group medical practices. By 1995 the Sutter network had grown to include

John Hummel, BS, is CIO and Vice President of Information Services at Sutter Health. Lee Marley, MHA, is CIO and Vice President of Technology Assessment at Mills-Peninsula Health Services, a Sutter Health Affiliate. Ed Kopetsky, MS, is Executive Vice President at Healthlink Incorporated.

16 acute care hospitals, 5 medical foundations, and 5 long-term care centers throughout Northern California. Sutter had also established a majority ownership position in Omni Healthcare, an HMO insurance plan, a business line Sutter would later abandon as it sought to focus on healthcare delivery services allowing it to work with all payers in its markets.

Under the leadership of Van Johnson, CEO since 1995, Sutter has continued a strategy of growth. In addition to market growth through expansion of its delivery network, Johnson placed increased emphasis on the operational performance of the system. He recognized that overall enterprise performance must be strong enough to extend and sustain the benefits of membership to local affiliates. As a result, Sutter was selected as the 12th best-integrated healthcare network in April 1999. This selection, by the Chicago-based SMG Marketing Group from a field of 600 systems, was based on quality of services, access, financial stability, and relationships with physicians.

Johnson and the board dramatically advanced the magnitude of Sutter Health in 1996 with the single biggest healthcare merger in California's history. Sutter's merger with California Healthcare System (CHS) resulted in an organization with total revenues of $2.5 billion and total assets of $2.7 billion. Operating income in 1996 totaled $38 million.

By 2002, continued growth under Johnson's leadership positioned Sutter as the largest healthcare delivery network in Northern California. With 26 acute care facilities, 5773 hospital beds, 4 physician practice foundations, and more than 36,000 employees, Sutter clearly had achieved comprehensive services and geographic presence in the market it serves. Today, Sutter Health has operating revenues in excess of $4 billion and an operating margin of 5 percent, exceptional when compared to its contemporaries.

Strategy and Regional Governance

Sutter Health's strategy and governance approach since the early 1980s has been to develop comprehensive medical services covering Northern California, a geography that provides economies of scale and negotiating clout. Enterprise resources and expertise supplement the local governance structures, which include community experts responding to local health and community needs.

Negotiating leverage with purchasers of provider services, commercial health insurers, is also a major advantage of being an affiliate within the Sutter Health system. Benefits of large provider networks include more than negotiating strength with commercial insurance plans and purchasing clout for goods and services. There is also improved access to capital markets. For example, the cost of bonds for Sutter is about half that of the typical stand-alone facility, saving millions of dollars in interest expense annually.

These advantages are rather obvious and have been available to other large provider networks. Johnson's management philosophy has been to set a general direction at the enterprise level, while maintaining a significant amount of local autonomy and accountability at the affiliate level. It is the combined roles of the "system" and "local affiliate" that Johnson focused on and, in many ways, it is at the heart of how Sutter has differentiated itself.

Community-based, not-for-profit, local affiliates participate in the planning, implementation, and support processes that directly affect operations. Local profit-and-loss accountabilities require that affiliates have a direct role in decision making. As described by Andy Pansini, Chairman of one of the affiliate boards, "Sutter allows us to run our hospital at the local level. It's not a cookie cutter system where word comes down from on high." (*California Medicine*, June/July 1999).

Beyond the direct financial advantages, Sutter also fosters opportunities to share best practice processes for clinical and administrative needs. Values adopted by Sutter stress that by working together, sharing expertise, and adopting best practices, the delivery of care is improved for the communities served.

Information Technology Strategy

The evolution of Sutter's IT strategy has been largely based on finding cultural fit. Sutter Health has grown through affiliation with multiple healthcare organizations, and this growth was promulgated based on local accountability combined with corporate leverage. Most of the new affiliates came into the Sutter Health organization with existing IT departments, capital plans, and vendor partners. At the same time, the need for corporate leverage would lead to the adoption of system standards to be adopted by the affiliates.

Sutter's IT strategy has changed over the past decade, moving from strong centralized control to a blended model emphasizing corporate standards and local affiliate planning and prioritization. This evolution has resulted in both centralized IT and processing resources and local affiliate-based IT support organizations.

An early attempt to dictate application standards and centrally control IT capital and operating budgets was modified in 1999 by incoming CIO John Hummel. Having served as Director of System Integration and Applications at Sutter, Hummel had seen firsthand how centrally crafted solutions and carte blanche mandates for adoption had led to adverse fiscal outcomes as well as failed application projects. Hummel tailored the approach to one of change adoption over time, as determined by the participation and prioritization of each affiliate. Promoting local accountability and corporate leverage was a strategy more in line with Sutter's philosophy. This approach contributed to Sutter's selection as 205th in the list of the top 500 companies with superior and innovative information technology solutions by *InfoWorld*.

Regions of IT Governance

To parallel Sutter's geographic division of business regions, Hummel created regions of IT governance: these included the Sierras, East Bay, West Bay, and Central Valley. Each of these regions varies, depending on affiliates within the region, existing state of information technologies, and the functional, political aspects of each. Some regions have a mature regional management structure, while others govern largely through the independent affiliate structure. The approach taken by each regional CIO reflects the "state of the region." Some Sutter regions have adopted regional IT governing committees, which include participation by each affiliate CEO. In less-structured regions, decisions are made at the affiliate level within the general guidelines of Sutter corporate IT. Like Sutter's overall approach, the IT governance structure is designed to be flexible with changing times and adaptable to local community-based needs.

At the same time, Hummel has recognized the importance of system standards and common technology platforms. Technical standards ranging from desktop standards to software application standards would ultimately lower acquisition and support cost

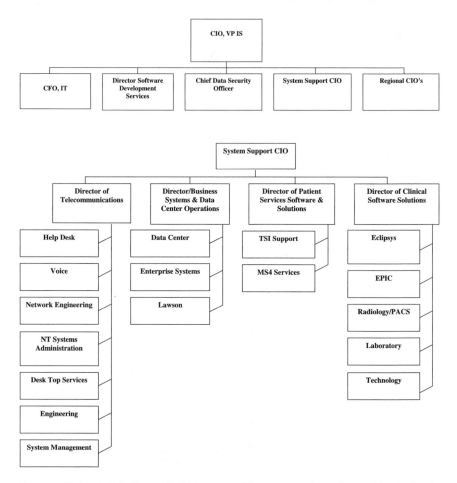

FIGURES 21.1 and 21.2. Sutter Health's current IT structure reflects the combined role of corporate and affiliate resources and teams. While maintaining close association with affiliate IT organizations, local IT organizations continue to have a direct reporting relationship locally.

across the Sutter enterprise. There were also certain corporate requirements for reporting and data consolidation, which would necessitate installing common financial systems across all of Sutter within prescribed timeframes. To ensure that major IT decisions are in keeping with the overall Sutter Health goals and executive direction, an Executive Information Technology Committee reviews and approves standard application system selection committees and capital project plans that exceed local spending authority.

The current IT organization structure within Sutter Health is depicted in Figures 21.1 and 21.2. This structure reflects the combined role of corporate and affiliate resources and teams. While there is close association with affiliate IT organizations, local IT organizations continue to have a direct reporting relationship on the local level. At the same time, corporate IT resources are organized to support both enterprise initiatives and systems and serve the local level through expertise and project management.

Ultimately, the value of IT is based on its ability to increase value to enterprise stakeholders. An example of recognizing information technology as a means of achieving competitive differentiation can be seen in Sutter's decision to implement Bridge Medical software for patient identification and screening during the administration of medications. This project supports Sutter patient safety initiatives and is expected to reduce medication errors significantly. In partnership with business process owners, IT professionals assist with process design and quantification of project objectives—activities well beyond the traditional role of hardware and network installation.

The mode of operation for IT within Sutter Health has become one of corporate direction on enterprise system standards, coupled with evolutionary adoption and self-support at the affiliate level. In rare instances are corporate decisions mandated, and only in the interest of achieving strategic objectives stated by the CEO's office. Otherwise, a course of affiliate self-determination is followed within the guidelines of standards needed to support operational efficiencies across the system.

22
INTERNATIONAL PERSPECTIVE
Wesley Hospital, Australia: Making IT Happen in a Private Setting

WARREN J. ARMITAGE

> *The goal at Wesley Hospital was to implement a clinical information system, whose main objective was to support patient care rather than administrative efficiency.*

The Australian Healthcare System

This project was an ambitious attempt to implement and integrate a leading Clinical Information System and an Enterprise Resource Planning System (ERP) within the context of the Australian healthcare system. The investment required for the implementation was approximately four times that ever previously devoted by an Australian private hospital to information systems.

Private hospitals in Australia compete against a "free" public hospital system. Every citizen pays a 1.5 percent tax levy used by the federal government to fund State-based hospitals. In return for payment of the levy, and, necessarily, other nonidentified taxes, citizens receive access to a high-quality public hospital system at no charge.

Private hospitals in our health system are typically smaller community facilities, with an average size of 80 beds. This is in part because the national population is small and geographically dispersed; only five cities have a population of more than 1 million from a total population of 19 million. In addition to the 1.5 percent tax levy, the federal government provides several incentives to citizens aimed at encouraging private health insurance. The most effective is a 30 percent rebate or subsidy toward the cost of insurance, managed through the tax system.

Although average facility size is small, the private hospital sector cares for 32 percent of all hospital patients and performs 56 percent of cardiac valve surgery. Despite the free public hospital system, 42 percent of the population holds private health insurance.

With 420 beds, the Wesley Hospital is the largest private hospital and specializes in cardiac and cancer care. The hospital is owned and operated as a "not-for-profit" hospital by the Uniting Church.

Warren J. Armitage, MBA, is General Manager for Strategy and Information for Uniting Health-Care and Director of IT Strategy for Uniting Care in Brisbane, Australia.

Implementation Goals

The Clinical Information Systems initiative at Wesley Hospital began in 1999. At that time, less than 1 percent of the hospital's recurrent expenditure was on information systems. After implementing Cerner's Millennium application suite and SAPs ERP system, this spending has risen to 4.5 percent of total costs.

The intent from the start at Wesley was to implement systems that support patient care, rather than administrative efficiency. Over its 25-year history, the hospital had implemented only one software application directly relevant to patient care, a patient dependency system used in reality more to force nurses to justify use of resources than to benefit care processes or outcomes.

Implementing Millennium was intended to:

- *Directly Support Care Processes.* Improving the quality of documentation, measurement of outcomes.
- *Automate Clinical Pathways.* Providing systems support for evidence-based practice and outcome review.
- *Effect Quality Improvement.* Reducing rates of medical error, improved falls assessment, and shorter length of stay for patients.
- *Clinical/ERP Integration.* Routine capture of clinical information to support the billing process as a by-product of care processes.
- *Attract the Best Physicians.* Offering information systems support for specialist physicians, frequently after their return from training positions in North American hospitals.

Project Scope

The first phase of the implementation was to replace a legacy application that had been in use at the hospital for more than two decades and to introduce the ERP system for financial/materials management and patient billing. Because of a Y2K imperative, the first-phase applications were implemented over only 9 months.

Phase One—Completed October 1999

- Person Management: basic Admission, Transfer, Discharge functionality.
- Enterprise Scheduling.
- Medical Record Management, Morbidity Coding.
- Perioperative Documentation.
- Interface to SAP for Patient Billing.

The second phase of the project involved the introduction of the clinical systems; initially in a busy obstetrical unit, followed by the emergency department, critical care, and other nursing units.

Phase Two—Completed October 2002

- Clinical Pathways.
- Medication Management.
- Orders/Results.
- Nurse Documentation.

- Emergency Department.
- Critical Care Unit.

Other Features

- *Multicampus.* Within 1 month of go-live on the main hospital campus, the implementation was extended to three much smaller community hospitals and an ambulatory care facility.
- *Centrally Hosted.* One configuration of the applications was to operate at all hospitals on a single IBM Unix server.
- *Thin Client.* End users at the remote hospitals (one more than 800 miles distant) and wireless local area network (LAN) notebook users all access the applications from Citrix-based thin clients.
- *Wireless LAN and Frame-Relay WAN.* Within the main hospital campus, a Symbol 802.11 wireless network was established, and for the remote hospitals, an extremely low bandwidth (maximum 256K) frame-relay wide area network (WAN) was created.

Resource Issues

The multidisciplinary project team for the implementation was surprisingly small, peaking at 23 staff/contractors. The team included information technology (IT) professionals, one medical officer, nursing professionals, and health information managers. Overall, more than half of the team came to the project from non-IT roles.

An early decision was taken to contract project management expertise from IBM. This externally sourced project management role began early, in fact, prior to the execution of the vendor contracts, and provided independent advice to the hospital. The role was used to enforce management discipline, and at various times to arbitrate minor disputes between the hospital and contracted parties. Issues were typically resolved quickly and amicably.

Two resource issues arose during implementation. First, the early involvement of medical staff on the project team led to some difficulties in expectation management. The initial rollout of applications provided for minimal functional use by medical staff, and yet physicians were well aware of the potential.

Second, the members of the project team were used to not only implementing new applications and functionality but also to providing second- and third-level support. Although cost-effective and efficient, this practice led to a tired project team over an extended period of time and almost certainly slowed the implementation.

Training

The majority of end users were provided with a maximum of 4 hours of classroom training, followed by a short period of mentoring by expert users in the work environment. The major training difficulty during the project related to the scheduling of staff to attend hands-on training as close as possible to Go Live. In our Obstetric unit, the first to implement Clinical Pathways, over 80 staff members were required to attend training in the week leading up to Go Live. Significant rostering difficulties resulted in the unit.

Other training difficulties were presented by the need to train "agency" or contract nursing staff, up to 10 percent of total staff numbers in some clinical units. The project team was also literally exhausted by the need to provide 24/7 second- and third-level support over the first month of use of the applications and then having to deal with problem rectification during business hours.

Medical Staff Involvement

More than 1000 specialist physicians have admitting rights at The Wesley Hospital. Fewer than 20 are salaried employees, and therefore the majority are far from a captive audience, receptive to new IT initiatives.

Our goal for medical practitioners was to communicate clearly with them about the progress of the project, but to resist implementing functionality unless we could clearly demonstrate it would not cause delay in their already busy practice. Consequently, in the final analysis, thus far into the project, we have implemented little of direct relevance to physicians.

Technical Issues

Downtime

Although unanticipated downtime has been minimal during the life of the project, planned downtime has caused considerable angst, because of both its frequency and its duration. Within the first year, systems were unavailable routinely due to software application updates, introduction of new applications, and the occasional software- or hardware-related failure. The maximum lost time was 32 hours in a single event. Unfortunately, this experience early in the life of the systems created unhappy users and loss of trust, which has taken a further 2 years to restore. After 3 years of use, we now have only two scheduled downtime events, less testing of software updates, and happier users.

Portable Devices

The only portable devices in use with the Cerner/SAP system are IBM notebooks operated from mobile trolleys. Despite great urging from the user community, we have not found any other practical devices offering use of the full functionality of the software and acceptable portability (weight), battery life, and durability. Handheld and tablet style devices offer great promise but only where very limited functionality is required and where user expectations can be well managed. On a more positive note, we have been very satisfied with our experience of a campuswide wireless network.

Lessons Learned

Data Migration

Unexciting as it may sound, our experience with data migration from a legacy application to Cerner/SAP has been salutary. Approximately 400,000 person records were migrated, with associated administrative and financial data. If there were to be a single regret with our approach to the original implementation, it would be that insufficient attention was paid to the testing of the data within the new environment. Many errors and inconsistencies were encountered in older data, and migration efforts frequently stalled. This took at least 2 months longer than anticipated, despite 24/7 data processing. The migration was completed nearly 1 month after go-live, leading to a much higher rate of duplicate person records than we ever anticipated.

Time Is the Enemy

Despite the pressure to deliver the predicted benefits that our experience strongly suggests, delaying implementation is a far preferable outcome to failure. Although major project milestones were met early on, we found that, over time, people tired, and users became less rather than more tolerant of disruptions and problems. From about 1 year into the project, we began to consciously delay introduction of new features or functionality to allow better testing and training. Alternatively, we chose to limit the number of clinical/administrative areas given early access to applications. Problems with complex systems and software *will* occur, and rolling back changes is embarrassing and sometimes downright dangerous.

After 3 years of very hard work from a small team, I have to conclude by saying that we would do it all again. We chose the right companies with which to partner, and the technology remains the best available. Our project has now delivered almost completely on its original functional scope. The remaining major challenge, over the coming years, is to provide engaging functionality for the medical staff.

Section 4
Patient-Centered Technologies

Section Introduction

Now that planning, implementation, and transformation have occurred, the focus shifts to the continuum of care, the stops along that continuum, and the support that information technologies lend along the way. At the forefront are issues that promise to shape the future of the industry. Creating a new delivery system encompasses topics such as outcomes management, the electronic medical record, physician practices, nursing, patient safety and medical errors, pharmacy delivery systems, and the Health Insurance Portability and Accountability Act (HIPAA).

Technology is the driver, but the message of this section is that the healthcare delivery system will always be patient centric. Technology and patients can coexist and collaborate to enhance both sides of the equation. One chapter, in particular, in this section introduces a new concept to this ever-changing equation—the consumer as owner of his or her health information and what this will portend for the healthcare delivery system. Another chapter focuses on how consumerism is enhancing efficiencies at the physician practice setting and truly creating a new method of outpatient healthcare delivery. As throughout the rest of this book, the domestic and international examples instill confidence that these concepts can be implemented and go from theory to practice.

23
Patient Outcomes of Health Care: Integrating Data into Management Information Systems

Donald M. Steinwachs

This chapter discusses the integration of patient outcomes data and the potential for using this information to improve cost and quality performance.

Striking changes are occurring in the American healthcare system. Public confidence in the quality of care provided by doctors and hospitals has been shaken. The Institute of Medicine report, *To Err is Human* [1], published in 2000, found that more people are killed annually by mistakes in medicine than by car accidents. The more recent report, *Crossing the Quality Chasm* [2] in 2001, calls for fundamental restructuring of American health care to assure high-quality chronic disease care. At the same time, substantial increases in healthcare costs are facing all payers, after a number of years of relatively flat costs associated with the growth of managed care. In many cases the increases in costs are being passed on to consumers through higher coinsurance and copayment rates for hospitals, doctors, and medications.

We appear to be paying more for less; however, the reality is mixed. New diagnostic tests, drugs, and treatments promise better survival and quality of life, yet generally drive up costs. While advances in treatment are readily adopted, much of the healthcare system has resisted organizational innovation and is trying to provide 21st century healthcare services in ways that have not changed much over the past 50 years.

Central to addressing these challenges is a new generation of information systems to support management, patient care, and public health needs. One critical aspect of new systems needs to be the linkage of patient health outcomes to information on services provided. In the following sections, the role of patient outcomes data in quality performance measurement is discussed, leading into an examination of issues that will have to be addressed if patient outcomes-based measures of quality performance are to be integrated into management information systems. The final section discusses the potential for using patient outcomes information to improve cost and quality performance in health care.

Donald M. Steinwachs, PhD, is a Professor and Chair of the Department of Health Policy and Management at the Johns Hopkins School of Public Health in Baltimore, MD.

Quality Performance

The measurement of quality performance is based on a well-developed paradigm that the healthcare *structure* (personnel, technology, and facilities) underpins the *process* of care (diagnosis, treatment, and management of disease and injury) that contributes to the health *outcomes* experienced by patients [3,4]. Historically, quality performance measurement has placed greater emphasis on structural and process characteristics than on the range of health outcomes experienced by patients. This is changing; health status outcome measures are emerging as the foundation for quality performance indices of the future. The rationale is simple. Healthcare services should lead to health status outcomes that patients value and payers think are worth purchasing, within resource and technology constraints. Patients value their functional capacity, that is, they are able to do what they want to do and are not limited by poor health, and most payers also value functional status, that is, people are able to be productive.

The technology for measuring quality performance in health care is well developed for many health problems. Systems for capturing quality performance measures for enrolled populations include the Health Plan Employer Data Information (HEDIS) that is required of HMOs seeking accreditation by the National Committee on Quality Assurance (NCQA). However, HEDIS provides limited information about outcomes and emphasizes structural and process measures of quality [5].

Patient Outcomes Measurement: State of the Technology

The measurement of patient outcomes should be broadly conceptualized and include:

- Disease status, including current status and end results of the disease process (e.g., mental and physical impairments).
- Health status as indicated by functional capacity, including physical, mental, and social.
- Satisfaction with healthcare services and satisfaction with health status outcomes, sometimes referred to as quality of life.

The importance of recognizing these three dimensions is illustrated by findings from research supported by the Agency for Healthcare Research and Quality (AHRQ; formerly Agency for Health Care Policy and Research, AHCPR) as part of their Patient Outcomes Research Teams (PORT). In the PORT on cataract surgery, patient satisfaction with vision is more highly correlated with visual functioning ($r = 0.34$) than with visual acuity ($r = 0.03$) [6]. Thus, the dimension the patient values is not significantly related to the clinical measurement (Snelling visual acuity) that is traditionally recorded in the medical record and has been used to measure outcomes. Furthermore, one might guess that most payers would also give greater importance to changes in functional capacity (e.g., ability to read, drive a car) than to changes in the ability to read a Snelling eye chart. This finding of differences between disease outcomes and health status is not unique. Another example is high blood pressure, which is generally asymptomatic and has little health status effect, but if uncontrolled places the person at increased risk of heart attack and stroke.

Health status measurement tools are currently available that meet rigorous criteria for validity, reliability, and sensitivity to the type of healthcare services being examined. In most cases, these instruments are designed to be self-administered or completed by an interviewer.

Health status measures can be divided into two broad categories. One category includes numerous condition-specific measures, such as the one cited above that was developed to measure visually related functioning, the VF-14 [6]. These measures tend to be brief, sensitive, and disease specific. Their major limitation is that they are applicable only to one set of conditions and cannot be used across a range of patients with different health problems.

The other category is referred to as generic health status measures because they can be applied to any person, independent of the condition or diagnosis they have. These measures include the Short-Form 36 or SF-36 [7], the Sickness Impact Profile or SIP [8], and the Quality of Well-Being Scale or QWB [9]. The SF-36 has the advantage of brevity, measuring 8 dimensions of functioning, whereas the longer SIP has the advantage of somewhat greater sensitivity and measures 12 dimensions of functioning, plus a summary total score. The QWB is comparable in length to the SIP and has the advantage of producing a single summary score based on utility weights, ranging from zero equals death to one equals the highest level of functioning.

Research comparing condition-specific to generic measures of outcome has found little difference in explanatory power [10,11]. The general conclusion is that generic measures perform as well as condition-specific measures in explaining functional outcomes, while having the advantage of being universally applicable. The advantage of disease-specific measures relates to the clinical relevance and interpretability of the information.

Another category of outcomes is satisfaction with the care received. An example of a rigorously developed instrument is the Consumer Assessment of Health Plans (CAHPS). This survey instrument has been used nationally to compare private and Medicaid health plans from the perspective of the enrollee [12]. This is now the most widely used instrument for assessing satisfaction with health plans.

Analyzing Patient Outcomes

A conceptual model utilized in many patient outcome and quality improvement studies is depicted in Table 23.1. There is a set of information sought at baseline that is intended to reflect the patient's characteristics and status before treatment; this includes sociodemographic characteristics, diagnosis, severity, extent of comorbidities, disease status (if different from the measure of severity), generic health status, and satisfaction. Other items that have been found useful may vary by condition, including knowledge of the condition, self-management capacity, and extent of social support.

At one or more specific time intervals after the baseline assessment, most of these same items of information need to be obtained. In addition, information is required on changes in treatment, if any, during the follow-up interval.

The analysis usually involves the application of multivariate statistical models in which baseline disease severity, comorbid conditions, health status, and intervening treatment is used to predict outcomes, including disease status, health status, and satisfaction at follow-up. Models with high predictive power over time and across variations in treatment and patient characteristics will provide more valid and useful information for management. If there is little or no variation in treatment, including variation associated with the extent of patient adherence to treatment, it is more difficult to know if the model is valid. Specifically, variability in treatment provides a test of the model's capacity to discriminate between outcomes associated with better or worse treatment (e.g., as defined by adherence to treatment guidelines, preferably evidence based).

TABLE 23.1. Conceptual model for analysis of patient outcomes related to a specific diagnosis.

Baseline	Intervening care	Outcomes[a]
Sociodemographic		
Diagnosis		Severity
Severity		Comorbid
Comorbid conditions		
Treatment	Change in treatment	Treatment
Clinical status		Clinical status
Health status		Health status
Satisfaction		Satisfaction
Patient knowledge[b]	Patient knowledge[b]	
Self-management capacity[b]	Self-management[b]	
Provider characteristics[b]	Changes[b]	
Managed care features[b]	Changes[b]	
Social support[b]	Changes[b]	

[a] Outcomes may be measured at one or multiple time intervals after the baseline; there are no accepted guidelines for timing of outcome measurements, nor whether timing should vary across different conditions and treatments.

[b] These categories of information may be optional, depending on the nature of the condition being examined and the types of management issues that are being addressed.

Where alternative appropriate treatments for a condition exist, it is desirable that there be variability in the sociodemographic, social support, and self-management capacity characteristics of patients who receive each treatment. Here, the statistical model should provide information regarding whether there are differences in outcomes for similar patients who get alternative treatments, as well as for dissimilar patients who get the same treatment.

The paradigm is built on the opportunity to exploit random and systematic variations in health care to gain information on patient, provider, and treatment characteristics related to patient outcomes; specifically, variability is desirable among:

- Patients and their characteristics.
- Provider decision making regarding treatment.
- Patient adherence to treatment.

Observing this natural variability provides a basis for statistically assessing the effectiveness of treatment(s) in terms of disease status, health status, and satisfaction outcomes. To achieve this objective involves choosing diseases for which clinically meaningful variations are likely to exist and choosing samples of patients that cut across diverse populations being served by different providers and healthcare organizations. The Institute of Medicine (IOM) suggested criteria for choosing specific diseases for effectiveness evaluation; these criteria are very useful [13]. Recently, an IOM committee recommended 20 conditions as targets for improving quality of care in America [14] and encouraged that progress be monitored through the National Healthcare Quality Report [15].

Integrating Outcomes into the MIS

The healthcare management information system (MIS) is usually structured to capture information at the time of patient enrollment or registration and at the time services are received. This potentially provides two of three key elements for analyzing patient outcomes; namely, the baseline characteristics of the patient, the patient's condition (e.g., diagnosis), and treatment prescribed and/or received, plus intervening treatment. However, baseline need not always be measured at the time of a visit or hospital admission. For chronic conditions it may be preferable to measure baseline independent of services to assess average status and not status at the time medical care is sought, which is probably worse than average if care was sought in response to symptoms or complications.

Most clinical information systems (CIS) capture similar information to MIS, with the important addition of clinical status measures at the time of diagnosis and at the time of follow-up care, if any is received. In both MIS and CIS, some information on treatment may be absent if the patient has received services from other providers, or other systems of care, including services obtained through out-of-pocket payment.

The critical third element missing from MIS and CIS is the routine capture of outcomes information on all patients, whether or not they return for follow-up care. In general, outcomes should be measured at the same time interval from baseline for all patients, otherwise patients will be at different points in the natural history of the disease (injury). This can be done by sending patients questionnaires by mail, or by interviewing patients by telephone or in person at a fixed interval after baseline. As the domestic information highway is extended into people's homes, this may provide a new modality for capturing outcomes information. Patient questionnaires/interviews can be an expensive process to do well, but statistical calculations can be used to determine the minimum sample size needed to examine the outcomes being evaluated. Also, healthcare organizations may want to come together to pool data on patients, further reducing sample size requirements and increasing variability in the overall patient group. One example of this is the Consortium on Outcomes Management formed by the Managed Health Care Association (MHCA). Sixteen managed care organizations are participating with 11 employers to examine patient outcomes for common and expensive conditions [16].

The links between MIS, CIS, medical record, and the development of a patient outcomes database are summarized in Table 23.2. It is evident that this is not a simple extension of MIS, but is a linked parallel system that augments traditional MIS and CIS to provide the information needed to understand cost and quality performance. In general, a combination of data sources is required that can make maximum use of MIS and CIS. In addition, there need to be patient questionnaires at baseline and follow-up. There are pros and cons for including a physician data form or questionnaire. The cons include the difficulty of gaining physician cooperation and the cost of the physician's time for completing questionnaires. The pros include the physician's capacity to provide reliable diagnostic, severity, comorbidity, and treatment information at the time the patient is being seen. How these are weighed in a final decision may vary by type of disease and treatment and by how the information is to be used (e.g., physician questionnaires may be more important if the purpose is to use the information to change physician practices).

TABLE 23.2. Data sources for patient outcome analysis.

Data elements	Data sources
Sociodemographic	MIS, CIS, PQ[a]
Diagnosis	MIS, CIS[a], PDF, PQ
Severity	CIS[a], PDF, PQ (?)
Comorbid conditions	MIS, CIS[a], PDF, PQ[a]
Treatment	MIS, CIS[a], PDF, PQ (adherence[a])
Clinical status	CIS[a], PDF, PQ (follow-up[a])
Health status	PQ[a]
Satisfaction	PQ[a]
Patient knowledge	PQ[a]
Self-management capacity	PQ[a], PDF
Provider characteristics	MIS, ADS, PDF[a]
Managed care features	MIS, ADS[a]
Social support	PQ[a]

Potential data sources include management information systems (MIS), clinical information systems (CIS) or medical records, physician (provider) data form (PDF), patient questionnaire (PQ), or other administrative data sources (ADS).
[a] Preferred source(s) considering cost, difficulty, and validity in the author's opinion.

What Management Questions Will Outcomes Data Answer?

From what has been discussed, it should be clear that patient outcomes analyses are designed to answer important clinical management questions (i.e., what types of patients benefit from which treatments and under what circumstances). These analyses also can address management concerns involving the structure of insurance benefit coverage, allocation of resources, design of system service capacity, and the management of cost and quality. There are relatively few concrete examples to cite, but one could anticipate several areas in which patient outcomes information might influence management decision making:

- When more expensive treatments, including specialty services, show little or no patient outcomes benefit over less costly treatment, the less costly treatment would be encouraged through staffing and resource allocation decisions.
- When patient outcomes do not meet payer (e.g., employer) expectations (e.g., return to work is delayed), management may seek to invest more resources toward improving specific patient outcomes.
- As new and expensive technologies are introduced into practice, outcomes information could provide a means to assess additional benefits and to identify types of patients who do not benefit and should not be referred.
- As high-cost providers, including teaching hospitals, seek to market their services to managed care organizations, outcomes information becomes critical in documenting the value of services to the purchaser.

These are some of the management targets for patient outcomes information, in addition to the more frequently cited applications in quality monitoring and quality improvement.

Value Performance

One definition of value is that it is equal to the ratio of cost to patient outcomes, adjusting for factors affecting the patient's prognosis that are outside the control of the provider or healthcare organization. Examples of this measure can be seen in some of the cost-effectiveness assessments of technologies that extend life. Here it is possible to calculate cost per additional year of life, or preferably quality-adjusted year of life.

Using this definition of value, greater value can be achieved by reducing costs, improving outcomes, or doing both. More complicated to evaluate are scenarios in which value is improved by reducing both cost and outcomes, but cost is decreased more substantially than outcomes, thus increasing overall value. In a competitive marketplace, the payers are searching for value and so are patients, although their view of cost is what comes out of pocket and not the total cost of care. By using the patient outcomes methodology (see Table 23.1) and including costs of care, value can be calculated. Further analysis can reveal sources of variation in value and suggest characteristics of patients, treatments, and providers associated with lower or higher value.

An Application of Outcomes Management to Adult Asthma

Quality improvement efforts all too often lack critical information regarding the full range of outcomes experienced by patients. To the extent this is applicable, they may miss opportunities. In an initiative led by the Managed Health Care Association (MHCA) Consortium on Outcomes Management, a patient outcomes monitoring and evaluation methodology was tested. Eleven major employers brought 16 of their managed healthcare providers together to collect treatment and outcomes information on adult asthma. The managed care organizations identified adult asthmatics using MIS or CIS and searching for enrollees with two or more asthma diagnoses over the past 2 years, inpatient, emergency room, or outpatient. Hospitalized asthmatics were oversampled. Adult asthmatics were sent three questionnaires at annual intervals and asked about treatment, symptoms, health status, work loss, and satisfaction. Their physicians were also sent questionnaires. The baseline data showed significant undertreatment of severe adult asthma based on existing treatment guidelines [17]. This was due, in part, to providers not prescribing corticosteroids (76 percent reported having corticosteroid inhalers) and, in part, due to patients not taking corticosteroid regularly (54 percent of those with inhalers reported using them less often than daily). Some of these individuals had been hospitalized in the previous 2 years for asthma; 34 percent of severe asthmatics reported missing 1 or more workdays in the previous 4 weeks due to health problems; and 44 percent reported canceling usual activities in the past 4 weeks due to asthma.

The managed care organizations were expected to take the findings from their plans and initiate quality improvement efforts. These varied across plans and included providing home peak flow meters to improve self-monitoring, patient education, home visits, and case management. After 2 years, there were significant increases in the possession of peak flow meters, their daily use, and in self-reported knowledge regarding how to manage asthma. These changes were associated with changes in outcomes, included reduced symptom severity and fewer canceled activities due to asthma, and higher health status (SF-36) and greater satisfaction [18].

Summary

The technology of patient outcomes management was characterized by Paul Ellwood (1988) as leading to ". . . a national data base containing information and analysis on clinical, financial, and health outcomes that estimate as best we can the relation between medical interventions and health outcomes, . . . (providing) an opportunity for each decision-maker to have access to the analyses that are relevant to the choices they must make" [19]. We remain a long way from this goal, but it is clearly an important goal. This is the direction in which we need to move. The challenges are numerous and include what do we measure, on whom, and when do we measure outcomes of health care? Once measured, how do we interpret the results in ways that can lead to better health care in the future? In summary, I would like to share one statement of caution and one strategy for meeting this challenge.

The caution about which I remind myself each time I begin an analysis of outcomes is—under circumstances of no care or inadequate care, some few patients experience good outcomes, whereas under the best of medical care available, some patients experience poor outcomes—biomedical and health services research continues to search for the answers as to why and mechanisms to intervene and improve outcomes. There are many reasons for variability in outcomes, ranging from treatments that are not uniformly efficacious to the unexplained recuperative powers of the human body. Using outcomes data from the actual experience of patients to assess comparative success of different treatments is more uncertain than the interpretation of a randomized control trial study, but it is equally important. Only in the analysis of patient experience can we understand if our healthcare system is achieving its goal of protecting, improving, and maintaining health.

There are two strategies that appear to be promising in the development of outcomes information. One strategy is to focus attention on high-volume and/or high-cost procedures to understand what factors contribute to better and worse outcomes. In the 1990s, the AHRQ PORT studies emphasized studies of high-volume and high-cost care provided in the the Medicare and Medicaid programs (e.g., cataract surgery). This strategy places a focus on value issues, assures adequate numbers of cases for study, and attracts interest from major stakeholders in the healthcare enterprise. The principal limitation to this strategy is that it generally does not focus on those at risk, but only on those who seek and receive a specific diagnostic procedure or treatment. Hospitals and providers who do focus on procedures and acute/intensive care can use this strategy on their patients.

The second strategy is to focus on high-cost or highly prevalent conditions (diagnoses) that contribute substantially to healthcare costs and/or disability (e.g., lost days of work or limitations in usual activities). These conditions are frequently chronic or recurrent and might best be studied by sampling individuals with the condition and tracking them at periodic intervals independent of the care they are receiving (e.g., adult asthma). This strategy can be applied in insured/enrolled populations and can be used to probe into how well patient care is managed over time.

Taken together, these two strategies begin to link the issues facing managed care and acute care institutions. The recent IOM report, *Priority Areas for National Action: Transforming Health Care Quality* [14], applies these criteria, plus others, to select promising targets for improving quality of care and patient outcomes. The challenge remains the implementation of routine systems for patient outcomes assessment by healthcare provider institutions. This is feasible to do, but it does require an investment. Based on the MHCA experience, there are efficiencies to be gained by forming consortiums to pool resources to adapt measurement, analysis, and interpretation technologies to their needs. In addition, there are advantages to pooling data across organizations; it increases variability within the sample and provides comparisons to judge relative performance.

References

1. Institute of Medicine. To err is human: building a safer health system. In: Donaldson M, Corrigan J, editors. Washington, DC: National Academy of Science Press; 2000.
2. Institute of Medicine. Crossing the quality chasm: a new health system for the 21st century. In: Donaldson M, Corrigan J, editors. Washington, DC: National Academy of Science Press; 2001.
3. Donabedian A. The role of outcomes in quality assessment and assurance [see comments]. Qual Rev Bull 1993;19(3):78.
4. Brook RH, Lohr KN. Monitoring quality of care in the Medicare program. JAMA 1987; 258(21):3138–3141.
5. National Committee on Quality Assurance. The state of health care quality: 2002. Washington, DC: The Committee; 2002.
6. Steinberg EP, Tielsch JM, Schein OD, et al. The VF-14—an index of functional impairment in cataract patients. Arch Ophthalmol 1994;112:630–638.
7. Ware JE, Sherbourne CD. The MOS 36-item short form health survey (SF-36): I. Conceptual framework and item selection. Med Care 1992;20:473–483.
8. Bergner M, Bobbitt RA, Carter WB, Gilson B.S. The sickness impact profile: development and final revision of a health status measure. Med Care 1981;19:787–805.
9. Kaplan RM, Anderson JP. The quality of well-being scale: rationale for a single quality of life index. In: Walker SR, Rosser RM, editors. Quality of life assessment and application. Lancaster, England: MTP Press; 1988. p. 51–78.
10. Bombardier C, Melfi CA, Paul J, et al. Comparison of a generic and a disease-specific measure of pain and physical function after knee replacement surgery. Med Care 1995;33(suppl 4): AS131–AS144.
11. Gliklich RE, Hilinski JM. Longitudinal sensitivity of generic and specific health measures in chronic sinusitis. Qual Life Res 1995;4(1):27–32.
12. Landon BE, Zaslavsky AM, Beaulieu ND, Shaul JA, Cleary PD. Health plan characteristics and consumers' assessments of quality. Health Affairs 2001;20(2):274–286.
13. Institute of Medicine. Clinical practice guidelines: directions for a new program. Field M, Lohr K, editors. Washington, DC: National Academy of Science Press; 1990.
14. Institute of Medicine. Priority areas for national action: transforming health care quality. Adams K, Corrigan J, editors. Washington, DC: National Academy of Science Press; 2003.
15. Agency for Healthcare Quality and Research. National healthcare quality report: update. Fact Sheet. AHRQ Publication No. 02-P028. Rockville, MD: AHQR; 2002.
16. Steinwachs DM, Wu AW, Skinner EA. How will outcomes management work? Health Affairs 1994;13(3):153–162.
17. Steinwachs DM, Wu AW, Skinner EA, Campbell D. Asthma patient outcomes study: baseline survey. Report prepared for Managed Health Care Association Outcomes Management System Project Consortium, Health Services Research and Development Center, Johns Hopkins University; 1995.
18. Steinwachs DM, Wu AW, Skinner EA, Young Y. Asthma outcomes in managed health care: outcomes management and quality improvement. Report prepared for Managed Health Care Association Outcomes Management System Project Consortium, Health Services Research and Development Center, Johns Hopkins University; 1996.
19. Ellwood PM. Shattuck lecture—outcomes management. A technology of patient experience. N Engl J Med 1988;318(23):1549–1556.

24
Measuring Outcomes: Bringing Six Sigma Excellence to Health Care

CHARLOTTE A. WEAVER and TONYA HONGSERMEIER

As new directions emerge in the management of healthcare quality in the United States, this chapter challenges the industry to look to Six Sigma for solutions.

The Institute of Medicine's (IOM) report on medical errors, *To Err is Human: Building a Safer Care System*, published in 2000, sent shock waves across the United States and across the healthcare industry [1]. As concern intensified, business coalitions, the insurance industry, state legislatures, health policy groups, and Congress have engaged to drive fundamental change in healthcare quality management in the U.S., focusing particularly on the measurement and analysis of care delivery practices and processes. Industry leaders acknowledge that this profound change will not come from within the industry but will be imposed upon the healthcare provider segment of the industry by external forces [2]. As they prepare to make this inevitable transformation, administrators and clinical leaders are looking for guidance as to the appropriate direction to take.

Measurement is not the issue. There is nothing new about collecting data to report on outcomes that reflect the quality of care provided. The healthcare industry has had mandatory reporting requirements for decades, imposed from the government, regulatory agencies, and healthcare plans. Despite these long-standing requirements, error rates within our medical system are still shockingly high by any quality standards. This awareness, resulting primarily from the work of the IOM's Committee on Quality of Health Care in America, has engendered new health policy imperatives for quality improvement that are now beginning to permeate the industry. The new direction emerging from these efforts is to *base process and system improvements on outcome measurements*. This means that organizations now need to set target goals for achieving best practices based on evidence generated from clinical interventions. They also need to use measurements on a regular basis to monitor their progress toward these goals and to guide process redesign. In this mode, decisions are based on knowledge derived from performance measurement.

Charlotte A. Weaver, RN, MSPH, PhD, is CNO and Vice President of Patient Care Systems for the Cerner Corporation in Kansas City, MO. Tonya Hongsermeier, MD, MBA, is Corporate Manager for Knowledge Management and Decision Support at Partners HealthCare System in Wellesley, MA.

In this context, administrators and clinical leaders are struggling to determine what to measure, within which quality framework, and what investments in resources and technology are required to implement these quality measurement initiatives. In addition, these externally imposed demands are coming on the heels of an unrelenting downward spiral in the national economy and cuts in government reimbursement to health care [3]. Consequently, investment dollars must be used judiciously to minimize risk and to gain maximum returns. Healthcare organizations are approaching these system/processes/technology investments with extreme caution. The theme is to "Go Forward," but to avoid taking the wrong quality management direction and avoid investing in technology infrastructures that will not position the organization for success in this new quality-driven marketplace.

This chapter is intended as a practical guide that will summarize the major initiatives, define the main players, and discuss the recommendations that are being generated by these policy-setting bodies. We will look at these national initiatives against the backdrop of the recommendations of the IOM's Committee on Quality of Health Care, the current status of quality measurements being proposed by regulatory agencies, Leapfrog standards, and legislation in process that will mandate public reporting. We also address advances in the information technologies that the IOM committee and other quality groups have recommended for adoption. We will explore the emergence of economic incentives for evidence-based practice as an integral component of safe, effective, and efficient care delivery, and we also discuss the clinical information systems necessary to support evidence-based care and the new standards to achieve quality reporting. Finally, we will examine four healthcare organizations that are leading the way in applying Six Sigma quality to health care.

Health Care Looks at Itself

Michael Millenson, author of *Demanding Medical Excellence*, points out that the tendencies toward error in our healthcare system have been reported in the literature since 1955 [4]. Millenson contends that the information in the Institute of Medicine's 2000 report did not come as anything new to the select few who are in the healthcare quality field [2]. However, the report did succeed in breaking into the media and grabbing the general public's attention. The report's conclusion, that preventable medical errors account for as many as 98,000 deaths in hospitalized patients and more than 1 million preventable injuries, at an estimated cost of $29 billion annually [5], shocked the nation and set many initiatives in motion [6].

Congress reacted swiftly to the IOM report. Hearings were held, and $50 million in funds was released for research on the causes and preventions of medical errors. In the Healthcare Research and Quality Act of 1999, Congress mandated that a national healthcare quality report be developed and published annually starting in 2003. In turn, the Agency for Healthcare Research and Quality (AHRQ) asked the Institute of Medicine's Committee on Quality of Health Care to undertake the planning effort for this national quality report on healthcare delivery. By early 2003, four bills about error reporting systems had been introduced in Congress and are under consideration at the time of this publication.

Congress's rapid response, both for funding research and mandating change, has enabled an amazing amount of research and activity by professional bodies. Since 1998, the IOM has published a total of six reports. The first of these came from The National Roundtable and focused on delineating the complexity behind the major causes of error and defects in quality across our medical system [7]. In 2001, the IOM published *Crossing the Quality Chasm*, which contains its recommendations for needed changes in healthcare delivery, payment, and education [8]. Finally, in late 2001, the IOM issued its vision on how standardized measurement systems should be introduced across the breadth of our healthcare systems at the state reporting level and its support of a national healthcare quality report [9].

So what has been the impact of the IOM report and of all the subsequent legislation and professional activities? From the consumer's perspective, what quality improvements have been achieved across our healthcare system in these intervening years? Mark Chassin and Don Berwick, two key leaders in healthcare quality, noted in late 2002 that, despite the extraordinary amount of activity generated by the IOM's 2000 report, not much has changed in the quality of care delivered across America [2]. Unfortunately, the reality is that participation in these initiatives from the provider side of the industry has been notably absent. Evidence even suggests that some community physicians and hospital administrators, citing medical/legal concerns, have resisted the mandatory reporting and standardized safety practices promoted by the IOM initiatives [2]. Cultural factors add to this resistance. Professional autonomy is central to physicians' sense of ethos and dates back to Hipprocrates. Adoption of changes that call for team collaboration, practice based on guidelines, and published reporting will not be easy to implement without incentives. Most importantly, resistance to implementing change stems from the lack of a business case imperative in health care strong enough to warrant the substantial investments required. In the U.S., we do not yet buy health services based on the quality of the product delivered. Without the demand from large purchasers of health care and the consumer public, administrators lack the business rationale to justify the investments needed to effect the major process and system changes called for by the recommendations of the IOM's Committee on Quality of Health Care.

The Emerging Business Case for Quality

The Public Relations Campaign

The IOM campaign for healthcare reform has been seen as an ongoing public relations initiative [10]. Keeping the issue of quality in health care in the public eye is a very deliberate strategy to build public and consumer demand for quality improvement, just as the public would do if these errors occurred in Firestone tires or in the aviation industry. Since the IOM report, "medical errors in health care" is a story that refuses to die. The media continues to run quality and safety stories as front-page news across the country on a weekly basis. In 2002, more than 5500 stories on medical errors in hospitals were published in U.S. newspapers and popular press magazines [11].

As every politician knows, winning the hearts and minds of the consumer public is critical to creating marketplace demand and financial incentives for change. In the U.S., consumer purchasing behavior has not been traditionally linked to quality outcome measures; thus, the healthcare industry has not felt a business imperative to pursue quality improvement [12]. In addition, consumers range from the individual to the megaindustry purchaser. This complexity in targeting the healthcare buyer has added to the challenge of sustaining public concern for quality health care. Furthermore, because there are 40 million uninsured individuals [13], a substantial percentage of consumers are merely seeking access, let alone quality. To cut through this complexity, health policy groups advocate the mutual cooperation of consumer consortiums, big business, and government purchasers to influence the linking of quality to purchasing decisions.

From Commodity to Value-Based Purchasing

Looking at the history of other industries, such as automobile manufacturing, we see that competitors were forced to pursue disciplined quality improvements to offer products or services at better quality and lower costs [14]. In the 1970s, cars from Toyota stole a rapid market share from U.S. car manufacturers based on their superior product quality and lower costs. Honda quickly followed Toyota into the U.S. market, and together they have maintained a dominant market share for the past 30 years. Both these auto manufacturers are famous in the industry for their pursuit of quality. They demonstrated that consumers' buying behavior was tied directly to both product quality and cost. They also proved that high quality was achievable with high productivity, a low defect rate, and, consequently, lowest cost. Competition from the Japanese car manufacturers forced the American auto industry to make quality improvements, standardization, measurement methodologies, and cost reduction a business survival imperative. Consumers buying Japanese cars forced this change in U.S. auto manufacturers.

Health care in the United States has long resisted the existence of a relationship between quality, defect rates, and cost. Consequently, quality issues aside, in 2002, our U.S. healthcare expenditures were about $1.5 trillion [15]. Not only is this the highest per capita or GDP spending of all Western nations, this figure also exceeds the size of the economies of most Western nations! The lack of normal business competition in the U.S. healthcare system has resulted in the highest costs and poorer health outcome indicators to consumers as compared to all other Western nations. Many thought that managed care would bring us into line with expenditures of other Western nations. But as some are fond of saying, managed care turned out to be neither managed nor appropriate care. The reason why the managed care movement failed was because it treated services largely as a commodity, competing only on the basis of cost efficiencies [16]. As a nation, we want to move away from commodity thinking and put value-based purchasing options before the consumer public. Our destination in this journey is to arrive at a point where individuals as well as large, employer-based purchasers select one organization over another based on quality measures including costs. When we arrive at this destination, our healthcare industry will be driven by the same quality incentives as other industries, and we will start to see lower costs and higher health outcomes as compared to other Western nations.

Big Business Leaps First

Within a year of the IOM's 2000 report, The Business Roundtable, with support from the Robert Wood Johnson Foundation, formed the Leapfrog Group, a consortium of more than 50 of the nation's largest employers. These Fortune 500 companies wanted assurance, in the face of ever-increasing healthcare costs, that they were getting value for their dollars spent. The Leapfrog Group banded together for the purpose of pressuring healthcare organizations to adopt three practices linked to optimum patient outcomes, error prevention, and significant cost savings.

These three practices are:

- Use of computerized medication order systems for physicians.
- Intensive Care Unit physician staffing (IPS).
- Evidence-based hospital referral (EHR) for high-risk surgery and neonatal intensive care.

Using their purchasing power, the Leapfrog companies were the first to link quality performance to purchasing decisions. Leapfrog began in 2000 with its coalition of companies covering seven metropolitan areas. As of April 2003, the Leapfrog Group has grown to more than 135 member companies that include Fortune 500 companies and other large, private and public sector healthcare purchasers across 22 regions, encompassing more than 950 urban and suburban hospitals [17].

Initially, the Leapfrog Group based its three safety practice standards on extensive review of published research and in consultation with leading experts in the respective three areas of practice. The standards apply to nonrural hospitals. Leapfrog estimated quality improvements, errors avoided, and lives saved, based on this same body of literature and information about the population at risk served by nonrural hospitals. Leapfrog estimates that implementing these three safety practices would result in the annual prevention of 522,000 serious medication errors, saving 2581 lives for five high-risk procedures, 1863 lives with high-risk deliveries, and 160,000 lives due to IPS staffing [18]. Leapfrog has continually revised its standards, based on data collected from hospitals and physician communities according to the latest standard revisions posted in April 2003. The criteria for the Leapfrog standards are cited below since they are being adopted as the benchmark for states and legislative bodies.

Leapfrog Standards

CPOE Standard
- Assures that physicians enter hospital medication orders via a computer system that includes prescribing error prevention software.
- Demonstrates that inpatient CPOE system can alert physicians of at least 50 percent of the common serious prescribing errors, using a testing protocol.
- Requires that physicians electronically document a reason for overriding an interception before doing so.

ICU Physician Staffing Standard
- Managed or comanaged by intensivists who:
  ○ Are present during daytime hours and provide clinical care exclusively in the ICU.
  ○ At other times (at least 95 percent of the time) can
    ▪ Return ICU pages within 5 minutes.
    ▪ Arrange for an FCCS-certified physician or physician extender to reach ICU patients within 5 minutes.

Evidence-Based Hospital Referral
- Volume Criteria:
  ○ Coronary artery bypass graft, ≥450/year
  ○ Percutaneous coronary intervention, ≥400/year
  ○ Abdominal aortic aneurysm repair, ≥50/year
  ○ Pancreatic resection, ≥11/year
  ○ Esophagectomy, ≥13/year

○ High-risk delivery, ≥15 average daily census
- Expected birth weight <1500 g in Neonatal ICU
- Gestational age <32 weeks
- Prenatal diagnosis of major
  congenital anomaly

In addition to volume criteria, the latest version of the standards has added outcome measures and specific process measures, which are available for review on the Leapfrog Web site (www.leapfroggroup.org). Any hospital organization wishing to participate can record their data on the Leapfrog site and receive recognition for meeting Leap standards both by the Leapfrog purchasers and by individuals looking up their local hospitals' quality ratings on the Leapfrog Web site.

In a first, the state of Wisconsin announced, in December 2002, that it is requiring public publication of the Leapfrog Group's quality indicators, as well as requiring the use of clinical physician order entry systems (CPOE) by the state's 124 hospitals as a condition of purchasing healthcare services for its employees [19]. The Wisconsin Business Group on Health estimated that adoption of this standard could save 853 lives and avoid 10,910 errors annually. Finally, both the Centers for Medicare and Medicaid Services (CMS, formerly HCFA) and Blue Cross/Blue Shield Insurance groups are offering higher reimbursement incentives to organizations that adopt quality improvement initiatives [20]. Together, these initiatives portend positive change and show that the alignment of quality, purchasing decision, and financial reward is finally beginning to take hold in health care (Figure 24.1).

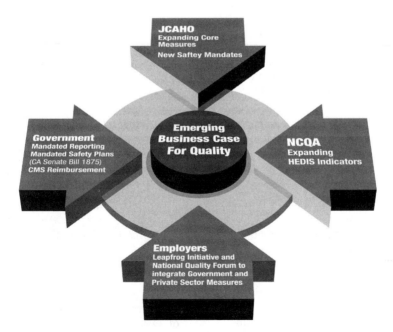

FIGURE 24.1. Pressures imposed on the healthcare provider industry by initiatives from government, regulatory agencies, and the business sector are beginning to cause a fundamental change in healthcare quality management and finally creating a business case imperative.

Understanding What to Measure

The Institute of Medicine's six published reports on the quality of health care in America began with the National Roundtable on Health Care Quality in October 1997. The National Roundtable report established a number of important points upon which the latter committee's work is based:

1. Quality can be measured in health care.
2. A significant gap exists between average quality of care and best available.
3. Gaps of overuse, underuse, and misuse exist in care delivery, regardless of financial structure [21].

These findings were substantiated by the work of the IOM's National Cancer Policy Board in an entirely different effort, looking at cancer care in the U.S. [22]. In addition to identifying the quality gaps for cancer care, the Committee showed that there was a positive correlation between volume and outcomes in terms of cancer care. Since that time, a substantial body of literature has been published relating volume to better outcomes, especially in the areas of highly technical procedures such as cardiac surgery and transplants [23–26]. These and other research findings served as the basis for Leapfrog's adoption of volume as a quality indicator. However, in research findings conducted by the VA National Surgical Quality Improvement Program, no positive correlation was found between surgical volume and outcomes for eight procedures of intermediate complexity [27]. The authors caution that their results may be unique to VHA hospitals due to the high rate of academic affiliation of VA faculty and resident care for patients.

The IOM's Committee on the Quality of Health Care in America was formed in 1998, charged with identifying strategies for improving the quality of health care delivered to Americans. The committee's first report, *To Err is Human*, focuses on the specific quality concern of patient safety and is based on evidence from about 30 publications from the past 12 years. The report emphasizes that the serious and widespread medical errors found are not due to individuals' shortcomings but rather "because of fundamental shortcomings in the way care is organized" [5, p. 13].

IOM's Six Aims as a Balanced Measurement Framework

The committee's second and final report, *Crossing the Quality Chasm*, provides the guiding framework, principles, and aims for a transformed, high-quality healthcare system [8]. Six aims are identified as the defining characteristics of an improved health system. These define a system that is safe, effective, patient centered, timely, efficient, and equitable. Subsequently, these aims have been incorporated into many of the quality measures and reporting recommendations of regulatory and health policy bodies, such as the Joint Commission of Accredited Hospital Organizations (JCAHO) and the National Quality Forum.

The IOM Committee has translated these six aims into 10 simple rules, or guiding principles, for ideal healthcare system design (Table 24.1). They are being reflected in health policy and new quality process measures.

As simple as these "Rules of Care" appear, they represent profound system and cultural change. Role relationships at the patient–provider level are shifted from the physician as authoritarian/expert to one of a peer-based collaboration with an informed, knowledgeable consumer. Similarly, the working relationships across the members of the care team shed the authoritarian nature of rank and privilege and

TABLE 24.1. Ten simple rules for the 21st century healthcare system.

Current approach	New rules
Care is based primarily on visits relationships.	Care is based on continuous healing.
Professional autonomy drives variability.	Care is customized according to patient needs and values.
Professionals control care.	The patient is the source of control.
Information is a record.	Knowledge is shared and information flows freely.
Decision making is based on training and experience.	Decision making is evidence based.
Do no harm is an individual responsibility.	Safety is a system property.
Secrecy is necessary.	Transparency is necessary.
The system reacts to needs.	Needs are anticipated.
Cost reduction is sought.	Waste is continuously decreased.
Preference is given to professional roles.	Cooperation among clinicians is a priority.

Source: Ref. 8, p. 71.

transform to emphasize teamwork, respect, and cooperation. Change of this magnitude requires not just a retraining of the workforce, but also a new beginning in the very basic way our future healthcare professionals are educated and trained. Notable thought leaders, such as Mark Chassin and Kenneth Shine, are pushing for a total over-haul of medical education [6,10]. Our current approach to physician education and training is based on an apprenticeship model developed more than 200 years ago. As Chassin and Shine note, the medical educational model is no longer appropriate, based as it is on the assumption of medicine as a learnable body of knowledge with the men-tored physician as sole decision maker. This care delivery approach neglects the impor-tance of how these decisions are enacted by the care delivery team and each discipline's contribution to patient care and outcomes. For health care to become patient centered, the physician decision must become a component of the care process that is delivered through the coordination and cooperation of multiple disciplines, multiple venues, and the patient himself or herself. According to Chassin and Shine, the new education par-adigm will train physicians as information management advocates on behalf of their patients, multidisciplinary team quarterbacks, and effective users of clinical decision support tools and quality measurement feedback.

Six Sigma as a Model for Evidence-Based Practice

Striking dichotomies mark our healthcare system. In spite of an explosion of scientific knowledge and technologies unimaginable only a short generation ago, our healthcare system delivers inconsistent quality of care. Never before has the knowledge base for medical practice been better supported than it is today, as evidenced by the exponen-tial rate of scientific publications. Take the example of clinical trials: in 1966 there were about 100 published papers on randomized, controlled trials, but by 1995 there were more than 10,000 published papers [10, p. 582]. With pharmacogenomics, the data requirements for accurate and safe decision making will further expand. And yet, there is much evidence that clinicians are not adhering to well-established identified best practices. In a recent study conducted by the RAND corporation and published in the *New England Journal of Medicine,* medical charts were reviewed for thousands of adults randomly selected from 12 metropolitan areas. It was found that, on average, patients received only about 55 percent of appropriate care recommended by commonly accepted quality indicators for diagnostic, preventive, and therapeutic interventions. Of eligible women, 45 percent did not receive their mammograms, 70 percent of children did not receive the chicken pox vaccine, 30 percent of patients with myocardial infarction were not discharged on beta-blockers, and 20 percent of diabetics had not had HgA1c monitored [28,29]. The challenges facing our clinicians is twofold: how to stay current with best practices, and how to put safety systems in place that protect from errors of omission, initiate reminders, perform checking, and send alerts. Clinical information systems have reached the technical maturity sufficient to support evidence-based practices and safety net systems to reduce error to a Six Sigma level.

Undoubtedly, the shift to evidence-based practice as the basis for how clinicians plan, make decisions, and evaluate their care will be a catalyst of profound system change. To assist with the multiple dimensions and the magnitude of systems change needed, the IOM Committee acknowledges the need to pull from the quality improvement successes of other safety and manufacturing industries, such as the aviation industry [30]. These quality improvement methodologies, especially Six Sigma, emphasize process-driven change and the careful use of measurements to accurately capture progress made [31,32]. In many ways, this shift to measuring process indicators of quality, defect rates, and outcomes is linked to the underlying assumptions in evidence-based practice. At the heart of evidence-based practice is the premise that a clinician's decisions are based on information. Information may be generated from queries against a single patient's electronic record or against an aggregate population database. Queries are launched to answer "Are we getting better or getting worse?" Information technology is key to the required data capture, summarizing, and statistical analysis that go together to generate new knowledge, identify cause and effect, and establish relationships to outcomes not previously known.

The National Healthcare Quality Report

As mentioned earlier, Congress mandated that the Agency for Healthcare Research and Quality (AHRQ) develop and publish an annual report on national healthcare quality starting in 2003. The aim of the proposed report is to serve as the "Consumer Price Index" for public reporting on health care. Healthcare organizations will have the responsibility of providing the data needed to populate the defined indicators. These data will be rolled up to the state level and from there to the national level to provide summarized reports. To anticipate how clinical outcomes and quality reporting requirements will change, it is helpful to look at the specifications put forward by the IOM Committee on the National Quality Report on Health Care Delivery. In the 2001 report "Envisioning the National Health Care Quality Report," the committee recommends that AHRQ select three to five key findings about healthcare quality and have enough measures to clearly support these key findings [33]. Ideally, only 3 to 5 measures per finding would be presented for a total of 9 to 25 measures in the report. For example, if one of the key findings were to be on the safety of surgery, this summary measure would be based on a number of measures for a variety of surgical procedures. The purpose of the Quality Report would be to highlight what the nation has achieved, where it has made progress, what needs improvement, and areas in which a high degree of variation exists [33, p. 141].

The committee recommended that the indicators reported should relate to the six aims outlined in *Crossing the Quality Chasm*. As an industry, health care does not have a tradition of collecting data that clearly reflects effectiveness, or patient-centeredness, and, harder still, equitability. These are concepts that are just beginning to permeate the U.S. healthcare system, and provider organizations are going to be hard pressed to redefine data capture and measurements that will quantitatively reflect their performance for these six aims. In many instances, before the data can be captured, fundamental system redesign will have to take place. "Effectiveness," for example, is an evidence-based practice metric and supposes the use of standard guidelines with levels of evidence embedded behind the recommendations. Since this set of practices is just beginning to be implemented in our most forward-thinking organizations, it is more an issue of being able to measure the clinical processes targeted and the progress made as an evolving journey toward total information-based practice.

The National Health Service Experience

In Great Britain, the National Health Service (NHS) has pursued a national health report with a consumer and quality focus since 1998 [34]. In Great Britain, however, the government is the sole purchaser of health care, and in contrast to the U.S., there is no excess of physicians or facilities. The U.K. has a nursing shortage similar to that of the United States, but their shortage of general practitioners is a more acute problem. In the U.K., as in all Commonwealth countries, entry into the health system is through the general practitioner, who then makes all referrals to specialists and, subsequently, for elective hospitalization. Thus, access to health care and wait times are critical quality indicators in all the Commonwealth countries. However, the privileged few with economic means to go outside the public healthcare system can buy immediate access to care. Although the economic structure of the healthcare systems differs between the U.K. and the U.S., the same dynamic is at play: "one gets the quality of care one can afford to buy." Equitable quality of care, regardless of the personal characteristics of the patient, is an issue in all health systems.

The NHS launched its quality initiative in 1998 and chose for its annual report a framework of six key areas that patients care most about:

1. Health improvement.
2. Fair access to services.
3. Effective delivery of health care.
4. Efficiency.
5. Patient and caregiver experience.
6. Health outcomes of NHS care.

The NHS annual report evaluates performance at local Trust level as well as presents a summarized national overview. The NHS prescribes to the Trusts a uniform set of measures on service utilization, patient satisfaction, care outcomes, and service performance. Work on the measures for patient satisfaction is continuing to evolve so that it migrates beyond the consumer service level into aspects of patient-centered care participation. Measures on effective care delivery are linked to the use of standards and best practices in clinical processes. The NHS is intensely focused on developing "National Service Frameworks" for guidelines for the care of specific conditions and population groups. This approach is especially targeted at the care of chronic, lifetime conditions. The programs developed to date include coronary heart disease, mental health, elder care, and diabetes. In its entirety, a National Service Framework serves as both guideline standard and service model because it develops the performance measures to track progress and establishes programs to carry out the new care guidelines [35,36].

Preparing for the National Quality Report

Healthcare organizations must prepare for the transition to measuring the discrete quality indicators currently mandated by regulatory and third-party payer groups, such as JCAHO, for hospitals, and the National Committee for Quality Assurance (NCQA-HEDIS), for ambulatory care. The new indicators will reflect performance measurement for clinical process and clinical outcomes against guidelines and benchmarks. Rather than posting static numbers or rates, future emphasis will be on reporting that defines what processes are being targeted for improvement, measurements against benchmarks, and progress made within a quality improvement framework.

For the National Quality Report, the IOM committee recommended that the measures defined in the National Health Care Quality Data Set reflect a balance of outcome-validated process measures and condition- or procedure-specific outcome measures. This recommendation may serve healthcare organizations well also and may be a useful guide in planning. The IOM committee also advised against using structural measures because such measures have not been shown to link to quality of care and desired outcomes [33, p. 13]. The IOM committee report states that "ultimately a balanced quality healthcare report will need to be a combination of process and outcome measures to satisfy the needs of policy makers, clinicians and consumers" [33, p. 13].

The new JCAHO safety and quality measures, effective January 2003, may provide hospital organizations with a start to this transition. JCAHO's new requirements include 6 National Patient Safety Goals and 11 recommendations to guide providers in achieving quality and safety in the care environment [37]. The core measures target the following areas:

- Accuracy of patient identification.
- Effective communication among caregivers.
- Safety of using high-alert medications.
- Wrong site, patient, or procedure surgery.
- Safety of using infusion pumps.
- Effectiveness of clinical alarm systems.

The purpose of the National Quality Forum is to establish a "set of voluntary consensus standards for the quality of hospital care," as well as a standardized process for implementing and maintaining these standards. The National Quality Forum (NQF) has published three reports since 2000 on the requirements for hospital performance evaluation. Their 2000 report was based on the description of a framework for hospital care performance evaluation [38]. In the NQF's 2002 report entitled "Hospital Care National Performance Measures," the NQF identified a set of well-known and widely used measures as the first group of national standards for hospital quality reporting [39]. The 2002 report represents a much-expanded version over their earlier performance measure recommendations for hospitals. Such rapid change has occurred over the past 3 years, however, that the reporting framework and quality measures were quickly found to be out of step with the industry. In their 2003 report, the NQF shifted the focus to hospital performance measurements and reports that are within a framework aligned with the six aims recommended by the IOM Quality Committee [40].

New Reporting Methods: User Friendly

In planning for the new quality reporting requirements, hospital-based health systems will want to consider the NQF recommendations, as well as some of the principles advocated by the IOM Quality Report committee. These are:

- Use benchmarks or standards.
- Present data on performance, processes, or outcomes and compare to established benchmarks.
- Use benchmark data established from previous year's performance or from regulatory bodies, clinical guidelines, or expert groups.
- Summarize or synthesize findings in ways that limit the number actually presented.

The use of benchmarks is key in this reporting and reflects the disciplined methodology advocated in the "Six Sigma Way" used by Motorola and General Electric [41]. Comparisons against benchmarks or standards make the data presented *"evaluable,"* meaning that it provides a context for understanding the information in a way that defines value, for example, good, better, or worse. Summarizing a set of measures into a single finding makes results "user friendly" and is advocated as the best format for reporting to consumer and public policy groups. Following this principle allows for a complex set of data to be viewed and comprehended at a glance. For example: an *evaluable* presentation on seven indicators of diabetes care would award a star for each measure that is clinically or statistically calculated as "good to adequate" care. If all seven measures achieve the "good to adequate" care rating, the "perfect star" rating would be easy to see at a glance. The IOM committee recommends that this principle be widely used to facilitate quality reporting that is easily understood and is actionable by wide audiences within organizations, the consumer public, and health policy groups, such as the AHRQ. Such measures should be of such simplicity and clinical relevance that consumers will make informed purchasing decisions and providers will know where and how to target performance improvement initiatives [33, p. 146].

Table 24.2 presents a hypothetical example of this *"evaluable"* presentation approach. The seven measures include care process and clinical outcomes with

TABLE 24.2. Hypothetical quality stars for diabetic care: comparison of actual to benchmark goal.

Indicator	Actual	Benchmark	Star
% w/≥ 1 lipid profile/yr	85%	82%	*
% w/annual foot exam	98%	95%	*
% w/≥ 1HbA1c test(s)/yr	90%	85%	*
% w/dilated eye exam/yr	100%	95%	*
% w/BP ≤ 140/90 mmhg	50%	90%	
% w/LDL ≤ 130 mg/dl	45%	85%	
% Smokers w/smoking cessation counseling	100%	95%	*
		Perfect Star	5 Stars

Source: American Diabetic Association and American Medical Association.

defined benchmarks as compared to actual performance. The star next to an indicator allows the reader to see at a glance the number of indicators meeting benchmark criteria, as well as the summary indicator of "5 Stars." If this report were to be monthly or annual, it could be compared at a high level against the goal of "the perfect star" rating and as a "star rating" trend over time to evaluate progress made. In the example presented here, we deliberately made the clinical outcomes below the benchmark target to suggest that counts of care interventions do not equate to effective disease management. The summary finding would be a "Five Star" rating for diabetic care management, which would fall short of the "Perfect Star" benchmark goal.

Information Technology as the Key Enabler

Clearly, reporting against each of the indicators listed in Table 24.2 as well as core measures emerging from JCAHO require computer-based patient record systems that cross the continuum of care. The maturity of clinical information systems with decision support makes this type of reporting feasible today. The indicators in Table 24.2 require the ability to do an aggregate analysis of an entire diabetic patient population for a given health clinic or practice. The feasibility of doing manual chart audits to extract the required data is unsustainable in most settings. Even if the charts were accessible for audit, completeness, legibility, and accurate documentation are problematic with paper records. Until recently, historical databases generated from financial systems have been used as the basis for "clinical reporting." These data included procedure data, medication and lab charges, utilization, length of stay, and costs and mortality rates by ICD-9 or DRG diagnosis codes.

In the example given for diabetes population management in Table 24.2, the first four measures may be obtained from financial and administrative data. However, the other three clinical indicators require a system for capturing discrete lab results, blood pressure measurements, medication results, and documented assessments for smoking cessation counseling. The most efficient way to capture this clinical information is through coded documentation and results stored in an electronic record that allows for retrievable summary analysis across thousands of patient records.

Advances in information technology today make it possible to discover how well we actually deliver care against benchmarks for an entire patient population. Importantly, this information technology enables organizations and practitioners to make the shift to practice, based on information. This shift to using information as the basis for decision making occurs as clinicians and organizations continually evaluate how well they are doing at delivering against guidelines and to discover clinical outcome trends over time. This detailed analysis of massive amounts of clinical data over time is only feasible with electronic medical records technology.

In this decade, clinical systems with repository, electronic patient record, and statistical reporting capabilities will be the backbone of quality and performance measurements. The current NQF and JACHO measures already require fields that must be extracted largely from the medical record and not from billing and administrative data alone. Investment in this enabling information technology will be basic to the strategic operations of the quality-savvy healthcare organization. The high-quality healthcare organizations of the future will use technology in the following ways: to capture performance data as a by-product of care delivery, to access expert knowledge databases, and to analyze data so that clinical and operating decisions are based on information.

Clearly, as we reflect on what will be required to report on the IOM's six aims of quality health care, it is apparent that this shift is really only feasible now with the highly sophisticated clinical information systems available in the marketplace today. The latest information technology provides powerful clinical decision support tools. Information may be pushed to the clinician at key points in the workflow, pulling from data in the patient's electronic record and from best practice guidelines. Quick-access, patient-specific clinical guidelines or reference information embedded in alerts allows clinicians to evaluate the evidence and decide appropriateness for the given patient. Systems for coordinating care across disciplines and across patient care venues have emerged that integrate orders, care plans, documentation, medication administration, and task completion into a common interdisciplinary application. These are essential to enabling measurement of process and clinical outcomes as a by-product of delivering care.

When these decision support capabilities are combined with the ability to capture all clinical information in a single database, the result is profound social and cultural change for medicine. Consider the ramifications of deriving measurements for the IOM aim of *equitable* health care. For a healthcare organization to be able to examine if they have different patterns of care delivery by ethnicity, socioeconomic status, sex, or religion requires longitudinal, cross-enterprise, and detailed clinical data in a single database. The basic rule is automation of work processes and integration of systems. *Effectiveness* is even more demanding as a quality measure. Based as it is on the assumption of a standard or guideline, organizations will have to adopt the use of best practice guidelines before they can address this aim. Measuring variance between identified standards of best practice and clinical outcomes is then possible with robust clinical systems. For these analyses to be feasible and affordable, the data capture needs to be a by-product of care delivery, the data need to be structured and codified for analysis, and system capacity needs to be sufficient to store lifetime, clinical records for large populations. Clinical databases are pivotal to our industry's ability to move forward and base decisions on information. Past approaches of using administrative databases and chart audits to derive clinical findings will no longer meet reporting needs nor support quality initiatives. Advances in information technology are allowing health care to redefine the basic constructs of how care should be delivered, evaluated, and redefined.

Four Case Studies on the Journey Toward Six Sigma

A number of healthcare organizations are engaged in quality improvement initiatives that serve as valuable case studies by demonstrating the power of these initiatives to deliver major improvements in the effectiveness and safety of patient care. These studies are all remarkable for being driven by leadership within the provider organizations. The four case studies are Clarian Healthcare System in Indianapolis, Indiana; Tallahassee Memorial Health System in Tallahassee, Florida; the Veterans Health Administration in Washington, D.C.; and the Northern New England Cardiovascular Disease Study Group with headquarters in Hanover, New Hampshire.

Clarian Health

Clarian Health in Indianapolis, Indiana, is an integrated delivery network organization that embarked on an administration-led, quality-focused journey in 2001. The Clarian story is covered in depth in a separate chapter in this book and includes a description of their strategies, approaches, and progress to date (see Chapter 5, this volume). Three hospital organizations make up Clarian Health: Methodist Hospital, Indiana University Academic Medical Center, and Riley Hospital for Children. Clarian's quality initiative began with a vision that focused exclusively on achieving clinical, operational, service, and financial excellence. The Clarian administrative team decided to focus on achieving levels of quality as their end goal, rather than focusing on costs or cost savings as the driver. As stated by Marvin Pember, Clarian's CFO and a key member of the executive team driving the "Quality Excellence" program, "Not only is focusing on clinical excellence the *right* thing to do, if you take care of quality, cost will take care of itself" [42].

The Clarian administrative and clinical leadership took a "back to basics" approach with the planning of their quality excellence mission. Guided by the belief that quality and effective medicine should produce cost-effective medicine as a by-product, the leadership team defined a comprehensive process improvement framework that addressed key work processes and patient safety areas across all clinical settings. Clarian's significant innovation, however, was their decision to focus also on the major disease categories that are treated within each of their three hospital organizations. This prioritization of disease/diagnostic categories was used to guide an intense redefinition of treatment approaches, standardization, and workflow redesign. In addition to this traditional process improvement initiative, Clarian made a commitment to base their care delivery on *evidence-based practice*. Once this framework was identified as the means to clinical excellence, the organization defined the information technology (IT) infrastructure and requirements for a clinical information system that would enable this evidence-based practice approach. Since their 2001 quality excellence kickoff, Clarian, in collaboration with their IT supplier/partner, has been developing evidence-based guidelines, implementing the clinical information system, and engaging in massive process redesign and measurement. Clarian's investment in resources to accomplish this quality transformation has been extensive. Their approach to achieving excellence encompasses the IOM Committee on Health Care Quality's recommendations, including that of using measurements to guide quality and process improvements. As Clarian Health begins to publish its results, it will clearly serve as a role model and benchmark in the industry for what is possible to achieve with best practices, borrowed from Six Sigma methods, and in alignment with the IOM's and AHRQ's recommendations for health care.

Tallahassee Memorial HealthCare and a Robert Woods Johnson Foundation Grant

Tallahassee Memorial HealthCare in Tallahassee, Florida, was selected as one of six healthcare organizations to receive a Robert Woods Johnson Foundation's "Pursuing Perfection" grant [43]. The selected organizations qualified for the grants based on their demonstrated commitment to develop quality initiatives in the key areas of patient safety identified in the IOM 2000 report. These site grants are administered by Don Berwick, president and CEO of the Institute for Healthcare Improvement (IHI), a nonprofit organization centered in Boston, Massachusetts [44].

Tallahassee Memorial HealthCare has had a long tradition of measurement driven, self improvement in all categories of the IOM's six aims for a transformed healthcare system. Within their Pursuing Perfection program, Tallahassee Memorial is focusing on perfecting their medication use processes and cardiovascular service line [45,46]. Tallahassee Memorial made significant investments in information technology as part of their transformation strategy. In line with the IOM's recommendations and the Leapfrog CPOE standard, Tallahassee Memorial is implementing an electronic patient record whereby physician order entry is integrated with the pharmacy system and the online medication administration record. Resources are dedicated to the regular reporting on adverse drug events, patient satisfaction, care processes, and clinical outcomes for key disease categories. Quality improvement teams assess current performance against goals and progress. These processes for medical management are similar to those in Six Sigma methodologies: benchmarking, measurement, relating measurements to processes, designing new processes, and creating clear structures for leadership and accountability. The results emerging from the work of Tallahassee Memorial and their Pursuing Perfection colleagues will create a self-improvement road map for other healthcare delivery organizations in the U.S.

Veterans Health Administration: NSQIP Program

The National Veterans Administration Surgical Quality Improvement Program (NSQIP) was started in 1994 at the direction of a peer group of chiefs of surgery in the VHA. The NSQIP was created to extend the methods and reporting developed in the National VA Surgical Risk Study (NVASRS) [47]. Importantly, the NVASRS study was driven by senior surgeons who recognized the need for risk-adjusted, outcomes data to enable quality management of the VA surgical centers. The NSQIP program was implemented to provide reliable, valid, and comparative information about surgical outcomes across the 123 VAMCs performing major surgery (95,000 to 100,000 operations annually) [48,49]. The data collected and reported include preoperative patient risk factors, key intraoperative process information, postoperative 30-day mortality and morbidity rates, and length of stay. The mortality and morbidity rates are risk adjusted and compared to observed-to-expected ratios. The VA maintains that the rationale for studying comparative outcomes of healthcare delivery is that the health status of patients after medical treatment mirrors the processes of care that they receive. The NSQIP reports improvements across their key outcome indicators since 1991, summarized in Table 24.3. Postoperative morbidity was tracked by NSQIP against 20 predefined postoperative complications.

The NVASRS and NSQIP attribute these quality improvements across the 123 participating VAMCs to better surgical and anesthesia techniques, improved supervision of residents in surgical training, and improvements in technology and equipment [50].

In addition, the NAVSRS visited 20 VAMC surgical service sites to understand better the characteristics of the best performers compared to the lowest performers.

TABLE 24.3. Improvements in NSQIP outcome measures for major surgery in VHA between 1991 and 1997.

Measurement	1991	1997	Percent change
30-day mortality rate	3.1	2.8	9.6%
30-day morbidity rate	14.8	10.3	30%[a]
Length of stay	10.2 days	5.1	5-day decrease

[a] Data from 1994 to 1997.
Source: Ref. 47.

Significantly, the NVASRS site visitors found that the surgical services with better-than-expected outcomes had higher levels of formal and informal communication among surgeons, nurses, and anesthesiologists in the administration of the surgical service as well as in the direct care of patients. The high-performing surgical centers also used protocols and best practice guidelines more often than surgical services with worse-than-expected outcomes; they also received higher patient satisfaction scores among surgical patients [51].

The distinguishing characteristic of the VAMCs quality improvement efforts is the fact that it is physician driven and has executive leadership support. Importantly, the IT infrastructure of the VA's progressive VISTA system has enabled the centralized storage of data from across their 123 participating VAMC centers with data summarization for the needed analyses. The VISTA system is a VHA-developed electronic medical record system that is deployed throughout the country.

The Northern New England Cardiovascular Disease Study Group

The Northern New England Cardiovascular Disease Study Group (NNECDSG) is a regional voluntary consortium that was founded in 1987 to share and provide information about the management of cardiovascular disease in Maine, New Hampshire, Vermont, and Massachusetts [52]. Members include cardiothoracic surgeons, cardiologists, nurses, anesthesiologists, perfusionists, and scientists associated with nine institutions that provide cardiac care across the region. They maintain registries for all patients receiving coronary artery bypass graft, heart valve surgery, and percutaneous coronary interventions. To date, data collected on paper forms for more than 113,000 consecutive procedures has been analyzed for key surgical processes and outcomes. This organization achieved dramatic reductions in mortality and morbidity through robust analysis of the etiology underlying the significant variability in outcomes among participating institutions. Together, they developed what are now widely used models for preoperative risk assessment and are continuously publishing new information and guidelines for surgical care processes that are associated with the best clinical outcomes. This consortium has demonstrated that accurate data can be collected and case-mix adjusted, and, more importantly, that the etiology of variability in outcomes can be understood and genuinely improved.

Summary

The six series reports produced by the Institute of Medicine build an eloquent and powerful case for the changes needed to address our healthcare system's deficiencies and for the high human costs they exact. It is clear that meaningful change will be driven from a business case imperative—and that imperative is still in the making. Health policy groups such as the Agency for Healthcare Research and Quality (AHRQ) and purchaser coalitions like the Leapfrog Group are implementing the public reporting of quality indicators in ways that will encourage consumers to base their choice of a clinic, hospital, or nursing home on those indicators. When the majority of consumers and purchasers base their buying decisions on published quality indicators, the business imperatives needed to drive change will be in place.

Hanging in the balance today is the question of what mixture of market forces, health policy, and legislative mandates will be required to drive implementation of the IOM

Committee on Health Care Quality's recommendations. Given our long history of resistance over correcting known sources of error, many think that for change to occur, it will need to be imposed from outside the provider industry. At the time of publication of this chapter, we see a growing linkage of powerful purchasing groups between the reimbursement incentives introduced by the government's CMS office, Leapfrog's ever-growing big business coalition, and the insurance industry. This pressure from payers and purchasers is occurring against the backdrop of state and national legislation requiring implementation of quality initiatives and compliance with new quality reporting. Despite this progress, our healthcare industry is beleaguered and stressed by the financial drain of implementing HIPAA, reduced CMS reimbursements, and the expense of the technology infrastructure these quality initiatives require. To implement the IOM's quality recommendations across all our healthcare organizations, government must come to the table in support of technology standards and funding support. Without such support, the American healthcare system will be at risk of becoming a two-tiered system: those organizations that can afford to invest in technology and major process change, and those organizations that are relegated to manual processes, paper charts, and poor quality as compared to their automated peers. As a society, we are all invested stakeholders in seeing that our healthcare industry achieves this quality transformation successfully. Partnerships between business, service organizations, and academia may well allow for expertise and resources to be brought to bear on these challenges in ways that expedite and achieve gains that are not as achievable with each segment of the industry acting alone [53]. Each of us can look for opportunities to build these cross-industry-segment partnerships and engage our respective organizations in these endeavors. We all own the challenge of helping to make the quality transformation of our healthcare industry happen—and it will happen best if we each participate.

References

1. Business Round Table. BRT-Sponsored inititiative focuses on patient safety. Press Release; 2000 Jan. 26. www.brtable.org/press.cfm/375.
2. Boodman SG. No end to errors. The Washington Post 2002 Dec 3; HE:01.
3. American Hospital Association. AHA White Paper: the state of hospitals' financial health 2002. AHA: Chicago; 2002.
4. Millenson ML. Demanding medical excellence, second ed. Chicago: University of Chicago Press; 1999.
5. Kohn LT, Corrigan JM, Donaldson MS, editors. Committee on Health Care Quality in America, Institute of Medicine. To err is human: building a safer health system. Washington, DC: National Academy Press; 2000.
6. Shine KI. Health care quality and how to achieve it. Robert H. Ebert Memorial Lecture. The Milbank Memorial Fund: 2001; p. 1–13. http://www.milbank.org/reports/020120Ebert/020130Ebert.html.
7. Chassin MR, Galvin RW, and the National Roundtable on Health Care Quality. The urgent need to improve health care quality. JAMA 1998;280(11):1000–1005.
8. Committee on Quality of Health Care in America, Institute of Medicine. Crossing the quality chasm: a new health system for the 21st century. Washington, DC: National Academy Press; 2001.
9. Hurtado MP, Swift EK, Corrigan JM, editors. Envisioning the National Health Care Quality Report. Washington, DC: National Academy Press; 2001.
10. Chassin MR. Is health care ready for Six Sigma quality? Milbank Q 1998;76(4):575–591.
11. Factiva Internet Search. 2002 Jan. to 2002 Dec. 31.
12. Coye MJ. No Toyotas in health care: why medical care has not evolved to meet patients' needs. Health Affairs 2001;20(6):44–55.

13. U.S. Census Bureau. Health insurance coverage: 1999. Current population survey. By Robert J. Mills. Washington, DC: U.S. Census Bureau; September 2000. Online at http://www.census.gov/hhes/www/hlthin99.html.

14. Berwick DM. As good as it should get: making health care better in the new millennium. Boston, MA: Institute for Healthcare Improvement; 1998. At www.ihi.org.

15. Goldsmith J, Blumenthal D, Rishel W. Federal health information policy: a case of arrested development. In process, April 2003. hfutures@healthfutures.net.

16. Coye MJ, Detmer DE. Quality at a crossroads. Milbank Q 1998;76(4):1–6. Available at: http://www.milbank.org/quarterly/764featcoye.html.

17. Leapfrog Group. 2003; April. http://www.leapfroggroup.org/about.htm.

18. Leapfrog Group FactSheets, 2003; April. http://www.leapfroggroup.org/FactSheets/CPOE_FactSheet.pdf; http://www.leapfroggroup.org/FactSheets/EHR_FactSheet.pdf; http://www.leapfroggroup.org/FactSheets/ICU_FactSheet.pdf.

19. State of Wisconsin. Press Release, 2002; December 6. http://www.wha.org/mo/wha/leapfrog.htm.

20. Coye MJ. No Toyotas in health care. Health Affairs 2001;20(6):44–55.

21. Chassin MR. Is health care ready for Six Sigma quality? Milbank Q 1998;76(4):575–591.

22. Hewitt M, Simone JV, editors. Ensuring quality cancer care. Washington, DC: National Academy Press; 1999.

23. Williams SV, Nash DB, Goldfarb N. Differences in mortality from coronary artery bypass graft surgery at five teaching hospitals. JAMA 1991;266:810–815.

24. Phibbs CS, Bronstein JM, Buxton E, et al. The effects of patient volume and level of care at the hospital of birth on neonatal mortality. JAMA 1996;276:1054–1059.

25. Begg CB, Cramer LD, Hoskins WJ, et al. Impact of hospital volume on operative mortality for major cancer surgery. JAMA 1998;280:1747–1751.

26. Roohan PJ, Bicknell NA, Baptiste MS, et al. Hospital volume differences and five-year survival from breast cancer. Am J Public Health 1998;88:454–457.

27. Khuri SF, Daley J, Henderson W, et al. Relation of surgical volume to outcome in eight common operations. Results from the VA National Surgical Quality Improvement Program. Ann Surg 1999;230(3):431–433.

28. Asch SM, Sloss EM, Hogan C, Brook RH, Kravitz RL. Measuring underuse of necessary care among elderly Medicare beneficiaries using inpatient and outpatient claims. JAMA 2000;284(18):2325–2333.

29. McGlynn EA, Asch SM, Adams J, et al. The quality of health care delivered to adults in the United States. N Engl J Med 2002;348:2635–2645.

30. Helmreich RL. Managing human error in aviation. Sci Am 1997;276:62–67.

31. Pande PS, Neuman RP, Cavanagh RR. The Six Sigma way. New York: McGraw-Hill; 2000.

32. Harry MJ. Six Sigma: a breakthrough strategy for profitability. Quality Progress 1998; 31(5):60–64.

33. Hurtado MP, Swift EK, Corrigan JM, editors. Designing the national health care quality report. In: Envisioning the National Health Care Quality Report. Washington, DC: National Academy Press; 2001. p. 139–158.

34. Department of Health. National Service Frameworks, and NHS Performance Indicators. Leeds, England: National Health Service (NHS) Executive. Available at: http://www.doh.gov.uk.nhsperformanceindicators 2000; and at: http://www.doh.gov.uk.hsf.about.htm (February 6, 2001).

35. Enthoven AC. In pursuit of an improving National Health Service. Health Affairs 2000;19(3):102–119.

36. Mulligan J, Appleby J, Harrison A. Measuring the performance of health systems. Br Med J 2000;321:191–192.

37. JCAHO's Patient Safety Goals 2002 Apr. Available at: http://www.jcaho.org/accredited+organizations/patient+safety/npsg/npsg_03.htm.

38. National Quality Forum. Hospital care national performance measures. Washington, DC: National Quality Forum; 2000.

39. National Quality Forum. A national framework for healthcare quality measurement and reporting. Washington, DC: National Quality Forum; 2003.
40. National Quality Forum. A comprehensive framework for hospital care performance evaluation; 2003 Apr. www.qualityforum.org/membersonly.
41. Arndt M. Where precision is life or death: the nuts and bolts of Six Sigma. Business Week 2002; July 22:72–73.
42. Pember M. Quality transformation: the journey. Conference Proceedings. Kansas City, MO: Cerner Healthcare Conference; October 12, 2002.
43. Robert Woods Johnson Foundation. Available at: www.rwjf.org or http://www.ihi.org/pursuingperfection/.
44. Berwick DM. Institute for Healthcare Improvement, Boston MA. Available at: http://www.ihi.org and DBerwick@IHI.org (April 2003).
45. Tallahassee Memorial Pursing Perfection Project Description. Available at: http://www.ihi.org/pursuingperfection/projectparticipants/tmh/TMHCReportAcuteApril03.pdf (April 2003).
46. Wysocki B Jr. Treatments—Medication Makeover: Tallahassee Memorial hospital is upending the way it prescribes and delivers drugs. Wall Street Journal 2002; Nov. 11.
47. Daley J. About the National VA Surgical Quality Improvement Program. Forum. VA Health Serv Res Dev 1998;Nov.:1–3.
48. Khuri SF, Daley J, Henderson W, et al. The Department of Veterans Affairs' NSQIP: the first national, validated, outcome-based, risk-adjusted, and peer-controlled program for the measurement and enhancement of the quality of surgical care. National VA Surgical Quality Improvement Program. Ann Surg 1998;228(4):491–507. PMID: 9790339 [PubMed-indexed for MEDLINE].
49. Best WR, Khuri SF, Phelan M, et al. Identifying patient preoperative risk factors and postoperative adverse events in administrative databases: results from the Department of Veterans Affairs National Surgical Quality Improvement Program. J Am Coll Surg 2002;194(3):257–266. PMID: 11893128 [PubMed-indexed for MEDLINE].
50. Neumayer L, Mastin M, Vanderhoof L, Hinson D. Using the Veterans Administration National Surgical Quality Improvement Program to improve patient outcomes. J Surg Res 2000; 88(1):58–61. PMID: 10644468 [PubMed-indexed for MEDLINE].
51. Khuri SF, Daley J, Henderson WG. The comparative assessment and improvement of quality of surgical care in the Department of Veterans Affairs. Arch Surg 2002;137(1):20–27. PMID: 11772210 [PubMed-indexed for MEDLINE].
52. Malenka DJ, O'Connor GT. The Northern New England Cardiovascular Disease Study Group: a regional collaborative effort for continuous quality improvement in cardiovascular disease. Jt Comm J Qual Improv 1998;24(10):594–600.
53. Connors HR, Weaver C, Warren J, Miller KL. An academic-business partnership for advancing clinical informatics. Nurs Educ Perspect 2002;23(5):228–233.

25
The Electronic Health Record: A New Form of Interaction

BETTY L. CHANG

The concept of a womb-to-tomb health record presents many benefits, challenges, and areas for future research, affecting both the industry and the consumer.

Information technologies, such as the Internet, the World Wide Web, interactive TV, and media kiosks have increased consumers' access to health information and have effected a paradigm shift in the delivery of health care. Privacy guidelines developed as a result of the Health Insurance Portability and Accountability Act (HIPAA) have also given consumers increased specific rights and powers [1]. Today's consumers have the right to access their health records, obtain copies of these records, amend and correct these records, and control access by third parties. The opportunity to obtain and exercise control over healthcare information has empowered consumers to become partners with their healthcare providers (HCP) in decision making. In short, information and communication technologies have transformed consumers (patients) from passive recipients to active participants [2]. This chapter describes ways in which consumers become owners of their health information. It will discuss the potential of the Electronic Health Record (EHR), as well as the benefits, challenges, and areas for future research that it presents. Various avenues by which consumers can access health information and communicate with their healthcare providers have been well characterized in other literature and are not detailed in this chapter.

The term Electronic Health Record refers to a longitudinal record of a patient's health care from "Womb to Tomb." It combines information derived from patient contacts with healthcare providers with other health data such as laboratory reports, health outcomes, disease management programs, and other data relevant to the consumer's health. More importantly, it emphasizes the consumer's involvement and control of the record [3]. The functionality of an EHR may vary from systems that support communication between and among various data repositories (e.g., clinical/hospital information systems, primary care practitioners, pharmacies) to a simple Web-based interface smart card for interactive data entry and data review by individual consumers.

Imagine this . . . A primary healthcare provider, who is seeing a pregnant patient, orders laboratory tests, medications, and a genetic consultation, all electronically to the

Betty L. Chang, DNSc, FNP-C, FAAN, is a Professor at the University of California at Los Angeles School of Nursing.

appropriate departments. The HCP's assessments and treatment plans for this consumer will be recorded in the patient's own EHR throughout her pregnancy, which may be available to her on the Internet or placed on a smart card or other medium for access via a home computer. When results from the tests and consultation report are sent to the HCP, the HCP will send the woman an interpretation for her EHR. The Web program or smart card contains appropriate Web site links to educate her about what to expect during pregnancy, recommendations about diet, exercise, and other relevant information. The woman may also belong to an online support group by which consumers will share their own experiences and advice for health care. At any time, the woman may seek clarification from the HCP via e-mail. She can expect to receive a response within a reasonable time frame.

This same EHR will contain a complete record of her health care throughout pregnancy and subsequent health encounters. When her baby is born, the baby will have his/her own electronic health record, which tracks condition at birth and all care provided. Moreover, the consumer (or a consumer's surrogate/deputy) will have control of information in her EHR and can give access to portions of it to selected healthcare personnel.

Functionalities of an EHR generally include these [4]:

a. Providing secure password-protected access.
b. Providing summaries of medical information (e.g., health history, medications).
c. Serving as a portal to consumer education.
d. Serving as a database for self-monitoring.
e. Providing for secure consumer–HCP communications.

In the near future, increased numbers of consumers will have access to EHRs. Researchers, healthcare organizations, and vendors are in the process of planning, developing, and evaluating systems that will make well-functioning EHR systems widely available.

Plans for a National EHR

Where do such systems exist, you may ask, and what would be the effect of such a system on consumers? In the United States, the National Committee on Vital and Health Statistics has taken on the task of creating a National Health Information Infrastructure (NHII). One of its working groups, the Personal Health Dimension, has been studying the information needs of consumers, healthcare professionals, and other health system stakeholders [5]. This working group seeks to manage health information such that consumers can participate in more informed healthcare decision making. Its health information system will contain information supplied by consumers for their own as well as their HCP's use; consumers will be able to select from among different levels of information to be accessed. It is anticipated that both longitudinal and cross-organizational health records will be compiled. Technologies such as the Internet and smart cards may be employed to provide easy access from various settings (e.g., clinics, home, while traveling), and during emergencies [5]. The goal is to create an EHR within primary care that is eventually universal, possibly with a Universal Identifier, which records the health care of individuals throughout their life. The approach adopted will need to take into account the type of information, its use, and overall trends in technology.

A number of other countries are developing initiatives for EHRs as well. In the United Kingdom, for instance, as part of an overall strategy to provide optimum health care for consumers, the government has laid the groundwork for developing a lifelong electronic health record for every citizen. Seamless patient care would be provided through HCPs, hospitals, and community services, while healthcare information would be available through online information services and telemedicine [3]. For example, a medical center may have an integrated healthcare system in which information about the patient would be recorded in a system networked from the HCP to laboratories, pharmacies, consulting physicians, insurance companies, and government organizations that accredit care and approve or examine costs. Although such systems may be seen by healthcare providers, administrators, researchers, and policy makers as essential for improving the quality of care, patients can also use subsets of the health record to enhance their own role in information seeking and decision making about their own health care. They may access information through their home computer via the Internet, or from libraries, offices, or a range of public service places.

Canada is also creating a pan-Canadian electronic record registry to foster collaboration and partnerships among provinces and private sectors to identify EHR solutions. The Australian government plans to introduce EHR by means of a national network [6,7]. Developing a fully integrated EHR for consumers (patients) would mean that the record will be available to the patient and updated with information at every health encounter. These encounters would include any hospitalization, emergency room admissions, visits to clinics, office visits, reports from special services, referrals, and long-term and hospice care. Healthcare information would be available on an around-the-clock basis.

Regional Projects

In the United States, a number of regional collaborations and partnerships have been formed to implement EHR solutions. Four examples are described in the section that follows.

Winona Health Online

Winona (Minnesota) Health Online (WHOL) and the Cerner Corporation are collaborating in a project to enhance the consumer–HCP partnership in health care. Using software developed by the University of Virginia and Cerner, the program provides comprehensive online personal records (PHR) such as personal family health history, medications, emotional state, stress, lifestyle factors (use of tobacco, alcohol, caffeine, illicit drugs, exercise), heart disease, stroke, diet, work-related illness, risk factors for injury, cancer, glaucoma, immunizations, sexual behavior, pregnancy, and other general information. Users fill out a survey and, on completion, are immediately given feedback based on their answers. Entered data are stored for comparison with future data. Members with certain chronic conditions are placed into online disease management programs [8]. Mammogram and Pap smear results along with their interpretation are sent directly to consumers (patients); refill medications can also be obtained online.

Membership to WHOL is being recruited by means of a grassroots, word-of-mouth marketing strategy. Special interest groups are also being targeted, including schools, employers, and elders. In addition, mass media is being utilized via advertisements, newspapers, billboards, and displays at point-of-purchase [9]. A later chapter in this book also presents a detailed case history of this project.

Santa Barbara

The Santa Barbara County Care Data Exchange, a collection of medical groups, hospitals, clinics, laboratories, pharmacies, payers, and other healthcare organizations, has committed to exchanging clinical data at the point of care. More than 70 percent of leading healthcare organizations in Santa Barbara are participating in the Santa Barbara Care Data Exchange Network. These groups of healthcare organizations have established mutual information technology goals and are addressing their information and technology challenges in unison. They are currently developing a set of initiatives that will demonstrate and deploy Internet-based technologies, including business rules and data standards to guarantee the appropriate and secure sharing of patient information throughout the county. They plan to have consumer clinical data available across enterprises that will be readily available under the control of local health managers and HCPs. Security and privacy protocols are employed to be compliant with HIPAA requirements. The 3-year project will create a fully operational peer-to-peer data exchange for healthcare providers in Santa Barbara County [10].

Michigan

A coalition of Michigan doctors, hospitals, insurance technology companies, and healthcare professionals has launched an electronic medical record initiative. The goal of this initiative is to improve medical treatment by providing immediate access to essential patient lab reports, medical charts, and X-rays, while eliminating the wasteful duplication of services and life-threatening delays and errors inherent in outdated paper systems.

According to David Ellis, the coalition's executive director, new software using a standardized data-reporting format has already been adopted by most of the state's major healthcare providers. Consumer information from different sources can be linked and made available over the Internet. Beaumont Hospital and University of Michigan Hospitals are among the larger facilities participating, along with an urgent-care clinic, a diagnostic lab, and a private doctor's office. The project has already signed up some major supporters and has been endorsed by cyber-state.org, an Ann Arbor-based nonprofit dedicated to improving access to technology in Michigan [11].

Eastern Maine Healthcare

In response to the findings of a study, Eastern Main Healthcare (EMH) is using a Web-based solution powered by IQHealth software from the Cerner Corporation. Called MyOnlineHealth, it allows residents to gain and send secure communication with their HCP. Consumers in about two thirds of the state (but containing only one third of the population) can access four components: a personal health record, secure online messaging and scheduling, clinical content for consumers, and a health assessment tool [12]. Consumers may complete online health risk assessments, receive feedback, be linked to other health content, or received tailored information from their HCP. They may also view their laboratory test results, obtain a prescription refill, or request an appointment [13].

Research and Evaluation Projects

Besides regional projects, a number of defined research projects have been conducted. Several of these projects have reported their evaluation data.

Patient Clinical Information System

Cimino and colleagues developed a patient clinical information system (PatCIS) to interface with the clinical repository at New York Presbyterian Hospital (NYPH) to allow consumers (patients) to add to and review their medical data [14]. The PatCIS was available through a Web browser; however, physicians primarily controlled access. Patients could also specify what they wished to view; however, they could not specify a higher level (e.g., greater amount of information) than that specified by the physician.

Patients were able to enter data (e.g., blood pressure, diabetic diary) and review data from the NYPH clinical data repository, such as laboratory test text reports, advice, customized educational materials based on the patient's data, and educational information from external sources. Cimino and colleagues provided access to the system to 13 subjects (enrollees) over a 36-month period and obtained evaluation data on 11 of the 13 subjects.

Of the eight patients who were in the study 9 months or more, five responded to the follow-up questionnaire, of whom one never used the system. The majority of the remaining four agreed that the use of the system had improved their interactions with their physicians, and that the system was easy to use, understand, and allowed them to take a more active role. All three physicians who provided subjects for the study thought that the patients' use of the PatCIS helped them to gain control over their own health care. The authors found that despite the variety of reasons patients stated for wanting to use the system, they were primarily interested in reviewing laboratory results.

Patient-Centered Access to Secure Online

Masys, Baker, Butros, and Cowles reported on a Patient-Centered Access to Secure Online (PCASSO) project, designed to apply state-of the-art security to the communication of clinical information over the Internet [15]. A total of 216 physicians and 41 patients were enrolled as users of the system; 68 physicians and 26 patients logged in one or more times.

The typical physician enrollee was male (78 percent) and had good computer skills (53 percent) and knowledge of the Internet (48 percent). The typical patient enrollee was female (73 percent), well-educated (71 percent with a college degree), had excellent computer skills (49 percent), and had excellent knowledge of the Internet (54 percent). A larger percentage of patient enrollees used the system than did physicians. A majority (68 percent) of the patients who provided feedback considered the security features as reasonable, whereas none of the physicians considered it so. Sixty percent of the physicians thought it was "reasonable," and 40 percent rated the system as "unreasonable" or "intolerable." Both physicians and patients rated the value of having records available to them over the Internet as "very high." This system was rated high on safety and compliant with HIPAA's (then interim) requirement for security services to guard integrity, confidentiality, and availability, and in guarding against unauthorized access to data transmitted over a communication network [14].

The high percentage of enrollee usage and favorable feedback of this small select group may have been related to consumer characteristics. A high percentage of enrollees were college educated and had excellent knowledge of computers and Internet skills.

Informatics for Diabetes Education and Telemedicine

A large-scale project, Informatics for Diabetes Education and Telemedicine (IdeaTel), was begun in February 2000 [16,17]. This 4-year project, funded by the Centers for Medicare and Medicaid Services, contains a component that would allow patients to enter data (e.g., blood pressure, glucose, diet) and review their clinical data. E-mail, video teleconferencing, and educational materials will also be available. As part of this demonstration project, primary care providers and nurse case managers will have interactive access to the system. It is anticipated that 1500 participants will be randomized into the intervention group ($n = 750$) and the usual care group ($n = 750$). Evaluation data are not yet available.

Baby Carelink

An example of a variation of an EHR, but nevertheless allowing consumers to actively access information and participate in decisions regarding consumer care, is a program called Baby Carelink, a secure collaborative environment for parents of premature infants in a Neonatal Intensive Care Unit (NICU). Parents are able to log into Baby Carelink and obtain daily clinical reports, doctor's notes, and a baby growth chart. Messaging capabilities, appointment scheduling, reminders, guidance to further educational materials, as well as the actual clinical content of educational materials are also available through this program. Feedback from consumers indicates a reduction in reports of quality of care problems, better communication, high satisfaction with care, and earlier discharge from the hospital [18].

Muenster University Hospital

At the Muenster University Hospital, Ueckert et al. initiated a project to design and develop an EHR called Akteonline. It provides functions for secure access by consumers via a standard browser. Currently, data structures have been implemented for the storage of basic personal data (contacts, next relatives, allergies, risk factors), outpatient visits, preventive care, hospital stays, medical conditions (history, diagnosis, treatment), and diagnostic tests and results. There are also provisions for context-sensitive patient information, importing/exporting of standardized clinical documents, and reminder-based disease management support [19]. The developers envision several types of security and access control. At the time of this writing, evaluation data were not available.

Commercial Tools

On a smaller scale, some tools are available for personal electronic patient record implementation (Table 25.1). Some industry watchers report that more than 60 percent of healthcare institutions are investigating this technology. Table 25.1 lists some examples of companies offering electronic health record products for consumers (often

TABLE 25.1. Examples of companies and consumer health record software.

Company	Web site address	Record
Capmed Inc.	http://www.capmed.com/	Personal Health Record
Cerner	http://www.cerner.com/	Vitality: IQHealth.com
Cuffs Planning & Models, Ltd, Health-Minder	http://www.health-minder.com/	Health-Minder
Dr I-Net	http://www.drinet.com/	Dr.I-Net (personal health record–free)
Epic Systems, Inc.	http://www.epicsystems.com/	MyChart
GE Medical Systems Information Technologies	http://www.medicalogic.com/	Aboutmyhealth (Personal Health Record)
HealthCare Data Inc.	http://www.healthprobe.com/	Personal Record, a portion of physician product
HealthRecordsOnline Inc. (Canada)	http://www.healthrecordsonline.com	Health Records Online
I-beacon Inc	http://www.i-beacon.com/	i-beacon (health record)
IDX systems Corp	http://www.idx.com/	Patient Online
i-Traxs Inc.	http://www.i-trax.com/	Myfamily md
K.I.S. Medical Record Solutions	http://kismedicalrecords.com/	Kismedical Records Solutions
Imetrikus	http://www.imetrikus.com/	Medicompas (health record)
McKesson	http://www.careenhance.com	Personal health profile
MOMR Inc.	http://myonlinemedicalrecord.com	MyOnline Medical Record (free basic easy tool for consumers)
PersonalMD	http://www.personalmd.com/	PersonalMD.com
PrimeCare: Your Own Health	https://www.yourownhealth.com/	Yourownhealth
PrimeTime Software	http://www.medicalhistory.com/	Instant Medical History
Resolution Health	http://www.resolutionhealth.com/	Wellpatient.com
Health Link and Vitality	http://www.dohealth.com/	Healthlink Online
Telemedical.com Inc	http://www.telemedical.com/	Personal Record System
Wellmed	http://www.wellmed.com	Personal Health
Your Diagnosis.com Australia	http://www.yourdiagnosis.com/yourdiagnosis/start.htm	Personal health record and self-diagnosis (recommended for specific problems)

Source: Accessed 1/29/03 (bchang).

called personal health records) on their Web sites found through the use of several search engines/directories (e.g., google.com; yahoo.com; and others). Individuals have access to the software, either through their HCP, through the company's Web-based portal, or by purchasing it independently to install on their own computers.

Although the offerings vary in function, in general, these applications allow consumers or HCPs to enter data and obtain updated information about their health.

Consumers may enter and/or access their health history and information about allergies, track medications, test results from hospital laboratories, and treatments, display laboratory reports, and store and organize digital images. In many instances, the HCP can provide the patient with the software that contains the patient's own clinical data and add prescribed Web links for the patient's use. This record will be updated by the HCP at each visit, or when new information about the consumer is obtained.

Some programs offer an online medical diagnosis personal health record program, which can guide the consumer through a comprehensive private history, including details difficult to obtain in standard medical consultation. Based on the user's responses, a set of custom-designed algorithms provides a list of possible problems, which should be discussed with the individual's HCP. The appropriate use of such a record is expected to lead to individual empowerment and improved health and health care. The creators of the programs emphasize that the use of their programs is not designed to replace the medical practitioner, or to offer advice, but it assists the consumer to become more knowledgeable about his/her condition (see Table 25.1).

An advantage is that the users have total control of their own record and information. Security measures are employed, and it is stated that measures are to be used to maintain privacy and anonymity. Although in their evaluation of 11 Web sites Kim and Johnson found that personal electronic health records varied widely in functionality and organization, they found that at the basic level each site provided access to personal medical information. The majority extended this capacity to provide access to emergency situations. Many of the limitations cited were related to the process of consumer (patient) data entry without much guidance or explanation [4]. However, one must keep in mind that products are continually being revised, and a comprehensive evaluation of the commercial record programs has not been conducted. Furthermore, with the rapid changes seen in technology and software vendor fields, some of the Web sites cited in Kim and Johnson were not accessible to date at the time of this writing.

Other Sources of Consumer Information

A plethora of health information sources has been developed for Internet (and Web) delivery, which can increase consumers' knowledge about their conditions. As mentioned in the introduction of this chapter, these sources of consumer health information and issues surrounding them are extensively covered elsewhere and are not part of this chapter. Web sites containing recommended literature, as well as tailored information for health promotion and disease management, are readily available. The National Library of Medicine's Medline-Plus was created specifically with consumers in mind. Reliable information here is targeted at consumers seeking information on numerous health topics. Healthpath, the U.S. Government's portal for health information, is also designed for consumer use. In addition, many academic centers maintain educational Web sites, as do disease-specific organizations, that are accessed by HCP and consumers alike. Numerous commercial sites are available and may be the most blatant in their attempt to capture the consumer's attention on the Web. The variability in quality of Web sites has been well documented [20].

Extensive reports also exist for various categories of Internet healthcare services and consumer opportunities that can be found online. At the 2002 Annual Symposium of the American Medical Informatics Association, Ferguson presented 11 levels of participation of patients online [21,22]. He reported on HCP–patient online communications (e-mail), tailored advice systems with or without coaching from a professional, online health professionals, e-patients conducting research, online support groups, and patient-to-patient support. Consumers can be most effective in sharing experiences in managing their symptoms, recommending providers, or seeking other sources of help. They have become partners in research in some instances. Literature on the effectiveness of e-mail communication with respect to patient satisfaction and physician experience [23] and the willingness of a few pioneer insurance companies to reimburse for such services also exists.

Consequences of EHR

Having a health record available on the Internet under the control of consumers will have numerous consequences. There are obvious benefits and challenges. There will be increased accountability by consumers, enhanced quality of health record, better management of chronic conditions, and ultimately improved healthcare delivery. At the same time, there will be increased attention to privacy because names or personal details are disclosed.

Moreover, using the Internet for consumer information may result in more knowledgeable consumers regarding the quality of information on the Web. Although numerous criteria are available for evaluations of Web sites, the Pew Foundation reported that consumers generally judge the content to be of good quality if they find the same information on several sites, or if the information confirms their preexisting beliefs [24]. With greater exposure to different kinds of Web site information, there will be increasing governmental and voluntary organizations to serve as "quality monitors." Although consumers may learn to discriminate among the quality of Web information, there are limitations, just as consumers are able to judge the quality of automobiles available to a limited extent.

Benefits and Challenges

Clearly, benefits can be seen for a womb-to-tomb EHR. Not only do consumers have access to their own health records, but they also may further control who receives specific types of information. There are benefits to the consumer, the HCP, public health professionals, and researchers. By the same token, there are challenges inherent in consumer issues such as security, privacy, and confidentiality. Not to be underestimated are variations in consumers' comprehension of health information, desire for responsibility in participation in decision making, and potential modification of behavior in HCP–consumer interactions.

Benefits for Consumers

The clarion call is for more knowledge to enable consumers to participate in decision making about their own health care. EHR will enable consumers to have more information about the possible significance of their signs and symptoms and choices in treatment given a definitive diagnosis. Consumers will receive interpretations of the meaning of their tests and receive reminders from their HCPs. They will be knowledgeable about their own medications, and thus may be able to avoid some of the polypharmacy and drug interactions currently common among consumers, especially in elders. They can compare medication actions and learn about contraindications. The possibility of cost comparison of medications will allow the consumer to decrease medication expenditure. It is reasonable to hypothesize that these capabilities will empower consumers and may result in improved health outcomes and higher consumer satisfaction.

Benefits for the Healthcare Provider

Cumulative health history including information available from various sources will provide the HCP with a comprehensive medical record. All necessary information will be available at all times, thus avoiding missing information for an evaluation of diagnosis. The HCPs will have information for diagnosis, treatment, emergencies, and for closer tracking of consumers' (patients') progress.

Documentations will be more efficient for the HCP. Specific templates may facilitate documentation; reminders may be embedded to remind the HCP of guidelines, protocols, and tests for specific conditions. The HCP can also query the database for specific information. Prescription writing will be simplified, with automatic documentation in the consumers' record and sending the order to a pharmacy. HCPs can provide customized consumer education information for consumers according to consumer needs and capabilities. Universal access to records now only provides information where needed, but it can also be reviewed by different types of service providers (for instance, primary HCP, pathologist, and surgeon) at the same time. There will be less time lost for transfer and searching for medical records from different offices.

Clinics and offices may be able to eliminate or reduce the need for transcription of services and repeated "pulling" of medical records, resulting in cost savings. One group practice, for example, reported that each physician generated about 1000 chart pulls a week to accommodate transcribing of notes, entering test results, and answering phone calls about the next day's appointments [25].

Benefits for Public Health and Researchers

There are benefits in having aggregated health data on large populations of consumers. Public health officials can use the information generated to guide health initiatives and programs and to evaluate the effectiveness of public health programs. Such data can serve as a basis for broad-based health outcomes research related to a variety of biological, physical, environmental, and psychosocial interventions. However, despite these potential benefits, there are challenges to this effort. Over the next few years, all medical records will be held in electronic form, according to the HIPAA. Such data must be compatible with federal standards and be treated to assure security and privacy. Although controversial, a unique identifier for consumers has been recommended.

Challenges

What are some of the challenges to the widespread use of longitudinal EHR? The challenges are many and vary from technical to human factors. Important challenges for developers and HCPs in standards, terminology, and interoperability across settings are addressed in other chapters. Major concerns that immediately impact consumers include issues of privacy/confidentiality, security, and modifications in behaviors of HCP and consumer interactions. These consumer issues are described below.

Privacy and Confidentiality

Privacy is viewed as freedom from intrusion, and it is closely related to the concept of confidentiality or that of not divulging information to others or to unauthorized persons. Ample evidence exists that Web-based systems amass detailed consumer information with the capability of identifying and tracking users for a variety of purposes, often without the person's knowledge or consent [26]. Privacy statements found on Web sites not only varied but also were inconsistent between their stated policy and actual practices. Moreover, personal consumer health information has been made widely available accidentally [27]. Without enforced, stringent privacy rules, many consumers will be unwilling to use a Web-based system for their EHR.

A national survey of e-health behavior found that (a) 75 percent of people are concerned about health Web sites sharing information without their permission, and (b) a significant percentage do not and will not engage in certain health-related activities online because of privacy and security concerns. For example, 40 percent will not give a doctor online access to their medical records; 25 percent will not buy or refill prescriptions online; and 16 percent will not register at Web sites. However, nearly 80 percent said that a privacy policy enabling them to make choices about whether and how their information is shared would make them more willing to use the Internet for their private health information [26].

To address these concerns, the U.S. Congress passed HIPAA in 1996, effective 2001, which, among its many provisions, gives consumers the right to their medical records, to limit disclosure, and to add or amend their records [28]. Providers must comply by April 2003. Covered entities include health insurers, physicians, hospitals, pharmacists, and alternative practitioners such as acupuncturists [29].

In addition, states may enact laws that are more protective of individual rights within the baseline set by the federal government [30]. E-health companies and industry organizations have also applied for "seals" as evidence of adhering to ethical principles that include privacy, confidentiality, and quality. Examples are Health on the Net Foundation (HON) and TRUST-e. Industry coalitions such as the Internet Healthcare Coalition (IHC) and the Health Internet Ethics Coalition (HI-Ethics) address privacy concerns. However, to date, privacy and confidentiality concerns have not yet been completely alleviated.

Security

Security and protection of unauthorized access of data in electronic systems is another challenge. Developers of EHR systems are embedding security measures as the systems are being designed. A variety of strategies have been implemented in the systems presented. Security features are variable depending on the functions of the EHR and expectations of the users. Integrated clinical projects have uniformly reported the use of strong enterprisewide authentication, transport security (encryption), several levels of role-based access control, auditing trails, computer misuse detection systems, protection of external communications, and disaster protection through system architecture as well as through physically different locations [14,18,31]. It goes without saying that systems provide consumers access only to their own data.

Where national uniform ID numbers are used, Uckert and colleagues, among other strategies, described a basic level of envisioning two databases to address security and access control. One database will have consumer identification (ID) geographic information linked to an ID number. The second database will have actual clinical information indexed by patient ID number but no personal data. Other management functions considered include controlled access, such as a one-time access where the consumer can give access to parts of the record to anyone for one session only, and a "read access" where consumers in an emergency situation can provide access to an emergency subset of the record.

A Pew report documented that 89 percent of health seekers were concerned about privacy issues, with fully 71 percent very concerned [24]. When people were made aware of the possibility of the issuance of universal medical ID numbers, a Gallup poll found that 91 percent opposed the plan; 96 percent opposed the placement on the Web of information about themselves held by their own doctor [32].

On the other hand, healthcare administrators are aware of security issues and have many safeguards in place. In a recent survey of healthcare information technology executives, participants ranked the protection of health data as their primary concern [33]. Hospitals, for example, indicate that current security technologies in use include antivirus software (100 percent), firewalls (96 percent), virtual private networks (83 percent), data encryption (65 percent), intrusion detection (60 percent), vulnerability assessment (57 percent), public key infractions (20 percent), and biometrics (10 percent). Virtually all respondents expected to use all these technologies to some degree during the next 2 years [34].

Modification of Behavior of HCP and Consumer Interactions

Increased participation in decision making is expected to change the nature of interaction between health consumers and medical health advisors, possibly in unexpected ways. Currently a small proportion of healthcare providers use electronic medical records that are integrated to obtain comprehensive health information of consumers. It is expected that a more empowered consumer will work as a partner with the HCP toward improved healthcare outcomes. However, such changes in behavior may present themselves as challenges as well.

Will the HCP believe the consumer's health care is enhanced by patient empowerment or will they feel threatened and uncomfortable? Many physicians who are accustomed to a more authoritarian approach to consumers may now need to become more egalitarian and allow consumers to take a more active role.

On the other hand, not all consumers will have the same level of knowledge or will want the same level of accountability. The twin elements of empowerment and responsibility cannot be divorced from each other. It is conceivable that not all consumers empowered with knowledge about their conditions and treatments would be willing to take responsibility with their HCP as a partner in decision making. Some may prefer to have others take responsibility in deciding on the "best" course of action. The process of consumer access control, while desirable in concept, may yield variable results when implemented.

The related question of health literacy needs to be taken into consideration in evaluating consumer knowledge. Some individuals who read English may not be familiar with medical and technical terminology. Although system designers have addressed this issue to some extent by developing glossaries and "context-specific" explanations, problems of health literacy have not been totally solved to date. An overassumption of knowledge may lead to unreasonable expectations of the consumer in consumer–HCP interactions.

Ideally, HCP will be interacting with more sophisticated consumers. Although consumers may approach the clinical interaction with more information, the HCP will need to help them in understanding and drawing conclusions from myriad reports. HCPs will continue to assume leadership in making diagnoses and in playing an important role in discussions with consumers about treatment options. Consumers will continue to seek their expertise and depend on them for information and guidance in therapy. The role of the HCP will be more collaborative, serving more as a partner and consultant to the consumer, rather than as an authority figure.

Summary

As can be seen from the foregoing, a unified EHR will allow for adequate information for HCP at any time, anywhere, with varying degrees of control residing with the consumer. Relevant information from patient history, medications prescribed by different HCPs, and lab work performed for different specialists can be readily available. Redundancies can be reduced or eliminated. Cumulative records for a community or regional level can provide public health agencies with information to address community or regional problems. Benefits accrue to both consumers and HCPs in terms of health outcomes, satisfaction, and adequacy of information for decision making, plus cost savings for healthcare facilities. A key concept of consumer-accessed systems is the consumer as a participant and partner in the flow of information resulting in consumer empowerment. This aim is accomplished while recognizing the rights and responsibilities of the consumers, healthcare professionals, and other stakeholders, such as insurance enterprises and healthcare organizations.

Numerous challenges remain in the implementation and evaluation of the EHR. These challenges relate not only to issues of privacy, confidentiality, and security of data but also to human behavior factors. For instance, some questions for future resolution may include: To what extent should consumers have control over healthcare providers' selective access to health information? How can a consumer's longitudinal record be best stored and saved? If a chip is used and given to the consumer, what actions would take place if the consumer lost the chip? Can methods suggested [35], such as that of archiving records or maintaining a complete audit trail from which records can be reconstructed, be successfully implemented?

Future research is suggested in several areas: More large-scale studies are needed to investigate to what extent "empowerment" results in better healthcare outcomes and for consumers with which characteristics. How best to match consumer expectations with HCP behavior? What would be the optimal level of participation for different consumers? How can consumer and HCP behavior be changed to effect more effective and cost-effective outcomes? How can aspects of health information literacy be incorporated into systems for individualized consumer education?

Security of consumer data must continually receive high priority. Methods will undoubtedly improve with technological advances and creative applications. The extent to which security is maintained, and privacy and confidentiality are safeguarded, will be highly related to the acceptability of EHR systems to consumers. It is critical that further research be conducted to address these and other related issues. With continued application of research and support from healthcare providers, organizations, and governmental agencies, these and other challenges to the use of "womb-to-tomb"

EHRs will be overcome. Ultimately, more widespread use of a lifelong EHR is expected to improve health care for all people.

References

1. USDHHS (U.S. Department of Health and Human Services). Standards for privacy of individually identifiable health information. Final rule, 45 CRF Parts 160 and 164, RIN 0991-AB14; 2002. www.hhs/gov/ocr/hipaa/privruletxt.txt. Accessed 12-1-02.
2. Ball MJ, Lillis J. E-health: transforming the physician/patient relationship. Int J Med Inform 2001;61(1).
3. NHS Information Authority. Information for health—an information strategy for the modern NHS; 2002. http://www.nhsia.nhs.uk/. Accessed Dec.2002.
4. Kim MI, Johnson KB. Personal health records: evaluation of functionality and utility. J A Med Inform Assoc 2002;9:171–180.
5. Baur C, Deering MJ, Hsu L. ehealth: federal issues and approaches. In: Rice RE, Katz JE, editors. The Internet and health communications. Thousand Oaks, CA: Sage Publications; 2001. pp. 355–384.
6. National Electronic Health Records Taskforce. Health Online Action-Plan, 2nd ed., 2002. http://www.health.gov.au/healthonline/. Accessed 2003.
7. Patton MA. Research to impact national electronic health record agenda. DSTC Media Release; 2003. DSTC: http://www.dstc.edu.au. Accessed 2003.
8. Nash DB, Shulkin D, Comite F, et al., and the Winona Health Online Outcome Group. Measurement of the impact of health online. Dis Manag 2001;4(1):15–18.
9. Morrissey J. Minn. town to get health data online. Week in Healthcare; 2002. http://www.modernhealthcare.com/. 12-3-02.
10. Santa Barbara County Care Data Exchange; 2003. http://www.carescience.com/healthcare_providers/cde/. Accessed 12-4-02
11. Wendland M. News Front, Press Press; Dec. 2002.
12. Hagland M. Finding the e in healthcare. Healthcare Informatics 2001;November.
13. Turisco F, Metzger J. Rural health care delivery: connecting communities through technology. ihealth Reports 2002 (prepared by First Consulting Group, 17).
14. Cimino JJ, Patel VL, Kushniruk AW. The patient clinical information system (PatCIS): technical solutions and experience with giving patients access to their electronic medical records. Int J Med Inform 2002;68(1–3):113–127.
15. Masys D, Baker D, Butros A, Cowles, KE. Giving patients access to their medical records via the Internet. J Am Med Inform Assoc 2002;9(2):181–192.
16. Shea S, Starren J. Columbia University's informatics for diabetes education and telemedicine project: rationale and design. J Am Med Inform Assoc 2002;9(1):49–62.
17. Starren J, et al. Columbia University's Informatics for diabetes education and telemedicine project: technical implementation. J Am Med Inform Assoc 2002;9(1):25–36.
18. Safran C. The collaborative edge: patient empowerment for vulnerable populations. Int J Med Inform 2003;69(2–3):185–190.
19. Ueckert FK, Prokosch H. Implementing security and access control mechanisms for an electronic healthcare record. In: Proceedings of the American Medical Informatics Annual Symposium 2002. Philadelphia: Hanley & Belfus; 2002.
20. Berland GK, Elliott MN, Morales LS, et al. Health information on the Internet: accessibility, quality, readability in English and Spanish. JAMA 2001;285(20):2621–2612.
21. Ferguson T. E-patients: Robert Wood Johnson White Paper. Presented at the Annual Symposium of the American Medical Informatics Association, Nov. 2002, San Antonio, TX.
22. Ferguson T. What e-patients do online: a tentative taxonomy. Ferguson Reports, #9, Nov. 2002. http://www.fergusonreport.com/. Accessed 1-16-03.
23. Sands D. Electronic patient centered communication resource center. http://www.e-pcc.org. Accessed 1-16-03.
24. Fox S. Vital decisions. Pew Internet & American Life Project. http://www.pewinternet.org. Accessed Nov. 2002.

25. Baldwin G. Automating patient records. Reprinted from Technology in Practice 2002;3(3).
26. Goldman J, Hudson Z. Virtually exposed: privacy and e-health. Health Affairs 2000; 19(6):140–148.
27. Brubaker B. Sensitive Kaiser E-mails go astray. Washington Post 2000;Aug.10; Sect. E1.
28. Health Insurance Portability and Accountability Act of 1996. Public Law No. 104-191. Section 1173, USC 201. 1996.
29. Fox S, Wilson R. HIPAA regulations: Final. HIPAA Regs 2003; <http://www.hipaadvisory.com/regs/>.
30. Pitts J. Implementing the Federal health privacy rule in California; 2003. http://www.chcf.org/topics/view.cfm?itemid=19670. Accessed 1/22/2003.
31. Baker DB, Masys DR. PCASSO: a design for secure communication of personal health information via the Internet. Int J Med Inform 1999;54(2):97–104
32. The Gallup Organization. Public attitudes towards medical privacy. The Institute for Health Freedom; 2000. http://www.forhealthfreedom.org/Gallupsurvey/.
33. iHealthbeat. 2001. Business & finance: survey. http://www.ihealthbeat.org/members/basecontent. Accessed 1/22/2003.
34. Thomson Corporation and Health Data Management. Survey: hospitals boosting data security. http://www.healthdatamanagement.com/html/. Accessed 1/22/2003.
35. Grimson J. Delivering the electronic healthcare record for the 21st century. Int J Med Inform 2001;64(2–3):111–127.

26
Transforming the Physician Practice: Interviewing Patients with a Computer

Allen R. Wenner and John W. Bachman

Replacing the patient interview with detailed, patient-entered data via computer is refocusing the office encounter on the patient.

Evolution of the Physician Practice

Physician practices have evolved dramatically from the solo operations of yesteryear consisting of the husband-physician and wife-nurse team. Today, most physician practices are members of a larger group practice, sometimes a group of three physicians and sometimes multispecialty conglomerates with several hundred physicians. Within these myriad possibilities, there exist a variety of managed care structures, such as health maintenance organizations (HMO), preferred provider organizations (PPO), and physician hospital organizations (PHO). This evolution has resulted in the emergence of physician practice management as a field of study and in the reorganization of physician practices, in such a manner that the quality of patient care is of utmost priority.

Many physician organizations have faced crisis situations, beginning a decade ago, when the responsibility for payment of services shifted from the patient to a third party. Third-party regulations ended in-house laboratory testing for all but large groups, required the establishment of sophisticated back-office systems for payment processing, and ushered in new requirements for documentation and record keeping. These changes also required adjustment in the office workflow to accommodate the new rules.

Sir William Osler once said, "Listen to the patient, he's telling you the answer"[1]. Medical professionals, likewise, believe that 90 percent of diagnoses are made on the basis of the subjective history, 5 percent are made on the basis of the physical examination, and 5 percent are made on the basis of laboratory or X-ray studies.

In modern medicine, however, few physicians have the time to ask a patient all the questions necessary to complete the history of the present illness. Pressures from

Allen R. Wenner, MD, is Content Designer for Primetime Medical Software at the University of South Carolina School of Medicine at Columbia. John W. Bachman, MD, is a Consultant with the Department of Family Medicine at the Mayo Clinic. He is also a Professor of Family Medicine at the Mayo Medical School in Rochester, MN. Nothing in this chapter implies that the Mayo Foundation endorses the products of Primetime Medical Software.

management organizations put a premium on efficiency, making it increasingly difficult for providers to hear the patient's answers and formulate a thorough subjective note. On the other hand, federal regulators are raising the standards of care to require the gathering and documenting of a complete history for all patients. This bidirectional constriction is forcing providers everywhere to seek solutions to the data crisis of modern medicine.

The Doctor–Patient Relationship

Electronic medical records (EMRs) have emerged, amid much fanfare, as tools for managing health care's data dilemma. The most powerful EMR systems are able to manage data discretely for outcomes studies and coordination with billing systems. However, many fail to improve efficiency for the same reason: they require physicians or staff to enter all the data. Although many advanced technologies are emerging to aid the process of data entry, requiring clinicians to enter data into any record is the fundamental obstacle to reaching maximum efficiency. The ultimate solution embraces a new source of energy for data entry: patients.

It is very hard for physicians to make the choice between the patient and the third-party documentation. Physicians treat patients, not paper. Third parties require verification of the circumstances of the office visit that, if thoroughly completed, would force the physician to choose between treating the patient and buffing the chart to get paid. Only by using information technology can this dichotomy be resolved. The office visit with the patient should take center stage.

The practice philosophy is important to patients who come to a specific medical office. Insurance is certainly paramount, but the concept of a "locus of control" is also important in determining a physician. There are three forms of doctor–patient relationships:

1. The doctor is paternalistic, telling the patient what to do.
2. The doctor gives the patient information and the patient decides what to do.
3. Patients and doctors share information to determine the best plan for given conditions. Patients will help the physician when they have some degree of control, as in forms 2 and 3.

A real case history from the clinical practice of Allen R. Werner, MD, aptly illustrates this last point. This incident was the inspiration for Dr. Wenner to develop Instant Medical History.™ In 1984, before his clinic became the official research clinic for Primetime Medical Software, Inc., Wenner received a visit from a 60-year-old woman presenting nonspecific weakness and vague complaints. She was referred to numerous local specialists who were similarly nonplussed. Finally she was sent to a tertiary care center where a third-year medical student made the diagnosis. Unlike his predecessors who were rushed, the medical student asked her questions for 2 full hours. His relentless questioning revealed dysguesia, xerostomia, and xeropthalmia. When the information was summarized and presented to the interns, residents, and attending physician on medical rounds in the hospital, one of the experienced clinicians said that it sounded like Sjøgren's syndrome. The attentive student had gathered the information that revealed the answer that had eluded 12 other physicians. Osler was right. Upon the patient's return, she recounted the interview and diagnosis to Dr. Wenner. Marveling at the time-consuming interview process, he speculated as to whether a computer could ask all the same questions that the medical student had asked. Thus began the development of Instant Medical History.™

After researching the successes and failures of the simple systems developed by early pioneers, Wenner shifted his focus to studying the primary care medical practices of rural family practitioners. This helped to provide insight into office practice at its maximum. Because of the scarcity of rural physicians, these doctors often saw 70 to 100 patients per day. The clinics were generally very busy, significantly overworked, had difficult patients, and were under considerable pressure. There was no time to use computer systems for isolated complaints of special patients. A total Review of Systems diagnostic approach for developing a functional clinical application was necessary. Wenner's examination of the methods of service in these rural clinics served as an example for a comprehensive computer application.

A clinic day is a constant stream of patients with acute illnesses mixed with patients returning for review of chronic disorders. It is very hard to predict exactly how long each patient will require for the highest level of care to be delivered, so doctors often run behind. In contrast, the opportunity to add information to the medical chart while waiting is accepted by patients. Patients from the morning often spill over into lunch, which is often abbreviated. Major challenges for the staff are keeping the patients from waiting too long in the waiting room or exam rooms by getting vital signs and laboratory studies done quickly. The clinic can be more efficient with patient-entered data, reducing the paperwork required by the staff, thereby speeding the patient throughput.

Nurses in many primary care offices function as physician extenders. Using their considerable clinical experience and personal knowledge of patients, they take present illness histories by talking with patients before the encounter. In the conversation, the nurse reviews the pertinent organ system, follows up each positive, checks the pertinent negatives, and inquires about other issues such as stress, diet, etc. Using a fund of knowledge "database," the nurse performs a repetitive, yet necessary, labor-intensive task for the physician. In doing so, the nurse aids the physician at arriving at a diagnosis by presenting critical information to the physician for review. It is important to observe that a nurse never tells a doctor the diagnosis. In other words, the nurse is an "expert system" that helps the physician to decide what is wrong with the patient. Wenner believed that a computer could also function in this capacity to extend the physician's ability to interview patients, and like the medical student, the computer could also have plenty of time to be thorough, tireless, inexpensive, and go without food or rest for days.

In emergency rooms, specially trained "triage nurses" screen patients to decide which patients need immediate attention. The emergency room triage nurse is also an "expert system" because he or she helps to decide how sick a patient really is and how long treatment can be delayed. This assessment function is based on a simple branching "database" of knowledge deduced each time from what patients say about their symptoms. The review is often a simplified, organ-specific review of systems like that performed by the clinic nurse. Also in like fashion, the physician is directed by this triage assessment to begin determining the diagnosis. Additional analysis of this interview process suggests that a computer could also be used to triage patients.

Encounter by Computer

A nurse walks a patient to a computer in an examination room. Using knowledge-based questioning, the computer collects the medical history and symptoms of the present illness directly from the patient. The questions gathered from a database of more than 50,000 questions are response driven so that each interview is personalized. In addition, standardized, published self-rating and self-assessment scales from the medical literature are administered and tabulated.

At the conclusion of the computer interview, the patient's complaints are succinctly presented, either on a printout or electronically, to a physician entering the examination room. The physician glances at the positive answers with graphically depicted scales and arrives at a working clinical impression in a few seconds. In the opening moments of the interview, confirmation of the diagnosis is possible with open-ended questions.

When the encounter begins, the physician and the patient are totally and instantly focused on the problems at hand. Time is provided for relationship building, patient education, and casual conversation. The majority of information needed to create a note has been obtained without any effort by the physician, so less time is spent on documenting the interview. With a few notes added by the physician, the record is complete when the patient leaves the examination room. The patient can even be given a copy of the documentation. The encounter is comprehensive, efficient, and compassionate.

The seeds of this effort were developed in 1949 at Cornell University. Patients answered questions on a punch card and inserted it into a massive, expensive computer. The conclusion of the experience was that "... It collects for appraisal a large and comprehensive body of information about the patient's medical history at no expenditure of the physician's time; it facilitates interview by making available to the physician a preliminary survey of the patient's total medical problems; its data, being systematically arranged, are easier to review than those on conventional medical histories, and, *by calling attention to the patient's symptoms and significant items of past history*, *it assures that their investigation will not be overlooked because the physician lacked time to elicit them*" [2]. Today, computers are interviewing patients in offices and on the Web. This chapter discusses the merits and practicalities of using computers for patient interviewing.

The Future Is Now

For 40 years, the computer software programs used for patient–computer studies were not available commercially. There has been one exception. During the past 15 years, Primetime Medical Software, Inc. (Columbia, SC; www.medicalhistory.com/) has introduced artificial intelligence medical interview software that enables patients to enter their own subjective complaints and populate their own medical records. Eliminating the bulk of transcription and dictation and replacing it with detailed, patient-entered data has transformed the office encounter from a data-gathering session into an opportunity to concentrate on the most important task at hand: caring for the patient.

Today, the Internet increases efficiency even more dramatically. The same patient can create his or her own subjective note from home before visiting the physician's office. The physician receives the information in advance through secure transmissions, schedules an appointment of the proper duration for the indicated complaints, and allocates the necessary personnel and equipment for any expected procedures. When all the patients follow the same routine, precision appointment management reaches its pinnacle.

Listening to the Patient

Recalling the words of Sir William Osler, "Listen to the patient, he's telling you the answer" [1] brings up the question: How do clinicians listen? The evidence indicates that they do not listen as well as they would like. Surveys of patient perceptions of physicians' skills rank communication as one of the poorest. Observations of medical interviews find that physicians often discourage the voicing of concerns, expectations, and requests for information, an approach that results in the loss of relevant information [3,4]. For example, during the standard interview, physicians interrupt a patient in less than 24 seconds. Physicians often use medical terminology that is not understood by patients [5]. Why? Physicians are pressed for time and need to get to the point quickly. There are increasing demands to document the encounter, which saps time away from the patient. Documentation is now not only for the healthcare provider but also for protection against malpractice claims and for remuneration. The entire phenomenon has been termed the "hamster effect" [6]. Physicians are running faster and faster on a treadmill to stay in the same place—just like a hamster. A better method is needed.

Slack et al. first described the use of a digital computer to obtain a medical history in 1966 at the University of Wisconsin [7]. The use of computers in medical interviewing has also been reviewed extensively [8]. The review has shown that computer–patient interviewing provided more information, especially about areas clinicians fail to investigate, such as review of systems, prevention, and psychiatric issues. The review also described numerous studies showing that the computer is more adept at obtaining socially sensitive information, such as alcoholism, abuse, and sexual behavior, because the computer is impersonal and makes no judgments. This experience has been described as follows [9]:

It (the computer) does not get tired, angry, or bored. It is always willing to listen and to provide evidence of having heard. It can work at any time of the day or night, every day of the week, every month of the year. Its performance does not vary from hour to hour or from day to day. It has no facial expression. It does not raise an eyebrow. It is very polite. It has perfect memory. It need not be morally judgmental. It has no superior social status. It does not seek money. It can provide the patient with a copy of the interview to study. It does what it is supposed to and no more (and no less).

Other advantages of patient interviewing by computer are these. Patients can review their histories and organize their thoughts for the physician. The computer produces legible output. The computer calculates well and can use the answers to several questions to form a scale or graph. Patients can complete the computer program at their own pace. Software can be used to provide questions in different languages or in spoken form.

The review also pointed out some shortcomings of patient–computer interaction. The computer generated more false-positive results than traditional interviewing. If a patient replied that he did not have a symptom, the answer was generally true. However, if the symptom response was positive, the symptom might have been trivial or of no consequence. Thus, clinicians should not check all the responses a computer has given but deal with only the positive responses. The computer–patient dialogue does not allow judgment of nonverbal behavior. A computer is unable to look at a patient and see sadness or anxiety. Generally, patient acceptance is very high, but a small group of patients will not want to use a computer.

The Computer–Clinician Partnership

With the advent and proliferation of the personal computer in the late 1980s, software engineers and clinical application experts at Primetime Medical Software, Inc., collaborated in the production of a comprehensive application capable of delivering artificial intelligence patient interviews from a branching knowledge base of thousands of questions. First called the "Review of Systems System," the technology used by Instant Medical History evolved with advancements in hardware. Over time, the first interactive review-of-systems interview software running on the Microsoft DOS platform became an extensible interview-component technology embedded in many electronic medical record applications and deliverable through the Internet. As a result, it became immediately possible to administer medical history interviews to patients at their homes before they visited their physicians' clinics [1,10].

The computer and the clinician are partners, not competitors. The human brain and the computer work best together when each is given the tasks that they do well. Computers do low-level thinking very fast. For example, repetitive, monotonous, or boring tasks lend themselves well to automation. Alternatively, people do high-level integrative tasks very fast. In 1968, John Mayne at the Mayo Clinic captured the spirit of this interaction:

... to relieve the physician from routine, although important, time-consuming activities, thereby extending his capabilities to provide medical care.

If the time physicians spend collecting, organizing, recording, and retrieving data could be reduced, at least in part, by information technology, more time would be available for actual delivery of medical care (and, thus, in effect increase the number of physicians) and at the same time the physician's capabilities for collecting information from patients would be extended [11].

Integrating information, making diagnoses, and forming summaries are done well by physicians who have been trained thoroughly in medical schools. Computers cannot infer diagnoses well from limited or excess information. Computers gather data and calculate. Clinicians integrate facts into conclusions. Early experimentation in patient interviewing emphasized the diagnostic possibilities of putting patients' complaints into differential diagnosis algorithms, but the tremendous number of diagnostic variables suggested that physicians could always integrate information better than software. A computer that interviews patients provides more data so the physician can integrate better.

Development of Instant Medical History

In the first attempt to develop the Instant Medical History, it was decided that the computer could ask all the necessary questions intelligently if it was given a limited set of initial information. On the basis of the functioning of a clinic nurse or an emergency room triage nurse, it was decided that a nurse could select age, sex, and any of an array of symptoms or organ systems for review from a menu on a software interface. At that point, the computer could pose questions that simulated a live patient interview. When the software was produced in the late 1980s, the nurse initiated it in this manner. Eventually, the Instant Medical History program allowed patients or the accompanying caregiver to conduct the triage function and load the necessary initial information set for the clinical interview. After the initialization information was obtained, extensive branching technology used a patient's responses to each question to initiate additional, more specific questions and thus generate a personalized interview.

Over time, the knowledge base was expanded, but to demonstrate its content, the simplest example is that of an interview for a patient presenting with both cold and flu symptoms. For example, if the nurse activated the URI and Sinus section, the patient would answer questions about nasal discharge, fever, allergies, and other related topics. If the patient indicated having a fever, then the computer asked several questions about the fever and followed up each positive response with questions that provided specific information about, for example, nature and duration. Wenner and his team of software developers determined that this process was most similar to the behavior of a physician in a live interview. As medicine becomes more complex, increasing information is required. For example, an interview about the upper respiratory tract and sinuses should include questions about prevention, use of tobacco, and risk for pregnancy. The clinician may forget or just not have enough time to ask these questions. A physician survey about another computerized general history program showed that the questions that were most valuable to clinicians were those related to psychiatry (100 percent), alternative care (93 percent), review of systems (80 percent), occupational exposures (67 percent), and prevention (60 percent) [12].

Patient-Entered Data: Efficiency and Point-of-Care Documentation

Once the patient had answered the questions, the recorded answers became the starting point for the encounter. The symptoms were put in an organized format. The output mechanism was designed to be succinct and easy to read to suggest a correct diagnosis to the skilled clinician at a glance. When the interview was complete, the positive and pertinent negative responses were presented in list form to the physician instead of being passed into a diagnostic algorithm. Headings such as Past Medical History or ENT were color-coded. The positive responses were in boldface and the negative responses were in light gray type. Specialists were allowed to adjust settings on the software so more detailed questions pertaining to their specialty could be asked. Generalists could adjust the settings to provide a broader set of questions with less depth. In addition, computers combine the answers to several questions and provide a scale for assessment of a condition. Examples include scales on sleep disturbances, depression, or severity of prostate symptoms. The output (minus the colored font) of a patient–computer interview is as follows:

Chief Complaint
DSC is a 20-year-old female. Her chief complaint is "neck pain."

History of Present Illness
#1 "neck pain"
She reported: neck pain with weakness and dizziness | neck stiffness | neck pain sometimes prevents sleep.
She denied: swelling of neck, arm, hand.
Location
She reported: neck pain radiation | neck pain radiates to shoulders | neck pain radiates to mid back | neck pain radiates to arms | neck pain radiates down arm | neck pain starts in shoulder | neck pain changed location | pain started between the shoulders.

Quality
She reported: neck pain description as sharp, cutting, or shooting | neck pain description as dull, sore, or aching | neck pain different this occurrence.

Severity
She reported: neck pain mild.
She denied: neck pain increasing severity.

Duration
She reported: neck pain present for days | neck pain present all the time | neck pain duration longer.

Time
She reported: neck pain recurrent | nocturnal neck pain | neck pain is sometimes worse in the morning | neck pain onset between 3 days and 3 weeks ago | neck pain recurrence less than once a month.

Context
She denied: recent sudden neck extension.

Modifying Factors
She reported: neck pain caused or exacerbated by activity | neck pain aggravated by neck extension | neck pain aggravated by motion.
She denied: neck pain caused or exacerbated by sitting or lying in certain positions | neck pain aggravated by cold | neck pain improved by head motion | neck pain improved by shaking arm | neck pain alleviated by heat.

Associated Signs and Symptoms
She reported: pain prevents enjoying family life.
She denied: neck pain has affected mental health | pain prevents leaving home | pain prevents work.

Past, Family, and Social History
Past Medical History
She denied: recent surgery or injury.

Pregnancy History
She denied: pregnant now | pregnancy.

Social History
She denied: repetitive motions | prolonged work above shoulders | recent new activity.

Activities for Daily Living
History of: difficulty with certain activities.

Alcohol
She denied: alcohol use this month.

Medication History
History of: analgesic use.

Ongoing Medications
History of: acetaminophen for pain | non-prescription non-steroidal anti-inflammatory medication for pain.
She denied: aspirin for pain | prescription non-steroidal anti-inflammatory medication for pain | steroids for pain | moderate analgesics for pain | strong analgesics for pain | narcotics for pain.

Review of Systems
Constitutional
She reported: fever in the past week | fever 3 to 4 days | pain sometimes prevents going to sleep | pain stops activities.
She denied: fever over 100.4°F (38°C) | rigor associated with fever.

Respiratory
She reported: neck pain is sometimes accompanied by dyspnea.
Cardiovascular
She denied: chest pain associated with neck pain.
Breast
She denied: currently breastfeeding a child.
Gastrointestinal
She reported: nausea associated with neck pain.
Neurological
She reported: frequent cephalgia | headaches more than twice a month | headache similar to previous headaches.
She denied: paresthesia associated with neck pain | worst headache ever | headache daily.
Psychiatric
She reported: recent stress | calm a good part of the time | sad some of the time | some of the time feeling happy.
She reported: nervous a little of the time | depressed a little of the time.

Self-Assessment Scales [13]
Title: **Mental Health Inventory Screening Test (MHI-5)**
Description: Short 5-item version of the 18-item Mental Health Inventory for detecting affective disorders. No level of severity is revealed because of the brevity of the scale.
Patient Score: **10—Passed mental health screen**
Scoring Key and Interpretation:
   0–17: Passed mental health screen
   18–30: Failed mental health screen

Reviewing this output is easy, and before going into the interview, the physician is armed with a great deal of useful information to help the patient efficiently. Also, the patient-provided information documents much of the information a clinician would need to type or dictate.

In reviewing the history, a physician learns a great deal in a minimal time. In this instance, the back pain was now absent. However, the interview was able to deal with the patient's smoking. The patient was ready to quit and needed a basic outline of how to do it. Also, the problem of alcoholism was identified. This sometimes is difficult for clinicians to address. In this interview, the clinician was able to say, "The computer states that you have a problem with alcohol. What do you think about this?" This question led to a dialogue, which resulted with the person getting additional help for chemical dependency.

Another important element of history taking is the depth to which a patient is asked questions. Perhaps the detail in the example given is too much, but this amount can be changed. The software developed by Primetime allows the clinician to select the intensity, or level of detail, of an interview. Consequently, a physician can eliminate the psychological testing that occurs if there is a lack of systems to deal with the issues. The use of computer interviews improves the quality of the information presented by the patient through standardized screening and allows a physician to converse casually with a patient while gathering the objective information needed to make a confident diagnosis. The amount of writing, typing, or dictation is reduced dramatically. More time is provided for explaining the diagnosis and educating the patient than during traditional encounters. Figure 26.1a,b compare time allocations for a 12-minute office visit with the allocations when the Instant Medical History is used. Examples of other patient outputs are available at www.medicalhistory.com.

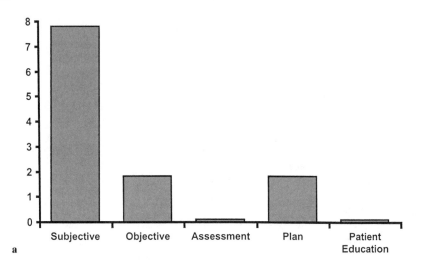

a

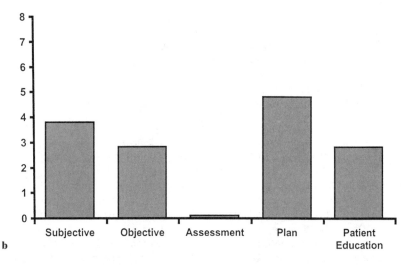

b

FIGURE 26.1a,b. a Allocations of a 12-minute traditional office visit; b shows allocations of a 12-minute office visit in which patient interview was conducted with Instant Medical History. The numbers on the vertical axis represent minutes. The amount of writing, typing, or dictation is reduced dramatically in b. More time is devoted to explaining the diagnosis and educating the patient than in the traditional encounter.

In addition to improving the quality of the encounter, the computer interview reduced the pressure to enter information into the computer by a clinician. In the late 1990s, because the output of the computer interview could be printed or copied into electronic medical records immediately, documenting the visit became as easy as annotating the subjective output with macros enabled by the electronic medical record application. Combining these technologies meant that the chart usually could be finished completely when the patient left the examination room. Realization of this workflow, called "point-of-care documentation," is the ultimate efficiency goal of clinicians.

Documenting an encounter at the point of care is the most efficient method of practicing medicine because the physician completes the medical record at the time of a patient's visit. Dictation time is saved (a primary care physician dictates for more than 50 minutes in an 8.2-hour workday) [14], and the need for personal dictation aides is eliminated. Thus, point-of-care documentation is less expensive than traditional dictation with its associated high cost of transcription. In addition, the physician can sign the note immediately. Patient care is improved because the patient can leave with a complete copy of the medical record, a step that stimulates compliance. The delivery process is improved with point-of-care documentation because referrals can be accomplished with full information available at the time that the referral is needed. For these benefits to occur, the clinical workflow changes to improve efficiency, increase data accuracy, and lower the overall cost of health care delivery. Finally, it provides transparency, one of the several goals advocated to improving our health care system [15].

For understanding point-of-care documentation, assessment of the typical office visit without the benefit of interview software is instructional. The traditional workflow requires that the physician enter the examination room and greet the patient. Because no information has been provided about the patient except for a few notes from the nurse, the physician begins by asking why the patient has sought care. After briefly listening to the patient describe a complaint, the clinician interrupts to clarify the story, often cutting off the patient's natural flow of narration. The physician then begins to ask questions that elucidate a medical problem indicated by the patient. The physician controls the duration of the interview. Because of time pressures, the physician tries to ask the fewest possible number of questions to arrive at the diagnosis. With experience, a physician will ask increasingly fewer questions to formulate a provisional diagnosis before proceeding to the physical examination. After completing the assessment, writing a prescription, explaining the treatment, and showing the patient out, the physician goes to a private area to complete the patient's record and dictates his or her recollection of the history as told by the patient, any other relevant data gleaned from the chart or encounter, information from the physical examination, diagnosis, prescription, and treatment plan. After the patient leaves the clinic, there is a delay of a few days for closure of the medical record while the dictation is transcribed, sent for signature, and filed in the patient's medical chart. If the patient needs care before the medical record is completed, the valuable information from this encounter is not available to the treating clinician except from memory, and it is not available at all if another clinician is summoned.

Interview software and electronic medical record technologies can dramatically improve this traditional workflow. Because interview software provides a structured, organized document before the encounter begins, two main avenues for improved efficiency result. First of all, the physician has the opportunity to formulate a diagnosis before seeing the patient. This allows the physician to ask fewer questions about the diagnosis and more about its effects on the patient. The clinician does not need to interrupt the rambling of a patient's story because the basics are already known. Second, after asking a few confirmatory questions, physicians can complete the medical history in the examination room while the patient is still present. This improves the accuracy of the record and enables point-of-care documentation. Data concerning prevention, abuse, or other screening are also documented and never forgotten because the interview software records them. Also, when the patient is being interviewed by a computer, the patient controls the speed of the interview.

Because interview software records subjective information from the patient, the data are a more complete and accurate reflection of a patient's complaints than a physician's dictation thereof after the visit. Also, because the physician can review the information already entered by the patient, the patient's time and effort to enter the data are rewarded and the physician can add additional information as necessary by editing and adding to the text provided. Physician annotations can be reviewed by the patient for accuracy at the point of care instead of weeks later.

Electronic medical record systems facilitate documentation of the rest of the visit at the point of care. First, autotext macros, common in word processors, allow the physician to document the physical examination rapidly, documenting only by exception. With this often completed in less than a minute and ready for the record, no dictation or transcription is necessary. Next, because most electronic medical records specialize in diagnosis, prescription, and treatment plan automation, these elements often can be completed with rapid clicks of the computer pointing device. In the most sophisticated practices, the completed chart is handed to patients as they exit the building. This is clearly only possible with point-of-care documentation.

Developing an Ultimate Knowledge Base

Obtaining a medical history with computer software is a form of artificial intelligence, and for a long time it has been recognized as a potentially efficient means of gathering patient data. Although Wenner and associates now deliver patient interview software over the Internet at high daily volumes, this was not possible during the early phases of knowledge base development because of the scarcity of personal computers capable of supporting such technology. It was not until the early 1990s that such advanced technology was successfully implemented in a clinical setting. Clinicians were not in environments where personal computers were available. The infrastructure to support networks has been developed only in the past few years.

These factors forced the development of patient questioning to be empirical in its earliest stages. Wenner and associates continuously revised and improved their knowledge base in thousands of clinical encounters. The process was time-consuming, difficult, and expensive. In fact, many years of the development process required private investment because of the lack of a market and the lack of an infrastructure that included personal computers and access to the Internet. However, these difficulties were not limited to the developers of interview software at Wenner's facility. As late as 1999, many electronic medical record software companies suffered great losses or even stopped their operations because of the same lack of penetration into the medical practice market.

The software developed versatility. For example, specialists want detailed information about a small area of complaint. Generalists want information that covers a wide spectrum. Consequently, settings were developed that allowed changes to the depth of questioning about a complaint. For the complaint of allergy, for example, a high setting might involve 60 questions and a low setting 10. Also, the ability to populate fields in an electronic medical record has been realized. In 2002, GE Medical Systems Logician (GE Medical Systems, Hillsboro, OR), an electronic medical record, entered coded text from Instant Medical History into its system. This was a very big step in history taking. The patient entered information in a codified, structured format that could be searched, retrieved, and studied from within a comprehensive electronic health record.

Designing Questions for Patients

Having interviewed about 100,000 patients since 1991, Wenner determined several rules for designing an interview for a patient. All the rules are based on his reinforced finding that because patients want their physicians to arrive at the best diagnosis, they are willing to answer questions, especially when they are posed in an interesting medium and in an efficient manner.

Respect for the Patient

Patients are sick. They usually have a specific reason for coming to the office. They want and expect to be asked questions about this reason. They do not want their time to be wasted. They want their physician to have enough information to treat them appropriately. Patients deserve respect throughout the medical process. They should be the center of care whether having their blood pressure determined or sitting in front of a computer. The computer should be in a place where no one else can see what the patient is entering into the computer.

Principle of Neutrality

Computers are nonjudgmental, impartial, and fair. Patients perceive that the computer will not judge them as a result of their answers because interview software makes no indication about the rectitude of responses. When every patient who visits a clinic routinely is asked to use the computer, the egalitarian nature of the computer interview is reinforced further. These factors allow the computer to gather information that would not be given to an interviewer and explain why patients provide more sensitive information to a computer than to a person.

Principle of Parsimony

There is a maximum number of questions that a person can tolerate answering on a computer. This number is not known. A weak, tired, and dizzy patient might answer numerous questions and be pleased that "someone is finally listening." Alternatively, a person with a sore throat might want to answer only a few questions. Software has been developed that provides either a short or a long list of questions for a particular symptom. Another obvious help is the ability to stop the computer program and retain the information gathered if the physician thinks that too much time is being spent on the interview.

Principle of Narcissism

People like to talk about themselves and their problems. Good listeners know this rule well. Computers should observe the same principle if they are to be successful. The design of software questionnaires must attend to the issues of the patient. If the percentage of negative answers increases as the patient continues through the program, then it is not addressing the patient's complaint. The patient does not have the problems about which questions are being asked. The converse of this principle is that patients do not like to talk about what is not wrong with them. Patients will tolerate several negative or irrelevant questions because the answers may be important to the physician. There is a short limit of perhaps a dozen or fewer questions that the patient will want to deny before questioning the pertinence of the interview.

Principle of Transference

Patients believe that the physician is really asking the questions being posed by the computer. This power of interview software increases a physician's productivity. By transferring some work to a computer, the physician can perform other tasks. Because the physician can review the results of the interview before seeing the patient, the physician can formulate open-ended questions related to the subjective prompts; this sequence encourages patients to perceive that the time they spent on the computer contributed directly to the physician's understanding of their complaints. During the time that one patient is completing the computer interview, the physician can be treating another patient, thus improving productivity.

Principle of Persistence

Computers are consistent and persistent. The computer can ask questions exactly the same at 5 P.M. as it did at 8 A.M. Humans tire; computers do not. Humans forget; computers do not. When a physician tires, he or she may forget to ask a question that is vital to a diagnosis. Without the proper information, the physician will not know the correct diagnosis and possibly not pursue the proper course of action. When all the information is always presented in the same consistent way, the job of the physician is simplified. This is the power of persistent interviewing of patients.

Branching to Responses

Screening should mimic human conversation in response time and logic sequences. In human conversation, one question leads to another; one thought may lead to multiple questions. Instant Medical History functions similarly: answers to initial questions determine subsequent questions. Because the software has a knowledge base of tens of thousands of questions, innumerable question patterns are possible, but certain packets are recognizable as Question Sets. Determining these question paths through its many Question Sets is the task of the software engine, and it is driven by triggers.

Triggering

The concept of triggering is important. A *trigger* is the stimulus that initiates the *response*: the next question, set of questions, or bank of questions. Questions are grouped in *sets* and *sequences*. A set of questions contains questions relating to the same symptom or organ system. A sequence of questions quantifies or qualifies a prior question. A *bank* of questions includes all the sets and all the branches from these sets. Primary questions occur in sets, and they trigger secondary, tertiary, and quaternary questions in sequence. Both question sets and sequences can be triggered by different patient input responses.

Patients can and will find themselves answering questions in various sets because the questions within the sets also branch. Only a physician should determine which questions were actually germane to the complaint about the present illness and which questions were purely confirmatory or supplemental to the history. Care must be taken to reduce the number of confirmatory questions to increase screening efficiency.

Instant Medical History Trigger Types

Four types of responses to triggers occur in Instant Medical History:

1. Simple trigger: questions trigger more specific follow-up questions

   Do you have a fever? ↵

   ⇨ Was your fever over 102°F?

   ⇨ Was the highest fever in the past 24 hours?

   ⇨ Have you had a fever for more than 5 days?

   ⇨ Did you have chills with your fever?

2. Bank trigger: questions trigger entire banks of questions

   Do you have any pain in your chest with activity or exercise? ↵

   Cardiovascular Review of Systems

3. Cascade trigger: specific questions trigger self-assessment evaluations

   Did you drink any alcohol in the last month? ↵

   CAGE Alcohol Screen ↵

   Michigan Alcohol Screening Test

   (In this case, a positive response led to confirmatory question and subsequently a standardized rating scale.)

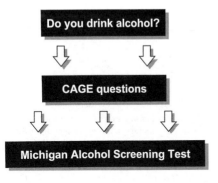

Exhibit of Common Instant Medical History™
Trigger Sequence:

Positive Response → Confirmatory Questions → Standardized Rating Scale

4. Pattern triggers: patterns of responses trigger banks of questions

   Positive or abnormal answers to 75% of questions ↵

   Mental health assessment ↵

   Self-rating scale for life stress ↵

   Self-rating anxiety scale ↵

   Self-rating depression (positive or abnormal answers to 7 or more organ systems) ↵

   General Health Questionnaire

Implementation

Physical Plant Considerations

Traditional clinical medicine (Table 26.1) is characterized by its interview process, in which a physician asks a patient several questions to formulate a diagnosis. A nurse may ask the patient a few screening questions to focus the physician on the patient's reasons for seeking a medical evaluation. After the examination, the physician dictates notes for a transcriber; after transcription, the notes are included in the medical record. Alternatively, records are handwritten and placed in a chart.

With computerized screening (see Table 26.1), however, the procedure allows physicians and nurses to concentrate their efforts on healthcare delivery instead of documentation. In Patient-Initiated mode, at the start of a patient's visit, the computer poses triage and subjective complaint questions directly to the patient, summarizing the patient's responses in medical jargon for the clinician. (If Nurse-Initiated mode is configured, the nurse does the primary triage and configures the software for specific questioning.) The nurse evaluates vital signs, enters results into the medical record, and presents the output summary to the provider. The provider reviews the summary before the medical interview, and then the examination begins. The provider should very quickly have a working clinical diagnosis on which to direct the patient encounter. At the end of the examination, the provider can quickly generate the output and close the chart. Documentation can be completed in several ways: by annotating the report generated, by copying the output to any electronic medical record already in place, by saving the subjective complaint information in a text file, or by printing the subjective information for inclusion in a paper chart system.

TABLE 26.1. Comparison of a traditional office visit with computerized screening office visit.

Traditional	Computerized screening
1. Patient checks in, waits to be called	1. Either the nurse or the patient initiates Instant Medical History computer questioning
2. Patient completes or updates paper forms	2. Patient enters own history into the computer
3. Nurse triages patient on basis of complaint	3. Computer separates the positive and important negative responses and translates the patient data into medical jargon for physician
4. Nurse makes notes to guide physician interview	
5. Nurse assesses and records vital signs	
6. Staff enters data from paper form	4. Nurse assesses and records vital signs in electronic medical record
7. Patient waits for physician in examination room	
8. Physician enters examination room	5. Physician reviews the data before interviewing the patient
9. Physician gathers SOAP data in interview*	
10. Patient pays at staff counter and exits	6. Physician formulates a working diagnosis before examination of patient
11. Physician records notes for chart or dictates, then sees next patient in next examination room	7. Physician finishes the OAP component of SOAP data while patient is in examination room
12. Transcriptionist completes chart	8. Physician sends output to electronic medical record, paper, or electronic file and then sees next patient
13. Staff handles reimbursements	
14. Reimbursement request denied by insurance agency because of lack of documentation	9. Patient arranges for payment at staff counter and exits
	10. Staff handles reimbursements, receives full rate because of thoroughness of documentation

* SOAP, subjective, objective, assessment, plan.

Offices implementing computerized screening should keep the education procedure changes in mind when considering how office flow will be affected by screening patients with a computer. Primarily, physicians should be ready to view the results when patients finish the questioning. This timing consideration has an impact on the visit scheduling because patients need to arrive 10 to 25 minutes (depending on the speed of the PC, PC availability, and the complexity of a patient's complaint) ahead of their appointment time (or schedule the appointments 10–25 minutes ahead of the attending physician's schedule). Wave scheduling, in which two patients arrive at the same time, is often useful. If the interview is done on the Internet by the patient at home, the information can be used to determine the duration of the office visit. Clinicians can receive structured histories obtained by interviewing software through e-mail and virtual office visits.

Administration Logistics

Deciding where and how to administer computer screening depends on the physical plant and equipment available to the practice. Medically, new patients require more time at the computer, and examination of complex complaints takes more time than that of simple complaints. The decision of where and how to administer the screening hinges on the factors of hardware and location.

Hardware Considerations

Interviewing software does not require expensive computers. Computers that are outdated by today's standards serve well. Generally, preference should be given to a computer that can be dedicated exclusively to patient screening if an electronic medical record is not in place. Touch tablets and point-and-click devices, although more expensive, work well for the interviewing process. Alternatively, Internet connections that interface to an electronic medical record system can be provided in waiting areas operated by the facility.

Location Considerations

Laptop or desktop computers at private consoles in the waiting or subwaiting area allow patients to spend unlimited time generating their subjective histories. Handheld screening units provide similar amenities. Output can either be printed for the user at the kiosk or sent to a printer in the examination room, aiding efficiency. If the screening is configured for interface with an electronic medical record, the data can be uploaded automatically to a network without prompting.

E-mail triage of scheduling concerns can be accomplished with patient screening. The interview occurs in a secured environment that allows it to be viewed by the healthcare providers. The data then can be transferred to the proper chart or electronic file well in advance of a patient's arrival, and the appointment time can be adjusted according to the complexity of the patient's complaints.

The ideal setting for the computer interview is in an examination room. This enhances the privacy of the interview and, on some systems, allows for interface with the electronic medical record at the point of care. Because both patient and physician appreciate these benefits, this approach is recommended. However, examination room administration requires a computer for each room and ample rooms for patients requiring additional screening time. For practices in which the physical plant affords the necessary space and staff to support examination room administration, particular attention should be paid to appointment scheduling (see "Physical Plant Considerations" above).

The use of interview software can be the first step to attaining an electronic environment. A clinician who handwrites notes will find that the output generated by Instant Medical History is a useful outline for editing with a pen or pencil.

Obtaining the Data

Data from patient screening are primarily useful for providing pertinent information that allows an immediate diagnosis. Not only does the physician have a reasonable idea of the patient's diagnosis before any examination begins, but also the data are instantly ready to become part of the medical record. The increased efficiency that computer screening allows makes office visits more enjoyable because the physician has more time to explain the diagnosis and educate the patient.

Ultimately, the combination of computer screening and an electronic medical record can provide the most efficient use of patient-entered data.

Preventive Health Screening

Because most patients wait 15 minutes to see a physician, it is medically appropriate to screen patients for compliance with health maintenance guidelines while they wait. For this reason, in 1997, Wenner implemented the Health Employment and Data Information Set (HEDIS) Prevention Guidelines for preventive procedures, vaccinations, and interventions as part of Instant Medical History. The implementation, called the Health Maintenance portion of the knowledge base, was designed for placement in the waiting area of clinical facilities. This specialized use of Instant Medical History poses questions about compliance with the HEDIS Guidelines and also about wellness and diet, which serve as reminders to exercise, drink water, eat fruits and vegetables, and not smoke.

In the course of a yearlong study that eventually continued into spring 1999, legacy systems (486–25MHz, 40MB HDD, laser printer) installed on $60 kiosks for under $350 were stationed in semiprivate corners of the waiting areas in 10 UCI Medical Affiliates' Doctor's Care clinics [12]. Patients were invited to answer a few questions on the computer when they spoke to the triage nurse, but screening was completely voluntary. Over time, the software revealed the need for hundreds of tetanus shots, varicella vaccinations, Papanicolaou smears, and other preventive measures by asking patients simple questions about the duration since their last assessment.

One case history in the HEDIS study particularly illustrates the power of interview software. One afternoon, J.G., a patient of Dr. Wenner's, visited the clinic to obtain a prescription for a refill for his wife, also Wenner's patient. In the lobby of the Doctor's Care Family Medical Center in West Columbia, South Carolina, he noticed one of the computer kiosks running the Instant Medical History program. A sign posted beside the system urged patients to "Stay Healthy: Take Our Prevention Questionnaire." Because J.G. was aware of some health risks for men older than 50, he decided to answer the questions while the prescription refill was being authorized. In addition to eating and exercise recommendations, the results of the interview suggested that J.G. needed the standard procedure to check for colon cancer because he could not recall having been checked within the timeframe suggested by HEDIS (the computer question was, "Have you had a lighted tube rectal exam [proctosigmoidoscopy] in the last five years?" and the output to the clinician was "PREVENTIVE PROCEDURES POSSIBLY NECESSARY: proctosigmoidoscopy").

At the suggestion of the computer, J.G. spoke with the triage nurse about the procedure. The nurse confirmed it as a wise preventive action to take and scheduled an appointment. A few weeks later, J.G. returned to the clinic and was waiting in the examination room when Dr. Wenner entered. Surprised about J.G.'s visit for such a specific health procedure months before his annual physical examination, Wenner asked who scheduled the appointment. In a tone reflecting his expectation that it was common for patients to schedule proctosigmoidoscopies on their own volition without a prior discussion with the physician, J.G. responded, "Well, your computer did."

Although J.G. had consulted with the nurse, Wenner had not been informed of his reasons for seeking the procedure. Because he could see that J.G. fit the risk category (although the software had acquired that information before posing the procedure as a needed item anyway) and was due for the test, Wenner performed the procedure. The large precancerous polyp that was discovered might have gone completely undetected without the intelligent prompting of the Instant Medical History program. The polyps were removed without complication, and J.G. was prevented from having colon cancer. J.G. strongly believed that Instant Medical History saved his life by interactively checking his status with federal prevention guidelines. He even volunteered to provide a testimonial to Wenner as a means to market the product and spoke at a plenary session of "Toward an Electronic Patient Record" in 1998 advocating patient interview software as an empowering medical technology for patients [14,15].

Another development in the preventive screening of patients was the purchase of a modified version of the Instant Medical History program by the Cooperative Ministries of Columbia, South Carolina. In 1998, at the urging of Wenner, Anne Derrick of the Cooperative Ministries and Duncan Belser of Primetime Medical Software developed a database of the providers of preventive procedures and counseling services. The database cataloged specific locations where each of the approximately 30 distinct preventive measures in the Instant Medical History program could be performed by charity hospitals in the greater Columbia area. The providers were divided into three categories for each procedure on the required ability of its clients to pay for services (able to pay, unable to pay, and eligible for veterans' benefits). In addition, the centers were grouped by zip code so that the facility closest to the primary residence of the Cooperative Ministries client could be determined.

As a result of the local provider database augmentation to the Instant Medical History application, indigent citizens visiting the Cooperative Ministries can make their own referrals based on their health needs for their age, sex, ability to pay, and zip code. This automation saves the Cooperative Ministries tremendous repetitive effort by automating the process of gathering "at-risk" category facts and supplying the necessary action-step information. Similar to the automating of the subjective portion of the visit note for the provider, automating this process of the encounter at the Cooperative Ministries allowed its employees to service the individual health needs of its clients more efficiently.

Outcome studies have shown the effectiveness of computer interviewing [16]. As quality control programs encompass more and more areas, clinicians will be rewarded for more complete histories. In the outcome study by Williams et al. [17], patients in 60 primary care practices in Virginia were interviewed with a computer about cancer prevention. The study showed an increase in screening mammography (6.6 percent) and clinical breast examinations (6.1 percent), the increase being in patients who had not had a preventive visit in the past year. Another study [18] in inner-city Chicago showed that 95 percent of patients who interacted with a computer program requested prevention information and that 62 percent, when telephoned later, recalled prevention intervention (versus 27 percent in the control group). Other favorable outcomes were found for predicting suicide [19] and risk factors for pregnancy [20,21].

Overview of Screening with Instant Medical History

Instant Medical History can be configured to operate in two screening modes: Nurse-Initiated and Patient-Initiated. In the Nurse-Initiated mode, a nurse or other clinician is responsible for the initial patient triage to determine the appropriate set or sets of questions for Instant Medical History to administer.

The Nurse-Initiated screening mode is ideal for providers with a computer in each examination room, but it also can be used on any office computer if personnel are available to initiate the screening. The secret to successful administration of Instant Medical History in the Nurse-Initiated mode is having enough examination rooms (or available computers) and coordinated appointment scheduling to accommodate patient computing time. Patients can spend as few as 5 or as many as 20 minutes answering questions, depending on the nature of the complaint, the complexity of the questions administered, and the computer hardware in use.

When Instant Medical History is operated in the Nurse-Initiated mode, the nurse leads each patient from the waiting room to an examination room, gathering primary triage information en route with casual, welcoming conversation. On entering the room, the nurse sets up patient screening to administer the appropriate questions, seats the patient at the computer, introduces the software to the patient, and allows time for the patient to answer the questions. After 10 minutes, or after the program notifies the patient that questioning is complete, the nurse returns to retrieve the output and to ready the patient for examination. Before entering the examination room, the provider reviews the computer-generated subjective note. Then the physician enters the examination room to complete the objective assessment and to plan and document the visit.

Instant Medical History also contains algorithms to automatically triage patients for administration of the appropriate questionnaire(s) for their complaints. Because this mode of screening does not require a nurse to initiate the screening, but only to introduce the patient to the computer, it is called Patient-Initiated mode.

In Patient-Initiated mode, Instant Medical History captures complaints from patients based on their responses to general, top-level triage questions. The software then processes the information provided, selects the proper set or sets of questions to administer, and screens the patient. The output can be printed, saved, viewed on screen by the provider, or passed automatically to an electronic medical record.

In Patient-Initiated mode, Instant Medical History can be rapidly deployed to screen patients in the waiting area if limited staff are available for assistance. In this case, Instant Medical History offers automatic printing, filing, and viewing capabilities that can all be leveraged for maximal efficiency. Instant Medical History in Patient-Initiated mode can be easily embedded in a practice Web site to allow patients to enter detailed previsit information about their reason for seeking care. The clinician can make medical treatment decisions without a face-to-face visit in many instances.

The Future of Medical Interview Software

The Internet is the enabling technology that allowed patients to enter their medical histories at home into their own personal, secure, online health record and gather tailored patient education materials. Since that time, other Internet healthcare providers have licensed the software for similar purposes. These developments offer several interesting possibilities for the future in medical communications, data storage, and electronic medical record use and management. The potential for enhancing the efficiency of providers and improving the quality of health care is dramatic.

Internet healthcare providers offer a channel for connecting patients and providers to facilitate better communication. Secure Internet Messaging, a technology that allows encrypted e-mail and other secure document transfers, provides the conduit through which the bulk of future medical correspondence may occur. The communication tool will dramatically change workflow in the clinical setting. Instead of scheduling an appointment at the provider's office in advance of the encounter for a standard block of time, the combination of Instant Medical History and the capabilities of Internet health care providers will refine the process.

The workflow will change such that patients will first access the Internet from their homes and log in to their online personal health record instead of calling the clinic. They will initiate an interview corresponding to their complaint from a list or through free-text entry, and the results of their session will be stored in their record enabled by the secure data repository provided by the Internet healthcare provider. Secure messaging then will transmit the subjective complaints to the provider's secure scheduling module, where the estimated time for the visit will be extracted from the subjective data and the complaints stored in the clinical electronic medical record.

The workflow changes as new options present. The patient may be notified of the appointment time and of any advance measures for which to prepare. For example, laboratory tests necessary for the encounter will be scheduled automatically, dietary changes for specific procedures will be recommended, and the patient will be reminded of the appointment in advance by the system. A second option is treatment recommendations without an office visit. Using the detailed and complete data entered by the patient, the experienced clinician could initiate a care plan. Because the Internet allows much closer follow-up through secure messaging, a treatment can be initiated more quickly than with the typical delay in care with the traditional workflow. In either case, the complete history of the present illness is automatically a part of the patient's electronic health record at the physician's office.

If a medical visit is indicated, the documentation is largely complete because the history of the complaint is a large part of a medical record. At the point of care, with his or her electronic medical record platform, the provider will review the patient's subjective complaints and the results of any standardized scales either through access to the patient's personal health record or through the data stored on the local system. When the patient arrives for the visit, the nurse will record the objective findings for the provider in the electronic record. On entering the examination room, the provider will immediately have time to ask open-ended questions and converse casually with the patient to make the assessment and plan because macro tools provided by the local system will enable point-of-care documentation. At the conclusion of the visit, the local electronic medical record system will transmit an update of the patient's record to the patient's online health record, thereby triggering the online record to send the patient by e-mail a page of links to patient education materials from its archive. Depending on the patient's health plan, his or her checking or credit accounts will automatically be debited with secure E-commerce technology. Meanwhile, the provider will already be seeing the next patient.

Instant Medical History provides the foundation for this future interactive health-care environment in several ways. Primarily, digital interviews record discrete data elements in a standardized language of patient complaints. This language is what will enable Internet healthcare providers to trigger patient education materials, provide appropriate drug advertisements, and efficiently conduct outcomes analyses.

The second chief benefit from interview software is the provision of discrete data. This language can be converted to various standardized vocabularies as alternative output formats. Note that in 1999, a powerful member of the pharmaceutical industry took an interest in electronic medical records. Experts in the field were not surprised because discrete data from patient interviews and electronic medical data repositories are the gold in the mines of the information age. Although data mining of the online health records will likely become a legal issue, many are hedging that it will likely be permitted with patient consent. This will allow direct marketing to consumers of specific products by region. As public health organizations take an interest in interview software, macro studies of presenting symptoms and outcomes analyses will be facilitated. Interventions, preventive care, and accurate measures of population risk factors will all be possible in the near future because the data will be provided directly from the patients in cost-effective ways. Patient data will be the basis of outcomes studies. Deidentified data will be used to shape the future of health care.

Perhaps the most important benefit from interview software to the future of health care comes from the standardization of expert interviews. When experts in their fields collaborate to develop a digital interview, the same expert questions can be posed to patients everywhere to distribute the highest quality of health care to the most remote areas. The standardized language of complaints will further play a role as physicians in remote areas are able to refer to their colleagues in the most developed metropolis the detailed subjective histories in a common language. With discrete data, even multiple languages are facilitated; thus, lingual barriers are transcended and patients who need care receive the standard patient interview, anywhere. With this powerful information provided directly by the patient in a form that can be used for research, a new era in evidence-based medicine will unfold. Comparing the same baseline patient information across a large population will answer many questions about the quality and cost of health care.

References

1. Osler William (Sir). Aphorism attributed to him, appearing on a medal designed for the Jikei Medical College, Tokyo, Japan. (See Osler B and Osler CS.) New York: Oxford University Press; 1997.
2. Brodman K, Erdmann AJ Jr, Lorge I, et al. The Cornell Medical Index: an adjunct to medical interview. JAMA 1949;140:530–534.
3. West C. Routine complications: troubles with talk between doctors and patients. Bloomington: Indiana University Press; 1984.
4. Beckman HB, Frankel RM. The effect of physician behavior on the collection of data. Ann Intern Med 1984;101:692–696.
5. Marvel MK, Epstein RM, Flowers K, et al. Soliciting the patient's agenda: have we improved? JAMA 1999;281:283–287.
6. Morrison I, Smith R. Hamster health care: time to stop running faster and redesign health care (editorial). Br Med J 2000;321:1541–1542.

7. Slack WV, Hicks GP, Reed CE, et al. A computer-based medical-history system. N Engl J Med 1966;274:194–198.

8. Bachman JW. The patient-computer interview: a neglected tool that can aid the clinician. Mayo Clin Proc 2003;78:67–78.

9. Colby KM. Cited by Erdman HP, Klein MH, Greist JH. Direct patient computer interviewing. J Consult Clin Psychol 1985;53:760–773.

10. Wenner A. EMR data input from the patient's home. Conference Proceedings—Toward an Electronic Patient Record '99, vol 3. Medical Record Institute: Newton, MA; 1999. p. 68–73.

11. Mayne JG, Weksel W, Sholtz PN. Toward automating the medical history. Mayo Clin Proc 1968;43:1–25.

12. Wald JS, Rind D, Safran C, et al. Patient entries in the electronic medical record: an interactive interview used in primary care. Proc Annu Symp Comput Appl Med Care 1995; 19:147–151.

13. Berwick DM, Murphy JM, Goldman PA, et al. Performance of a five-item mental health screening test. Med Care 1991;29:169–176.

14. Jancin B. Two hours a day of unreimbursed time. Fam Pract News, June 1, 2001.

15. Committee of Quality of Healthcare in America, Institute of Medicine. Crossing the quality chasm: a new health system for the 21st century. Washington, DC: National Academy Press; 2001.

16. Krishna S, Balas EA, Spencer DC, et al. Clinical trials of interactive computerized patient education: implications for family practice. J Fam Pract 1997;45:25–33.

17. Williams RB, Boles M, Johnson RE. A patient-initiated system for preventive health care: a randomized trial in community-based primary care practices. Arch Fam Med 1998;7:338–345.

18. Rhodes KV, Lauderdale DS, Stocking CB, et al. Better health while you wait: a controlled trial of a computer-based intervention for screening and health promotion in the emergency department. Ann Emerg Med 2001;37:284–291.

19. Erdman HP, Greist JH, Gustafson DH, et al. Suicide risk prediction by computer interview: a prospective study. J Clin Psychiatry 1987;48:464–467.

20. Lapham SC, Kring MK, Skipper B. Prenatal behavioral risk screening by computer in a health maintenance organization-based prenatal care clinic. Am J Obstet Gynecol 1991;165:506–514.

21. C'De Baca J, Lapham SC, Skipper BJ, et al. Use of computer interview data to test associations between risk factors and pregnancy outcomes. Comput Biomed Res 1997;30:232–243.

27
Nursing Administration: A Growing Role in Systems Development

Mary Etta Mills

Nurse administrators have a key role to play in the development of systems by which data will be converted into useful information.

Healthcare systems are dependent on high-quality information collection, integration, and accessibility of data for clinical and administrative decision making. Information systems must provide data able to be used to evaluate and predict utilization of human and material resources, determine effectiveness of care through patient outcomes, develop budget projections, support the analysis of comparative health services, and project trends on which plans of action can be formulated.

The shortage of nursing staff; high acuity of patients; growth of technology in the healthcare system; stringent regulations for privacy of health information and the transmission of that information; and the demand for comparative data, demonstrative of evidence-based practice, and quality outcomes are driving requirements for computer-based information management. Nurse administrators must do more than support the development of computer-based data collection. They must work directly with the Chief Information Officer and Nurse Informatics Specialist to develop systems by which data will be converted into useful information.

Information Requirements

Accreditation

The Joint Commission for Accreditation of Healthcare Organizations promotes standards directed at identifying processes to ensure the effective management of information as a resource [1]. Toward this end, there is an emphasis on five broad categories of information management standards:

- Processes by which organizations plan and manage their information needs.
- Management of patient-specific data.

Mary Etta Mills, RN, ScD, CNAA, FAAN, is Associate Professor of Nursing Informatics and Administration and Assistant Dean for Graduate Studies at the University of Maryland School of Nursing, Baltimore, MD.

- Aggregate data collection.
- Accessibility of knowledge-based information.
- Collection and use of comparative data.

Planning anticipates that the information management processes meet the organization's needs, provide for data confidentiality and security, use uniform data definitions and quality control systems, are managed by appropriately prepared individuals, provide timely and accurate transmission of data, and enable integration of data from various sources. The expectation is that the information system will enable the collection, transformation, and communication of data, addressing individual *patient data* specific to processes and outcomes of care. Furthermore, the information system must provide *aggregate data* to support managerial decision making and operations. In support of patient care and organizational processes, there must be availability of *knowledge-based information* such as reference information. Finally, *comparative data* on which to evaluate performance must be provided.

As the capability to network information systems becomes more sophisticated, and as the demand to provide systems integration in support of continuity of care and coordination of services across settings becomes a greater expectation, administrators will need to consider how standards will be addressed in a broader, systemwide, context. The development of uniform definitions and unified data systems that allow secure transmission of healthcare information is key to this process.

Legislation

The Health Insurance Portability and Accountability Act (HIPAA) of 1996 has given rise to far-reaching issues for the field of healthcare informatics and for health services administrators [2]. These national standards represent the initial development of federal policy for the way providers and payers process, secure, and electronically transfer health information. They address the electronic collection, storage, updating, and integration of healthcare data.

The first set of HIPAA final rules went into effect in 2002 and addressed the electronic exchange of health data. The rules include standards with regard to collection of data, including national provider, payer, employer, plan and individual identifiers, claims attachments, and security and privacy rules and enforcement. HIPAA regulation seeks to restrict data access only to authorized individuals and includes an expectation for the physical security of information stored in file rooms and on computer monitors and the training of staff in how to maintain information privacy and security.

Implementation of the security and privacy standards will require that a number of technical measures be put in place, such as authentication procedures, audit trails, and automatic log-off of inactive equipment [3].

In considering the application of electronic transfer of information within an integrated healthcare delivery system, administrative procedures must be developed to guard the confidentiality of data. This principle also extends to telehealth services that may be offered by the healthcare organization. Telehealth services may provide the transmission of visual, auditory, and physiological monitoring data across geographic distances where specialized consultative services are not readily available [4]. While the necessary partnership agreements that ensure nondisclosure of electronically transmitted information must be developed at the legal counsel administrative level of the organization, nurse administrators must ensure that a review system is established to provide ongoing evaluation of information security. This may involve everything from policies regarding password protections to actions to be taken following termination of an employee. Health providers must have exposure to educational programs addressing security controls and personal responsibilities. Client information must also be made available with regard to rights pertaining to the management of individual health information.

Applications for Key Management Functions

Organizational Structuring

The availability of integrated databases and analytic models provides opportunities for nurse administrators to acquire and organize data not only to monitor and coordinate activities of nursing and patient care services but to support future-oriented administrative decision making. Key performance indicators can be accessed in real time as well as consolidated over standard reporting periods. These reports allow for timely decision making regarding systems operations as well as strategic planning. Some fundamental systems support nursing department operations: workforce management systems, financial management systems, and quality management systems.

Workforce Management Systems

There will be an estimated shortage of more than 400,000 registered nurses by the year 2020 [5]. An increased demand for nurses due to higher patient acuity, an aging nursing workforce, and a shortfall of new nurses entering the field to replace those retiring makes the efficient use and adequate support of those nurses in practice of key importance. The organization and work of hospital-based nurses has been criticized as needing redesign to reduce excessive paperwork and correct inefficient communication systems [5]. In some instances, unrealistic nurse workloads have compounded the problem of workforce shortage [6].

Nurse administrators are compelled to determine the level of care needed in a given area at a given time by analyzing patient acuity levels and applying patient classification systems. In addition, the Joint Commission on Accreditation of Healthcare Organizations has drafted a model for the assessment of staffing effectiveness [7] that may be combined with workload demand models and analysis.

The model is designed to screen for possible staffing problems through the use of sets of resource indicators. The JCAHO leaves it to the healthcare organization to define a method for determining staffing effectiveness for the population served and to conduct self-monitoring. Measures include outcomes such as overtime usage and agency staff and patient outcomes such as falls and medication errors. Other variables such as skill level of professionals may be considered.

Automated methodologies facilitate the collection, storage, manipulation, and retrieval of large volumes of this type of workload and effectiveness data. When used in planning for and evaluating the result of the allocation of human resources, these data can be used to:

- Identify workload by diagnostic category or center of excellence.
- Facilitate analysis of workload trends and resultant patient outcomes.
- Serve as a means of evaluating the cost of care and value of the expenditures related to efficiency and effectiveness of care services.

Nursing personnel systems can track all human resource planning information necessary to manage the nursing workforce with database architecture created specifically for that purpose. Personnel databases can include information regarding every position (availability, specifications) and each individual (employment history, performance tracking, wage and salary history, professional registration, credentials, and educational preparation). Comprehensive, up-to-date information facilitates effective management of nursing personnel, assists in the recruitment and retention of nurses, and documents their career paths. Nursing personnel systems can also assist in providing career counseling, monitoring licensure and continuing education attendance, meeting hospital accreditation requirements, and developing manpower contingency plans in the event of disaster.

The staff scheduling system uses the database provided by the personnel management system and functions in conjunction with the patient classification system to generate staff schedules based on specific patient care requirements. Because schedules are based on the personnel management and patient classification systems, staffing systems can take into account patient need, staff expertise, staff scheduling preferences, and personnel policies. However, the complexity of such systems varies widely, with intelligent systems capable of adjusting staff schedules in an interactive manner on a shift-by-shift basis.

Scheduling systems assist the nurse manager in maintaining records, monitoring attendance, ensuring compliance with personnel policies, and scheduling time off for personnel. Information is readily available to document work patterns of all nursing personnel.

Financial Management Systems

Operating budgets for nursing departments account for approximately 40 percent of the typical hospital's operating budget. Information systems are essential if managers are to effectively control the nursing department budget and accurately plan for new programs. The primary advantage provided by financial management systems lies in their ability to organize, track, trend, forecast, store, and retrieve data in preparing departmental budgets and analyzing budgetary variances.

Budget preparation for nursing departments is often a tedious, time-consuming, number-intensive process. By linking patient classification data, staffing requirements, and evidence-based practice data to a budget methodology, the preparation of an annual operating budget can be expedited and justified. Necessary reallocations and adjustments for new programs are facilitated by the use of spreadsheets. "What if" scenarios can be tested to ensure that the budget provides a realistic plan for managers.

Financial management systems provide managers with up-to-date reports that focus their attention on major variances and potential problems. Nursing financial management systems allow a great deal of flexibility while linking reports to responsibility centers. Reporting can be tailored to the organizational level as well as to individual nursing units. These capabilities are critical in today's competitive environment; they make it possible for nursing to respond effectively to the demands for cost control.

By integrating patient classification data, personnel management data, and budgetary data, managers are able to analyze variances and explain budgetary deviations due to price, volume, staffing, or acuity variances. Nurse managers are able to target management interventions, designed to produce the desired performance results and to achieve organizational goals.

Automated information systems support linking administrative and clinical data in unique ways within and across organizational boundaries. Potentials for economies of scale and quality of care can be analyzed and services organized to promote the most efficient and effective patient care delivery systems configurations.

Quality Management Systems

Care quality and fiscal success of the healthcare system are critical outcomes. Benchmark patient outcomes data are an important means of comparing best practices among peer institutions [8]. Information systems provide a means of analyzing comparative data from which performance improvement plans can be suggested. In an integrated system, indicators can also be selected that can be collected both on-site and across settings. Data can then be analyzed across the healthcare system as a means of evaluating overall system effectiveness and can result in making changes to care processes [9].

Performance improvement also involves examination of operating structures such as achievement of goals and consistency of performance across the patient care service continuum. Systematic data collection and analysis are central to this process. Nursing-sensitive quality indicators for acute care and for community-based nonacute care settings developed by the American Nurses Association [10,11] provide a set of indicators designed to link nursing actions and patient outcomes. Acute care nurse staffing quality indicators include:

- The percent of RN care hours as a total of all nursing care hours.
- Total number of productive hours worked by nursing staff with direct patient care responsibilities on acute care units per patient day.
- RN contracted hours.
- Total contracted hours.
- RN nursing care hours per 1000 patient days.
- Nurse satisfaction.

Patient-oriented indicators include:

- Pressure ulcers.
- Rate of patient falls.
- Patient satisfaction with pain management, educational information, overall care, and nursing care.
- Nosocomial infections.

Many of these indicators can be captured from existing databases, such as automated staffing and scheduling systems, infection control, risk management, and customer satisfaction monitoring systems.

Community-based settings also have quality indicators such as pain management, consistent RN provider; total number of direct care hours, or encounters provided by an RN; client satisfaction; and number of clients attending educational sessions regarding tobacco use and cardiovascular disease.

Since 2001, Magnet hospitals have been required by the American Nurses Credentialing Center Magnet Recognition Program to submit quality indicator data to the National Database of Nursing-Sensitive Quality Indicators developed in 1998 [10, p. 3]. Participation in this project and information systems development to collect this data for internal use as well as benchmarking can provide administrative decision support to prevent or correct system-level problems.

Integrated Systems

The collection, coordination, and communication of information to support complex patient care, organizational, and regulatory requirements are of growing importance. Integration provides a cost-effective approach to systemwide coverage and an effective way to access and manage information that supports complex decision making.

In an era of resource limitations, including both financial constriction and personnel shortages, efficiency and effectiveness have become increasingly important. Having data automatically distributed into multiple programs for analysis specific to given output generation and perhaps redistribution into still other programs becomes an essential conservator of valuable staff time. Elimination of duplicate information recording, collection, and analysis by nursing staff can reduce the almost 40 percent of nursing time currently spent on paperwork. This in itself will facilitate the use of professional staff in directly delivering or supervising patient care.

In a truly integrated system, all the functions are designed from the outset to work together. Although fully integrated software development continues in this area, interfacing that connects unrelated automated systems has had more success. As a result, some nursing management systems such as patient classification, staffing requirements, scheduling systems, and productivity analysis have been interfaced for automated sequential analysis. The interrelationship of these programs provides the nurse administrator with information specific to correlated administrative issues. In addition to providing an immediate image of key operational issues, this type of program networking allows planning and forecasting with the use of data-based simulations.

Information systems integration also extends beyond the boundary of a single organization to include all parts of the integrated or organized healthcare delivery system. An integrated system creates one unified entity composed of many organizations. The organized delivery system provides a coordinated continuum of services, but the system components may not have common ownership [9].

Organizations are beginning to incorporate evidence-based clinical knowledge, integrated clinical and financial information systems, point-of-care technology, and related work process redesign [12]. Initiatives being implemented include an integrated electronic medical record, clinical data repository, embedded knowledge-driven order sets and clinical tools, a clinical decision support tool to benchmark outcomes, and financial system. The end result should be designed to ensure that patients have an automatic ongoing evaluation of progress against expected outcomes based on preestablished patterns of outcome expectations [13]. The nurse administrator must be involved in the development of an information system strategic vision to identify hardware and software necessary to support applications that can be used in many units or linked with applications in other facilities. Administrative and clinical data should be linked through information systems in an interactive circle of communication that defines and evaluates resources, service planning, adherence to legal and regulatory requirements, patient care needs, clinical interventions, and outcomes and patterns of care across the service continuum of the organized delivery system.

Information Access and Dissemination

Wireless local area networking and personal digital assistants offer the ability to document interactions and to "provide health care organizations with the ability to establish fixed connections between buildings where the installation of new wires proves either impractical or impossible" [14]. This permits information to be sent by radio signals instead of hardwired systems and allows staff the flexibility of documenting patient care on the spot and in real time.

Electronic bulletin boards, calendar, filing, and mail provide a means by which nursing administration can communicate basic announcements, notices, and sets of information to a broad array of nursing managers and staff as well as to support departments. This means of rapid information transfer has provided an ability to manage basic systems communication rapidly, in the short term, and without expensive and lengthy paper generation and distribution. Groupware can be used to combine input from multiple individuals or groups into a quantifiable summary for use in gaining feedback on issues and plans.

Administrative computing further encompasses word processing, graphics, and database management. At this time, most businesses consider word processing basic to their office routine as a means to rapidly produce documents that can be modified without redundant work effort. Graphics capabilities allow the administrator to manipulate and display data. These are especially useful in determining and depicting trends relative to budget management, productivity, and resource flow. For example, critical data elements such as key expenditures, productivity figures from automated management systems, and personnel recruitment and turnover can be routinely input or downloaded from existing databases. Using this base of information, the administrator can visually depict both experiential and predictive trends for use in planning and management.

Local area network technology that links micro/mini/mainframe computers can further enhance both computing and communication technologies by integrating departmental healthcare computing systems to allow use of distributed data management techniques. This system can help meet informational needs by providing access to clinical research databases, patient management systems, and patient charges.

Telecommunications such as voice messaging services, interactive video conferencing, and linkages to the health science library further expedite administrative functions. Time available to plan and creatively conceptualize is often a luxury, making the availability of these types of technology an asset.

System Design Goals

Ten system design goals are important to the development or selection of computer systems that support integrated data management:

1. *A Single-Patient Database.* There should be a single-patient database. This single database should be exclusive of the geographic location in which the patient is seen clinically. With data in a single central repository, redundancy of documentation will be reduced; care and treatment plans will be cohesive across episodes of health care.
2. *Integration of Clinical and Financial Data.* Integration of clinical and financial data should be accomplished so that episodes of care can be reflected in a single, integrated picture.
3. *One-Time Entry of Information.* There should be one-time entry of information. For example, a patient's demographic data should be entered into the admitting/registration system and used across all locations of care.
4. *Easy Retrieval of Data from the Database in a Form Defined by the User.* Easy retrieval of data from the database in a form defined by the user should be possible.

5. *Flexibility.* The system should be flexible. It should be easily modified to meet changing user needs and regulatory requirements and should allow users to easily tailor the input and output components of the system.
6. *Easy Expansion.* The system should be easily and cost-effectively expandable to accommodate increasing terminals, users, applications, and data, including those in diverse geographic locations.
7. *Reliability.* The system should be reliable and operational 24-hours-per-day, 7-days-a-week. Contingency backup should be available for all electronically based patient care applications.
8. *Security.* The system should provide for extremely tight data, program, and terminal security, and should be able to restrict access on multiple levels.
9. *Data Analysis Capability.* The system should support the examination of data through descriptive statistics, use of benchmarks, comparisons (as time series comparisons; cross-sectional comparison; comparison of cost, and quality outcomes).
10. *Data Reporting.* The system should provide the display of data in graphs, bar charts, and matrices for easy visualization of results.

Data Needs

Data must be provided that are required to plan, analyze, monitor, and control individual departments, divisions, and the organization as a whole. Information systems should support and reflect integrated and related functions in the following broad administrative and financial areas:

- Patient billing, review reports, volume statistics.
- Budget, purchasing, general ledger.
- Personnel, payroll, full-time equivalents, cost center reports.
- Capital planning, expenditure.
- Quality improvement, utilization review, case mix, severity, acuity.
- New systems to support data analysis as a routine effort.
- Budgeting process (planning, development, control).
- Financial statements and all related reports.
- Cash report, inventory reports, investment report.
- Census/patient volume report.
- Project management reports.
- Productivity.

Clinical data not addressed here also need to be integrated with financial and administrative data to provide a complete system information base.

Full information access for the nurse administrator enhances systemwide planning. The administrator generates decision support questions for data retrieval and display by information managers or personally accesses the database to obtain information. Given the paucity of planning time available in most daily administrative schedules, it is unrealistic to expect the nurse administrator to directly generate analytical reports. Information system coordinators are especially useful in this role in addition to systems design, implementation, and operation toward optimally supporting nursing.

Future Directions

Major Research Challenges: What Lies Ahead

The Federal Government has identified several research focus areas that have implications for health care. For fiscal year 2003, the Networking and Information Technology Research and Development initiatives [15] include:

- Technologies and services to enable wireless, optical, mobile, and hybrid communications.
- Networking software to enable information to be disseminated to individuals, multicast to select groups, or broadcast to an entire network.
- Research on modeling and simulation of the Internet.
- Improved end-to-end performance and performance measurement.
- Software components for distributed applications such as digital libraries and health care.

The National Institutes of Health's National Library of Medicine plans to extend its leading edge in telemedicine and security technologies to networked healthcare environments. Project proposals will focus on applications for healthcare delivery systems, medical decision making, public health networks, large-scale emergencies, health education, and medical research [15, p. 19]. Among the major research challenges identified were:

- Trust: security, privacy, and reliability.
- Adaptive, dynamic, and smart networking.
- Measurement and modeling of network performance.
- Networking applications, including vertical integration and supporting tools and services such as middleware.

Middleware is vertical integration software that enables networked resources and multiple applications to work smoothly together to provide end-user services such as those sought in integrated healthcare delivery systems. Additional research will have a focus on multiple modalities of human–computer interaction, such as by voice, touch, and vision. Development of systems integrating multimodal forms of interaction will have application in supporting emergency and critical care where staff must have their hands free. Awareness of these initiatives can assist the nurse administrator in anticipating the possibilities of information management and contribute to strategic planning and flexibility in supporting innovative applications of information technology.

Organizational Priorities for the Nursing Information Specialist

The challenge for the nurse administrator is how to best organize, coordinate, and develop information system management. The Nursing Information Specialist (NIS) is frequently in a direct reporting relationship to the Chief Information Officer of the institution. While this is a reasonable organizational alignment, it elevates in importance the need for the information specialist to also communicate directly with the Chief Nurse Administrator to ensure that nursing priorities for clinical and administrative decision support across the organization are addressed.

Systems planning, implementation of clinical nursing systems to support nursing staff and facilitate monitoring and evaluation of clinical and budgetary outcomes, and strategic planning are priorities. For the nurse administrator, this implies a need for clear articulation of key initiatives, resource support, and involvement of the NIS in meetings that establish information expectations.

Systems Development

Systems Integration and Networking

The future standard against which administrators judge computer systems will be the ability to acquire data and display information that optimally represents the status of sets of a large number of interacting variables, the outcomes of these interactions, and the probability of future outcomes based on changes in the variables. Ultimately, system integration must go beyond systems internal to the organization to include network capability linking those internal systems to external environments (i.e., care providers, social and support services, benchmark databases, and regulatory bodies). These expanded systems will serve to increase resources available for healthcare service and administration.

Data compilation and integration are critical to the effort to control cost and provide high-quality care in the face of escalating staffing shortages and increasingly expensive technology. Opportunities exist to link networks to external information bases, including statistics on staffing levels, mix, and cost analysis; compensation for distinct local and regional areas; turnover and employment; and patient care outcomes [16]. The comparison of such data will be critical to the formulation of program plans and strategic direction.

Patient Record

Input to the patient record will combine automated patient physiological monitoring and manual or voice data entry of clinical information. Key physiological indicators will be monitored against preestablished standards and analyzed for trends and interactions predictive of health status intervention needs. This information will become part of the integrated patient record—a unified record that documents a continuum of care.

Information specific to patient care orders and process and outcome of care documentation will be entered into the record. This primary database will automatically service programs designed to generate required corollary information. This includes patient classification and acuity analysis, staffing requirements, personnel scheduling, productivity, payroll data, specific patient service charges, practice patterns, quality of care management, and risk management monitoring.

Quality Management

As a key program component for clinicians, administrators, and regulators, quality management will focus increasingly on automated monitoring of predetermined variations (thresholds) indicative of trends in patient care. These trends may be positive or negative and may be specific to individual patients or reflective of patient group experience (e.g., diagnostic categories). Providing a qualitative base (quality) against which quantitative experience (resource use and expenditure) can be assessed is important. Even more valuable is the early identification of problems, creating the opportunity to intervene to achieve optimal patient care.

Eventually, much qualitative data will be formatted to be compatible with regulatory reporting requirements such as those of the Joint Commission for Accreditation of Healthcare Organizations and federal legislation. This will include programming software to systematically collect, track, analyze, and report clinical and organizational data.

A continuing emphasis on organizational and management effectiveness will expand the current concept of quality to include organizational variables as affecting patient care. The development of integrated systems will facilitate automated collection and reporting of these variables for internal and external use.

Managed Care

The healthcare system will continue to focus on cost and quality with attention to competitive environments and their ability to effect positive patient outcomes. Health insurers and public payer systems (such as Medicare and Medicaid) will emphasize the authorization of reimbursement levels with only modest interest in the coordination of services. To the extent that the creation of integrated systems and networks that allow systems to interface are developed to ease patient movement through various types and levels of care providers, cost-effective cohesive care may yet be made a priority. This includes such features as appointment systems, progress tracking, clinical paths, outcome measurement, and cost reporting and analysis. Decision makers will need data-based guidance in evaluating and reconciling cost and quality considerations.

Resource Utilization

Every system entails costs and benefits. Many hospital administrators assume automated systems will pay for themselves by reducing costs, mostly from changes in workforce requirements (either in numbers or in function). Many of these same administrators further assume enhanced patient care and increased provider effectiveness. Future development of computer systems, however, will need careful study of the impact of automated information systems on workers. The results may provide guidance for job restructuring before the system is implemented. This approach would enable the manager to effectively reduce costs while conserving staff and improving productivity and patient care.

Summary

Nurse administrators have an opportunity to use computer-based information management resources to maximum effect in administrative decision support. These systems must be used in compliance with increasingly stringent accreditation standards and legislative requirements in the area of systems integration and information security.

Integrated system elements are critical to optimal administrative functioning. Single-entry data sets that directly support multiple reporting requirements (some analytically based) will conserve valuable staff time. Programs supported by integrated systems include, for example, patient classification, acuity, productivity, quality of care, and financial analyses.

In the future, computer systems will support both intraorganizational systems integration and interorganizational networking. Computer-based patient records will serve as a primary generation point for data required by administrative systems. Quality management at the patient and organizational level will be an area of increased emphasis. Computer systems will be developed to coordinate services offered in the diversified care settings created by healthcare restructuring. Systemwide analyses will extend to include the cost/benefit ratio of computer implementation and the effectiveness of job restructuring in reducing costs while improving patient care.

References

1. Joint Commission on Accreditation of Healthcare Organizations. Management of information. In: 2002 Hospital Accreditation Standards. Oakbrook Terrace, IL: Joint Commission Resources, Inc.; 2002. p. 239–256.
2. Health Insurance Portability and Accountability Act of 1996, Pub. L. No. 104.191, F of Title II. 45 CFR Parts 160 and 162 (HCFA-0149F) RIN 0938-A158 (pp. 60313–50372); 1996 August 21.
3. Mills ME. Computer-based health care data and the Health Insurance Portability and Accountability Act: implications for informatics. Policy Politics Nurs Pract 2001;(2):33–38.
4. Quade G, Novotny J, Burde B, et al. Worldwide telemedicine services based on distributed multimedia electronic patient records by using the second generation Web server Hyperwave. In: Lorenzi NM, editor. Journal of the American Medical Informatics Association, Proceedings '99. Philadelphia: Hanley & Belfus; 1999. p. 916–920.
5. Buerhaus, PI, Needleman J, Mattke S, et al. Strengthening hospital nursing. Health Affairs 2002;21:123–132.
6. Aiken LH, Clarke SP, Sloane DM, et al. Hospital nurse staffing and patient mortality, nurse burnout, and job dissatisfaction. JAMA 2002;288:1987–1993.
7. Mercer TA. JCAHO staffing model. Adv Nurses 2001;31–32.
8. Rudy EB, Lucke JF, Whitman GR, et al. Benchmarking patient outcomes. J Nurs Scholar 2001;2:185–189.
9. Newhouse RP, Mills ME. Nursing leadership in the organized delivery system for the acute care setting. Washington DC: American Nurses Association; 2002, p. 35.
10. American Nurses Association. Nursing-sensitive quality indicators for acute care settings and ANA's safety and quality initiative. Washington DC: American Nurses Association; 2002.
11. American Nurses Association. Nursing-sensitive indicators for non-acute care settings and ANA's safety and quality initiative. Washington, DC: American Nurses Association; 2002.
12. Kerfoot K, Simpson R. Knowledge-driven care: powerful medicine. Reflections on Nursing Leadership 2002;3:22–24,44.
13. Stead WW, Miller RA, Musen MA, et al. Integration and beyond: linking information from disparate sources and into workflow. J Am Med Inform Assoc 2000;7:135–145.
14. Simpson RL. Eyeing IT trends and challenges. Nurs Manag 2002;33:46–47.
15. National Science and Technology Council. Networking and Information Technology Research and Development Supplement to the President's FY 2003 Budget. Arlington, VA: National Coordination Office for Information Technology and Research and Development; 2003. p. 19.
16. Gregg AC. Performance management data systems for nursing service organizations. JONA 2002;32:71–78.

28
Pharmacy Systems: An Emerging Role in Drug Treatment Management

Peter L. Steere

Pharmacy, a profession that has long relied on computer support, is enjoying the maturation of systems that will further enhance its value.

Evolution of Pharmacy Systems

The practice of pharmacy is essentially composed of three very different activities:

- The determination and administration of appropriate drug therapies.
- The distributive elements of moving products from the wholesaler through the pharmacy and, eventually, to the patient.
- The billing and reimbursement of dispensed prescriptions.

At various points in time, one aspect of pharmacy service may have had greater priority over the others. In more recent years, however, the *pharmacist-as-drug-treatment-manager* is the role on which the profession has set its sights.

In the early 1900s when pharmacy was considered more of a shopkeeping profession, focus on the compounding elements of prescription preparation occupied the time of most pharmacists, or druggists, as they might have been called [1]. Volumes of prescriptions were very small by today's standards, and, until commercially prepared products became more prevalent, dispensing activity was, in some ways, limited to the ability of the pharmacist to measure, mix, and mold those prescriptions that made their way to the store.

As the numbers of prescriptions increased, pharmacists sought to reduce the time spent on the technical aspects of dispensing by incorporating devices such as the Shake and Roll[®1] and various other special counting trays for getting prescribed amounts of drugs from a bulk container to the vial to be handed to the patient.

During the 1970s and 1980s, prescriptions were increasingly covered by third-party insurance programs. Rising numbers of prescriptions, coupled with a need to efficiently bill pharmacy benefit management (PBM) companies[2] on behalf of insured patients,

---

Peter L. Steere, MBA, RPh, is Assistant Professor of Healthcare Administration at the Massachusetts College of Pharmacy and Health Sciences in Boston, MA.

[1] The *Shake and Roll*, a device invented to help pharmacists more quickly count and prepare tablets and capsules for dispensing, continues to be distributed by the Chem-Pharm Corp., West Palm Beach, FL.

[2] An example of a PBM is *AdvancePCS*, based in Irving, TX.

brought about a widespread use of computers in even the most average-sized pharmacies. Initially developed as patient profile, drug dispensing record, and invoice generating systems, one of the more valuable early applications of computers was to provide hard copy bills, on "universal claims forms" (UCFs), of weekly or monthly filling activities.

Growth of the PBM industry continued, and, with it, strong competition by pharmacies for enrollees who would be eligible for coverage of their prescription claims. As drug costs rose, the need to reduce costs to the insurer for prescription medications meant, at least in some way, that reimbursement to pharmacies would be negotiated downward. In return for such discounts, systems that helped to reduce the time necessary to dispense, invoice, and be paid were instituted, so that, for example, a pharmacist could eventually know, upon being presented with a prescription, whether the individual was covered on the date of service, whether the drug was included on the PBM's formulary, the amount of the patient's copayment, and how much the pharmacy would be reimbursed by the payer.

From here, the pharmacy software industry began a series of systems enhancements that would offer workflow and managerial improvements, counseling efficiencies, and mechanisms to ensure safety in the filling process.

Tasks Accommodated

The insertion and expansion of computer systems in pharmacy has allowed pharmacy managers to move from using early programs to sequentially numbering new prescriptions and track refills (something previously done manually using various numbering devices) to be capable of some or all of the following tasks:

- Time-in-motion studies of prescription fill processes.
- Prescription claim generation, submission, and payment tracking.
- Determining staff clinical, technical, and other interventions on prescription activities.
- Make automatic substitutions of products that are multisourced (e.g., available as generic versions of branded prescription medications), to accommodate contractual and regulatory requirements.
- Track inventory costs, turnover, and price changes.
- Determine drug–drug or other interactions that relate to the dispensing of a prescription.
- Allow consumer-input refill data to be supplied electronically.
- Limit, in some cases, the products available for use by clinicians.
- Allow diminished dependence on staffing in the technical aspects of prescription filling.
- Many other service enhancements.

Segmentation of Systems: Software Versus Hardware

Ambulatory

The marketplace for pharmacy software, when the industry was moving from manually processed activities toward online adjudication and systems-based inventory management, was largely made up of independent pharmacies. Chain operators, with their

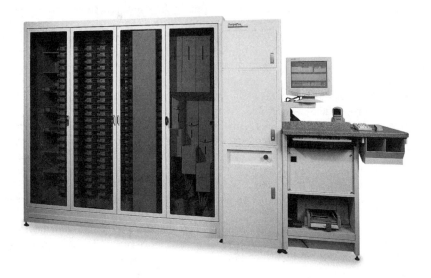

FIGURE 28.1. Automation distributors are creating store-based patient- and dispensing-management systems, such as this ScriptPro 200, which hold the potential for communicating more effectively with prescription filling equipment.

proprietary pharmacy software programs, represented a growing, albeit limited, outlet for most of the upstart systems developers.

As independent pharmacies became less and less prevalent, the market for smaller, off-the-shelf pharmacy systems shrank. Until recently, the trend within the pharmacy systems industry appeared to some to be in steep decline. Pharmacy software vendors were downsizing or even abandoning their sales staffs and, perhaps more critically, were often diminishing the support available to systems still operating in the field. Those that have and continue to offer products for this application include QS/1,[3] Rx30,[4] and Condor.[5]

Because of this market vacuum, the emerging automation distributor industry has begun integrating *backward*, creating store-based patient- and dispensing-management capabilities that hold the potential for communicating more effectively with prescription-filling equipment[6] (Figure 28.1).

Automation, on the other hand, tended to come from a very different sort of expertise. Robotics manufacturers, seeking to find new applications for their technologies (e.g., product security in the case of Diebold[7]) began experimenting with pharmacy, realizing that product storage, selection, and distribution were very repetitive in pharmacy, much as they were in other industries in which they had years of experience.

---

[3] QS/1 is a product of J.M. Smith Corp., Spartanburg, NC.
[4] Rx30 is a product of Transaction Data Systems, Inc., Ocoee, FL.
[5] Condor is a product of The SCO Group, Lindon, UT.
[6] For example, ScriptPro, LLC.
[7] Diebold's MedSelect division has since been sold to Medecorx, L.L.C. (renamed MedSelect, Inc), based in Alpharetta, GA.

Innovations more recently pertain to enhancing pharmacists' clinical and managerial capabilities. As pharmacy liability and scope of practice have expanded, documenting compliance with laws, regulations and, quite simply, appropriate practice standards has become a more complex and time-consuming process. Before clinical support functions in early pharmacy dispensing systems, pharmacists made notations on the back of the prescription or on a separate, customized note card. Eventually, systems were developed to detect drug–drug interactions, although early versions did not always provide automatic or in-process documentation of any pharmacist intervention. Today, capturing and attributing clinical activities by pharmacist or technician is standard.

More and more information is being converted from paper or interpersonal communications methods to formats that allow for electronic demonstration of compliance, including such tasks as a pharmacist's offer to counsel. While not yet standard practice, companies such as Opus Core Corp.'s electronic signature capture indicate one example of the use of technology for more definitively demonstrating a pharmacy's offer and the client's decision to accept in a more immediately retrievable (and usable) form. Many similar expectations of documentation and management of consent are also leveled on pharmacists (e.g., notice of a patient's desire for childproof caps on a prescription vial). In cases such as these, electronic data capture will hold greater value, allow for better use of staff time, and create opportunities for substantially more customized services to occur (Figure 28.2).

Hospital or Health System

The separation of software and hardware is perhaps most obvious in hospital systems. Understandably, hospitals have integrative needs, unlike retailers whose businesses

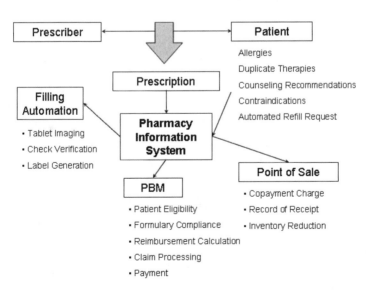

FIGURE 28.2. Electronic data capture is changing the pharmacy landscape and affecting factors such as ambulatory workflow, allowing for better use of staff time enabling the tailoring of customer services. (From P. Steere, 2003.)

tend to be more homogeneous from store to store. Laboratory values, patient charge capture, and even up-to-the-minute census information have more acknowledged value (historically) to the hospital pharmacist as intravenous admixtures and other products intended for a relatively high acuity patient are dispensed. As a result of this interdepartmental dependence on information, hospital pharmacy functionality has, traditionally, been less tied to packaged hardware and instead might be more likely served from a multitasking mainframe.

Cerner, McKesson HBOC, and other makers of hospital pharmacy operating systems typically offer similar programs for collateral departments within the institutions they serve, such as share-capable medical records, facility financial management, imaging record keeping, and product and materiel sourcing as an attempt to consolidate and standardize hospitalwide information processing.

Because of these multidepartmental service capabilities, selecting a system that provides comprehensive clinical data exchange along with broad-based ease-of-use functionality is a tricky, expensive, and time-consuming initiative. Attempts to incorporate the needs and opinions of such varying users as pharmacy, nursing, medicine, laboratory, and administration often reveal perceptions of handicapping less politically robust departments in favor of systems that support stronger constituencies' applications.

Tasks requiring accommodation within the hospital setting include the following:

- Cost capture or charging capabilities including automation-dispensed medications.
- Patient medical profiling.
- Price and inventory management planning.
- Clinical intervention and outcomes monitoring.
- Formulary adherence and protocol administration.
- Medical information including drug database access.
- Dosage calculator(s).
- Sterile admixture batch tracking.
- Support of decentralized drug distribution, including nurse-based product administration.

Due, in part, to persistent pharmacy labor shortages, hospitals appear eager to move away from people-based drug distribution and toward systems that limit the amount of time needed for drug handling by staff members. This trend has interesting benefits that are, in part, the result of regulations intended to allow pharmacists to maintain control of medication management. While pharmacists are physically touching the drug less and less, the automation that has been developed by such organizations as Pyxis Corp., McKesson's Baker APS, and AutoMed allows greater access, safety, and savings, due to the ability to carefully select those products that will be available for equipment-based dispensing.

Automation, and, of course, the patient and operations management software that support it, including AccuDose-Rx® and MedStation®,[8] have allowed controlled substances to be distributed and tracked even in the absence of pharmacists [2]. Importantly, because pharmacy is not only responsible for determining and making available appropriate drug therapies, such applications of technology are enhancing the protection and security of products that have abuse potential, even while moving them away from the pharmacy and toward patient care areas.

---

[8] AccuDose-Rx and MedStation are products of Pyxis Corp.

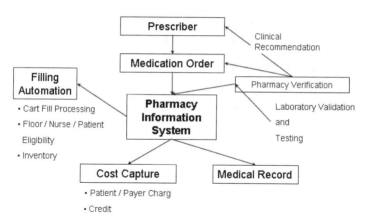

FIGURE 28.3. Institutional workflow. Systems capabilities are enabling centralized pharmacy clinical services across several hospitals.

Interestingly, while these information and product distribution technologies were designed primarily to help lessen nonclinical tasks of pharmacists, the transition of drug supplies from the pharmacy to the patient unit has been very well received by other healthcare professionals, namely, nursing. Having a nearby drug inventory, enhanced availability, and patient information integration in a comaintained unit can substantially enhance nursing satisfaction with their role in drug therapy management [3].

Also, due to pharmacist labor shortages, as well as perhaps the availability and systems capabilities of leveraging certain operating costs, entrepreneurial pharmacy leaders have begun demonstrating centralized pharmacy clinical services across several hospitals. In an effort to offer pharmacy oversight and access to clinical decision makers, organizations such as MedNovations[9] have begun using remote access to hospitals' pharmacy systems to provide overnight services [4]. Although initially it would make sense for smaller hospitals that have difficulty justifying the cost of around-the-clock care, larger, more automated facilities may also benefit if they are able to shift evening and nighttime pharmacy responsibilities to be more purely checking, validating, and approving of medication orders on a more consultative basis (Figure 28.3).

Mail Order or Distributive

Large-scale mail order distribution facilities development is somewhat subject to swings in the prescription marketplace characterized either by an abundance of investment dollars (e.g., Medco Containment Services, Inc., now part of Merck-Medco, Inc.), new market share opportunities (online prescription fulfillment), or both combined (**note:** benefit and provider-based pharmacy services such as through CVS, Inc. and its integrated CVS.com, ProCare, and PharmaCare divisions). Such systems, to offer meaningful and sought-after operational efficiencies, typically limit tasks performed or prompted by humans. Receipt of the prescription or patient-generated refill request,

---

[9] MedNovations, Inc. is a pharmacy management services provider based in Greenbelt, MD.

clinical screening, determination of patient eligibility, claims generation, and filling could all conceivably occur before any technical or clinical staff interventions. Even checking functions, usually consisting of a visual comparison of the filled product with that of a computer-held image, can be streamlined, yet still comply with most regulatory requirements of dispensed-product verification.

Unlike situations where automation is added to staffed pharmacy operations (e.g., in hospital and community-based programs), large-scale mail order services are designed from the beginning to reduce dependence on people in the filling process. As one might expect, there is less of a perceived threat by employees that positions will be eliminated in favor of automated fulfillment functions, as have been experienced, for example, by health system staff [5].

These systems tend to be large and custom built, although perhaps with certain components available to store-based providers, such as any of a variety of robotics, including AutoMed's OptiFill products as well as Baker's AutoScript III^{TM}. Smaller-scale adaptations, used to extend the service area of a pharmacy or simply to enhance patient convenience offered as an extension to the traditional practice model (e.g., community pharmacy), typically incorporate some of the workflow concepts used by the large distributors, but rely on technicians, rather than conveyor belts, and on store-based picking stations and automated dispensing systems instead of more warehouse-appropriate product selection and labeling equipment.

Infusion

Infusion services, whether as part of a health system pharmacy program (hospital-based) or within ambulatory clinic and home care vendor portfolios, carry their own specific set of system needs. In addition to the profiling and medical record-keeping requirements of any pharmacy software application, infusion information also includes batch and compounding tracking, laboratory value monitoring, and care planning.

Although increasingly infusion pharmacy providers are billing PBMs for products dispensed, they also depend on other components of a patient's health coverage for reimbursement. Further, unlike the routine business seen in most mainstream pharmacies, certain products in home or ambulatory infusion are covered by Medicare, and so cost and invoicing mechanisms, as well as claims tracking capabilities for these sorts of services, can be unique to infusion provider needs.

While most pharmacy software packages accommodate the cost capture and charges relating to extemporaneous compounding, infusion-focused pharmacies have long sought their own unique systems for their special services applications. Because infusion providers often are also engaged in durable medical equipment (e.g., wheelchairs, hospital beds) and oxygen therapy, and because the service and billing functions of these service lines are similar, most software vendors to this industry offer products that accommodate them. Healthcare Automation,[10] for example, offers products that accommodate separate prescription component charges, calculations/mixing records support for sterile preparations, and deliveries scheduling, as these steps are unique service features of the home infusion industry.

Infusion and respiratory services involve rather unique inventory management processes in that, unlike more traditional pharmacy services, supplies that *support* the

---

[10] Healthcare Automation is a niche pharmacy services system vendor based in Providence, RI.

dispensed prescription—in the case of infusion, pumps, tubes, alcohol swabs, gauze, etc.—require attention due to cost and other concerns. Pharmacies that are more mainstream and that use standard pharmacy systems may occasionally have to adapt certain functions of their program's compounding capabilities or create manual processes that duplicate some of the functions of a more specialized infusion-based package. Furthermore, because more traditional pharmacy products use the medication's unique National Drug Code (NDC) to identify the medication dispensed (and determine reimbursement rates), billing for infusion services may require the use of various code systems meant to describe not only the type of product but also to suggest what *services* were delivered in the course of dispensing the prescription.

Use of Systems

Information-Based

Therapy

Pharmacy software systems are—at their most basic application, whether hospital-based, community-based, or used for distributive purposes—vehicles that capture and track changes in drug therapy. When originally developed, therapy management applications were little more than lists of drugs prescribed for patients, along with dates of dispensing. Today, new prescriptions are weighed against many relevant sources of information, from simply checking allergies to evaluating seemingly overlapping treatment regimens. Patient age and weight flags are now possible, and programming body surface area (BSA) dosing schedules will allow either verification of a prescribed dose or recommendations for dosing when drug strength is in question.

In addition to in-pharmacy systems capabilities, and due, in large part, to the rapid growth of scientific knowledge available to guide drug therapy, a number of Internet-based information service providers are available to pharmacies in both free and subscriber formats [6]. Medline, IPA (International Pharmaceutical Abstracts), and other databases capture, consolidate, and rate information for use by healthcare practitioners. Other organizations, such as AHRQ (Agency for Healthcare Research and Quality), provide online clinical practice guidelines and, through its CONQUEST systems, offer clinical performance benchmarks and indicators [6].

The value of data availability should not be considered limited to clinical decisions or the ability to anticipate drug–drug or other interactions. It should also be considered that pharmacies can now truly begin to use the results of other providers in decision-making processes from standard-of-care issues to cost determination and benchmark outcomes establishment [7]. Importantly, when considering the creation, extension, and management of clinical decision-making processes, information systems leaders must acknowledge the quality of the many, many sources of data, the preparedness of the pharmacist-user, legal and liability-based aspects of such considerations as demonstration of standards of practice, and, of course, how readily information gained from both "owned" (in-house platform information) and "gained" (e.g., via the Internet), can be incorporated into clinical practice [8].

Allergy Record Keeping

Allergy and adverse drug reaction (ADR) data have, until recent years, been reported to manufacturers and regulatory agencies (e.g., the Food and Drug Administration) mostly by physicians, as they witnessed what seemed to be unusual effects of drugs in their patients. For perhaps many reasons, including pharmacy's rise in capturing, monitoring, and using this information when dispensing, a number of system-based methods of tracking and reporting observations of adverse medication events are arriving at the pharmacy level [9]. This seems particularly important, given, among other things, the increase in prescription-to-over-the-counter shifts of drug products that are occurring in the industry, leaving the doctor—heretofore the traditional point for reporting these events—unaware of some of the issues with which their patients may be dealing.

Patient Demographics

As pharmacists assume greater roles in the provision of healthcare services, they are finding an increased need for and dependence on patient demographic data. At one time, due to patient confidentiality guidelines, a patient's address and telephone number were, essentially, the extent of data collected regarding his or her background. More sophisticated systems are now able to track ethnicity, family medical history, and other relevant information that could be used to predict and prevent illness.

Prescriber Management

A number of issues have conspired to make prescribing a more complicated and often costly endeavor. Rising drug costs, managed care oversight, controlled substance reporting, and other factors have led to data capture requirements, either by pharmacies, state agencies, or insurers, that not only add layers of oversight to prescription-related patient care but threaten the privacy expectations of physicians, pharmacists, and patients.

For example, certain states require reporting controlled substance prescriptions (e.g., those medications found in Schedule II) electronically, for the purpose of monitoring activities that may suggest overuse or abuse of narcotic prescriptions. Pharmacy systems long ago were adapted to be able to comply with this reporting expectation, although, interestingly, the process is unique in that patient and prescribers are often identified in ways that permit tracking to occur. The Health Insurance Portability and Accountability Act of 1996 (HIPAA) could be seen to undermine certain components of this reporting process, although legal testing of the requirement to report has not proved conclusively how the regulation will affect controlled substance prescription monitoring.

A more frequent and pervasive form of prescriber management might be in the way managed care organizations collect and disseminate cost information relative to physician prescription writing. Comparing product selection, formulary compliance, prescribing volume, and other factors when determining the "costliness" of a physician has become a standard procedure in "ranking" doctors on the basis of drug expense, production, care acuity, and, to the extent that it can be measured in this method, quality.

Pharmacy reporting capabilities, via in-store systems and their electronic claims submissions to third-party processors, have long included the ability to accurately capture and send the prescriber information necessary to be able to track cost and drug utilization. Even so, because identifiers such as a physician's Drug Enforcement Agency-provided number are not required on noncontrolled prescriptions (e.g., nonnarcotic prescriptions), this method of tying prescriptions to prescriber has, to date, produced only fair results at best.

Inventory and Sales Activity

Pharmacy systems, in addition to being patient and drug therapy tools, also are expected to perform important business management functions. If there is an area where systems are underutilized, it is typically this back-office processing.

Using pharmacy software to value and track inventory, capture sales, and determine variances in reimbursement as it is received can require a significant commitment of time. There are, in any given pharmacy, as many as 4000 stockkeeping units (SKUs), or products held in inventory. An actual inventory level of each product must be entered into the system—a process made difficult by "broken" quantities common in pharmacies, meaning bulk packaging of as many as 1000 or more doses that have been previously and partially used to fill prior prescriptions. The balance needs to be determined and entered to initiate a founding inventory. Also, because some products are "multisourced," such as generics that may be purchased from several manufacturers, different, equivalent versions of the same medication may be in inventory, but not available to the computer for filling, due to the NDC system of identifying products, packaging, and manufacturer. Although, for example, two interchangeable products may sit on the shelf or in a piece of dispensing equipment (separately), the computer can only—logically and legally—select one for dispensing and labeling purposes. This tends to lead to increases in inventory duplication and an aging inventory of small, less-than-required remaining quantities of product.

Pharmacy practices also contribute to errors or imbalances in stated inventories. For example, patients will frequently call in for prescription refills, as might prescribers with new orders. Days may pass following the preparation of the prescription, and, in some cases, it may never be picked up at all. A "return-to-stock" process occurs, where a pharmacy employee credits the prescription to any third-party payer and places the product back in inventory. In the past, some systems have considered the payer management and the inventory management two separate functions, and the inventory adjustment often did not occur due to the added step it required. Furthermore, if it was a prescription for a cash-paying patient, added steps were often required to place the prescription "on hold" or undispensed and the drug back into inventory, steps that were not always followed.

Because of these failures to complete the in-process tasks required to keep inventory values current, business managers find that they can have only limited, if any, faith in the resulting figures. An error of as little as 1 or 2 percent in inventory value, within pharmacies experiencing that as their year's margin, is meaningful.

Contributing to all these difficulties are the well-meaning intentions of the wholesalers, who attempt to make disk-delivered or online cost/price updates reflect more accurately the cost of products bought and sold within the pharmacy. While the ability to establish "par" levels of products in the pharmacy exists, and interfaces are readily available that tie online purchase orders by the pharmacy to the wholesaler, proprietary contracts that influence product costs are to date infrequently capable of updating actual drug prices following order confirmation.

Chain/Regional Patient/Drug Availability

Whether to help reduce dependence on pharmacists during a period of significant shortage or to institute efficiencies into a prescription fulfillment process, centralized refill processing and, in some cases, initial prescription processing have been piloted in certain markets.

Unlike independent pharmacies or, similarly, institutional systems where patient data are held in-house for provider, billing, and medical record purposes, chain pharmacies centralize certain systems-based activities, including some claims generation and submission tasks, and, more simply, software management functions. Rather than manage information in several thousand stores individually, chain pharmacy operators consolidate certain aspects, such as patient demographic and medical information. This makes legal and clinical decisions simpler for the in-store staff, as well as more basic tasks such as inputting data upon a patient's arrival at the pharmacy.

Centralization of this information makes for other efficiencies as well, including the ability to shift filling (and refilling) prescriptions at a designated location—free of customer and other store-based distractions—and with the use of filling automation for greater economies in the distribution aspects of pharmacy service. To a certain extent, these same advantages are also available to hospital systems, and other methods of implementing these capabilities, but using a different "filler" can be seen in instances where wholesalers are picking up patient-specific order filling and distribution activities.

Centralized hospital cart filling services are being accommodated in a number of ways, freeing staff at the hospital level to provide clinical services rather than lose efficiency to the distribution process. Wholesalers, realizing that logistics and "picking" are two of their strengths, are promoting a fulfillment function to hospitals that includes patient or equipment-specific drug dispensing. If the program is offered on a patient basis, census and medical information is made available under contract to the wholesaler that includes therapy specifics, and carts are filled with individualized treatments for delivery to the hospital for cart exchange.

In other versions, and particularly in cases where multiple facilities are members of a single provider organization, pharmacy departments may consolidate cart filling functions—or other filling activities such as intravenous admixture services—to a central operation, taking advantage of the capacity of a piece of dispensing equipment without making multiple investments. Automation capable of this sort of leverage includes Baker's AutoScript III and AutoMed's Optifill line Others.

Patient-Triggered Filling/Therapy Management (e.g., Compliance, Refills)

Pharmacies generally operate on the basis of patient demand for products and services; in other words, prescriptions often do not get filled unless requested by a patient. A number of programs have attempted to enhance refill frequency, with at least one goal being better therapy adherence or compliance, leading, logically, to improved outcomes [10]. There is also an economic benefit for pharmacies regarding high refill rates—they usually mean "sales" to the vendor.

A number of diseases respond well to drug therapy but depend heavily on good patient adherence, including those treated with anticonvulsants. Studies examining compliance have found a number of methods effective in prompting a patient to renew or continue their medication, ranging from informational leaflets [11], to blister-packing [12], to system-managed refill reminder programs [13].

Most pharmacy information and management systems come with report writing tools that would generate lists of soon-to-be-due prescriptions. Use of the data could enhance sales, create opportunities for pharmacy interventions, and shift workload to less-busy periods of the day. What pharmacies do with this information remains subject to their available time spent disseminating the data and notifying the patient, which, additionally, could present privacy issues depending on how refill queries are presented.

Claims Processing/Adjudication

Claims preparation and submission is, by now, a very straightforward function, although from time to time format changes requested by PBM for adjudication purposes require accommodation. The National Council for Prescription Drug Programs (NCPDP) is the organization charged with creating, among other things, the data standards for pharmacy invoicing to payers. The recipients of these charges tend to be large, broadly contracted claims managers, including AdvancePCS, PAID Prescriptions, and Express Scripts, handling the patient eligibility, formulary, and network development requirements on behalf of indemnity or managed care insurance organizations.

Prescriber Order Entry

Prescriber order entry is, among other things, a rather obvious efficiency to the prescribe-fill-consume process and is an important attempt at making prescribing safer and more error free [14]. Insurers, systems developers, and the pharmacy and medical industries understand what hospitals and other institutional setting administrators have believed for some time: prescriber input of the medication order (prescription) is a critical step in reducing errors that could range from such simple (but real) issues as illegibility to, more importantly, dosage verification and therapeutic effectiveness [15].

Because the prescriber components of prescription writing have been developed, to date, separately from pharmacy input and dispensing systems, the process of online writing and delivery of a prescription to a pharmacy happens infrequently. Still, the actual process of sending private, patient-specific prescription information to the pharmacy is not difficult (healthcare providers have grown tremendously dependent on such similar functions as electronic mail), but it has been held up more due to regulatory issues, including those described by HIPAA. In addition, boards of regulation in pharmacy, in their historical attempts to avoid "deals" between doctors and pharmacists, have frowned on any process that would seem to be an unusual or inappropriate advantage of one pharmacy over another, and office-to-pharmacy prescriptions at one time might have created this sort of "uneven playing field." A compromise (one that helped to get prescriptions filled before a patient arrived at the store, or, instead, that would get a prescription to a mail-order facility), was that pharmacies could use significantly older, and, arguably, less-safe facsimile systems to get written prescriptions to the pharmacy, still, except for the duplication, in written form.

Today, pharmacy systems are, with very few changes necessary, ready to begin (if they are not already) accepting systems-sent electronic prescriptions. Policy issues continue to challenge the process of sending private data to the pharmacy, as do proprietary interfaces, but most physician practice software manufacturers, pharmacy vendors, and regulators understand the important gains in safety and efficiency held by physician-input prescribing. A number of services, such as those by SureMed, are actively attempting to tie the physician's office to the pharmacy and make simpler such prescribing steps as product choice, patient eligibility, cost and legal issues before the order arrives at the pharmacy, making the prescription cleaner, essentially preadjudicated, and less vulnerable to pharmacy interpretation errors.

Formulary Management

Formulary management is, for outpatient purposes, a task normally handled and administered by pharmacy benefits managers. Making information available for prescribers and pharmacies, as well as patients, who may be making financial decisions regarding their prescriptions, has been largely a paper process. Prescriber-input technology manufacturers are now very focused on getting formulary information loaded into the software provided to doctors by benefits carriers, because among other reasons and in many cases, the physician has at least some financial risk for the cost of the prescription. The issues of prior authorization for drugs restricted by a PBM, as well as alternative recommendations of various therapies, seem best done at the point of prescribing rather than downstream at the pharmacy.

For those payers that do not yet have formularies loaded or available for view by the physician, the pharmacy, in fact, becomes the conduit of information regarding appropriate selection of medications from the list of accepted drugs. Again, because of the contractual nature of drug costs that allow or deny a drug's inclusion on a formulary, approved drugs may vary from PBM to PBM. It is not always known, until the claim is generated electronically, whether a prescription is covered for a given patient at the time of service. If so, the benefits manager approves the prescription for payment, or, if not, recommends action by the pharmacist for resolving problems associated with the order.

Hospital pharmacies usually provide the products as well as determine their own accepted drug lists or any limitations they may put on drug use. Pharmacy systems, therefore, frequently allow hard-stops when doctors request drugs on restricted lists. Those barriers may include requirements that specific physicians be involved in the prescribing and/or that certain laboratory tests be completed and recorded before drug release. Otherwise, drugs with no restrictions would immediately be available for patient distribution, whether through handpicked means or via remote or nursing unit-based distribution.

Sampling, Indigent Care, and Various Web-Served Applications

Many hospital-centered health systems, as well as community-oriented services designed to help uninsured patients receive appropriate care, are struggling with financial issues associated with patients' comprehensive needs. Medication management, done properly, may possess the ability to help prescribers avoid other, more expensive forms of health care such as hospitalization. Those systems that experience large numbers of emergency room visits for needs such as asthma, for example, are realizing that the cost of providing chronic drug therapy is often cheaper than offering more sophisticated and possibly unnecessary services during periods of higher patient acuity if better care management were available instead [16].

Indicare[TM11] is one example of a software program designed to support the tracking, dispensing, and replacement of medications provided to uninsured patients. Most drug manufacturers maintain compassionate use or patient assistance programs that make their single-source products available to financially qualified patients.[12] The filing requirements for the programs vary significantly. Indicare[TM] seeks to consolidate the data processing portion of this service by providing templates that pharmacies, physicians, and health systems can use to sort relevant data in preparation of claims for their patients' medication.

---

[11] Indicare[TM] is a service of Pharmacy Healthcare Solutions, a division of AmerisourceBergen, Inc.
[12] A number of generic manufacturers or entities responsible for cost of drug care (insurance companies) are also experimenting with indigent drug distribution.

A practice that is related but not intended to be a version of compassionate use pharmaceutical services is *sample management*. Doctors' offices, clinics, emergency rooms, and other places where prescriptions are written frequently use medication samples to initiate or maintain drug therapy. While most sites, whether for accreditation purposes or more simply to ensure better patient care and control of its medication distribution practices, have adapted paper-and-pen systems for tracking sample prescribing, new technologies, including actual dispensing equipment, are available to better facilitate the process.

The Automated Drug Dispensing Systems (ADDS) by Telepharmacy Solutions is a cabinet designed for use in clinics and emergency rooms, allowing more comprehensive pharmacy practice activities to be incorporated into the dispensing of samples. Rather than simply giving a patient 3 or 4 days of "starter" doses, and counseling verbally on their use, the ADDS technology allows for patient-specific labeling, quantity monitoring, and inventory management, as well as generates patient-appropriate medical information and checks (and records) required information, such as product lot numbers and expiration dates. An interesting advance within pharmacy and Telepharmacy Solution's answer to the control issues associated with drug sample management is the cabinet's security access system; it utilizes fingerprint technology to identify approved users.

Outcomes Management

As pharmacy has assumed a greater role in the therapy component of healthcare management (e.g., clinical monitoring and use-of-data issues), its practitioners seek information that would be indicators for success or failure of their patients' therapies. Regulatory agencies do not consistently require relevant information to appear on a prescription or in any format that would allow pharmacists greater information of a patient's condition or need before filling and dispensing a medication. Therefore, until recently, much of the outcomes data was provided to pharmacy by drug manufacturers, in journals, and through other means, which would most likely not include information on the pharmacist's own patients.

Survey processes, general observations, and reliance on the prescriber to monitor outcomes historically has been the manner of participation of pharmacists in the results observation of the products they distribute. Realizing, that, whether for liability or for reasons of appropriateness, pharmacy needs to have greater access to outcomes information, a number of pharmacy software vendors have enhanced their systems' ability to record and use information stemming from all data-gathering sources. The value of knowing, for example, which antibiotic worked most effectively, was safest, and provided the most economically viable result would be important if gathered appropriately. PBMs use these data extensively in developing formularies, as do drug manufacturers for use in the marketing initiatives of their products.

Pharmacists, too, since having legal and professional obligations to the pharmaceutical care of their patients [17], are interested in either using purchased software for capturing and measuring outcomes data or developing in-house systems (paper-based or electronic) that help them with future clinical decision making. Information relating to outcomes, due to the various interactions patients may have with healthcare professionals, is somewhat fragmented, as could be expected, although a number of pharmacy software vendors are working to develop meaningful outcomes data tools.

Automated Dispensing

Storage and Retrieval

Variations on storage and retrieval applications depend significantly on the extent of counting and dispensing equipment used within the pharmacy. For example, the Pharmacy 2000[13] system will identify locations of bulk storage products (those products bottled in large quantity but are used by pharmacists for patient-specific dispensing) based on frequency of use, with those products used most often placed nearer the dispensing bench. Historically and still more typically, pharmacists distribute drugs around the pharmacy department alphabetically (by brand name, generic name, and, occasionally, by manufacturer), separating "fast movers," or frequently dispensed medications, from others. One interesting example of a method of exploiting limited space for drug storage is Omnicell's *Pharmacy Central* system, a rotating, escalator-like shelving system capable of being manually keyed to bring needed drugs to the practitioner, or, automatically, when prompted to do so via prescription-input product selection. Variations on this and shelf-based drug storage can also be seen in systems that put shelving on tracks that collapse "picking bays" when sections are not in use, maximizing circulation space within the department.

Remote Dispensing

Whether because of workflow, space constraints, proximity to clinics (and prescribers), or other reasons, a need to dispense medications remotely occasionally arises. Pharmacies are more rapidly deploying clinicians into areas usually associated with diagnosis and treatment to perform tasks ranging from formulary-based drug selection to disease management counseling services. When necessary to reduce filling pressures on the central pharmacy, certain elements of a prescription filling process can be done elsewhere [18]. Telepharmacy Solutions' remote cabinetry stocks prepackaged medications and labels and can help facilitate the clinic discharge process by getting drugs into a patient's hands before leaving the office, but, in any case, away from the pharmacy. Furthermore, because the equipment has limitations on the number of items that can be stocked, it can be used very effectively to monitor the drugs used by a prescriber, limiting cost and maximizing contract and market share-oriented purchasing compliance by selecting only those products preferred for use by the facility, prescriber, or formulary manager.

On an outpatient basis, in part due to staffing shortages and the resulting in-store inefficiencies, some chain pharmacies have centralized their prescription refill (and, in some cases, the original fill) processing. Moving filling or clinical review services to where efficiencies exist, or creating efficiencies by adding systems and resources to a central site, may help unburden outlying stores of those activities, while also producing certain managerial economies of scale (Figure 28.4).

Error Reduction and Checking Functionality

Bar Coding

Most, if not all, pharmacy systems, whether informational or mechanical in their use, incorporate bar-coding technology as a means to track and record various in-pharmacy processes, streamline product selection, and reduce human error. Unlike the incorpo-

---

[13] Pharmacy 2000 is the trade name of a workflow processing system of Baker APS, Inc.

FIGURE 28.4. Telepharmacy Solutions' remote cabinetry stocks prepackaged medications and labels and helps facilitate the clinic discharge process by getting drugs into a patient's hands before leaving the office but away from the pharmacy.

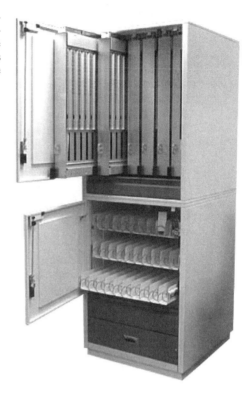

ration of certain forms of information and automation strategies that provide workaround opportunities (risking operations failures), bar-coding processes tend to more effectively standardize filling, checking, and dispensing functions [19]. Additionally, they are capable of providing management with important staff productivity information, used among other things to provide measurable efficiency benchmarks.

At its most basic application, bar coding allows pharmacists and pharmacy supervisors to track a prescription, as it is processed in either paper or electronic form, from input and insurance verification through labeling and, eventually, checkout. Common but more complex use of bar-coding technology includes validation of the medication selected, as manufacturers also identify their specific products with individual bar-code identifiers.

In hospital settings, bar-code matches may also include patients, by nursing, for determining their eligibility and approval to receive prescribed and verified medications. Bridge Medical's MedPoint medication management systems, for example, requires that the patient be identified by the drug distribution software before receiving medications that have been authorized for her care (Figure 28.5).

Pill Imaging

A second, important advance that has made its way into pharmacy practice is the opportunity to verify that the product prescribed is the same as the one that reaches the patient at the point of dispensing. Pill imaging and, relatedly, electronic imaging of the original prescription or order is a critical capability of the checking pharmacist

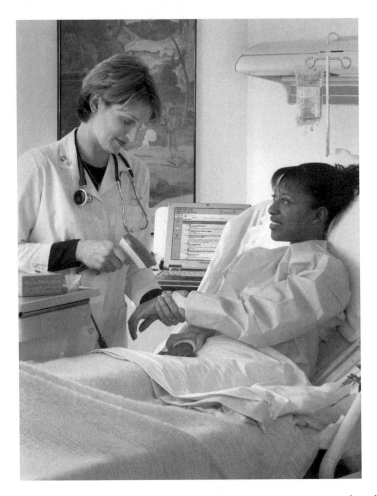

FIGURE 28.5. Bridge Medical's MedPoint medication management system requires that the patient be identified by the drug distribution software before receiving medications that have been authorized. (Photo courtesy of Rick Starkman, San Diego, and Bridge Medical, Solana Beach, CA, an AmerisourceBergen company.)

working in a high-volume practice, or in any practice where the processing, filling, and dispensing of prescriptions is segmented. Because the image is related by NDC number, even generic products appear on the checking screen exactly as they should be in a properly filled vial.

Task Assignment and Management

Relative to safety (i.e., rather than for productivity and other managerial applications explained later), segmenting job tasks within high-volume facilities is often the most practical method of moving prescriptions and medication orders through the department. While repetition could, over time, create new opportunities for error, limiting prescription-processing tasks by general category of activity usually helps to reduce filling and checking mistakes. A combination of bar coding (in this case, of actual staff members), reduced travel (and traffic) throughout the pharmacy, and using individuals for discrete tasks allows for enhanced productivity, greater focus on line-related job completion, and with supporting systems capabilities, more opportunities for work checks to occur by professionals along the filling continuum.

Interface with Prescriber Systems

Because of the unique needs of any of the various healthcare professionals who interface, personally or electronically, with pharmacy, there are rapidly developing information systems tools helping to bridge these interdisciplinary segments. Physician-input prescribing, for example, is now well advanced (albeit, not yet widespread in practice), with most software packages attempting to add efficiencies and clinical value to formulary issues, product selection, and outcomes monitoring. Innovators such as Allscripts, from Libertyville, Illinois, have helped to make "writing" a prescription as simple as three touches to an electronic screen [14].

In a community-based setting, prescribing is made easier through desktop or personal digital assistant (PDA) software, allowing wireless transfer of pharmacy, patient, prescription, and physician information. Once allowed under boards of pharmacy regulations, a pharmacy with automated intake capabilities could, conceivably, receive the prescription, process the medical information against known allergies, current therapies, and any other medical contraindications. Furthermore, if no clinical intervention were necessary at the pharmacy (excepting counseling requirements), the prescription could be adjudicated, and with equipment in place for the technical filling functions, a completed order made ready for checking and inspection. If done at the prescriber level, formulary (preferred product) management promises to substantially reduce the in-process time of a prescription in the pharmacy and dramatically lower time spent by pharmacy staff on payer-related issues. More important, perhaps, are reductions in error due to misinterpretation of a prescription, shelf selection, and complications due to polypharmacy [20].

It is in these exchanges, however, as well as with those relating to third-party payers (and other entities), that patient confidentiality issues may result and where compliance protocols need consideration. Consideration of managerial issues and gains resulting from physician-input prescriptions should also include the following:

- The simplicity of the transaction becoming automatically incorporated into the medical record.
- Time savings.
- Increased patient compliance.
- Elimination of drug waste in hospitals and clinics from overuse, formulary errors, and drug abuse.
- Cost savings from decreased inventory storage.
- Pharmaceutical companies can obtain real-time information about product utilization and modify shipping and production, as needed, among other benefits [14].

Further discussion on physician systems, including physician prescribing tools, is found elsewhere in this text.

Managerial Applications for Systems

Volume/Physical Plant

The initiation and use of sophisticated information systems and automation in pharmacy services is seemingly intended to accomplish at least one of three goals: to increase the utility of a small space, to limit the "human touch" in larger facilities, or to suggest a fix to problems that management has not been able to correct in any size operation.

Frequently, pharmacies built to support a certain volume grow to a point where they are processing more than that for which they were designed. Increases in the number of pharmaceutical products means that more space must be dedicated simply to storage. This, combined with an aging population and strong demand from patients for access to medications, has led to overcrowded pharmacies, poor workflow patterns, and in some cases, less than ideal situations to ensure the safety of the dispensing process.

More space or space reconfiguration is not always a possibility, and the promise of continued volume growth has suggested to pharmacy managers a need for investments in systems that safely extend the life of the space they already occupy.

Worker Productivity/Appropriate Delineation of Workload

Typically, pharmacies have added staff to dispensing processes when signs of worker failure, whether systemic or individual failure, became visible. Limitations on staff have to do with certain regulatory requirements—the technician-to-pharmacist ratio, for example—but also on such practical things as available space and workstations. Smaller pharmacies tend to see diminishing value of adding staff when volume rises, due usually to employees simply getting in each other's way.

Pharmacy managers frequently seek benchmark data on pharmacist productivity based on volume, dispensing errors, and other measurements, often en route to disciplinary action, although first steps for correction should, perhaps, include analysis of the workflow. As described earlier, there are systems available that help pharmacy staff do things from remapping their product storage within the pharmacy to, more extensively, completing the mechanical elements of prescription filling, unassisted by a staff member. While performance issues may often result from continuing faulty practices within the pharmacy, the manager should also consider the impact of physical space on the quality of an individual's work contribution.

Efficiencies are not exclusive to the dispensing process, however. In clinical (nondispensing) circumstances, and particularly in high-acuity settings (i.e., intensive care units), putting relevant drug information, literally, in pharmacists' hands allows them to be more available immediately for clinical decision making, and—critical to justifying the time and expense of equipping pharmacy staff with this technology—for capturing the clinical and economic implications of their actions [21,22].

Fiscal Management

Pharmacy systems have, historically, possessed adequate (or better) financial management capabilities. These system attributes were enhanced significantly when point-of-sale processes were introduced, particularly for retail applications. Still, unless the entire business is made up of pharmacies using selected and integrated pharmacy-based systems, financial managers frequently find certain finance-based pharmacy activities cumbersome to handle. This issue may have more to do with the nature of pharmacy charges, sales, and reimbursement than with failures of any integration of pharmacy finance software with more mainstream accounting systems.

For example, identical prescriptions may be charged out and paid for at any number of rates, depending on the nature of a given third-party insurance contract. Inventory changes—*first in, first out*, for example—are somewhat difficult to track given the way products arrive in the pharmacy, are put into inventory, and then eventually dispensed, not necessarily due to process, but due to lack of actual cost data from products having separate contract implications. Because the wholesaler is aware of its prices but still be unable to update drug costs by pharmacy-specific contracts at the store level, actual *cost of goods sold* data may not be available, requiring inventory adjustments at various intervals to determine profits or losses. In fact, since there are so many variations on price (e.g., wholesaler acquisition cost (WAC), average wholesale price (AWP), and actual acquisition price (AAC), which varies by pharmacy), broadly disseminated pricing information by the wholesaler has at best only limited value to the pharmacy manager.

It is important to point out that sales, accounts receivable, prescription filling, and other critical data are historically very accurate. Cost information, due to purchasing contracts that are negotiated pharmacy-to-wholesaler and pharmacy-to-group-purchasing-organization (GPO), is the component that tends to vary, yet has significant value in determining such things as operating margins and, ultimately, profitability

This sort of variability, frustrating to accounting and finance managers, is routine in pharmacy and is made worse because its near-term correction often requires human resource time within the pharmacy, tracking and updating prices within the pharmacy computer.

As wholesalers, pharmacies, systems manufacturers, and other holders of various cost and sales data continue to make efforts to get more accurate information into the pharmacy's dispensing system, the use of pharmacy-generated financial performance information will become more reliable and more acceptable to managers using it for real-time managerial decision making.

Current State of the Art

Underutilization of Systems

As information systems people know, technology frequently is applied to far fewer problems than it typically has capacity to support. Pharmacy information and automation systems are no different. Many capabilities built into pharmacy software packages are ignored either for being perceived as too cumbersome to commit upfront investment time or because they support tasks that have no corporate or regulatory directive for completion.

Most software programs, for example, come with reasonably sophisticated inventory management applications. Proper use of such back-office tools has been difficult, due to the need to load an initial inventory—perhaps including as many as 3000 stock-keeping units (SKUs)—and then maintaining that inventory as new product is received at the pharmacy, sold, or returned to stock, and adjusted for variances.

Proprietary Nature of Systems Integration

As with any situation where multiple systems vendors have products as components in a single task-based network, interfaces all become programming challenges. Integrating data and mechanical functionality, for example, clinical screening and subsequently tablet counting, require many individual software and hardware products that need some degree of universal compatibility. Because automation manufacturers also typically offer or are affiliated with profile management software vendors, smoothly integrated connections are most likely found in family systems.

Even so, end users, rather than suffering performance failures of lesser equipment in a company's portfolio, may prefer to buy the technology best suited for their application, which may again require the potential creation of an interface. Inevitably, costs associated with writing interfaces either rise uncontrollably or lend such fears of expense that system implementation never occurs in the first place.

Some manufacturers of automated dispensing equipment have noted that broad acceptance of their product has as much to do with its utility as it does with ease of adding on. ScriptPro®, for example, is known for its connectivity with a number of legacy pharmacy systems. Rather than having a complicated interface requiring profile, pricing, and other data access, it works instead by accepting the labeling information from the processing unit, triggering vial and product selection, tablet counting, label generation, and application.

The Future of Pharmacy

Pharmacy, a profession that has now long relied on computer support, is enjoying the maturation of systems that will further enhance its efficiency, its safety, and, perhaps as important, its value. From days when early programs were designed to essentially capture and hold billing information to now—when patient care products check compatibilities of admixtures, duplications, overlaps in therapy, eligibility under insurance or facility formularies, and further, select, count, label, and distribute medications virtually unaided by pharmacy staff and according to a prescriber's order—borrowed technologies from other industries have truly advanced the practice of pharmacy.

To support pharmacy during what is expected to be an extended shortage of licensed professionals, shifts in the way technicians are used and considered are legally under way. Traditionally limited to one to two technical staff members per licensed pharmacist, states are simultaneously loosening the ratios of "filler-to-pharmacist," while also stiffening the job requirements of the technician. Certification and eventually some form of licensure is expected for pharmacy technicians, efforts aimed at qualifying them for more of the critical elements of the distribution process, including, potentially, the checking and noncounseling-based dispensing of prescriptions. Despite such measures, there still is expected to be a very variably prepared technician workforce.

If such a workplace evolves in pharmacy—where pharmacists are disengaged from the filling functions of a patient's prescription—highly integrated technology needs to be capable of assuring the prescriber, the pharmacist, and the patient that the dispensed product is appropriate, effective, and accurate.

These human needs issues, coupled with the rapidly growing prescription marketplace, suggest strongly the need for closed, highly automated, highly integrated systems—systems that accept the medication order from a physician, allow pharmacist interventions to occur, produce error-free filled prescriptions, and create opportunities to capture, measure, and report outcomes on the basis of all given drug treatments.

References

1. Tebbe JL. Healthcare delivery in America: historical and policy perspectives. In: McCarthy RL, Schafermey TK, editors. Introduction to health care delivery. 2nd ed. Gaithersburg, MD: Aspen; 2001.
2. Wellman GS, Hammond RL, Talmage R. Computer controlled-substance surveillance: application involving automated storage and distribution cabinets. Am J Health Systems Pharmacy 2001;58:19.
3. Meyer C. Equipment nurses like. Am J Nurs 1992;92:32–36.
4. Keeys CA, et al. Providing nighttime pharmaceutical services through telepharmacy. Am J Health Systems Pharmacy 2002 Apr 15;59:8.
5. Crawford S, et al. Staff attitudes about the use of robots in pharmacy before implementation of a robotic dispensing system. Am J Health System Pharmacists 1998;55:18.
6. Lin SJ, Warren SJ. Researching managed care pharmacy using Internet searches. J Managed Care Pharmacy 2001;7:3.
7. Else BA, Armstrong EP, Cox ER, Data sources for pharmacoeconomic and health services research. Am J Health-System Pharmacists 1977;54:22.
8. Ponedal SA, Tucker M. Understanding decision support systems. J Managed Care Pharmacy 2002;8:2.
9. Levy S. FDA to launch ADR reporting system for dietary supplements. Drug Topics 2002; Sept.16.
10. White TJ, et al. Patient adherence with HMG reductase inhibitor therapy among users of two types of prescription services. J Managed Care Pharmacy 2002;8:3.
11. Seals TD, Keith MR. Influence of patient information leaflets on anticonvulsant drug compliance in prison. Am J Health System Pharmacy 1997;54:22.
12. Ukens C. Patient compliance tool boosts profits. Drug Topics 2002;Sept.16.
13. Levy S. Reliable refill program debuts at Familymeds. Drug Topics 2002;Sept.16.
14. Managing health care cost and quality with office-based information systems. The Aventis Risk Report: The Business of Health Care; Summer 2000.
15. Bad penmanship can lead to medical errors. Institute for the Study of Healthcare Organizations and Transactions, http://www.institute-shot.com/bad_penmanship_can_lead_to_medical_errors.htm. December 2, 2002.
16. Marcille JA. Remaking the hospital ambulatory pharmacy. Managed Care Pharmacy Pract 1996;May/June.
17. Ponedal SA, Tucker M. Understanding decision support systems. J Managed Care Pharmacy 2002;8:2.
18. Angaran D. Telemedicine and telepharmacy: current status and future implications. Am J Health Systems Pharmacy 1999;56:14.
19. Vecchione A. Bar-coding: a new future for some old technology. Hospital Pharmacist Report 1999;July.
20. Elson B. Electronic prescribing in ambulatory care: a market primer and implications for managed care pharmacy. J Managed Care Pharmacy 2001;7:2.
21. Reilly JC, Wallace M, Campbell M. Tracking pharmacist interventions with a hand-held computer. Am J Health Systems Pharmacists 2001;58:2.
22. Lau A, et al. Using a personal digital assistant to document clinical pharmacy services in an intensive care unit. Am J Health Systems Pharmacists 2001;58:13.

29
Computer-Enhanced Radiology: Imaging Transformed

ROGER H. SHANNON

> *Both imagers and computers continue to get smarter and to share the many tasks of communication that are emerging in this dramatically evolving field.*

Radiology is an information business. It is one of the core specialties of scientific medicine. In a sense, it is also a part of every direct care specialty, but it has differentiated into a separate field because of the special skills and knowledge that are required to correctly create and interpret images. In the early years, contrast materials dominated research in methodology. In 1953, S.I. Seldinger introduced the percutaneous catheter, giving easy, safer access to the recesses of the body. These catheters have become instruments of therapy as well as diagnosis. In 1972, Hounsfield launched computed tomography (CT) and digital imaging joined the armamentarium. From this platform and the stimulus that WWII gave technology, in general, other modalities such as ultrasound (US) and magnetic resonance imaging (MRI) were added to X-ray as means to probe the secrets of hidden tissues. From Roentgen's straightforward imaging of extremities, there has grown, in little more than a century, an immensely complex, technology-intensive specialty. The technology has enabled visualization of three-dimensional virtual organs in motion. By superimposing the image on body parts, they can be viewed as if they were semitransparent. Interventionalists can then guide catheters and other instruments to destinations that were completely elusive just a few years ago.

Physicians other than radiologists have also become skilled in aspects of imaging and fill important niches, but few have the fundamental training to appreciate the context in which radiology is practiced or have a sufficient command of the subject to enable them to choose the most efficacious, cost-beneficial course of study from a full set of alternatives. Even the most skilled clinical subspecialists rarely see the number and variety of cases that a radiologist encounters in serving a multitude of referring physicians. The mental library acquired by the intense practice of radiology becomes an asset that enhances every aspect of the art.

Because performing "procedures" is such an apparent feature of imaging, it is easy to assume mistakenly that radiologists are merely journeymen. To the contrary, imaging demands intense cognitive activity to analyze, synthesize, and constantly evaluate the immediate problem in full context. The radiologist is a critical link in the decision chain

---

Roger H. Shannon, MD, FACR, FACMI, is a Health System Consultant.

that determines patient outcome. A procedure is only a single aspect of a sequence that picks up the patient in one clinical state and ends with the patient in another state.

Radiological consultation, therefore, is best practiced in an environment of good communication between radiologists and referring physicians, however skilled at image interpretation the latter may be. Good communication in this technical world consists of intercomputer exchange in addition to the many forms of interpersonal exchange to which we have become accustomed. Both imagers and computers continue to get smarter and to share the tasks of communication discussed in this chapter.

Computers are used in two distinctly different ways by diagnostic imagers. The first, as components of acquisition devices, will be considered only in passing. Computers in one form or another are critical to nearly every modern imaging device—computed tomographic units (CT), ultrasound (US), computed radiography (CR), digital radiography (DR), gamma cameras, positron emission tomography (PET) scanners, nuclear medicine, and others. The more completely a department is converted to digital technology, the more pervasive is the computer as an acquisition device component.

The second class of computer applications embraces information management. The Medical or Hospital Information System (MIS/HIS) is the umbrella computer support system for radiology. As a diagnostic consultant or referral therapist, the radiologist is intimately embedded in the chain of patient care. The MIS, therefore, bears a parent position to the Radiology Information System (RIS). The latter uses information that is redundant to the MIS but also generates additional information that is logically subsumed by the MIS. The RIS can stand alone if it duplicates relevant information of the MIS, either by downloading or by independent collection. (The latter may introduce discrepancy that reduces record reliability.) It is clearly in the best interest of both patient and provider to have the MIS and RIS interoperable, functionally and regarding content.

A Picture Archiving and Communication System (PACS) is a second radiology system that is related to both MIS and RIS in one of the configurations described above. A PACS exists to manage radiology images. It, too, contains sufficient redundant information to support its functions independently. Full interoperability among the systems—MIS, RIS, PACS—is the ideal.

This chapter focuses on the second complex use of computers to manage information and comments on computers as integral to acquisition devices only to clarify the primary discussion.

The Major Function of Diagnostic Radiology

The purpose of diagnostic radiology is to render quality consultation. It will be easier to appreciate comments about information systems if the process of radiology consultation is clear. Although there is some self-referral, patients traditionally come to the radiologist by request of another physician. Thereby, a relationship is established with both referring physician and patient. This is characteristic of a consultation.

The ideal consultation incorporates several processes. First, one must choose what study or intervention to perform. Commonly the choice is straightforward, but often it is not. Choosing may require evaluation of complicated clinical information with preliminary consultation between referring physician and radiologist. Weighing benefits, risks, and costs is frequently difficult. The sequencing of tests and determining when they should be done may be issues. Second, the selected examination(s) must be excellently performed. Good equipment, competent personnel, and individually validated procedures are each critical factors. Third, images resulting from a study should be assembled with all relevant supporting material. Clinical information, previous similar examinations or other concurrent studies, and reference materials are frequently important. These constitute what may be called the selective clinical radiology information package (SCRIP) [1]. Finally, a timely report should be produced and communicated to the physician(s) who will incorporate the radiological results into the clinical decision stream.

The report has traditionally been rendered in hardcopy text, but it is becoming more common to make it available in electronic form. Everyday use of graphic annotation and voice notes is just around the corner. Regardless of final report form, communication of results, opinions, correlations, probabilities, and suggestions for resolving conflicting conclusions may require immediate personal communication on the part of the radiologist. Phone and e-mail are commonly used. Formal daily conferences between radiologists and clinicians have also become a highly successful way to achieve rapid, quality communication. Since the previous edition of this chapter, as we shall see, initiatives to enhance the process of SCRIP assembly have entered the marketplace, and reporting is becoming a more sophisticated communication process.

Consulting with excellence is the professional essence of diagnostic radiology. It is a complex process that occurs in a complex setting. There are two parts of that setting that must be appreciated by the manager, or administrator, of radiology. The radiology department itself—an involved, extremely technical, capital-intensive portion of the hospital—is the immediate environment in which the radiologist operates. Included in this concept of the radiology department are the main department and satellite operations in locations such as the emergency room, outpatient clinic, and surgery. Teleradiology also belongs in the imaging domain. It is clearly a technical extension of familiar territory. A workstation to take calls at home is teleradiology. A remote chest line or a cardiac care unit is not significantly different, nor is a clinic across the state. Teleradiology is more a notion than a distinct entity. No clear line marks its boundary.

What has been described as "department" exists in a larger setting characterized by direct care providers. Viewing stations, either light boxes or cathode ray tubes (CRT), are scattered throughout wards, conference rooms, surgery, and other service areas. They exist in remote clinics. Clinicians receive reports in their offices. All are elements of the second part of the setting—the "environment," or context—with which radiology communicates conclusions and evaluations. Discussions involving radiological images and reports are legion. Clinical decisions and procedures are continually influenced by radiology. New information leads to new radiological studies. It is largely outside of the formal radiology areas that clinicians assimilate consultations and the radiologist's efforts acquire meaning for the patient. The better the communication, the more powerful is the contribution the radiologist makes.

In review, the imager operates in an environment that he or she largely controls. This formal radiology system is embedded in the medical environment where the clinician holds sway. It is in this clinical context that the radiologist becomes meaningful. The radiology manager must be fully sensitive to the implications of this general systems principle that only in the environment does any system acquire meaning. The clinical process and the patient reside in the larger environment where consultations are generated and implemented [2].

Trends and Transition

Rapid Growth

The proliferation of computer support for radiology has been stimulated by two trends. First, enabling technology has mushroomed. Second, medical knowledge has also grown exponentially. The resulting complexity has demanded that computers be enlisted just to keep track of what transpires. Manual procedures are no longer sufficient to deal with the volume of detail. The RIS is the workhorse system that watches over people, process, and money.

Changing Technology

Seminal technology was introduced with CT in 1972 [3]. CT relies on a computer to capture and analyze thousands of measurements that are arrayed in planes, or slices, that portray cross sections of the body parts examined. More recently, techniques have emerged to generate volumetric data arrays that expand analytical possibilities and can be stacked along the fourth dimension of time. Other modalities using similar graphic methods have followed. Each has its strengths and may be combined with others to produce hybrid images that better depict certain types of body information.

Computed radiography (CR) and digital radiography (DR), relatively recent developments, are digital technologies that are able to replace all general film radiography with computed images. CR uses a light-stimulable phosphor that can be scanned by laser, erased, and reused many times. Its output is usually a film print. DR uses a storage phosphor or electronic detectors to replace film as the X-ray sensor. The images so obtained are usually presented electronically as "soft copy" on CRTs. They can be stored digitally in PACS. These systems fill the gap that prevented complete migration to filmless radiography. Advances in storage media permit archiving of many terabytes of information. Newer management techniques, such as Hierarchical Storage Management (HSM), optimize storage media to assure that needed data are nearly always quickly and cost-effectively accessible.

Support Systems

The grandfather computer system for health information management was the Hospital Information System (HIS), which dates back to the 1960s. These systems integrated clinical material by virtue of the mainframe technology used then. Later, minicomputers allowed specialties to become independent, and the concept of integrated records suffered a setback. There was always a faction among developers that held to the holistic approach. As the concept evolved, names changed to reflect scope. Medical information systems, healthcare information systems, and other names have been used. Early focus tended to be on provider and administrative needs. Recent systems have shifted emphasis to the patient. Again, new names have appeared. The computerized patient record (CPR) is currently a popular designation. The radiology information system (RIS) achieved respectability during the minicomputer era. More recently, the need to integrate has been recognized along with acceptance of the patient as a dominant driving force. Integrity of the patient record requires interoperability, and that requires standards.

RIS were fairly mature and were established in the market before PACS emerged in the early 1990s. PACS were conceived as a natural consequence of increasing sophistication and use of digital imaging. Again, special applications appeared before general ones. Cardiac care and intensive care units employed CRT displays of chest films, first for catheter placement and later for pathology. In 1992–1993, large-scale PACS were implemented in the United States at several military hospitals, at least two universities, and at the Baltimore Veterans Affairs Medical Center (VAMC) [4]. The Baltimore VAMC has achieved the goal of providing full electronic operation, including routine interpretation from CRTs. PACS sites continue to multiply, and development efforts are being focused on integration of information in the various types of patient record and administrative support systems.

Several synonyms have been used to designate digital imaging networks: PACS (picture archiving and communications systems), DIN (digital imaging networks), IMACS (image management and communication systems), and MDIS (medical diagnostic imaging system). PACS is most widespread. MDIS has been used by the military.

In 1983, the American College of Radiology and the National Electrical Manufacturers Association formed a joint committee (ACR-NEMA) to develop standards for interfacing digital acquisition devices to PACS networks. Proprietary imaging protocols unique to each vendor had tied the hands of buyers. The first version of the ACR-NEMA standard was published in 1985. It gained widespread use, evolved with increased scope, and changed its name to something more acceptable internationally for the version 3.0 publication in 1993. The resulting Digital Imaging and Communications in Medicine (DICOM) standard is now universally incorporated in industrial design, and contracts specify DICOM as a requirement. Since the last edition of this book, DICOM has achieved worldwide acceptance and has established a formal relationship with HL7 with the objective of collaborating to establish full compatibility between the two standards. This will enhance the interfacing of PACS with RIS and HIS systems.

RIS and PACS Functions

Radiology Information Systems

The typical RIS offers several sets of functions. These include:

1. Registration of patients.
2. Scheduling.
3. Patient tracking.
4. Film library management.
5. Reporting of results.
6. Department management.

Electronic mail, teaching applications, and research functions may be added. Various forms of decision support are also beginning to appear. Although the basic RIS is fairly mature, these systems continue to expand and evolve.

Registration

Registration is the demographic module. If the RIS is interfaced to the hospital information system (HIS), demographic information is passed to radiology from the hospital master record. If not otherwise available, patient information is entered directly.

Scheduling

Scheduling examinations may vary from a simple computer version of standard paper forms requiring a maximum of clerical effort to sophisticated systems with numerous automated functions that, after checking for conflicts and hazards, automatically schedule at appropriate times. They record examination-specific material, notify relevant action centers in the department, produce forms, allocate resources, and create pull notices to retrieve previous studies from film libraries, or implement archive retrieval procedures for PACS storage systems.

Patient Tracking

The patient-tracking module follows each patient from arrival to departmental discharge, showing at any moment where the patient is and how close the examination is to being completed. Often technical factors, number and type of views acquired, and other operational and resource use data are coincidentally collected.

Film Libraries

Film libraries are notoriously complicated and difficult to control. These are the centers of coordination for all medically important patient information. Not only are all images, past and present, retrieved, matched, sometimes duplicated, distributed, loaned and recovered, stored, and perhaps displayed, but also associated information that may include demographics, clinical findings, workup consultations, formal interpretations, codes, and follow-up with quality assurance (Q/A) information must be assembled together with the images. Film libraries collect and link the record elements that fully informed radiologists should have at their fingertips to perform the highest quality professional work. It is convenient to think of these image and information items as the selective clinical radiology information package (SCRIP) [3]. As each item is created, it ideally should be integrated into the SCRIP. Because material is acquired during the sequence of workup, examination, interpretation, decision, and follow-up, the professional user would never receive less than the current SCRIP with which to work. Information systems automate some of the tasks.

Reporting

The notion of clinical information packages naturally leads to consideration of the classic endpoint of diagnostic radiology—the written report of the radiologist's findings and interpretation. In traditional manual operations, the report is typed on the requisition form, thereby retaining whatever demographic and clinical information has been entered by the requester. With the advent of electronic systems, many combinations of automated and manual functions were implemented. Independent word processors gained popularity early. Some of these used the submitted paper requisitions, just as did typewriter operations. Others used continuous forms requiring that information on the requisition be reentered. As medical information networks have proliferated, it has become clear that work volume and error rates rise if identical information must be entered more than once. To take advantage of source entry and to ensure continuity of patient data, HIS, RIS, and PACS must be interoperable.

Modern RIS include good word processing modules and often provide electronic means of distributing reports to wards or other remote request sites. Progressively more complex and satisfactory integration of functional modules, like word processing, with RIS and hospitalwide systems is becoming commonplace. More sophisticated reporting has been followed by such ancillary functions as communication with billing systems, case coding, interesting case cataloguing, and capture of departmental management data. One solid entry into the clinical arena during the past several years is speech recognition for reporting. Systems of the late 1980s [5] have been considerably improved and are in regular clinical use.

Management

The final basic RIS module deals with management information. These modules vary widely but usually provide examination volume and distribution, resource utilization, statistics on timeliness of important functions, and financial information including revenues. Sorting of reports by source, referring physician, or interpreter can be used in support of quality improvement and privileging requirements.

These six functions—registration of patients, scheduling, patient tracking, film library management, reporting of results, and department management—together with electronic mail and support functions constitute the basic RIS.

Picture Archiving and Communications Systems

As RIS have matured, PACS have been evolving from somewhat different roots. However, both types of system appear to be converging to form an integrated multimedia information complex that will be a seamless combination of specialized medical devices and computer-based utilities.

One origin of image management systems can be found in the increasing use of digital acquisition devices, which have demanded that systems be developed to store, manipulate, and communicate electronic images throughout the radiology department and a growing variety of other sections of the medical community. A second origin of image management is found in the development of multimedia HIS [6]. These have been important for distribution of images and for integration of the medical record. PACS, however, are intimately linked to radiology. PACS and electronic imaging devices are an inseparable combination that has become recognized as an integral and essential component of the coming computer-based communications environment on which health care of the future will rely. PACS will do a number of interesting things that derive from antecedent image acquisition systems.

Image Manipulation

In a sense, individual digital imaging devices like CT have always embraced the rudimentary functions of PACS. Computer-generated images are displayed on television-like CRTs where they can be manipulated and altered in a variety of ways. For instance, one can adjust exposures or choose only a portion of the full range of exposure and expand it to examine the segment in detail. Edges can be sharpened or black and white can be reversed to produce a negative image. Future possibilities seem endless. Some will be important new diagnostic tools; others will prove merely curiosities. Display stations foreshadowed the full-blown PACS workstations entering the workplace today.

Communication

Frequently, acquisition devices have a second display station that communicates with the main viewing device, allowing monitored image acquisition to continue while previous examinations are reviewed simultaneously at the second site. These multiple viewer configurations constitute rudimentary communication systems, a second element of PACS. This concept now extends to entire hospitals, and teleradiology systems transmit images anywhere.

Archiving

Image storage, or archiving (a third element of PACS), has been achieved with magnetic discs in display stations to provide rapid retrieval of a limited number of active cases or with magnetic tape for longer-term retention of images that do not need to be so accessible. Although these images are fully manageable electronically, convention, an initial need for portability, diminishing but real technological limitations, and a cautious approach to new methods have resulted in recording these same images, for interpretation and storage, on film. The practice is redundant and expensive, and is becoming ever less justifiable in the face of competitive cost for quality electronic images. As the number and types of individual digital acquisition devices have increased, and as more complex and expensive storage technology, such as optical discs, has become available, sharing of support devices and expectation of easier access to images at distributed sites have been natural consequences. PACS consolidate these functions for entire medical communities. Emerging application service providers (ASP) enable outsourcing of these services. New hierarchical management techniques enable cost-effective accessibility.

Computed and Digital Radiography

CR and DR have become viable clinical tools that allow closure on the goal of fully digital imaging environments. Total electronic management has much appeal. Images need never be inaccessible or lost. Records can be organized and combined in the best manner to suit a clinical need, and they can be used simultaneously at different sites served by institutionwide networks. Retrieval time is minimized, and one can perform a wide variety of image adjustments and manipulations not possible with film. Furthermore, a redundant system duplicating electronic and film images is expensive, making full migration to a filmless system economically as well as functionally attractive to many PACS proponents.

Transition

In spite of pressures to transfer from film to digital electronics, PACS have encountered some resistance from the workplace for several reasons. First, properly exposed and developed films are very good [7]. Second, the ever-powerful inclination of people to avoid change generates resistance. This is in part justified by knowing that to learn even the best of new ways requires that one tolerate degraded performance until the new skills are adequately developed. Third, until recently there was not a fully developed filmless medical practice environment, but PACS have advanced to a point where the quality of patient care can be protected, and several filmless hospitals or departments exist or are in the process of implementation. In the meantime, sections of PACS—certain storage devices, simple workstations, image transmission networks, etc.—are also entering the market and seeing clinical use.

Finally, the economics and best strategy of transition are still not clear, but much is being learned from each new installation. Although costs will likely be greater than hindsight will indicate they might have been, evidence suggests that once the transition to filmless departments has been accomplished, costs of the new image support systems will be competitive with the old [8]. The transition will require the addition of a well-developed program for technology assessment (TA) and a strategy for dealing with human factors, operations, and economics. The fairly recently recognized need for "technology management" will become of major importance.

Technology Assessment

The problem of assessing whether or not a technology accomplishes what it is purported to do is relatively simple. To detect its unforeseen effects, particularly those that are indirect, is more difficult. Replacement economics also can be microcosted and adequately compared. Here, too, the indirect economic effects are more elusive. Perhaps the most difficult, but in the last analysis most important, is the assessment of a technology in terms of its impact on outcome of care to the patient [9]. This concept of technology validation in terms of the quality of results has achieved general recognition only recently. Support technology is particularly difficult to assess in this manner because, unlike the direct connection between the patient and individual tests and treatments, the effects of support technology are mediated through many channels, and, therefore, are more general and stochastically more subtle [10].

PACS in diagnostic radiology, as currently conceived and segmentally implemented, consist of shared digital storage devices, communications networks ranging from local connections to wide area use of satellites, workstations for image manipulation and display, and well-managed databases for facile handling of images and associated information. The concept is intriguing, but the future holds more.

Steps to the Future

Even as PACS mature, a vision is developing that will serve as the organizing principle for information systems. PACS will become integrated with the other forms of information systems in the healthcare setting. There will be qualitative enhancements of their functionality, and management concepts regarding information systems will become better understood and implemented in creative ways. We are on the verge of highly sophisticated technology management.

Organizational Support

Application service providers have augmented the many available ways to outsource. They make sophisticated offerings and promise to become more appealing as practitioners face the overburden of increasing technology, administration and regulation. They use off-site technology and infrastructure to serve an imaging practice through broadband linkages. Digital imaging and alphanumeric information is managed and stored by a central service site. Technology is provided as leased equipment that is rolled over to protect against obsolescence and avoid front-end capital outlay. Security, including encryption capability, is professionally handled with economy of scale. The ASP is a viable option as of this writing.

Integration

Many current systems are converging toward an integrated, computer-supported information environment that recognizes the whole patient. Full integration requires infrastructure, application, and clinical unification.

Technical Integration

Systems are coming together in three ways. First, currently separate systems with similar functional characteristics will be intricately interfaced. Personal computers and their workstation cousins will interact with departmental systems. These in turn will communicate with HIS and the last will participate in still wider area networks, including the Internet, that reach out to other offices and institutions with much the same ease as telephone and telefax systems. Wireless solutions will be ubiquitous.

Particularly influential in development of wide area support are the progressing activities generated by the High Performance Computing Act of 1991 written by Senator Al Gore [11]. Ten federal agencies participate in the High Performance Computing and Communication Program (HPCC). In 1993, legislation called for a National Information Infrastructure (NII) that would influence not only networks but also the enhancement of functionality to be discussed below in the section on "Functional Enhancements." Second, standards developments of the past several years have been encouraging in providing a basis for *open systems*. By opening systems, integrators are supported in combining diverse technologies and multiple vendors in seamless harmony. A third trend that is well established in the PC market is multimodality computing. We can expect to see a growing application of these techniques bringing together symbols, images, and voice in professional settings [12].

Initiatives are under way to ease and accelerate system integration. Three are of note:

1. HIMSS (Healthcare Information and Management Systems Society) has launched a national health information infrastructure (NHII) task force.
2. HIMSS and the Radiologic Society of North America (RSNA) have collaborated on an initiative for "Integrating the Healthcare Enterprise" (IHE).
3. The previously mentioned collaboration between DICOM and HL7.

On October 16, 2002, HIMSS announced the launching of their new NHII task force. The release stated that ". . . the task force envisions this infrastructure as a comprehensive system capable of providing trustworthy information to all healthcare decision makers" [13]. The task force is in its formative stages at this writing, but it carries the weight of a major organization with broad aspirations. It should contribute significantly to the underpinnings necessary for any synthesis of systems at the level of clinical content. The IHE initiative was aired publicly first at RSNA 1999 where vendors came together to demonstrate how products could provide a step up in integration [14]. The project is cyclical, each year adding to a set of integrating "profiles" of clinical functions that are critical for optimizing patient care. The profiles are negotiated cooperatively and specified in a detailed technical framework. As of 2001–2002, seven IHE profiles were in place: Scheduled Workflow, Patient Information Reconciliation, Consistent Presentation of Images, Presentation of Grouped Procedures, Access to Radiology Information, Key Image Notes, Simple Image, and Numeric Reports. These profiles incorporate aspects of HIS, RIS, and PACS. IHE is a powerful, ongoing public initiative to open systems for the benefit of the final consumer—the patient.

There is a fourth initiative that is an almost paradoxical force for integrity—the Healthcare Insurance and Accountability Act of 1996 (HIPAA). By federal legislation, HIPAA imposes privacy and security requirements that force radiology to pay careful attention to information that crosses the boundary with its environment. The key is protected health information (PHI). Wherever PHI goes, wherever it comes from, wherever it could be accessed, responsibility to see that PHI remains safe rests with whoever may have had responsibility for it. That is the tall order with which compliance is law as of April 14, 2003. The subject is covered in some detail elsewhere in this volume (see Chapter 30). However, it is worth noting that radiology practices are affected in a multitude of ways. The following is a checklist of the operational areas affected [15].

- Administration and oversight.
- Operations.
- Contracting.
- Information services.
- Human resources.
- Billing and collections.
- Compliance.
- Physical site security.

Cross-cutting the foregoing areas of operation are several lists of interest to information technology (IT). Types of vendors are those dealing with radiology information systems:

- Billing systems.
- Computer networks.
- Medical equipment that utilizes remote diagnostics services.
- PACS and teleradiology.
- Transcription systems.
- Connectivity and Internet access, especially if patients or referring physicians currently have access to patient information.

Security management tasks for IT include:

- Implementation of security mechanisms for downloads and data transfer.
- Implementation of network security mechanisms and audits programs.
- Installation of virus checking programs and management of virus checking processes.
- Development of virtual private network or similar network security process.
- Ensuring security on the practice's Web site.
- Setting up workstation time-out intervals.
- Ensuring workstation physical site security, including teleradiology/PSCS workstations.
- Ensuring the security of off-site connections including management access to systems/software laptop computers and report delivery mechanism.

Policies and procedures that IT may be asked to develop include:

- Granting and terminating system access.
- Workstation use.
- Removal and addition of hardware and software.
- Off-site access to systems.
- E-mail and Internet use.
- Tracking of upgrades and maintenance.
- Retention and destruction of electronic media.

These lists are imposing, but they are not to be ignored. The old dictum that responsibility cannot be delegated applies here. When responsibility must be shared with outsiders, a "chain of trust" is essential. Some relief from having to obtain patient consent for use of information has been conferred by the regulators to facilitate the referral process. Nevertheless, responsibility for privacy and security remain.

Domain Integration

The second type of system convergence involves systems that are functionally sepa-rated because they focus on subject matter that we often think of as tools. Ordinarily these must be accessed independently, often on dedicated terminals at a limited number of sites. Literature and other reference services, decision support systems, sta-tistics packages, and programs to do specialized analysis and graphics are examples of important functions currently inaccessible through most RIS or HIS systems. The Inter-net has done much to lower the barriers and to foster easy access to the "tools" domain. The World Wide Web is a fact of life.

Integration of systems in each of the described ways is beginning, but no well-developed model is yet available in a clinical setting. Integrating these systems requires research and development in cognition, linguistics, logic, and both software and hard-ware technology. Planning and analysis can accomplish some of the work, but other portions of the necessary knowledge can be gained only from experience. The path to integrated systems is neither short nor easy to travel, but it is destined to be traversed.

Clinical Integration

For diagnostic radiology, assuming that its niche in clinical practice remains substan-tially intact, integrated systems will provide the opportunity to enter the mainstream of practice in a way that has never been possible. The SCRIP, or information package, can be a practical reality. Participation in workup strategies, performance of examina-tions and interpretations with full access to relevant information, and the ability to be part of the clinical decision team will bring the full talents of the radiologist to bear on patient problems. The developed potential of radiologic diagnosis and management will contribute to maximizing the clinical efficacy of the medical team. Full realization of this goal will require cultural changes—a daunting challenge.

Functional Enhancements

Beyond the promise of integrating existing systems, there lie some promising, new func-tional developments.

Computer-Aided Diagnosis

Computer-aided diagnosis (CAD) is becoming viable as an adjunct to perception. It has caught imagination in mammography where it helps with detection and charac-terization of calcification and there is work involving lung and liver masses and colonic polyps [16]. Dr. Giger suggests that computers are showing potential as providers of a "second opinion" and support as a "second reader."

Image-Guided Surgery

Much work has been done in developing the technology necessary to fuse and recon-struct images from a wide variety of sources. Work continues and is being further encouraged by the NII program. Research has reached a point where it is feasible to impose the virtual reality of images on the reality of the human body. Fusion of dif-ferent presentations of reality enables physical procedures for diagnosis and therapy that were not imaginable just a few years ago. Image-guided surgery describes one of the most dramatic applications of these new developments, carrying with it a promise of new levels of collaboration among now disparate specialties [17].

Imaging Databases

A long-standing interest of many in being able to develop a database of visual information has been rather well examined and set forth by a National Institutes of Health group [18].The extension of databases beyond alphanumerics promises great enrichment of the integrated environment described in the previous section. Service, research, and education should all benefit.

Intelligent Systems

PACS have crossed the watershed to prove the feasibility of the "filmless" hospital. The contribution to image and information management is immense, but success in implementation immediately shifts the focus to improving operations. The application of techniques of "computer intelligence" to operations and image presentation is under way [19].

Management Issues

The notion that information systems are incidental to the real business of healthcare delivery must be replaced by full understanding that an integrated information system is pervasive, and that it must seamlessly permeate most of the operations in health care. On one hand, management must understand the big picture, the full system. On the other hand, because of its complex relationship to operations, different portions of the information system necessarily have different significance and different roles in relation to vested interests and responsibilities. These differences affect "ownership," management, funding, development, maintenance priority, and legal and regulatory status. For example, PACS in radiology are an essential element of the functions through which the radiologist fulfills his or her primary responsibility. The PACS role in this sense is qualitatively different from its function as a utility to distribute images remotely. The latter function is more nearly like that of the telephone. If these differences are not balanced with the larger view, managerial headaches will be legion [20].

Conclusion

Diagnostic radiology is currently so specialized and complex that it has become significantly differentiated from the mainstream of medical practice. Both the practice and the management of diagnostic radiology are too complicated to function properly with manual methods. RIS have provided excellent assistance with organization, monitoring, and communication. PACS are emerging as a by-product of digital imaging modalities and are becoming support systems of importance in their own right. The "filmless hospital" has been demonstrated as a model for the future. Integration of computer-driven information systems is now recognized as a general need of medical practice. Integration of RIS with PACS is receiving much attention. More recently, general recognition that the RIS/PACS combination must be folded into hospital information systems with access to other information domains has become established [19,21]. This technology, of proven value to patient outcome, can restore and enhance the patient's confidence in medical organizations. This will be an accomplishment of great importance as this nation assimilates the reality of managed care. At the center of the medical complex, however, imaging will be ever more critical to patient welfare.

References

1. Shannon RH. Computer enhanced radiology: a transformation to imaging. In: Ball MJ, Douglas JV, O'Desky RI, Albright JW, editors. Healthcare Information Management Systems. New York: Springer-Verlag; 1991. p. 81–91.
2. Grobstein C. Hierarchical order and neogenesis. In: Pattee HH, editor. Hierarchy theory: the challenge of complex systems. New York: George Braziller; 1973. p. 31–47.
3. Hounsfield GN. A method of and apparatus for examination of a body by radiation such as x or gamma radiation. Patent specification 1283915. London, 1972.
4. Gell G, Bauman RA. Large-scale PAC systems. In: Siegel EL, Kolodner RM, editors. Filmless radiology. New York: Springer-Verlag; 1999. p. 21–32.
5. Robbins AH, Vincent, ME, Shaffer, K, Maietta, R, Srinivasan MK. Radiology reports: assessment of a 5,000 word speech recognizer. Radiology 1988;167:853–855.
6. Dayhoff, RE, Maloney DL, Kenney JT, Fletcher RD. Providing an integrated clinical data view in a hospital information system that manages multimedia data. In: Clayton PD, editor. Fifteenth annual symposium on computer applications in medical care. New York: McGraw-Hill; 1992. p. 501–505.
7. Vizy KN. The roles of film in an increasingly computerized world. Invest Radiol 1989;24: 503–506.
8. Flagle CD. Economic analysis of filmless radiology. In: Siegel EL, Kolodner RM, editors. Filmless radiology. New York: Springer-Verlag; 1999. p. 113–136.
9. Lohr KN, Rettig RA. Quality of care and technology assessment. Washington, DC: Institute of Medicine, National Academy Press. 1988.
10. Shannon RH, Allman RA. Technology assessment using an informatics framework for medical imaging. In: Arenson RL, editor. Proceedings of the Ninth Conference on Computer Applications in Radiology. Philadelphia: RISC; 1988.
11. Lindberg DAB. Global information infrastructure. Int J Bio-Med Comput 1994;34:13–19.
12. Schramm C, Goldberg M. Multimedia radiological reports: creation and playback. J Digit Imaging 1989;2:106–113.
13. HIMSS. 2002. HIMSS News. http://www.himss.org.
14. Siegel EL, Channin DS. Integrating the healthcare enterprise: a primer. RadioGraphics 2001; 21:1339–1341.
15. Kroken P. HIPAA: administrative requirements for privacy and security. ACR Bulletin; Sept. 2002.
16. Giger ML. Computer aided diagnosis in radiology. Acad Radiol 2002;9:1–3.
17. Jolesz FJ, Shtern F. The operating room of the future. Report of the National Cancer Institute Workshop. Imaging-guided stereotactic tumor diagnosis and treatment. Invest Radiol 1992;27:326–328.
18. Zink S, Jaffe CC. Medical imaging databases. A National Institutes of Health Workshop. Invest Radiol 1993;28:366–372.
19. Stewart BK. Next-generation PACS focus on intelligence. Diagn Imaging 1994;81–84.
20. Shannon RH, Allman RA. Picture archiving and communication systems (PACS): a medical device. In: Brody WR, Johnston GS, editors. Computer applications to assist radiology. Proceedings of the Society for Computer Applications in Radiology (SCAR). Symposia Foundation; 1992. p. 48–54.
21. Shannon RH. IMACS and radiology: defining the problems. In: Mun SK, Greberman M, Hendee WR, Shannon RH, editors. Proceedings of the First International Conference on Image Management and Communication. New York: IEEE; 1989.

30
The Health Insurance Portability and Accountability Act: Confidentiality, Privacy, and Security

JOAN M. KIEL

HIPAA provisions relating to electronic transactions, security, and privacy must be integrated, not only to protect information, but also to deliver quality health care.

Leading Up to HIPAA

On average, $180 million could pay for 90,000 intensive care unit days, 225,000 regular inpatient days, or an extraordinary amount of outpatient care. Yet, that is the amount of money that the federal government, on behalf of the Veterans Affairs Healthcare System, may be spending—not on health care—but to settle a healthcare lawsuit. Filed in the fall of 2000, the lawsuit claims that, due to a lack of security, the computer system at any Veterans Affairs Healthcare facility has enabled workers to access personal and medical information about any patient or employee. Although the Veterans Affairs has installed a "software patch," one can override this and still gain access to the information. Individuals also cite that their personal information is already noted and being used for criminal activity such as opening up credit cards in their names [1].

As information technology use in health care continues to grow, lawsuits such as this are not uncommon. In addition, some incidents do not make it to the courts because patients never realize just how their medical information is being used. For example, with "medical record brokering," a pharmacy may sell its information to a hospital or insurance company, who then markets services to the patient that are analogous to the medications they are taking. A patient on a cardiac medication may be marketed exercise and diet products, or a person on insulin may be marketed foot care services. This chain of events all occurs because a patient's health information was passed on. One side claims breach of privacy, while the other side claims that they are acting in the best interest of the patient by introducing them to useful products and services. The judgment comes with the Health Insurance Portability and Accountability Act of 1996.

Joan M. Kiel, PhD, MPA, MPhil, is Chairman of the Department of Health Management Systems at the John G. Rangos, Sr., School of Health Science at Duquesne University in Pittsburgh.

History of HIPAA

The Health Insurance Portability and Accountability Act (HIPAA) of 1996 was instituted to provide health insurance portability for individuals, to protect the privacy and security of patient health information, and to eradicate fraud and abuse. Also known as the Kennedy–Kassebaum Act, or the Administrative Simplification Act, HIPAA was enacted on August 21, 1996. The law applies to all healthcare providers, clearinghouses, and healthcare plans, any organizations that transmit healthcare information electronically, and any organization that delivers, bills, or receives money for healthcare services.

The impetus for HIPAA came from both providers and consumers. Providers wanted standardization and simplification of healthcare claims. Presently multiple healthcare claim forms exist, both paper and electronic. Thus, many times when transmitting claims data, the data first must be passed through a clearinghouse that formulates the outgoing data from the provider to the receiving payer organization, and vice versa. This "added step" adds both time and cost to the process. HIPAA standardizes claim submission so the sender and the receiver will have the same format. Consumers have demanded privacy and security of their patient health information to include all oral, paper, and electronic notations. Healthcare information can be utilized to discriminate in employment settings and insurance buying. With wide-ranging implication, HIPAA is integral throughout the delivery of quality health care.

The HIPAA Format

The Health Insurance Portability and Accountability Act is composed of five parts called Titles. Titles 1 through 5 include Health Insurance Access, Portability, and Renewal (Title 1), Prevention of Healthcare Fraud and Abuse (Title 2), Tax Related Provisions (Title 3), Group Health Plan Requirements (Title 4), and Revenue Offsets (Title 5). Title 2, Prevention of Healthcare Fraud and Abuse, contains Subtitle F, which is Administrative Simplification. Within Subtitle F, there are six components as follows: Electronic Transaction Standards, Unique Health Identifiers, Standard Code Sets, Privacy Legislation, Electronic Signature Standards, and Information Security. Further delineation of the six components of the Health Insurance Portability and Accountability Act results in eleven Rules (Table 30.1).

1. Claims Attachment Rule: Will establish national standards for the format and content of electronic claims attachment transactions.
2. Clinical Data Rules: Will establish national standards for clinical data. This will include clinical messaging standards.
3. Data Security Rule: Will establish technical and administrative protocols for the security and integrity of electronic health data.
4. Enforcement Rule: Will establish rules on how the Government will enforce HIPAA.
5. First Report of Injury Rule: Will establish national standards for the format and content of electronic first report of injury transactions used in workers' compensation cases.
6. National Employer Identifier Rule: Will establish the federal tax identification number as an employer's national identifier.
7. National Individual Identifier Rule: Will establish one patient identifier for all of one's individual patient health information.

TABLE 30.1. The HIPAA format.

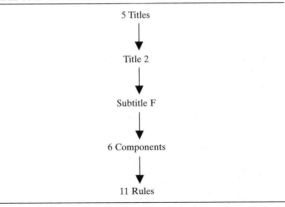

The three main foci of the Health Insurance Portability and Accountability Act are Electronic Transactions and Code Sets, Security, and Privacy; these are found under the 11 rules outlined here.

8. National Payer Identifier Rule: Will establish a national identifier for each health insurer.
9. National Provider Identifier Rule: Will establish a national identifier for each provider and the mechanisms for disseminating, storing, and updating the identifier.
10. Privacy Rule: Will establish guidelines for the use and disclosure of patient health information.
11. Transactions and Code Sets: Will establish standard formats and coding of electronic claims and related transactions [2].

Electronic Transactions and Code Sets Rule

With a variety of electronic medical records and healthcare software, transmitting information along the continuum of care within a healthcare system or between healthcare systems and providers necessitates that the sender and the receiver be able to communicate electronically with each other. But with upgrades and different variations of software and operating systems, this is not always the case. In fact, many times conversion software is needed to allow the sender software to work with the recipient software. Thinking of this on a grand scale between hundreds of insurance plans and hundreds of providers, the opportunities for errors and the time and cost involved in the conversions are numerous. The Standards for Electronic Transactions and Code Sets hopes to alleviate these issues.

The Standards for Electronic Transactions and Code Sets (Title 45: 162.900) require uniform transmittal forms and codes for electronic submissions. Here the sender and receiver will be able to communicate directly; thus, the "subtitle" of HIPAA, the Administrative Simplification Act. All submissions such as claim encounters, claims payment, eligibility inquiry and response, claims status inquiry and response, benefit enrollment, premium payment, and referral and certification, must follow the ANSI ASC X12 standard [3]. Providers who use a clearinghouse or third-party administrator are accountable that they are HIPAA compliant and can send and receive the electronic transactions. The Standardized Code Sets are the ICD-9, CPT-4, HCPCS for products and supplies, and CDT for dental services.

How do The Standards for Electronic Transactions and Code Sets affect a provider, payer, or clearinghouse? What needs to be accomplished to meet this HIPAA standard? Payers, providers, and clearinghouses need to first and foremost assess if their information systems are compliant with the ANSI standards: Are they using the mandated standards? (Table 30.2). They can do this on their own or by consulting with their information technology vendor. Given the recent rise in the utilization of information technology in health care, most systems in place now are compliant. It is similar to the Y2K issue; if one bought a system in the mid- to late 1990s, it was Y2K compliant. If the system is not compliant, then an investment needs to be made to upgrade or to purchase a new system. Although there is an upfront cost, with the projected simplification, it is predicted that money will be recouped over time.

Given that the system is ANSI compliant, one then needs to assess if the payers, providers, and clearinghouses that one communicates with are compliant. A simple call or e-mail is all that is needed. Given that there is a 2-year leeway to be compliant, some will choose earlier and some later dates to meet the standard. Testing is the next phase for this standard. Ensure that the system has interoperability with all those entities with which the system communicates electronic transactions.

The transactions that are covered by the Electronic Transactions and Code Sets Rule are [4]:

• Health claims or encounter information.
• Healthcare payment and remittance advice.
• Coordination of benefits.
• Healthcare claim status.
• Health plan enrollment and disenrollment.
• Eligibility for a health plan.
• Health plan premium payments.
• Referral certification and authorization.
• First report of injury.
• Health claims attachments.

To meet the standards of the Transactions and Code Sets, one must first determine their compliance level. The security officer, along with the facility's vendors and billing department, does this most often. Assess if the information technology system is compliant with the above-mentioned ANSI standard. Second, assess in which transaction(s) listed above one participates. Last, draft a compliance plan/letter. On December 18, 2001, President Bush signed HR 3323, which extended the compliance date from

TABLE 30.2. Electronic Transactions and Code Sets ASC X12N Version.

Standard	ASC X12N Version
1. Enrollment/disenrollment	834
2. Premium payment	820
3. Eligibility request and response	270/271
4. Authorization/certification request and response from the insurer	278
5. Claim or encounter (COB)	837
6. Coordination of benefits	837
7. Claim status inquiry and response (to check status of third-party payment)	276/277

All submissions must follow the ANSI ASC X12N standard [10].

October 16, 2002 to October 16, 2003. But to take advantage of this extension, entities must have sent their plan for compliance to the Department of Health and Human Services (HSS) by October 16, 2002. The letter/compliance plan should have included a description of why the provider was not in compliance; a strategy plan to reach compliance, which included a budget, schedule, work plan, and implementation schedule; a description of the contractor or vendor that the provider will use, if one at all; and a timeframe for testing and evaluating that began no later than April 16, 2003.

Security

Patient health information security refers to the prevention of having data and information accessed by those without a "need to know." The security and integrity of electronic health data must be protected from unauthorized users. Many people believe that HIPAA security involves only "computers," but as is discussed here, it encompasses both physical and electronic access, such as administrative policies and procedures, and physical and technical security measures.

The Security Rule challenges that all electronic transmissions maintain a balance between being accessible, but also being secure and confidential. Information technology systems will follow the ANSI (American National Standards Institute) Standards for interfacing with all systems, including storing, accessing, and transmitting data. In addition, the Security Rule encompasses various technical and operational policies and procedures such as password maintenance and management, incident reporting, periodic reminders to ensure a secure environment, virus protection, and monitoring of log-in and user access.

Organizations and providers begin by appointing a Security Officer. This does not have to be a dedicated, full-time person, but rather can be someone already in-house who will assume the HIPAA security responsibilities. The first responsibility of the Security Officer is to conduct an information technology security audit. The audit examines how compliant the software and hardware are with the HIPAA-mandated ANSI standards. Also, physical security changes, such as locked cabinets and storage areas not in the main work location, are to be examined. The Security Officer will also determine the employees who have a "need to know" and have access to patient health information; they must then undergo training and adhere to the various HIPAA policies.

The Security Rule also recommends a disaster recovery plan and routine backups for all electronic information. Facilities must identify a contingency plan to restore any loss of data and to identify safe storage locations such as an off-site mine. Disaster plan testing and recovery should be performed.

The HIPAA Security Rule is more than information technology. More so, the Security Rule must become a part of daily operations through policies, procedures, and standard operating practices.

Information Technology Security Audit

The Information Technology Security Audit is the framework for an organization to embark on their HIPAA security plan. The audit follows an interdisciplinary approach and involves those from medical records, information systems, finance, physical plant, and clinical departments. The audit focuses on the technical and physical safeguards and includes examination of the following areas [5]:

A. Monitoring access with audit trails, policies and procedures, and audit reports.
B. User Authentication with unique, individual identifiers, routine changing of passwords, and automatic terminal shutdown after a specified time of inactivity.
C. Surveillance of data integrity with digital signatures, encryption, and audits.
D. Physical Security with secure terminals and monitors away from the public, destruction of data no longer needed, off-site backup storage, and a disaster recovery plan.
E. Security for remote access with user authentication, firewall security, and security testing.
F. Software security with controls on software installation, virus scans on all computers, and virus monitoring.

The information security audit serves as the framework for designing policies and procedures for technology and personnel. Four major policies and procedures for personnel working with patient health information are the Organization Code of Conduct, Employee Code of Ethics, Access to Health Information Code of Conduct, and Computer Usage Policy. Employees may feel that they are "signing their life away," but each serves a specific purpose.

Codes of Conduct and Ethics

The Organization Code of Conduct expresses the entity's values on health information. A sample clause follows:

"This organization values each person as an individual with rights and dignity: the right to quality healthcare; the right to privacy; and the right to an assurance that health information is both confidential and secure. The individual and family members have the right to question their patient health information and the use of it. It is in the values of this facility to assure our individual and families that no breach of patient health information privacy, security, or confidentiality will be tolerated." [6]

The Employee Code of Ethics is read and signed by each employee so that they are aware of their responsibilities in regard to health information. As with all HIPAA documentation it is retained for 6 years. A sample clause follows:

"It is in the values of this organization to assure our patients and families, and fellow employees that no violation of law or breach of patient health information privacy, security, or confidentiality will be tolerated. There exists disciplinary measures, up to and including termination, for those found in violation.
In support of this, all employees will agree to:

• Document and bill accurately
• Not accept payment outside of your salary for completed work
• Comply with all audits" [7]

The Access to Patient Health Information Code of Conduct is a more specific statement of health information practices than the above employee code of ethics. This Code operationalizes HIPAA on an employees access to health information based on the "need to know" principle. Only those employees whose job description and role specifies that they will have access to health information to fulfill their work responsibilities are allowed the access. Once that access is granted, this code mandates how the user interacts with the health information. A sample clause follows:

"In the healthcare environment, it is best to consider *all* information transferred by any media (voice, text, symbol, etc.) to be confidential. You will not copy, talk about, release, change, or destroy any information. In regards to computerized information, you will not share passwords, alter programs, or participate in hacking" [8].

An interesting note on this Code is that it remains in effect even after a person has separated from the organization.

Computer Usage Policy

The last major mandate is the Computer Usage Policy. Again based on the "need to know" principle, this code specifies how the information technology system is to be used in an organization. A sample clause follows:

"This facility authorizes specific individuals who have a "need to know" health information, access to computers, information technology, and information. With this access though comes a responsibility that computer, information technology, and information will be used with strict security and confidentiality." Employees also agree to certain restrictions such as not accessing information for personal gain, preventing others from using your system, and cooperating with audits and monitoring of technology usage [9].

The Security Officer must then embark on the analysis and protection of both the physical health information and physical technology. Now, a technology inventory must be completed. Here, every piece of software and hardware must be inventoried to the degree of location, age, and type. Being very specific is key, as HIPAA requires, for example, that monitors be out of view of the public. Therefore, in completing the inventory, one must state, "16-inch monitor in second floor nursing station faces west wing elevator 2." Technology that is in storage, perhaps awaiting disposal, must also be inventoried.

After the technology inventory, the Security Officer must complete the data inventory. Here the facility must specify who has access to what type of data. This again is based on the "need to know" principle. The challenge here, especially for large organizations, is to keep up with the constantly changing workforce. Between hires, promotions, transfers, and separations, this data inventory must be maintained.

Last, the medical record location inventory must be completed. Just as with the technology inventory, specificity is paramount. All active, archived, and off-site records must be accounted for. The inventory must include whether the records are locked or in the open, such as a rack in an open nurses station. If the organization utilizes an off-site storage location, it must be specified if the organization owns the storage facility, since this will have liability and insurance implications.

The information technology security audit and the aforementioned inventories are based on HIPAA-mandated ANSI standards (see Table 30.2). The ANSI standards for each transaction, as required by the Electronic Transactions and Code Sets Ruling, demonstrate to organizations that they cannot use a silo approach to arrive at HIPAA planning. Rather, organizations will find that the various sections of HIPAA were meant to be operationalized into daily work functions; thus, they must be integrated.

In terms of complying with ANSI standards, the organization must first determine what transactions it performs. Then the standards are shared with the organization's computer vendor to determine if the current information systems *meet* the standards. If they do, a written letter stating their compliance must be obtained. If the information systems *do not meet* the standards, the vendors will suggest what is needed to have them meet the standards. Then upon upgrades, and, most importantly, testing, one can obtain the written letter of compliance.

Destruction and Disposal

Thus far, the security topic has focused on protecting patient health information. But what happens when a facility no longer has to save the health information, either as mandated by law or organizational policies and procedures? The answer lies in the destruction and disposal mandates for health information. When disposing of health information, one must ensure that the data are destroyed and cannot be resurrected. Simply removing it from the property or deleting computer files is not adequate. What are needed are strict mandates on the internal and external destruction of health information, and disposal of physical computers and health information. Keep in mind that since healthcare organizations may contract this task to an outside vendor this vendor must also abide by HIPAA regulations. Here, the outside vendor cannot use or disclose the patient health information before destruction. In addition, the vendor will use safeguards to ensure that the patient health information is not disclosed, but if disclosure does occur, the vendor will notify the facility immediately. If the vendor subcontracts to another agent, that agent must be known to the facility and must abide by the HIPAA regulations [11]. Patient health information shall be permanently destroyed, so that there is no possibility of reconstructing the data. Paper records can be destroyed by burning, cross-shredding, pulping, and pulverizing. Microfilm and microfiche can be destroyed by recycling and pulverizing. Magnetic data can be destroyed by degaussing [11]. A Certificate of Destruction must then be completed and retained by the organization.

As with the external destruction of health information, under HIPAA all patient health information that is to be internally discarded is to follow a procedure of destruction that will comply with the HIPAA regulation and ensure privacy, security, and confidentiality of all patient health information. Because patient health information is a component of normal business operations, the internal destruction policy mandates that the organization destroy patient health information that no longer has a business function and can rightfully be destroyed under law. Facilities can utilize shredders at the end of each shift or as the information to be destroyed is found. Ensure that the print queue is empty, so that health information is not being printed when proper personnel are not attending to it [11].

The last measure of health information destruction is computer disposal, the actual physical hardware being rendered clear of all health information. Also included here is when a computer is moved and used by another person who does not have "need to know" privileges for health information. When information is saved on a computer hard disk, the magnetic characteristics of that disk change in two ways. The first way is with the information that is stored on it, that is, the written file. The second way is with the address or the location of the file being stored on the magnetic disk; thus, the disk holds two identifying elements for each file stored. When a file is "deleted," the only part that is erased on the magnetic disk is the address or location. The information remains. Even though the disk is used over or formatted, the magnetic characteristics of the disk still hold the information, and, therefore it is accessible with certain technology tools. The only way to ensure that both the information and address are removed, that is, change the magnetic characteristics of the disk back to their original format, is to overwrite the disk with specific technology tools [12]. The technology tool for overwriting must meet the Defense Department Standard DoD 5220.22, whereby the overwriting takes place in several iterations [12]. After the overwriting is completed, the computer will be dated and initialed as to when and who did the overwrite procedure. The information technology department will also log the information.

The Security Rule of HIPAA involves both information technology and organizational policies and procedures. The key is for an organization to operationalize the HIPAA aspects, so that it becomes a "normal way of doing business."

Privacy

The HIPAA Privacy Rule is the area that is drawing the most attention because it directly affects both providers and patients. Patients are not going to be too concerned whether their insurance company's software cannot interface with their provider's software or whether it adheres to the Transactions and Code Sets Rule. However, if the patient's medical record information is shared with telemarketers or the office staff, the patient would be very concerned and may even sue; thus, the Privacy Rule's heightened status.

The HIPAA Privacy Rule concerns itself with the use and disclosure of identifiable patient health information and seeks to maintain its confidentiality. The Privacy Rule encompasses protecting the privacy with business associates and vendors, allowing patients to request to amend their medical records, and receiving consent and authorization before sharing information. Providers must also publicize their information practices in a "Notice." All personnel who have access to patient health information must be trained on the requirements.

Similar to the Security Rule, the Privacy Rule goes beyond medical records per se, as it also includes policies and procedures that affect one's standard operating procedures. Healthcare providers must designate a privacy officer. This person will be responsible for implementing the safeguards to maintain the confidentiality of the information. In addition, this will be the person who performs routine audits and investigates any breaches of privacy and ultimately disciplines those who have committed the breach. The breaches can surface in two ways—either through an anonymous complaint line or through the audits.

With the Privacy Rule, patients will be able to request to amend their medical records. The key here is that they can make a request, which will then be considered, but it does not guarantee that the change will take place. The patient would contact the author of the medical note and request that a change be made and also submit what the change should be. The provider or a committee will consider the request and make a ruling.

Statement of Confidentiality

Organizations must issue a Statement of Confidentiality for Patient Health Information. This statement is the organization's mission toward how they operationalize privacy of health information. Some of the issues that an organization will want to include are these:

- Only speak to individuals about confidential matters in private areas.
- Never discuss health information in a social setting.
- Never call out to an individual or staff member about tests, appointments, etc., that a patient will be having.
- Never ask the individual in public about a specific test; rather, just ask them "how they are doing."

- When transporting a resident inside or outside of the facility, always place the medical record face down.
- Always place test requests, resident notes, or any chart entries face down before placing them in the medical record.
- Never have a computer terminal face in the direction of public traffic.
- Medical record access is based on a "need to know basis" only for legitimate business as deemed by the facility.

This statement of confidentiality drives how the organization will handle private health information [9, p. 4:33].

Notice of Use and Disclosure

Emanating from the statement of confidentiality is the Notice Of Health Information Practices. This notice describes how health information about an individual may be used and disclosed and how one can get access to this health information. Many people routinely think that health information is mainly shared with insurers and other healthcare facilities for treatment decisions and payment. The Notice, though, covers many other entities that have an interest in one's health information for business purposes. Facility departments such as risk management, quality assurance, and disease management receive information to analyze the care, treatment, and outcomes of procedures and tests. This health information is used to continually improve the care by analyzing best practices. Information can be extrapolated by physician, procedure, or demographic characteristic. Healthcare facilities also maintain a directory used mainly by visiting clergy. Patients can now opt out of being in the directory by stating that before signing the notice. Business associates such as pharmacy, medical equipment, and medical laboratories receive patient health information. Business associates must follow HIPAA standards and certify that in writing to the healthcare facility.

In predominantly teaching hospitals and academic medical centers, health information may be disclosed to researchers if they have appropriate consent forms and the research has been approved by the institution's review process. The researchers will be held to the facility's health information privacy standards. Funeral directors will receive health information in accordance with state laws and for professional purposes only. Consistent with applicable laws, health information may be disclosed to organ procurement organizations or organizations involved in the transplantation of and related services for organs, tissue donation, and transplant [13].

A controversial area is marketing purposes. Health information can be disclosed to remind patients about treatments and services that may benefit them given their medical condition. Some healthcare entities, such as homecare organizations, sell data to insurers, therapists, and other providers to market services. This practice of "medical record brokering" can be stopped if the individual notes their disagreement to it before signing the notice. Federal government agencies such as the Food and Drug Administration may be required to disclose health information related to a food recall or outbreak of a food-related condition. State government agencies, such as workman's compensation, will share health information as it becomes necessary by law and to render a decision on a compensation case. The federal and state governments may require health information to be disclosed for public health purposes, such as for communicable disease tracking and injury prevention. The Notice specifies, in general, to whom health information can be disclosed.

For specific disclosures, an individual must sign an "authorization to disclosure" form. This form specifies who, by name, not general category, can receive the health information, what type of health information (such as history and physical, laboratory tests, allergy list) can be released, and for what purpose, and for how long a period of time (usually not more than 6 months). Organizations then must track the disclosures and retain the records for 6 years. Databases are most useful here because querying can retrieve information by patient name, and information, such as patient name, information disclosed, date, information recipient, and expiration, can be tracked in individual fields. Last, the expiration date field can be queried to assess which authorizations need to be updated.

Right to Inspect, Copy, and Amend

One of the most heralded parts of the HIPAA Privacy Rule is the Right to Request to Inspect, Copy, and Amend Medical Records section. In fact, one of the main purposes of HIPAA, from a consumer's point of view, is the right to look at and possibly amend records. The physical medical record belongs to the provider, but what many do not know is that the information contained within belongs to the individual; therefore, under State Privacy Laws, patients have had the right to examine their medical records. HIPAA corroborates this and states that an individual has a right to *request* to inspect, copy, and amend their medical record under most circumstance. Exceptions to this are psychotherapy notes; information to be used in legal proceedings or for forensic matters; information that could cause harm to oneself or to another, especially when inmates are involved; research information when a patient is in the sample; and if the requestor is judged that he or she may be further harmed by having seen the information [14].

The facility has the requesting party complete a request form and validate their identification (Table 30.3). The request form asks the patient what needs to be changed,

TABLE 30.3. Sample amendment form.

Request Form to Amend Health Information

Name: _____

Record Number: _____

Birthdate: _____

Address: _____

Date of information to be amended: _____

Type of information to be amended: _____

Why should the information be amended? _____

What should the amended information say? _____

_____   _____
Signature of Patient   Date

One of the main purposes of HIPAA, from the consumer's point of view, is the right to look at and possibly amend records [14, p. 64u].

why, and what the new wording should say. The healthcare facility must rule on the matter in a timely manner, generally 60 days. If the request is denied, the patient can appeal, whereby the facility will have an additional 30 days to review the case further. If the request to amend the record is granted, the healthcare facility will inform the requestor that the amendment was granted, then insert the amended language next to the changed language. The amendment must then be shared with all those who have a "right to know" about the changed language.

If the healthcare provider denies the request to amend the record, a written statement in laymen's terms of the reason for denial is given to the requestor. The requestor can then counter by writing a statement of disagreement. If it is again denied, the facility must alert the requestor that they can further appeal to the Secretary of Health and Human Services and the facility's complaint line. Also, the facility must make known the denied request in the medical record with any future disclosures of the patient's health information. One point for providers to keep in mind—there is no limit as to how many times a request can be made [14, p. 64S–T].

Monitoring Compliance

The authors of HIPAA wanted to ensure that providers would not simply put HIPAA in place and then forget about it. Rather, the authors wanted HIPAA to be operationalized into a provider's daily operations. To do this, they required that an organization institute operational audits, a reporting mechanism, and discipline procedures. Operational audits are an evaluation mechanism to measure compliance with the stated policies and regulations of HIPAA. The Compliance Officer and staff will conduct monthly (or more frequent) audits on various measures such as computer logins, medical record documentation, coding and billing, adherence to confidentiality policies, adherence to security policies, HIPAA training for employees, and a review of personnel access to patient health information. These steps, among others, will be conducted to assess system weaknesses so that corrective action can be taken to ensure that HIPAA is being followed. Audits can be announced or unannounced, but predominantly they will become a part of the facility's operations so that employees will see them as a part of routine business. First, if the audit detects problems, then an action plan must be specified on how to reeducate the affected employee(s) and/or department(s). Second, employee(s) and/or department(s) must be reaudited. Even if a problem is not found on the next audit, routine reaudits must continue so that a problem does not reoccur. All this must be documented on the audit forms. If the facility fails to reeducate and reaudit, or fails to document, it can be held liable for not correcting a situation of which it is aware [15].

Another way to detect nonadherence to HIPAA is via a reporting mechanism. Here, employees and other constituents can confidentially report violations or suspected violations of HIPAA, without retaliation. The facility must publicly advertise its reporting mechanism in all its locations. The reporting mechanism system can include a hotline telephone number, paper reporting system, or an electronic reporting system. The most important criterion is that the reporting system must be conducive for all levels of employees to use [16]. The employee and/or constituent can only report violations of credible, suspected violations of criminal conduct in relation to HIPAA; thus, this is not a general complaint line. Employees must also know that HIPAA is a federal mandate and that false reporting can lead to a criminal penalty. The reporting system must maintain the confidentiality of the reporting individual, and no retribution can be taken against the reporting individual. If the reporting individual complains of any retribution, the facility must document it and have a follow-up investigation immediately. When an employee or constituent files a complaint, the reporting mechanism call log is to be completed immediately. The complaint has a statute of limitations of 180 days. An initial investigation on the complaint must begin immediately, with the action and response being documented. After the investigation is complete, follow-up must ensure that credible violations are not repeated. In addition, the facility must cooperate with any outside investigation including sharing records in a timely manner and allowing access to pertinent records [17].

Disciplinary Measures

The last part of operationalizing HIPAA is to develop and implement a disciplinary system for HIPAA violations. With this, all breaches must be fully investigated, and, if warranted, disciplinary measures taken, including termination from and nonrehire to the organization. Disciplinary measures are taken on those who violate the HIPAA mandate and those who are responsible for monitoring, detecting, and reporting an offense but fail to do so; therefore, this covers acts of commission and omission.

A breach of patient health information confidentiality is defined as any or all of these [18]:

a. When a person accesses patient health information for any reason not related to *his or her* job responsibilities; therefore, it is a breach if a person is looking it up for another person, except in an emergency healthcare situation as warranted by the Administrator or Physician in Charge.
b. Conducts oral communication with another or others for purposes not related to patient care.
c. Uses individual health information in a manner of malice to the resident(s) and /or facility(ies) and/or any of its holdings.
d. Uses patient health information for personal gain whether it be monetary or nonmonetary.
e. Uses patient health information as an intimidation.

All breaches and sanctions in violation of HIPAA must be clearly documented and substantiated. During the investigation, as warranted by the Compliance Officer, the employee(s) under investigation can be moved to another position or facility, whereby access to patient health information is not warranted. If the investigation reveals a violation of civil or criminal, federal or state law, the violation must be reported to government authorities immediately. If the investigation reveals an overpayment to a facility, the overpayment must be returned immediately. Organizations must then discipline the individual according to their chain of discipline. For example, individuals who use health information for malice, personal gain, and/or intimidation will be terminated. Breaches that involve accessing patient health information not related to one's job responsibilities will be suspended without pay for 3 weeks, put on a 90-working-day probationary period, and undergo HIPAA training. A second offense will result in immediate termination. Organizations will need to determine if their present discipline procedures are stringent enough for the violation of health information privacy.

HIPAA violations need not occur if the organization develops a "campaign" to advertise HIPAA and its policies and procedures to all employees. This can occur through orientation sessions, yearly updates meetings as mandated by accreditors and inspectors, routine staff meetings, payroll reminders, and diligence among all employees.

Summary

The key for adherence to the Health Insurance Portability and Accountability Act is to operationalize it into the organization's daily operations. Transactions and Code Sets, Security, and Privacy must all be integrated not only to protect information, but also to deliver quality health care. With so much in health care depending on accurate information, HIPAA will become a standard practice.

References

1. Hopper ID. Employees sue Veterans Affairs, claiming breach of their privacy. Pittsburgh Post Gazette 2000 November 3. Sect A:16.
2. A guide to the HIPAA rules, technology in practice. EC Media Group 2002 January/February. p. 26.
3. Moynihan J, McLure M. HIPAA brings new requirements, new opportunities. Healthcare Financial Management 2000 March. p. 53–54.
4. Weiss SJ. Countdown to HIPAA compliance, managed care interface. Medicon International 2002 April. p. 57.
5. http://www.3com.com/Securitynet. "Information Security—It's Up to You." Accessed August 22, 2002.
6. Thieleman W. A patient-friendly approach to the record amendment process. J AHIMA 2002 May. p. 44.
7. Standards for privacy of individually identifiable health information. Department of Health and Human Services, Office of the Secretary; 2000 December 28; 45 CFR 164.530 j(2).
8. CPRI Toolkit. Computer-Based Patient Record Institute; 1999 February 1. p. 4:3
9. CPRI Toolkit. Computer and information usage agreement. Computer-Based Patient Record Institute; 1999. p. 4:3.
10. Bushman J, Krupp A. HIPAA implementation: a step-by-step guide. MGMA Legislative Conference, Washington, DC, April 22, 2002.
11. Hughes G. Practice brief—destruction of patient health information. J AHIMA 2000 April. p. 64A–64B.
12. http://www.hipaaadvisory.com/actionsecureqa/secure.htm. Accessed August 22, 2002.
13. Hughes G. Practice brief—notice of information practices. J AHIMA 2001 May. p. 64L.
14. Hughes G. Practice brief—patient access and amendment to health records. J AHIMA 2001 May. p. 64S–T.
15. Neville D. Six steps to compliance for small practices. J AHIMA 2001. p. 42.
16. Naughton-Travers J. Key to developing a regulatory compliance program. Behavioral Health Management 2001 July/August. p. 36.
17. Standards for privacy of individually identifiable health information. Department of Health and Human Services, Office of the Secretary; 2000 December 28; 45 CFR 160.306(b)(3).
18. CPRI Toolkit. Harvard Vanguard Policy on the disciplinary process for breach of patient confidentiality. Computer-Based Patient Record Institute; 1999. p. 4–46.

31
Information Technology and the New Culture of Patient Safety

JOYCE SENSMEIER and KATHLEEN COVERT KIMMEL

More than ever before, the healthcare industry is embracing information technology as a viable solution for promoting a culture of safety.

The New Culture of Patient Safety

Despite having unparalleled technology and resources, the U.S. healthcare system has room for improvement. Impressive advancements in medical knowledge have accelerated at a mind-boggling rate, but access to patient information and knowledge resources is limited and not readily available to the majority of providers. Innovative surgical procedures using advanced diagnostic equipment offer a sophisticated understanding of a patient's condition; however, information distribution and communication are hampered by the manual, paper-based charts present in most healthcare organizations. Handwritten medication orders are error prone, and deciphering handwriting is frequently a challenge for those processing orders. Medications with similar names but different action classes, effects, and dose ranges further complicate the medication management process. Front-line employees make high-risk decisions that require judgment and choices involving many variables with minimal system support [1].

The good news is that technologies are available to rectify these challenges. Information technology can contribute to a culture of patient safety. Decision support systems include knowledge resources to assist clinicians as they evaluate, diagnose, and treat patients. Integrated, enterprisewide electronic medical records offer real-time access to clinical notes, images, test results, vital signs, allergies, medication history, and other information to the entire gamut of caregivers. Computerized physician order entry (CPOE), combined with sophisticated alerts, can detect potential negative drug interactions and conflicts with other medical problems and greatly reduce errors [2].

Computerization in the clinical setting has focused on single-purpose applications. The proliferation of computerized clinical applications created an awkward collection of systems wherein pieces of data were stored in a variety of isolated silo-like systems.

Joyce Sensmeier, MS, RN, BC, CPHIMS, is Director of Professional Services for the Healthcare Information and Management Systems Society. Kathleen Covert Kimmel, RN, MHA, CHE, is Director of Clinical Information Systems at Catholic Health Initiatives.

As technology advancements occurred, new systems were often stacked on top of the old. Although this was originally intended to preserve familiar work processes, adding layers of functionality to already cumbersome and isolated legacy systems was similar to building a house of sticks; under the weight of additional layers, the system began to crumble and collapse. The work processes related to these systems became burdensome and enhanced the potential for errors.

Healthcare organizations have begun to take stock of their technology and applications and to evaluate clinical workflow. Clinical information systems have emerged as the most important healthcare application for organizations in the next 2 years [3]. If technology is applied to an inefficient manual process, however, it will retain its inefficiencies when automated. Information technology, combined with clinical process transformation, holds the most promise for improvement.

Given the expense of an electronic medical record system, which includes physician order entry, medication administration records, and decision support systems, funding by healthcare organizations supplemented by the federal government is needed. The events of September 11, 2001, and the subsequent threats of bioterrorism, have placed a spotlight on the inability of our nation's local healthcare delivery model to rapidly move patient-specific and organism/treatment-related data between and among hospitals and private physician practices. Just as the development of the U.S. highway system laid the foundation for interstate travel and commerce, a national health information infrastructure (NHII) is needed. This NHII will provide the "rules of the road" for the connection of distributed health data and integration of systems within the framework of a secure network, acting as a medical communication highway to protect citizens [4].

Building a Culture of Safety

Processes to detect and reduce medical errors in hospitals and healthcare systems have been hampered by the lack of integrated technology and decision support applications. As a result, for many years the extent of medical errors was unknown. Uncovering the degree of the problem was fueled by the medical error-related death of Boston Globe health columnist Betsy Lehman in 1994, which triggered a landslide of government hearings, meetings, and reports. Lehman, who was being treated for breast cancer at Boston's Dana Farber Cancer Institute, mistakenly received the cumulative dose of the cancer drug cisplatin, instead of the daily dose for 4 days. The overdose caused heart failure, which led to her well-publicized death. Postevent findings and analysis culminated in the release of the Institute of Medicine's (IOM) first report by the Committee on Quality of Health Care in America, titled *To Err is Human: Building a Safer Health System* [5]. This report shocked the nation by exposing a quality crisis, stating that between 44,000 and 98,000 deaths in hospitals each year are related to preventable medical errors. The report concluded that:

- The extent of harm that results from medical errors is great.
- Errors result from system failures, not people failures.
- Achieving acceptable levels of patient safety will require major systems changes.
- A concerted national effort is needed to improve patient safety.

The IOM report recommendations set a 50 percent reduction in medical errors as a goal within 5 years, which could be achieved by:

- Creating a Center for Patient Safety.
- Mandating a reporting system for medical errors.
- Encouraging voluntary reporting.
- Providing greater legal protection for data collected for patient safety and quality improvement purposes.
- Promoting performance standards (people and organizations) that emphasize safety.
- Emphasizing safe use of drugs through the Food and Drug Administration (FDA).

The Public Sector Response

Although there continues to be great debate about the actual number of errors, this report galvanized strong reaction from both the public and private sector. Within 2 weeks after release of the report, the U.S. Congress began a series of hearings. President Clinton ordered a governmentwide feasibility study, which was followed in February 2000 by a presidential mandate to implement the IOM recommendations, specifically, to reduce medical errors by 50 percent within the next 5 years. The President's mandate requires all 6000 hospitals participating in the Medicare program to implement patient safety initiatives, including medications and safety-oriented approaches [6].

A Medicare Patient Advisory Commission report suggested that the Centers for Medicare and Medicaid Services (CMS), formerly known as HCFA, consider providing financial incentives to hospitals that adopt CPOE systems [7]. The Agency for Healthcare Research and Quality (AHRQ) received $50 million to fund error reduction research, including information-related strategies. The AHRQ produced a report, "Making Healthcare Safer: A Critical Analysis of Patient Safety Practices," in July 2001 that represented a first effort to approach the field of patient safety through the lens of evidence-based medicine [8].

State governments have also responded. For example, the state of California passed a bill mandating that all nonrural hospitals implement technology that has been shown to eliminate or substantially reduce medication-related errors such as CPOE or bar coding by 2005 [9]. Wisconsin has announced that it will use its $710 million annual healthcare expenditures to encourage hospitals to implement patient safety methods and disclose quality information. Under the plan, state hospitals will be required to adopt CPOE and other patient safety strategies advocated by the Leapfrog Group, a coalition of large healthcare purchasers [10].

In the 2 years since the IOM report, the government has attempted to address the problem. In May 2001, Senators Bob Graham (D-FL) and Olympia Snowe (R-MN) introduced legislation to provide grants to hospitals and nursing facilities to implement technology that reduces medication errors. The Medication Errors Reduction Act of 2001 calls for nearly $1 billion in grants during the next 10 years, with $93 million available to hospitals and $4.5 million to skilled-nursing facilities each year. Under the bill, individual hospitals will be eligible for grants of up to $750,000, with grants for nursing facilities capped at $200,000.

In September 2002 the House Ways and Means Committee approved a bill, sponsored by Representative Nancy Johnson (R-CT), to improve patient safety. Under the bill, hospitals would voluntarily collect and submit data on medical errors. A new Center for Quality Improvement and Patient Safety, operated by AHRQ, would certify and coordinate compilation of the patient safety information. A Senate version of the patient safety bill was introduced in June 2002 by Senators James Jeffords

(I-VT), John Breaux (D-LA), Bill Frist (R-TN), and Judd Gregg (R-NH). This bill also includes voluntary reporting and prohibits the punishment of individuals who either report or commit errors [11]. Also in June 2002, Senator Edward Kennedy (D-MA) introduced legislation that would force providers to adopt CPOE. This legislation would include $350 million in grants for providers to upgrade equipment.

The Centers for Medicare and Medicaid (CMS) are currently emphasizing consumer-oriented outcomes, primarily focusing on two areas:

1. Quality measurements for hospital that aim to tie hospital payments to quality performance, and
2. Patient satisfaction surveys.

According to CMS administrator, Thomas Scully, "People who perform better will be paid more." Currently, officials at CMS are in discussions with Premier, an alliance of 1600 hospitals regarding conducting a joint demonstration project [12].

The Fiscal Year '02 Appropriations Bill includes a 10 percent increase in funding for the Department of Health and Human Services, with $55 million set aside for AHRQ to determine ways to reduce medical errors. Additionally, $15 million has been appropriated for rural hospitals and designated for medical errors' reduction and systems improvement to comply with provisions of the Health Insurance Portability and Accountability Act [13].

The FDA is implementing changes for the labeling of existing drugs, as well as testing new drugs before they hit the market [14]. Mixups with look-alike or sound-alike drug names are a major source of medication-caused injuries and death. This combination of eye-catching changes, which includes a mix of upper and lower case as well as different colored letters, should more easily gain the attention of pharmacists. In addition, FDA workers will begin testing groups of volunteer physicians, nurses, and pharmacists about potential confusion of new drug names before the drugs hit the market. The FDA is also considering mandating bar-code labels on drug packaging down to each unit-of-use. Announcement of the proposed rule is expected by year-end [15].

The Centers for Disease Control and Prevention (CDC) is collaborating with the E-Health Initiative to develop an information technology (IT) infrastructure to combat bioterrorism. The initiative joins the public and private sector wherein the CDC is working with a consortium of healthcare IT vendors and organizations to link legacy IT systems in hospitals, pharmacies, and labs with the CDC National Electronic Disease Surveillance System (NEDSS). This effort is an important first step in facilitating the capture of critical data at the point of initial contact and transmitting disease surveillance information to the government [16].

The Private Sector Response

In addition to government agencies, the private sector has also responded to the IOM report. The Leapfrog Group, a coalition of many of the nation's leading companies sponsored by the Business Roundtable, seeks to create meaningful, marketplace incentives to encourage the healthcare sector to adopt systemic quality improvement processes. The employer marketplace is responding to Leapfrog's message. As of June 2003, the Leapfrog Group represents 140 companies and 34 million employees, spending approximately $53 billion/year on employee healthcare. Leapfrog also has three healthcare industry members—the Joint Commission on Accreditation of Healthcare Organizations (JCAHO), HCA, and Promina.

The Leapfrog Group has identified three initial patient safety standards as the focus for consumer education and information and hospital recognition and reward:

- Reduce medication prescribing errors using CPOE.
- Evidence-based hospital referral.
- Staff Intensive Care Units (ICUs) with intensivists (i.e., physicians certified in critical care medicine).

Originally Leapfrog focused on encouraging providers to voluntarily adopt their recommendations. In June 2001, Leapfrog began taking action by using its economic clout to influence provider acceptance of the three recommendations. Approximately 900 hospitals in seven targeted markets around the country (Atlanta, California, Eastern Tennessee, Michigan, Minnesota, Seattle, and St. Louis), were being asked how they process medication orders, staff their ICUs, and how many open heart surgeries they perform each year. This information was made available to millions of hospital-seeking beneficiaries via their Web site [17]. In April 2002, Leapfrog added an additional 12 markets to target for patient safety, including Central Florida, Colorado, Dallas-Fort Worth, Kansas City (MO), Massachusetts, Memphis, New Jersey, New York City, Rochester (NY), Savannah (GA), Wichita, and South Central Wisconsin. As of June 2003, Leapfrog has expanded to 22 regions. These regions account for almost half of the U.S. population.

The Leapfrog Group and First Consulting Group have released two reports on CPOE. The first report is a guide to help hospitals assess the effectiveness of their CPOE systems in intercepting erroneous medication orders. The second provides starter-set information for hospital decision makers to help organize their CPOE effort and launch the search for an appropriate CPOE solution [18]. Leapfrog's report card-like summary of a hospital's IT infrastructure is expected to help spark action by many providers. Financial analysts are anticipating a profound impact on healthcare IT spending as employers begin to shift market share toward providers who adopt Leapfrog's patient safety standards [19].

The Leapfrog Group's efforts to impose economic sanctions to drive compliance are coming to fruition. In fact, by year-end 2001, General Motors rewrote their payer contracts to include patient safety requirements within their hospital provider contracts [19]. This action puts the onus of responsibility of obtaining provider compliance on health plans. Recently, a major health plan began encouraging compliance by presenting financial rewards to providers who meet the safety standards. Three Fortune 500 companies joined Empire Blue Cross to recognize and reward hospitals that achieve the Leapfrog safety standards. Beginning January 1, 2002, hospitals in Empire Blue Cross and Blue Shield's networks will receive a 4 percent bonus for meeting two quality standards—CPOE and ICU staffing with intensivists. Hospitals that meet this standard beginning in 2003 will receive a 3 percent bonus and those which wait until 2004 will receive a 2 percent bonus [20].

A study reported in the *Archives of Internal Medicine* found that physicians believe that reducing medical errors should be a national priority, but they are much less likely than the public to believe quality of care is a problem [21]. The survey, which included 1000 Colorado physicians ($n = 594$), 1000 national physicians ($n = 304$), and 500 Colorado households, assessed agreement with several proposals and conclusions from the IOM report. Perhaps demonstrating the persistence of a culture of blame, physicians believed that fear of medical malpractice is a barrier to reporting of errors and that greater legal safeguards are necessary for a mandatory reporting system to be successful.

The Second IOM Report: Crossing the Quality Chasm

In March 2001, the IOM Committee on Quality of Health Care in America produced a second report, *Crossing the Quality Chasm: A New Health System for the 21st Century*. This report presented a call for action to improve the U.S. healthcare delivery system [22]. Emphasis was placed on the critical role of IT in designing systems that produce safe, effective, patient-centered, timely, efficient, and equitable care.

This second IOM report decries a medical system where physician groups, hospitals, and other organizations "operate as silos, often providing care without the benefit of complete information about the patient's condition, medical history, services provided in other settings, or medications prescribed by other physicians" [22]. Harking back to the first report, this report again addresses patient safety problems, stating that the cause is a system that "relies on outmoded systems of work." The solution for safer, high-quality care is to "redesign systems of care, including the use of information technology to support clinical and administrative processes."

IOM Recommendations on Restructuring the U.S. Healthcare System

The report includes 13 recommendations for restructuring the U.S. healthcare system. While some recommendations pertain to quality of care, others discuss funding for monitoring and tracking existing solutions for quality of care. Also included are recommendations for mutual efforts between payers and providers to work toward a care system where patients and providers cooperate, collaborate, and share information that is current and evidence-based. Additionally, because 40 percent of all care is directed toward chronically ill patients, there are recommendations to identify at least 15 of the most prevalent chronic diseases and to develop strategies for improving quality of care for each.

The report also requests the AHRQ to facilitate further thinking by convening workshops designed to promote guidelines in specific topic areas. These areas include redesigning care practices, using IT to improve access to clinical information, supporting clinical decision making in an electronic environment, and coordinating care across patient conditions, services, and settings, over time.

In response to this second IOM report, the First Consulting Group (FCG) has published a summary of case examples that demonstrates how currently available technology is being used by care providers in ways that support the goals of the IOM [23]. The FCG report features applications that support clinical processes and emphasizes the organizational challenges that must be dealt with when implementing these technologies.

Medical Error Statistics

The IOM's first report not only highlighted the number of deaths in hospitals due to medical errors, it also estimated the costs generated by those errors. National healthcare costs attributable to preventable adverse events were estimated to be $17 billion [24]. How extensive are medical errors? The National Committee on Vital and Health Statistics (NCVHS) reports the following statistics [25]:

- One in 25 hospital admissions results in an injured patient.
- Three percent of adverse effects cause permanent disabling injury; of these, one in seven leads to a patient death.
- Preventable medical errors account for 12 to 15 percent of hospital costs.
- About 23,000 hospital patients die each year from injuries linked to medication use.
- Eighty percent of nurses calculate dosages incorrectly 10 percent of the time, and 40 percent of nurses make mistakes more than 30 percent of the time.
- In the United States, approximately 180,000 unnecessary deaths and 1.3 million injuries occur from medical treatment.

Besides the IOM and the NCVHS, The Advisory Board Company in Washington, D.C. is another source for information on medical errors. The Advisory Board divides adverse effects into several categories. Each category is listed with the number of times they occur per 1000 hospital visits:

- 65 incidents are due to adverse drug events.
- 60 incidents are due to nosocomial (hospital-acquired) infections.
- 51 incidents are due to procedural complications.
- 15 incidents are due to falls.

Adverse drug events (ADE) top the list in frequency of occurrences. ADEs have a wide range of causes and careful measurement is a complex process [26]. The second and third categories, nosocomial infections and procedural complications, may be related to provider training or experience and hospital infection control policies and procedures. The final category, falls, is usually related to unstable patients, including elderly patients, and can be traced to policies and procedures.

The average cost of an ADE is $4700 per admission. When ADEs, which account for more than 25 percent of all adverse hospital incidents, are studied, the following results are found [27]:

- 56 percent are attributed to physicians.
- 34 percent are attributed to nurses.
- 6 percent are attributed to unit secretaries.
- 4 percent are attributed to pharmacy staff.

ADEs, the largest single category of medical errors, can be immediately affected by information technology. CPOE and bar-code medication administration are two proven technology-supported work processes that can reduce medical errors in three of the categories listed above [24].

While technology is a critical component to patient safety management, it should also be a part of an organizationwide strategy that includes workflow process redesign. Decreasing the number of ADEs requires the combination of clinical workflow transformation with selective implementation of technology. Systems can be integrated and processes automated without solving the problem. Traditional workflows must be reevaluated to harness technology and assist in information capture, flow, analysis, transmission, and trending.

The Role of Technology

A common theme throughout the IOM reports is the critical role IT plays in reducing medical errors. In his statement before the subcommittee on Labor, Health and Human Services, and Education of the Senate Committee on Appropriations, Dennis O'Leary, president of JCAHO, stated, "Medical error reduction is fundamentally an information problem. The solution to reducing the number of medical errors resides in developing mechanisms for collecting, analyzing, and applying existing information. If we are going to make significant strides in enhancing patient safety, we must think in terms of the information we need to obtain, create, and disseminate" [28]. JCAHO is also providing leadership in creating an environment that is no longer focused on secrecy and blame by requiring institutions to inform patients whose treatment has included medical errors [29].

Other industry-based organizations are promoting the use of information technology to improve patient safety. The Healthcare Information and Management Systems Society (HIMSS) advocates the use of IT for point of care, unit-of-use bar coding to reduce medical errors and improve productivity [30]. According to a recent study, medication errors are frequent, occurring at a rate of nearly one of every five doses in the typical hospital and skilled nursing facility [31]. The most frequent errors by category were wrong time (43%), omission (30%), wrong dose (17%), and unauthorized drug (4%), many of which can be prevented by the use of bar-coded medication administration. Evidence of the impact of this technology is demonstrated by the Veterans Health Administration, which has seen a systemwide 75 percent reduction in medication errors since implementing Bar Code Medication Administration software [32].

The American Medical Informatics Association has published a white paper contending that errors can be prevented by computer systems which provide electronic patient records, physician order entry, practice standards, medical vocabularies, and computerized decision support [33]. General recommendations for reducing errors using IT include implementing clinical decision support; considering design consequences; adequately testing systems; promoting the adoption of data and system standards; developing systems that communicate; and using systems in new ways to measure and prevent adverse consequences.

Perceived Impact of Technology on Care Delivery

Any discussion of the role of technology in improving patient safety must take into consideration the effectiveness of technology in achieving this intended outcome. When implementations are not thoroughly planned down to the detail work process and operational workflow level, technology can backfire, creating time-draining duplicative work, clinician dissatisfaction, and may even increase the potential for medical errors. A study conducted jointly by VHA (Voluntary Hospitals of America) and IBM in the Spring of 2002 asked 1100 chief nursing officers (CNO) the following questions:
Would technology:

- Improve efficiency?
- Decrease paperwork?
- Increase nursing satisfaction and recruitment?
- Facilitate providing a higher level of quality patient care?
- Allow nurses to have more time for patient care?

A surprisingly high number of nurses did not agree that technology would improve patient care. Although 79 percent of the 236 respondents agreed that IT would improve quality and decrease costs, 40 percent did not agree that it would improve efficiency and reduce paperwork. Also, 50 percent did not agree that technology could increase nurses' satisfaction or recruitment, allow more time for direct patient care, or improve clinical quality.

The Barriers Offer Some Insight

Answers on types of barriers encountered offer some insight into why CNOs are leery of technology. Although they believe technology holds promise for improvements, many nurse executives have experienced obstacles that cause implementations to fail, be stalled, or become difficult. The top barriers reported were:

- Cost.
- Push-back from physicians and/or administration.
- Lack of willingness to set clinical process transformation as a top priority.
- Tendency to seek a "quick fix" versus developing an integrated solution.
- Lack of tried-and-true products and implementation processes that are integrated, easy to install, and easy to use.

The "Real Barriers" Said Differently

Review of the survey results with VHA CNOs who have implemented technology successfully provides additional insight [34]. In summary:

- It is not a software issue but a cultural issue. Change management is a strong component of a successful implementation.
- There is lack of an integrated approach. Piecemeal implementations that do not take the entire workflow process and related systems into consideration can lead to scenarios wherein nurses must enter the same data in multiple standalone systems as well as on the paper chart. This lack of an integrated approach creates a situation in which technology hampers efficiency and productivity—the very opposite of the intended outcome.
- Clinical transformation, implementation, and training are a tremendous drain on both time and resources.
- Technology implementations represent a "hard road," requiring persistence, leadership, and fortitude to overcome resistance to change.
- Many hospitals and healthcare organizations, already lacking nursing resources, simply do not have nurses with the required skills to tackle technology implementations.

Economic Justification for Information Systems Technology

Given the significant capital restraints now burdening healthcare organizations, purchasing this technology requires a demonstrable return on investment. The good news for hospitals is that positive return on investment data related to some of these technologies already exist. An early study at an academic medical center estimated that CPOE generated savings of $5 to $10 million annually on a $500 million budget [35]. A more recent study provides evidence from Montefiore Medical Center, a 1100-bed academic health system, of tremendous savings for CPOE and medication administra-

TABLE 31.1. Return on investment data substantiate the value of investing in technology.

Attribute		Technologically advanced hospitals
Average length of stay		0.091 days shorter than U.S. median
Difference in Medicare cost per discharge		$1,517 less than U.S. median

Financial attributes	Most wired hospitals	All U.S. hospitals
Highest AA credit rating	41.4%	13.3%
Total margin	4.5%	2.9%
Days cash on hand	78	46
Long-term debt to equity	41.2%	29.5%
Average age of plant	9.7 years	9.5 years
Net patient revenue per FTE	$91,183	$86,411
Percent of capital budget to IT	18.3%	16%

Patient safety attributes	Most wired hospitals	Less wired hospitals
UPN code for pharmaceuticals	61%	30.6%
Web-based clinician pharmacy order entry	39%	7.8%
Web-based provider consultation	51%	14.6
Web-based patient communication	39%	8.3%

Source: Ref. 37.

tion record, roughly $6 million annually. This figure combines the time savings for nurses, unit secretaries, and pharmacists [36].

As demonstrated in Table 31.1, the results of the fourth annual Hospitals and Health Network's survey indicate that the nation's "most wired" hospitals and health systems, namely those that have embraced technology solutions, have better control of expenses, higher productivity, and more efficient utilization management than their peers [37]. Data also demonstrate that the most wired have a 3.5 percent advantage in operating costs, adjusting for both case-mix differences and cost variations from market to market. One additional theme emerged: the most wired hospitals and health systems appear to have lower mortality and complication rates than the nation as a whole.

Realizing the Benefits

According to a report from Cerner Corporation, Samaritan Regional Medical Center saved $3 million annually and avoided 36 deaths by using a computerized data repository that was populated with medication rules [38]. A study by the Gartner Group estimated a positive return on investment for ambulatory computer-based patient records. This report produced a formula for calculating the amount of savings per year/per physician by multiplying $41,400 per year/per practitioner to calculate the savings in an ambulatory environment [39].

Several industry groups are working toward documenting the benefits of technology and evaluating the claims made by vendors. Information-collection projects include the following initiatives [40]:

- HIMSS has recently launched a Web-based Solutions Tool Kit™, a comprehensive healthcare IT database, which provides an aggregation of competitive vendor and product information.

- The Center for Information Technology Leadership (CITL), Boston, is researching the value of emerging technologies. Founded by Partners Healthcare, the CITL is collaborating with HIMSS as the distribution channel for research findings.
- The Institute for Medical Knowledge Implementation (IMKI), San Francisco, was formed to create a national library of clinical rules, easily uploaded in commercial systems and available to the public. IMKI is a not-for-profit organization dedicated to translating the best of medical care into common clinical practice by enhancing and expediting the adoption of healthcare information systems and other technologies.

Technology is rapidly progressing. Electronic medical record systems with decision support at the point of order entry are improving each year in their features, functions, and capabilities. These systems are justifying themselves in terms of saved dollars and saved lives. Accessibility to mobile computing devices at the point of care is evolving. Wireless computing devices enable physicians, other ordering clinicians, and nurses to enter patient data at the point of care. Disease management systems provide caregivers with information on efficacy of drugs and treatments at various stages of a medical condition. Use of bar-code technology in combination with decision support assures that patients are receiving the correct medication or treatment. Utilizing CPOE, physicians are able to review up-to-date test results and access knowledge resources to inform their decisions before entering orders.

More than ever before, the healthcare industry is embracing IT as a viable solution for promoting a culture of safety. Using Web-based technology, the healthcare team can also include the patient, who must be an informed decision maker and active participant in his or her care. When all healthcare stakeholders recognize their responsibility and work together to address patient safety issues, the quality of healthcare in this nation and all over the world will be greatly improved.

References

1. Valusek JR. Decision support: a paradigm addition for patient safety. J Healthcare Inform Manag 2002;16(1):33–39.
2. Bates DW, Teich JM, Lee J, Seger D, Kuperman GJ, Ma'Luf N, Boyle D, Leape L. The impact of computerized physician order entry on medication error prevention. J Am Med Inform Assoc 1999;6(4):331–321.
3. 13th Annual HIMSS Leadership Survey. Sponsored by Superior Consultant Company; 2002.
4. National Committee on Vital and Health Statistics. Information for health: a strategy for building the national health information infrastructure. Washington, DC: U.S. Department of Health and Human Services; 2001.
5. Institute of Medicine Committee on Quality of Health Care in America. To err is human: building a safer health system. Washington, DC: National Academy Press; 2000.
6. The White House Office of the Press Secretary. Press Briefing by Senior Administrative Officials on President's Initiative to Reduce Medical Errors, February 22, 2000. http://www.pub.whitehouse.gov.
7. Medicare Payment Advisory Commission. Report to Congress: selected medical issues. 1999; June.
8. Shojannia KG, Duncan BF, McDonald KM, Wachter RM. Making health care safer: a critical analysis of patient safety practices. AHRQ Publication 01-E058. 2001; July 20.
9. California Senate Bill No. 1875. Chapter 816, Statutes of 2000.
10. Manning J. State will ask hospitals for details on quality of care, Milwaukee Journal Sentinel 2002 November 30; http://www.jsonline.com/bym/News/nov02/99987.asp.

11. Tieman J. Racing to the finish: House passes bills, but it still has a tough battle. Modern Healthcare 2002; September 23:12–13.
12. Morrissey J. Making IT compute. Modern Healthcare 2002; September 16:6–7.
13. Healthcare Information and Management Systems Society. 2001 Congressional Review. Advocacy Dispatch 2001 January 18; www.himss.org/about/advocacy.asp.
14. Daily Dose E-Mail. FDA implementing changes with new labels. Modern Healthcare 2002; January 2.
15. FDA public meeting on bar code labeling for drugs; 2002 July 26; http://www.fda.gov/oc/speeches/2002/barcode0726.html.
16. Healthcare Information and Management Systems Society. CDC's ongoing push to create a national bioterrorism early warning system. HIMSS NewsBreak 2001; December 24.
17. Lovern E. Minding hospitals' business: purchasing coalition pushes hospitals to improve patient safety through process measures, but industry says standards are too expensive. Modern Healthcare 2001; May 28.
18. Kilbridge P, Welebob E, Classen D. Overview of the Leapfrog Group evaluation tool for computerized physician order entry. Leapfrog Group and First Consulting Group. 2001.
19. Falci RG, Steward RT, Weinberger A. An update on the Leapfrog movement: a macro catalyst is maturing into a fundamental change agent. Bear Stearns Equity Research White Paper. 2001; September 6.
20. Media Release Three Fortune 500 companies join Empire Blue Cross and Blue Shield to recognize and reward hospitals that achieve Leapfrog safety standards. Empire BCBS 2001; October 19.
21. Robinson AR, Hohmann KB, Rifkin JI, et al. Physician and public opinions on quality of health care and the problem of medical errors. Arch Intern Med 2002;162:19.
22. Institute of Medicine Committee on Quality of Health Care in America. Crossing the quality chasm: a new health system for the 21st century. Washington, DC: National Academy Press; 2001.
23. Kilbridge P. Crossing the chasm with information technology: bridging the quality gap in health care. California Healthcare Foundation; 2002 July.
24. Beers JB, Berger MA. Medical errors: sources and solutions. Proceedings of 2001 Annual HIMSS Conference and Exhibition, session 17, 2001.
25. National Committee on Vital and Health Statistics. Testimony. 1999; June 23–24.
26. Bates DW, Leape LL, Cullen DJ, et al. Effect of computerized physician order entry and a team intervention on prevention of serious medication errors. JAMA 1998;280:1311–1316.
27. Clinical Initiatives Center Prescription for Change. Best practices for medication management. Washington, DC.; The Advisory Board Company. 2000.
28. O'Leary D. Statement of the Joint Commission on Accreditation of Healthcare Organizations before the U.S. Senate and the Subcommittee on Labor, Health and Human Services and Education of the Senate Committee on Appropriations. 2001 February 22. http://www.jcaho.org/govt/oleary_02220.html.
29. Ball MJ, Douglas JV. IT, patient safety, and quality care. J Healthcare Inform Manag 2002;16(1):28–33.
30. Simpson N. Advocacy White Paper: Bar coding for patient safety. Healthcare Information and Management Systems Society; 2001 December. http://www.himss.org/advocacy/about/advocacy.asp.
31. Barker KN, Flynn EA, Pepper GA, Bates DW, Mikeal RL. Medication error observed in 36 health care facilities. Arch Intern Med 2002;162:1897–1903.
32. Johnson CL, Carlson RA, Tucker CL, Willette C. Using BCMA software to improve patient safety in Veterans Administration Medical Centers. J Healthcare Inform Manag 2002; 16(1):46–51.
33. Bates DW, Cohen M, Leape LL, Overhage JM, Shabot MM, Sheridan T. Reducing the frequency of errors in medicine using information technology. J Am Inform Assoc, August 2001;8:299–308.
34. Ricci R, Barr N, Hamilton S. Proceedings from the VHA Annual Meeting. Pain management for healthcare executives: IT solutions for healthcare. 2002 April 24. Courtesy of the VHA.

35. Glaser J, Teich JM, Kumperman G. Impact of information events on medical care. Proceedings of the 1996 Annual HIMSS Conference and Exhibition, 1996.
36. Manzo J, Taylor RG, Cusick D. Measuring medication related ROI; a process improvement after implementing POE. HIMSS News 2001 February.
37. Solovy A. Healthcare's most wired 2002. Hospitals & Health Networks 2002 July; 38–48.
38. Dennings EH. Healthcare management consultants. Cerner Corporation. 2001 June 22.
39. Duncan MA. Simplified financial ROI for an ambulatory CPR. Gartner Group; 1998 October.
40. Scalise D. Physician order entry: IMKI to success. Hospitals and Health Networks 2002; Oct:24–26.

32
INTERNATIONAL PERSPECTIVE
Pompidou University Hospital in France: A Component-Based Clinical Information and Electronic Health Record System

PATRICE DEGOULET, LISE MARIN, PIERRE BOIRON,
and ELISABETH DELBECKE

Created by merging three hospitals into one, Pompidou University Hospital employs a component-based clinical information system with integrated EHR.

The creation of the Pompidou University Hospital [or the Hôpital Européen Georges Pompidou (HEGP), as it is known in French], in southwest Paris, from the merging of three aging facilities presented an opportunity to conceive and deploy COHERENCE, a brand-new component-based clinical information system (CIS). COHERENCE features generic healthcare-related and generic components. The healthcare-related components include the patient healthcare record, the activity, and the resource scheduler components. Major functions of the CIS were operational when the hospital opened in July 2000. The generic components include a reference manager, a security manager, a document manager, a Corba bus, and various mediation and supervision tools. Three years later, the unique patient record and the provider order entry systems are being used in 100 percent of relevant healthcare units. Seventy-four percent of biological orders and 66 percent of imaging orders are being entered directly by physicians. Sharing by physicians and nurses of the common, multimedia lifelong health record, including online availability of images, is being achieved in 100 percent of the units.

Background

A long-term goal for healthcare institutions is the deployment of lifelong, longitudinal electronic health records (EHRs) that include all types of structured and unstructured information (i.e., coded information, free text, waveforms, voice, images) [1,2]. Such

Patrice Degoulet, MD, PhD, is CIO of the Georges Pompidou University Hospital and Cochair of the Public Health and Medical Informatics Department at the Broussais Faculty of Medicine in Paris, France. Lise Marin, MD, is Vice Director of the Information Systems Program at the Hospital Informatics Department of the Georges Pompidou University Hospital. Pierre Boiron, PhD, is Chief Engineer of Laboratory and Imaging Systems. Elisabeth Delbecke, RN, is Head of the Education and Training Programme.

EHRs offer many advantages when compared to paper-based records. These include more availability, accessibility, and legibility; the possible integration with decision support tools (knowledge coupling, alarms, reminders, or hypothesis formulation); improved security and confidentiality; and the regrouping of information for clinical or outcomes research [3–7].

Economic pressures to improve healthcare efficiency have become a strong incentive for healthcare institutions to collaborate and, eventually, to merge, stressing again the key role of the patient record in ensuring continuity of care [1,8]. More recently, EHRs have been proposed as one means to support patient empowerment and patient control over health problems [9]. This trend toward consumer empowerment has been translated into acts such as the Healthcare Information Portability and Accessibility Act (HIPAA) in the United States or the March 2002 law in France that allows patients to get a copy of their full medical record directly without going through a physician.

Attitudes about patient record systems, however, differ from one country to the next, from one institution to the other, and even among individuals in the same institution [10–12]. Examples of completely successful computerizations of the patient record remain rare [13]. Barriers to the development of the EHR include lack of understanding of the nature of clinical practice, overly high expectations of obtaining immediate benefits, lack of agreement on the underlying structure of the EHR, lack of involvement of health professionals, introduction of technologies that disrupt the physician's workflow, and lack of understanding of the impact on the organization.

When incorporated into a hospital information system, EHR functions need to be integrated with provider order entry (POE), resource scheduling, and decision support to provide efficient patient management and minimize medical errors [14–19]. Details of orders and appointments generated by the POE and scheduling systems are elements found in the patient's EHR. Decision support modules also need to be instantiated from the EHR content to avoid redundant data entry.

In this chapter, we describe and discuss implementation of the EHR component at the new Georges Pompidou University Hospital and its relationship to other components in the integrated clinical information system, and we include some data on its current use 3 years after its opening. Administrative and decision support functions, at the hospital level, are not covered in this chapter.

Material and Methods

The Georges Pompidou University Hospital

HEGP, located in southwest Paris, is one of 39 state-owned university hospital groups of the "Assistance Publique-Hôpitaux de Paris" (AP-HP). HEGP officially opened in July 2000 as a replacement for three aging facilities, the Boucicaut, Broussais, and Laennec hospitals (BBL), which totaled 1100 beds and 4000 employees at the end of 1999. HEGP currently has a capacity of 825 beds, although only 803 are currently open to the public (Table 32.1).

The hospital is organized around six major healthcare cooperating centers: cardiovascular, cancer, internal medicine (including an emergency and trauma center), anesthesia, imaging, and biology-pharmacy. Close to 3000 employees, including the equivalent of 1100 registered nurses and 370 full-time-equivalent physicians, staff the hospital. Observed activity in 2002, the second full year of hospital operation, is summarized in Table 32.1. In 2002 a total of 49,241 admissions were registered of which

TABLE 32.1. Pompidou University Hospital: main figures for 2002.

Characteristics	Number
Total number of active beds	803
Number (%) of 1-day hospital beds	69 (8.6%)
Number of operating rooms	24
Number of nurses	1,100
Number of physicians (full-time equivalent)	390
Total number of inpatient admissions	49,241
Number of outpatient visits	228,794
Number of visits at the Emergency Department	41,924

41 percent were for multiday inpatient care, 18 percent for 1-day medical or surgical investigations, and 40 percent for radiotherapy or chemotherapy sessions. On a daily basis, about 115 patients are routinely examined at the emergency and trauma center.

Component-Based Architecture

Component Selection Process

Strategic planning for the project took place during 1995 and 1996, and the project was started in December 1996. A best-of-breed approach was adopted, with a focus on integration and communication between predefined business components [20]. Preliminary extracts from the HISA model (European prestandard PrEnv 12967-1) were included in the technical documentation [21]. After an 18-month selection process, a consortium was selected, headed by SYSECA®, a branch of the French Alcatel company (now belonging to THALES®), with Hewlett Packard as the major hardware vendor and MEDASYS® and Per-Sé Technologies® as software component providers. A 5-year contract was signed in April 1998, which included a 24 × 7 guarantee that integrated solutions would be operational at the opening of the hospital and thereafter. The role of the prime contractor was to provide project support for the duration of the contract; to provide the necessary healthcare-related components, either directly or through subcontracts; and to provide the middleware tools for the integration of the different components into a three-layered architecture.

Figure 32.1 shows the basic architecture of the information system, called COHER-ENCE (Component-Based HEealth REference architecture for Networked CarE). Components were not only selected for their intrinsic capabilities and functionalities but also for their ability to be integrated into the overall architecture. Basic requirements for a component in the request for proposals included:

- A published application program interface (API).
- External exchanges through standardized messages.
- Immediate compliance or commitment to comply with the CCOW (Clinical Context Object Workgroup) recommendations for components involved with patient data management, now driven by the HL7 group [22].
- Existence of import or synchronization facilities to load the component data dictionaries from a terminology/reference component.
- Capacity to use an external authorization component and/or to synchronize user profile tables with an authorization component.
- Access to the detailed model of the component to allow easy access to tables through SQL queries and to allow integration through data when necessary.

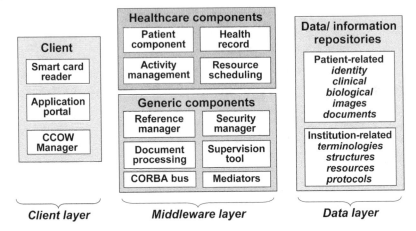

FIGURE 32.1. Functional architecture of the COHERENCE Hôpital Européen Georges Pompidou (HEGP) information system.

Healthcare-Related Components

Basic healthcare-related application components provided by the main contractor or subcontractors included:

- MEDASYS IMS®, a patient management component with functions for identification, admission, discharge, and transfer (ADT).
- MEDASYS DxCare®, which encompasses the functions of provider order entry and patient record components as requested in the initial call for proposals.
- ONE CALL® from Per-Sé Technologies for appointments and scheduling.

Each unique, longitudinal, and permanent (lifelong) EHR incorporates both inpatient and outpatient care (Figure 32.2). Created for new patients during their first visit to HEGP, it contains administrative data, clinical data (patient history, physical exam, follow-up notes), biological results, images, nursing transmissions notes, vital signs, orders and order status, appointments dates, and all reports. To enable change tracking, all items of information are permanently stored with the identification of the source of information and a time stamp. Clinical information can be entered as free text, semi-structured documents, or standardized questionnaires. Inpatient and outpatient reports are stored as Microsoft Word® documents produced by merging information extracted from the patient records, directly entered by the health professionals and/or dictated and transcribed by secretaries. Recorded elements cannot be deleted.

Activities can be described as single activities (blood count), repeated acts (blood pressure control), or sets (acts to be performed during the admission process for a coronary dilation protocol) with their time constraints. Acts and protocols are edited in the THALIS-Reference component.

The scheduling of appointments is managed by the Per-Sé OneCall component and shared by all HEGP units, including radiology, functional respiratory, and cardiac investigation units. Appointments are stored in the patient's permanent and unique scheduler, which is part of the EHR. Schedules for the different providers are either open (pulmonary radiography) or closed, requiring the agreement of the radiologist (e.g., MRI).

Generic Components

Generic components include a security manager, a reference manager, a document manager, a communications manager (CORBA bus), and a supervision and workflow manager. They constitute the HEGP Enterprise Application Integration platform, which is part of the COHERENCE overall information system [23,24].

The THALIS-Security® component manages the user profiles for the different health professionals entitled to access part or all of the system's functions. Access rights depend on the nature of accessible functions through the application components (e.g., provider order entry, transmission reports), the geographic coverage (e.g., cardiology unit 2), and the type of data accessed (e.g., clinical notes, biological results). Rights must be individually defined but inherit from general rights described for the different professional profiles (e.g., senior physician, registered nurse). A delegation mechanism has been developed to manage short-time use of the system (e.g., an intern on call to the emergency or intensive care unit or a physician replacement for a vacation period).

The THALIS-Reference® component stores the different concepts and nomenclature dictionaries shared by the various components. For example, the patient order entry system shares the same dictionary of exams with the health record component and the laboratory and radiology legacy applications (see below). The list of pharmaceutical drugs available to the hospital is shared by the provider order entry component, the health record component, and the pharmacy legacy application.

All interactions between components are achieved through standardized messages carried over a CORBA bus from Ionix®. Exchange message syntax formats include EDIFACT for patient transfer messages and laboratory orders and results, HL7 for drugs orders, and DICOM for image work lists and results.

The THALIS-Supervisor® is a graphical Java-based component developed to track and optimize the transmission of messages over the local area network. A persistence database of all transmitted messages facilitates the debugging of applications, the processing of rejected messages, and the management of recoveries.

All workstations provide access to the Microsoft Office® suite and the Internet. All end users have a personal e-mail account managed by a Microsoft Exchange® server and Outlook®.

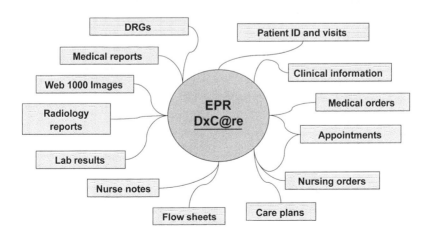

FIGURE 32.2. Content of the electronic health record (EHR).

Departmental Legacy Applications

Departmental applications (legacy systems) already in use in the AP-HP group were maintained active in ancillary departments and integrated through message communication with the previous components. They include:

- The MEDASYS Netlab® laboratory subsystem used for biochemistry, hematology, and microbiology.
- The SOPRA APIX® pathology subsystem, recently acquired by MEDASYS.
- The SIB (Syndicat Interhôpitalier de Bretagne) Phedra® pharmacy subsystem.
- The PHILIPS RADOS® radiology information subsystem and the AGFA IMPAX® picture archiving and communication system with the Web1000 image browser in the ward units. All images are produced as digital images. Results are encapsulated as DICOM reports. Both the reports and the images can be visualized on the workstations of the ward unit through a Web-enabled interface.

The Information System Portal

The THALIS-Portal® component from THALES is the general access interface module to the HEGP clinical information system. It displays the functions that are available to an end user according to his or her profile. It uses a Java thin-client architecture developed on top of an EJB/J2EE application server (Orbix Application Server Platform from Iona® Technology). Access to the system is provided through a single sign-on procedure. The user identification and passwords shared by the different components are managed by the Thalis-Security component. An implementation of the CCOW/HL7 standard allows the automatic transmission of patient context from one component to the other [25].

Several views of the same record are accessible to the health professional by type of event (inpatient, outpatient), by domain (digestive or cardiology units), and by time intervals. Individual preferences follow the end user when moving from one terminal to the user and are stored in his or her individualized profile.

The Hardware Infrastructure

Application components can be accessed both from fixed PCs and wireless portable units running under the NT operating system (Table 32.2). HEGP opened in July 2000 with a fleet of peripherals consisting of 1300 active, fixed PCs and 350 shared printers.

TABLE 32.2. Hôpital Européen Georges Pompidou (HEGP) HCIS figures: first quarter 2003.

HCIS use	Number
Hardware architecture	
• Number of Unix servers	17
• Number of Windows NT servers-2	45
• Number of fixed PCs	1800
• Number of mobile wireless PCs	85
• Number of networked printers	400
System load	
• Mean number of concurrent users at 11:00 A.M.	900

At the beginning of 2003, there were 1800 workstations and 400 network printers installed. In addition, 85 portable computers, connected through IEEE 803.11b wireless transmissions from Lucent Technology® and secured on a specially designed care cart, were deployed.

The application databases are managed by Hewlett Packard or SUN Unix servers with Oracle as the main database management system. Key components rely on redundant hardware (processors, disk space, cabling, etc.). Data tables are stored on disk repositories shared by the different UNIX or NT servers (Symmetrix EMC2). Application logic is hosted by Unix or NT servers. A complete and separate environment is used for integration and test procedures.

Blood samples are transported by automatic carrying suitcases between the healthcare units and the central reception area of the biology-pharmacy cooperative center.

Results

Professional Use of the System

The patient ADT component was operational at the opening of the hospital with 700,000 patient identifications prestored from the three closing BBL hospitals. Textual reports shared in the unique common record for both inpatients and outpatients was the easiest goal to achieve with more than 90 percent participation of units within the first 3 months. In 2001, 110,571 reports were registered through the patient record component, and 141,121 reports in 2002 (a 28 percent increase).

Consultation of laboratory results and images by physicians was readily available and well accepted (Table 32.3). During the first quarter of 2003, 100 percent of the relevant inpatient care units were using the POE component. Direct order entry by physicians was 73.6 percent for laboratory and 65.7 percent for image orders (Table 32.4). Deployment of wireless portable computers was considered highly effective in allowing physicians to enter their orders at the bedside, consult investigation results, and discuss them with the patient.

TABLE 32.3. Current use of the HIS function as a percentage of inpatient healthcare units: first quarter of 2003.

Function	Number using/number concerned	Percent
Admission, discharge, transfer (ADT)	35/35	100
Secretaries		
• In/outpatient reports	35/35	100
Physicians		
• Access to laboratory data	35/35	100
• Access to digital images (PACS)	35/35	100
• Laboratory order entry	35/35	100
• Radiology order entry	35/35	100
• Routine clinical notes	14/32	44
Nurses		
• Transmissions (inpatient care)	27/28	96
• Charts (inpatient care)	13/28	46

TABLE 32.4. HEGP POE figures: first quarter 2003.

Provider Entry Use	Number
Laboratory order entries (no./month)	45,147
Direct entry by physicians (%)	73.6%
Delegate entry (%)	36.4%
Imaging orders/month	8,170
Direct entry by physicians (%)	65.7%
Delegate entry (%)	44.3%

Economic Impact

HEGP is the product of the largest reorganization within the AP-HP administration. The implementation of an operational information system at the opening of the hospital was considered one of the key factors in increased productivity, with a reduction in the ratio of staff to number of beds from 3.10 to 2.95.

The installation of automation and information systems also supports innovative management principles like the redirection of human resources and the increase of nursing staff at the bedside (from 1.43 to 1.52/bed), reductions in the mean length of stay from 6.6 days in 1999 to 5.6 in 2002 for several days per inpatient stay, and gains in productivity and cost containment. Despite the rapid increase of medical costs for diagnosis and treatment (BBL Hospitals, 1999: 42 million Euros; HEGP 2002: 57 million Euros) and the improved healthcare offerings (10 percent are intensive care beds and 8 percent are 1-day hospital beds), overall operating costs are expected to stabilize (from 237 million Euros for BBL Hospitals in 1999 to an anticipated 240 million Euros for HEGP in 2003).

HEGP was built on a fixed contract, with a total budget of $249 million and an initial hospital information systems investment budget of $17 million, including material/software/hardware. This budget is in the low range for similar experiences in Europe and North America. Anticipated operating costs for the information system (including financial and management applications) are for 4.63 million Euros in 2003. This represents 1.93 percent of HEGP's overall operating budget. Salaries represent 49.9 percent of this budget.

Optimizing information workflow and care processes has improved the efficiency of the medical team. The global information system allows handing out "just in time" objects (automated conveying systems) and information (single multimedia patient records via the intranet).

The next gain in productivity will come with the extension of computerized physician order entry (biology, imaging, nursing) to drug prescribing, which started at the end of 2002, and with the breakdown of barriers between information systems inside and outside the hospital.

Discussion and Conclusion

All over the world, the technical infrastructure for health information systems has followed the same path observed in the computer industry: the monolithic mainframe systems of the 1970s, the distributed midframes of the 1980s, the client/server approach of the 1990s, and the current network-centric systems of years 2000 and above [25,26].

In the healthcare domain, Margulies et al. at Boston's Children's Hospital were among the first to build an integrated hospital information system from a set of inter-related departmental applications, including a clinical ordering module, a scheduler, and a medical record manager [27]. Integration techniques through data (Oracle Data-bases), interfaces (X Window terminals), and communications (HL7 messages) were considered key issues in this context.

In the mid-1990s several European projects pushed the idea of applications middle-ware and frameworks to foster health information systems integration [28–30]. The European prestandard prENV 12967-1 proposed in 1997 by the CEN organization is a reference architecture organized around three layers: the application, the middle-ware, and the bitways layers [21,31]. The HISA middleware layer is made of generic and healthcare-specific common services (including authorization, subjects of care, health data, activities, resources, and concepts and terminologies services). The AZVUB clinical information system in Brussels is one of the first instances of a hos-pitalwide implementation of the HISA model through a set of business components [2,30].

The HEGP fixed budget, the tight timeframe between the decision to invest in infor-mation technology, and the guarantee that a relatively extensive clinical information system would be operational at the opening of the hospital made the choice of an archi-tecture based on best-of-breed components the only achievable solution. Based on the state of the market at the time of decision (1998), pragmatic decisions were made to allow the industrial partners to progressively adapt their applications to the target architecture defined during the specification phases of the project (mid-1998 to mid-1999). In the current HEGP COHERENCE system, the activity component of the HISA model appears as a virtual component built on top of two different vendor com-ponents, the DxCare component from Medasys® and the OneCall resource schedul-ing component from Per-Sé. The RADOS appointment module from Philips is deactivated and the corresponding functions taken charge of by the PerSé OneCall component. The Medasys® DxCare component that currently combines the POE and EHR functions of the HISA models will be progressively split into two distinct components.

Despite strict criteria for the selection and integration of business components, several difficulties were encountered that need to be stressed:

- The complexity of the elaboration of the reference tables common to the different components (hospital structures, patient orders nomenclature, drug formulary) that required a strict development and testing process including:
  ○ The analysis of the needs of each component.
  ○ The makeup of the common reference tables taking into account semantic mismatches.
  ○ The development and test of the synchronization or import processes.
  ○ The development and test of strict updating procedures.
- The optimization of the workflow of messages between components. For example, the improvement of the output performance of a component (the production of output messages from the laboratory subsystem) may generate a bottleneck at the input point of a related component (the integration of results into the patient records).
- The fine-tuning of all the clinical information to guarantee performance and stability.

Except for the need for extra disk capacity, the management of the persistent database of exchanged messages with the THALIS-Supervisor component was found particularly useful during all optimization and tuning phases.

Presentation heterogeneity was not found to be a limiting factor insofar as the fluidity (timeliness) of transition between components from the different vendors could be achieved. This allows for the temporary use of traditional interfaces, giving industrial partners more flexibility in evolving toward generalized navigator-based application interfaces. Also, the two necessary adaptations of the components to ensure their compliance with the overall architecture were not difficult to achieve:

- The deactivation of the log-in and authorization procedures replaced, respectively, by the single sign-on and the common authorization component provided by THALES.
- The conformance of each component with the CCOW/HL7 standard.

Like many other European countries, France is grappling with serious problems of over-capacity at state-owned hospitals. Too many primary care hospitals and inadequate physician demography are part of the problem. The aim behind the decision to build a brand-new hospital to serve a residential population of 600,000 in southwestern Paris was to:

- Reduce costs by optimizing resources (staff, beds, infrastructure, etc.).
- Use this opportunity to take advantage of new technologies and information technology (IT) implementations to deliver improved health services.

When planning the hospital, two clear priorities emerged. The first was to develop not only the IT infrastructure but also the entire physical facility around the needs of the patient and to create IT solutions that would support the flow of patient care. The second priority was to provide decision makers, during the second phase, with medical/economic indicators to measure the efficiency of their new information and communication system. Hospital management, therefore, was faced with the challenge of building a user-friendly hospital information and communication system that would give all administrative and clinical staff access to a unique multimedia patient record that captures each and every clinical interaction.

HEGP opened with approximately 900 fewer staff than the three hospitals that were closing. A very progressive increase in activity was important in getting the professional staff involved in the new organization and IT. During this transition period, it was essential to put an emphasis on the computer education and staff training that had been started 1 year before the opening of the hospital. A 2-day training program had been offered to every future employee in the year preceding the opening of the hospital. Initial training was effected by a group of 14 trainers recruited from members of the IT department and from future end users. Seven parallel sessions spread out in classrooms over the three closing hospitals were necessary to handle the heavy time schedules and constraints of the healthcare personnel. This program culminated with a 4-day enhanced training session for an initial group of 50 end users (coaches) from their corresponding medical units. After 24 months of activity, the induction program has now been reduced to a 1-day program for each new nurse or secretary. Three years after the opening of the hospital, the training staff has been reduced to 7 health professionals who are also in charge of maintaining the references tables (drug formulary, protocols, etc.). A half-day presentation is now considered sufficient for new arriving physicians, such as interns or residents. Thirty additional coaches have been trained.

The objectives of Assistance Publique were to modernize obsolete medical services and reorganize the beds to improve healthcare offerings. The single multimedia patient record, used in 100 percent of the healthcare units, is the core of daily activity. Medical information is recorded by the physician at the bedside (through wireless portable computers), and medical prescriptions are distributed to the different technical platforms together with a minimum medical file attached. The appointment system, currently shared by 96 percent of the healthcare units, optimizes the use of the different modalities and generates a personalized care plan, which can be followed by authorized professionals on any of the 1800 computers. Waiting lists are reduced; patients' conflicting appointments are highlighted. The documented investigations are more focused.

Another important proven benefit is the reality of the multidisciplinary medical approach during a short hospital stay. Most elderly, chronically ill patients suffer from several pathologies: for example, approximately 60 inpatients per day have diabetes, although the diabetes unit only has eight beds. For these patients, the shared medical record is an added value in updating their diabetes treatment and accessing specialist advice. The information system is useful in offering therapeutic education to these patients and in implementing best practices. The information system breaks down the division in work organization and allows large team-based care, a cultural change that needs to be fostered.

As has been observed in most situations and countries, the major challenge remains the direct use by physicians of the POE system [32–36]. In a recent survey, Ash et al. reported that approximately one third of American hospitals use a partial or complete POE system and that only 20 percent of the systems have physician participation that is greater than 50 percent of the staff [30]. A rapid increase in physician participation was observed in the first year of HEGP's operation, with a much slower increase in the following months. At the beginning of 2003, approximately 75 percent of laboratory orders were directly entered by physicians, and a goal of 80 to 85 percent is targeted for 2004. System flexibility in enabling the customizing of protocols for individual departments was considered a necessary condition for health professional participation. However, interviews with physicians have indicated that further improvement is contingent on the extensive deployment of portable wireless computers allowing direct entry at the bedside, combined with strong and renewed incentives from the management board of the hospital.

Current efforts revolve around the development and deployment of the therapeutic parts of the POE component, including the nursing, medical, and educational portions of the protocols used by the different units; the migration of preexisting specialized records into the structured questionnaires of the medical record component; the installation of decision support tools; and progressive access to the information system by affiliated institutions and practitioners.

Acknowledgments. Deployment of the Pompidou hospital information system would not have been possible without the personal involvement of the managerial board of the hospital and its leading physicians. In particular, we would like to thank the hospital executive director, Louis Omnes, and Prof. Jean-Yves Fagon, the hospital medical director, for their personal and renewed commitment.

References

1. Iakovidis I. Toward personal health record: current situation, obstacles and trends in implementation of electronic healthcare record in Europe. Int J Med Inform 1998;52:105–115.

2. Van de Velde R, Degoulet P. Clinical information systems: a component-based approach. New York: Springer-Verlag; 2003.
3. Dick RS, Steen EB, editors. The computerized-based patient record. An essential technology for health care. Institute of Medicine. Washington, DC: National Academy Press; 1991.
4. McDonald CJ, Tierney WM. Computer-stored medical records. JAMA 1988;259:3433–3440.
5. Chute CG. Clinical data retrieval and analysis. I've seen a case like that before. Ann N Y Acad Sci 1992;670:133–140.
6. Safran C, Chute CG. Exploration and exploitation of clinical databases. Int J Biomed Comput 1995;39(1):151–156.
7. Uckert FK, Prokosch H. Implementing security and access control mechanisms for an electronic record. Proc AMIA Symp 2002;825–829.
8. Kuhn KA, Giuse DA. From hospital information systems to health information systems. Methods Inform Med 2001;40:275–287.
9. Ross SE, Lin CT. The effects of promoting patient access to medical records: a review. J Am Med Inform Assoc 2003;10:129–138.
10. Sittig DF, Kuperman GJ, Fiskio J. Evaluating physician satisfaction regarding user interactions with an electronic medical record system. Proc AMIA Symp 1999;400–404.
11. Gadd CS, Penrod LE. Dichotomy between physicians' and patient's attitudes regarding EMR use during outpatient encounters. Proc AMIA Symp 2000;275–279.
12. Penrod LE, Gadd CS. Attitudes of academic-based and community-based physicians regarding EMR use during outpatient encounters. Proc AMIA Symp 2001;528–532.
13. Doolan DF, Bates DW, James BC. The use of computers for clinical care: a case series of advanced US sites. J Am Med Inform Assoc 2003;10:94–107.
14. Dayhoff RE, Kuzmak PM, Kirin G, Frank S. Providing a complete on-line multimedia patient record. Proc AMIA Symp 1999;241–245.
15. Clayton PD, Narus SP, Huff SM, et al. Building a comprehensive information system from components. The approach at Intermountain Health Care. Methods Inform Med 2003;42:1–7.
16. Borst F, Appel R, Baud R, Ligier Y, Scherrer JR. Happy birthday DIOGENE: a hospital information system born 20 years ago. Int J Med Inform 1999;54:157–167.
17. Bleich HL, Slack WV. The CCC system in two teaching hospitals: a progress report. Int J Med Inform 1999;54:183–196.
18. McDonald C, Overhage JM, Tierney WM, et al. The Regenstrief medical record system: a quarter century experience. Int J Med Inform 1999;54:225–253.
19. Bates D, Teich J, Lee J, et al. The impact of computerized order entry on medical error prevention. JAMIA 1999;6(4):313–321.
20. Herzum P, Sims O. Business component factory. New York: Wiley; 2000.
21. CEN TC251. Healthcare information system architecture. Part 1 (HISA). Healthcare middleware layer. prENV 12967-1. Brussels: CEN TC251, March 1997. [http:// www.centc251.org/].
22. HL7. Health level seven context management standard. Version 1.4, May 2001. [http://www.hl7.org/special/Committees/ccow_sigvi.htm].
23. Zahavi R, David S. Linthicum DS. Enterprise application integration with CORBA component and Web-based solutions. New York: Wiley; 1999.
24. Lee J, Siau K, Hong S. Enterprise integration with ERP and EAI. Commun ACM 2003; 46(2):54–60.
25. HL7. Health level seven context management standard. Version 1.4, May 2001. [http://www.hl7.org/special/Committees/ccow_sigvi.htm].
26. Orfali R, Harkey D, Edwards J. client/server survival guide, 3rd ed. New York: Wiley; 1999.
27. Margulies D, McCallie D, Elkowitz A, Ribitzky R. An integrated hospital information system at Children's Hospital. Proc SCAMC 1990;699–703.
28. Degoulet P, Jean FC, Engelmann U, et al. The component-based architecture of the HELIOS medical software engineering environment. Comput Methods Programs Biomed 1994;45 (Suppl):S1–S11.
29. Spahni S, Scherrer JR, Sauquet D, Sottile PA. Towards specialised middleware for healthcare information systems. Int J Med Inform 1999;53:193–201.

30. Van de Velde R. Framework for a clinical information system. Int J Med Inform 2000; 57(1):57–72.
31. Ferrara FM. The standard "Healthcare Information Systems Architecture" and the DHE middleware. Int J Med Inform. 1998;52(1–3):39–51.
32. Sittig DF, Stead WW. Computer-based physician order entry. JAMIA 1994;1:108–123.
33. Ash J, Gorman P, Lavelle M, Lyman J, Fournier L. Investigating physician order entry in the field: lessons learned in a multi-center study. MEDINFO 2001;1107–1111.
34. Shu K, Boyle D, Spurr C, et al. Comparison of time spent writing orders on paper with computerized physician order entry. MEDINFO 2001;1207–1211.
35. Tonnesen AS, LeMaistre A, Tucker D. Electronic medical record implementation barriers encountered during implementation. Proc AMIA Symp 1999;624–626.
36. Weir C, McCarthy C, Gohlinghorst S, Crockett R. Assessing the implementation process. Proc AMIA Symp 2000;908–912.

Section 5
Outlook on Future Technologies

Section Introduction

The first four sections of this book present the here and now. Readers can take these ideas with them and apply them immediately. Section 5, on the other hand, offers readers the future to ponder. Of course, with technology and Moore's law, this future is now—from data tracking to telehealth to decision support systems to Web-enabled medicine to health surveillance to bioterrorism. These are the technologies that will lead us into the next revolution. As the beginning of one chapter in this section states, "The Internet changes everything!" The author then elaborates on the potential of the Internet as the technology that will continue to revolutionize the healthcare industry. That chapter, which underscores the power of information technology as an agent of change, epitomizes the theme of this book.

This book also has a decided emphasis on the patient as center. As the title of Neal Patterson's chapter promises, the mission of information technology in health care is to create a system that cares. This book is a testament that that mission is well under way.

33
Technologies in Progress: CPOE, Wireless Computing, and Biometrics

ROBERT J. CAMPBELL

CPOE, wireless computing, and biometrics are new and developing technologies that have the potential to shape the healthcare industry over the next decade.

Heralding of New Technologies

In the late 1960s, a generation of television viewers was introduced to the television show "Star Trek." What made "Star Trek" so interesting was its ability to forecast many of the technologies that are now coming into use in health care. For example, did not the communicator that Captain Kirk used to frequently ask Scotty to beam him up look strikingly familiar to the cell phones, or handsets, that many physicians and hospital administrators carry around with them today? And what about the tricorder? It could easily be mistaken for a personal digital assistant. The "Star Trek" technology, much like the technology we are seeing today, foreshadowed the breakdown of the barriers between data collection and data storage by newer handheld technologies. When Dr. McCoy wanted to know a patient's vital signs, all he did was run a little sensor over the patient's body. Devices now exist that literally do the same thing for physicians, who, incidentally, may or may not be in the same room with the patient. Finally, in "Star Trek," access to information was almost ubiquitous. When Captain Kirk needed important information, all he did was make a request of the computer, and the information was quickly and efficiently displayed. Systems such as computerized physician order entry (CPOE) hold the same promise for physicians who need immediate access to patient information, laboratory results, or the latest information on a new medication's dosage levels. This chapter will discuss some of the new and developing technologies that have the potential to shape the healthcare industry over the next decade. These technologies include CPOE, wireless/pervasive computing, biometrics, and customer relationship management.

Robert J. Campbell, BA, MLS, EdD, is Assistant Professor in the Department of Health Management Systems at the John G. Rangos Sr. School of Health Science at Duquesne University in Pittsburgh, PA.

A Need for Change?

The healthcare industry has come under pressure to eliminate medical errors, reduce utilization and cost, and alleviate the variability of health care across the nation. The Institute of Medicine [1] reports that each year 98,000 people lose their lives due to medical errors, making medical errors the eighth leading cause of death in the United States. Joanne E. Turnbull, Executive Director of the National Patient Safety Foundation, states that each medical error costs a healthcare facility "$5000 a piece and increases overall utilization of resources by 10 percent" [2]. Research by Wennberg [3] describes how physician "practice style factors" lead to a great deal of variation among physicians in terms of the frequency that treatments and diagnostic tests are used across the U.S. For example, the Dartmouth Atlas of Health Care [4] points out that men living in Baton Rouge, Louisiana, who are diagnosed with prostate cancer are more than twice as likely to receive a radical prostatectomy than men living in Pittsburgh, Pennsylvania, even though Pittsburgh has the second largest population of seniors next to Daytona County, Florida. Wennberg goes on to state that practice style factors or "local medical opinions regularly differ to the point that four times more people in one region get a surgery than do their neighbors" [5]. Variation differences tell us that many health consumers are receiving treatments that can be based more on doctor preferences and less on evidence that the treatment works and is the best course of action for the patient.

To apply a tourniquet to these problems and literally stop the bleeding, healthcare facilities in the next 2 to 10 years [6] will begin to adopt the use of computerized physician order entry systems (CPOE) to help eliminate medical errors, reduce utilization and cost, and eliminate unnecessary variability. Research [7,8] shows that only 2 to 12 percent of hospitals in the U.S. are using some form of CPOE, and with most of these systems, use by staff physicians is very limited.

What is CPOE?

Eisenberg describes a CPOE system as more than just a software application, or even a set of applications. "Rather, it is a process—a set of tools, which, properly implemented, can enable the desired outcome—safe, efficient, and effective patient care" [9]. The process being alluded to is physician decision making about patient management—a process identified by the Leapfrog Group as being "the single most critical and complex one in health care" [10].

To ensure that this process is safe, efficient, and effective, CPOE systems are most successful when they help offload the cognitive tasks that require physicians to make appropriate choices in terms of patient care. Teich [11] notes that when treating a patient, a physician can do one of three things: perform a procedure or operation, communicate with and educate the patient, or write orders for medications, tests, and other therapies. Orders become what Teich calls the "primary means of directing therapy for the patient." To make the proper choices, a physician must perform a great deal of cognitive processing in terms of connecting patient data, such as vital statistics, laboratory results, current medications, and previous conditions, with knowledge that supports and confirms the decisions he or she needs to make. As the number of patients the physician must treat grows, the amount of cognitive processing required to make appropriate decisions grows exponentially. And so does the odds that an error will occur. At the heart of a well-designed CPOE is a clinical decision support (CDS) system. The CDS contains a set of modules that guide and direct the physician's decision-making processes by presenting relevant patient information, recommendations for proper care (clinical guidelines and evidence-based medicine), and alerts for when a chosen action could cause a medical error or deviates from recommended practice. The Leapfrog Group has identified nine categories that structure and organize the functionality of an ideal CPOE system:

1. The most elemental category is *Basic Field Edits*. For each order generated, physicians are provided with default values, predefined selection lists, and required fields that guide them in "entering the order accurately and completely" [10]. This feature helps to reduce errors by making sure that erroneous information is not entered into order fields.

2. The second category, *Structured Orders*, provides a set of templates for each service ordered. Templates alert physicians to fields that require input and the allowable and default values for each field. The templates help physicians to create more complete orders, avoid medication errors (wrong dosage, or route of administration), and make sure their decisions follow approved hospital practice.

3. The next category, *Groups of Predefined Orders*, represents an order set or clinical pathway identified by the healthcare facility as the "recommended care for a particular diagnosis, procedure, or patient management strategy" [10]. Included in this category is the activation of an alert when a specific medication order requires that a blood test be performed to check for proper titrate levels. This action ensures that physicians are complying with approved hospital procedure, while reducing variation, utilization, cost, and medication errors.

4. A fourth category, *Order Checking*, checks medication orders for drug interactions, contraindications, proper dosing, and possible duplicate orders. What is not explicit here is that the CDS system works intuitively to check basic patient information: laboratory results, age, weight, and medication knowledge databases to ensure that a medication order does not trigger an adverse drug event.

5. Category Five, *Complex Order with Specialized Tools*, presents the physician with a set of tools—dose calculators, taper dosing, sliding scale, alternate day dosing, custom TPN, and chemotherapy—to use to complete complex medication orders.

6. Category Six, *Order Relevant Patient Data Display*, guarantees that relevant patient data are displayed that guides the physician's decision making. The amount of cognitive strain placed on the physician is reduced, leaving the physician to concentrate on the task at hand.

7. Category Seven, *Order-Relevant Patient Data Capture*, prompts or asks the physician to supply critical information to complete an order. For example, if the doctor is creating a medication order, the system could ask if the patient has any allergies, or if the patient has had a loss of weight since the last time this field was updated. This acts as a quality assurance check on all orders being entered into the system.

8. Category Eight, *Rules-Based Prompting and Alerts With Order Entry*, provides physicians with an alert informing them of specific rules they should follow in terms of dosing levels of medications being described for specific patients. This provides another quality assurance check to help reduce medication errors.

9. The final category, *Rules-Based Surveillance With Alerts Outside of Order Entry*, presents the physician with new information about the patient, such as laboratory results or significant changes in patient vital signs. These alerts prompt the physician

to consider generating new orders, or canceling orders in process, based on the new information.

From the description above, it is easy to identify the potential value a CPOE system can have within a healthcare facility: reduction in medication errors; greater compliance to standard practice; and reduction in utilization by the elimination of unnecessary tests and procedures, therefore leading to both a reduction in cost for the consumer as well as the healthcare organization. Theoretically, it is easy to see how a CPOE system can enhance healthcare delivery, but does it really work?

Turning Theory into Practice

In 2001 the Boston Medical Center (BMC), in an effort to eliminate medical errors while increasing patient safety, implemented the Eclipsys Corporation Sunrise Clinical Manager System [12]. Initially, this system allowed BMC physicians to generate medication orders that were electronically transferred to the pharmacy. This capability provided the facility with several unique benefits, including elimination of the need to have orders physically transported to their destination, the use of ancillary staff to enter orders into the computer, the need to clarify problems associated with interpretation and transcription, and alerts that let physicians know immediately when an ordering problem occurred.

During the creation and submission process, each medication order must adhere to a series of rules or checks for the order to be generated. These checks include inspection for duplicate orders, whether the order is for a patient under care at the facility, and checks for the following adverse drug reactions: drug–drug, drug–allergy, and food–drug interactions. Furthermore, the CPOE system allowed BMC staff to make modifications to orders based upon the type of drug being ordered. Modifications included the setting of defaults and limitation of alternatives; defining sets of required fields; creation of fields providing therapeutic drug interchange and educational information to the ordering physician; sets of warnings, for instance, informing the physician that no allergy information was defined; and the ability to filter lists of drugs that have been ordered to view only those medications currently being taken by the patient. Preliminary findings by BMC staff show a major decrease in indecipherable and incomplete orders, decreases Medication Administration Record (MAR) transcription errors, and a decrease in the time between order generation and order delivery.

Another CPOE implementation found researchers at Ohio State University Health System (OSUHS) [10] measuring the impact an electronic system had on medication turnaround times, radiology procedure completion times, laboratory reporting times, and severity length of stay [13]. These researchers also looked at the impact that the CPOE had when it was linked directly to an electronic medication administration record system (eMAR). Results show that CPOE implementation had a dramatic impact. For example, without CPOE medication turnaround times measured 5.28 hours, compared to 1.51 hours with CPOE. For radiology orders, turnaround times measured 7.37 hours (pre-CPOE) compared to 4.21 hours (post-CPOE). Laboratory results reporting times were reduced from 31.3 minutes (pre-CPOE) to 23.4 minutes (post-CPOE). In terms of length of stay severity adjusted cases, the OSUHS reports a decrease from 3.91 (pre-CPOE) to 3.71 (post-CPOE) days. The combination of CPOE with eMAR eliminated all physician and nursing transcription errors [13]. These results highlight the positive impact that a properly implemented CPOE system can have on the way a healthcare facility cares for its patients.

Barriers to Installing CPOE

CPOE systems present a golden opportunity to dynamically streamline the healthcare process. However, several barriers exist that can strain the implementation process. Scalise [14] notes that high cost and complexity are associated with most CPOE systems. In terms of cost, the Leapfrog Group states that, for a 200-bed hospital, the price tag will run somewhere between 1.2 and 7.4 million dollars over a 5-year period [10]. The AHA describes how a 250-bed hospital will need to spend between 1 and 5 million dollars on the system and then the same amount to make the system operational [15]. Additional costs accrued include the purchase of the hardware infrastructure needed to support the implementation. For example, each facility will need a significant number of PC workstations so that doctors can move seamlessly from patient interview and examination to order generation. Hospitals also need to have the proper networking technologies in place so that generated orders reach their destination, whether it is the pharmacy or the radiology department, in an expeditious fashion. Finally, resources need to be earmarked for product development, support, and training.

Implementing CPOE is not only costly, it is complex. CPOE systems can dramatically affect the processes physicians use to perform their jobs. For physicians to effectively use CPOE, they need immediate access to the system upon examining each patient. Without this capability the possibility exists for switching orders and patients [16]. Furthermore, implementing CPOE requires a great deal of time, coordination between healthcare professionals (physicians-nurses, physicians-radiologists), and communication between departments. Eskew notes that the timeframe from selection to full implementation of the product took 3 years (1999–2001) [12], while the OSUHS project took a total of 8 years from initial needs analysis to full implementation [17]. Thus far, the benefits and barriers as they relate to CPOE have been highlighted. However, what have not been discussed are the factors that determine whether an implementation is a success or failure? These factors will be identified and explicated in the following section.

The Difference Between Success and Failure

Research shows that the number one factor leading to successful implementation of a CPOE system is careful attention to physician workflow [18]. To achieve this goal, Chan recommends involving physicians in all aspects of a CPOE project including design, implementation, and evaluation [19]. The Leapfrog Group [10] goes further by stating that to successfully implement a CPOE system, a healthcare facility must have:

1. A deliberate strategy.
2. Strong leadership commitment and involvement.
3. Organized project structure to work through the many phases and accomplish many tasks.
4. Extraordinary efforts on the part of facility staff. Examination of the implementation efforts employed by the staff at OSUHS bear out the wisdom behind these implementation criteria.

Hospital Must Have a Deliberate Strategy

The OSUHS CPOE implementation was broken down into five separate phases that included needs analysis and clinical system selection, system analysis and design, system modification, initial system implementation, and complete system deployment. Ahmad [17] provides a more detailed description of each phase and how it contributed to the success of the project.

Leadership Commitment and Involvement

In the early 1990s OSUHS developed a strategic plan to implement a computerized patient record. This initiative had the backing of the Chief Medical Officer, the Chief Executive Officer, as well as the Hospital Board of Trustees and the Medical Staff Administrative Committee. Furthermore, it was agreed that implementation of CPOE would help realize the goal of having a functional CPR within the healthcare system.

Organized Project Structure

To usher CPOE implementation through each of the five phases, OSUHS staff established a design team that consisted of a lab technician, pharmacist, nurse, respiratory therapist, radiology technician, and traditional information technology personnel. This group represented the "core CPOE development team" [17].

To guarantee that physicians would be the primary users of CPOE and ensure that the system was customized to meet their needs, a "formalized physician consultant team" was established [17]. This team was made up of 10 physicians representing specific areas of clinical expertise within the healthcare system (emergency medicine, gynecology, cardiology). Each team member was required to sign a contract outlining his or her responsibilities and, where given, the power to approve "systems designs and policy" related to the CPOE project. Furthermore, the physician–consultant team worked together to reach an agreement on specific design elements, system policies, implementation plans, and the methods used for training. Ahmad states that physician involvement "had a positive effect on physician satisfaction and system success following implementation" [17]. This action also fulfilled the number one requirement to insure CPOE success: Get the physicians who will be using the system involved in the implementation process.

Extraordinary Efforts

From the information technology staff to the physicians, OSUHS received a number of extraordinary efforts that were essential to successful CPOE implementation. Case in point, to ensure that staff received support when using the system, OSUHS administrators created several permanent specialized support positions. Clinical staff provided support in these positions from 6 A.M. to 11 P.M., 7 days a week.

CPOE, with its power to provide physicians with the latest information on the status of a patient, guide clinical decision making, and provide alerts to possible medication errors, has the potential to become the backbone to the way a healthcare facility provides treatment in the next 2 to 10 years. However, as Bergeron points out, healthcare facilities and the physicians who staff them do not always gather, acquire, store, and access patient information from within the facility [20]. In fact, due to the rapid growth of information technology, these activities can happen, quite literally, from any part of the world. The new demands being placed on healthcare information has led to the growth of a new field called wireless/pervasive computing, and it could change the way health care is delivered within the next decade.

Wireless and Pervasive Computing

The growth of wireless computing in health care will take place for two reasons: (1) For CPOE and other electronic medical record systems to work, physicians cannot be tied down to wired PC workstations. They will need to use some type of wireless device that allows them access to the CPOE system and other relevant hospital databases. More importantly, physicians, not only the attending, but referring physicians, nurses, and other support staff, may need to access patient information from home, while traveling to work, eating dinner in a restaurant, or attending a conference in the Pacific Rim. Current wired networks do not afford these capabilities. (2) As the cost of health care continues to rise, many individuals are being treated on an outpatient basis. To keep track of an outpatient's vital statistics or signal when the patient needs immediate medical attention, many pervasive devices, such as toilet seats, scales, smart shirts, smart socks, and pacemakers, are being developed that collect relevant patient information. Collected data can then be transmitted via a wireless device using a wireless or mobile network to the patient's physician, who can then decide on possible interventions.

The problem with adopting wireless technology is that wireless devices, and the standards that support them are in constant flux. In the span of 6 months, devices such as personal digital assistants (PDAs), laptops, or cellular phones can support a wireless standard that is now being replaced. Furthermore, as Bergeron points out, the long-term viability of "wireless service providers, hardware manufacturers, and supported standards is uncertain" [20]. To combat this uncertainty, Bergeron advises healthcare administrators considering adopting wireless and pervasive computing to continually ask themselves the following questions: (1) what technology is available, (2) how can it be used to improve the care the facility provides or set the facility apart from the competition, (3) what are the costs, and (4) what are the costs to maintain and upgrade the facilities infrastructure and equipment?

To come to grips with wireless, it is important to know the types of devices available and the methods used to transfer data back and forth across both a wired and wireless network. Furthermore, when examining a device and its method of communication, Bergeron recommends that administrators become familiar with the following concepts: antennas, attenuation, range, bandwidth, encryption, field strength, frequency, interference, and modulation [20]. Before delving into the plethora of available wireless devices and their communication methodologies, each of the nine concepts identified above will be briefly discussed. For a more detailed discussion on each of these concepts, please see Bergeron [20] and Comer [21].

Antennas allow a wireless device to send and receive data using radiofrequency signals. Most antennas on wireless devices are relatively compact, are housed within the device, or contained in a card that plugs into a slotted connection on the device.

Attenuation is the amount of the radiofrequency signal that can be absorbed by buildings, walls, elevator shafts, and other natural or freestanding structures. The best way to determine whether attenuation is going to be a problem within a healthcare facility is to test the equipment or the wireless services offered in the area.

Range: wireless devices use access points (AP) or cells to propagate signals to either another access point or the destination source, which can be a server on a local wireless/wired network. Once the device moves out of range of the nearest access point, all communication is lost. Administrators must consider the range of the devices being used on a network and how many access points will be needed to propagate and receive signals to and from the main information source.

Bandwidth refers to the amount of information that can be sent from one device to another on a wireless network. Also included is the time it takes to transfer the information. Most home users have modems that transfer 56 kilobytes of data per second (Kbps). A standard laptop with wireless capability can transfer information at 11 megabits of data per second (Mbps).

Encryption deals with the security of the data being transferred across the network. With the new HIPAA privacy and security laws, administrators need to ensure that data on a wireless network are secure. Encryption can be provided at the operating system or application level, or special encryption programs, such as Virtual Private Networking, can be used to ensure data integrity.

Field strength: the intensity of the radio signal emitted from the transmitting device will decrease as distance increases. Increasing the strength of the signal will increase the distance the signal can travel, which affects range, battery life, creates possible health hazards to the end user, and interferes with the operation of other devices within the facility.

Frequency: wireless devices communicate using radiofrequency signals that can be defined by how much the amplitude of the electromagnetic energy varies with time. Frequency can be defined in KHz (thousands), MHz (millions), and GHz (billions). The government regulates the bands of frequencies that are allowable by wireless devices.

Interference: many devices, such as electronic monitoring equipment, cell phones, PDAs, automobile engines, and fluorescent light fixtures can affect the range and bandwidth of a wireless device. Furthermore, wireless devices and other hospital monitoring equipment can share the same frequency or multiples of that frequency that can create interference not only between each device but with other devices within the facility. Administrators must be careful not to use wireless devices that interfere with the operation of devices whose failure could be life threatening.

Modulation is the method used to turn voice and data into a wireless signal. The wireless signal carries the data from the transmitter to the receiver. Cellular, or what is called mobile computing, uses several different modulation techniques. The robustness of the techniques being used determines what type of information (mobile ecommerce, online multimedia, video on demand, voice) can be transferred across the network.

Wireless devices: the types of wireless devices available are abundant and include the personal digital assistant (PDA), laptops, tablets, Web pads, handheld OCR pens, wireless cameras, bar-code scanners, pagers, and even personal computers equipped with a wireless communication network card. Furthermore, cellular phones, which are now called handsets, come is several different varieties: analog or digital, PCS, Web-enabled, or smart. Each of these different handsets can provide voice access, and depending on the modulation technique or standard the device supports, it can provide access to the Internet or to the healthcare facility's wireless/wired network. As stated above, Bergeron admonishes healthcare administrators to be not only aware of what wireless devices are available, but also how those devices can be used to support current or future healthcare practices. It is important to realize that each wireless device has inherent limitations: PDAs and handsets have small screens, and Web content, to be used effectively, must be tailored for each individual device. These limitations will be discussed further when the topic turns to examples of how wireless is being utilized in health care. With the most prominent wireless devices identified, this discussion will now examine how these devices communicate with one another.

No Standard Protocols

One of the disconcerting facts surrounding wireless is that there is no standard protocol being used to allow devices to communicate. In fact, wireless communication standards can be tenuously divided into two camps: wireless local area networks (WLANs), which can be subdivided into personal area networks (PANs) and mobile computing, or what many call cellular communication. WLANs include laptops, notebooks, personal computers, PDAs, and standard PCs, while mobile computing consists of PDAs and handsets. PANs represent a hybrid network created from the combined use of handsets and WLAN devices. Each of the standards used to create a WLAN, PAN, and mobile computing wireless network is addressed below.

WiFi

WiFi, or wireless fidelity, can be used to create what Bergeron calls a fixed WLAN [20]. The term fixed means that the wireless network is located in a hospital department or ward. To create a WLAN, each device, whether it is a PC, laptop, or PDA, needs to have WiFi capability. WiFi capability can be integrated with the device, as in the case of most laptops, where the WiFi access is built into the sides of the display, or a WiFi network card can be installed within a slot on the device. The network card contains the antenna that allows the device to transmit and receive signals to and from an access point (AP), which can be directly connected to the hospital's local area network, the Internet, or a server running within the department. The most common standard of WiFi being used in North America is IEEE 802.11*b*, which has a range of 100 to 300 feet and transfers data at a maximum throughput of 11 Mbps. Again, when referring to range, this means that a physician using a laptop to enter patient information can stray no further than 300 feet from the nearest AP. If he does, all communication will be lost. For a big department, or long hallway, several APs can be spaced 300 feet apart, and then configured so they pass information on to the final destination, say, a CPOE system running on the hospital's wired network. IEEE 802.11*b* converts data into a wireless signal using direct sequence spread spectrum (DSSS) modulation, which operates at the frequency range of 2.4 GHz. The 2.4 GHz frequency is a common, unlicensed band also used by microwaves, cordless phones, and medical and scientific equipment, which could lead to potential interference problems. Material contained in walls, such as metal, stone, brick, and heavy wood, can inhibit the transmission of signals from room to room. Fortunately, WiFi comes in several different varieties.

WiFi 802.11*a* can transfer data at 54 Mbps using orthogonal frequency division modulation (OFDM) on the 5 GHz frequency band. The 5 GHz frequency band is not as crowded as the 2.4 GHz frequency band, and it is not susceptible to microwave and medical device interference. The problem lies in the fact that the 802.11*a* standard is not compatible with the 802.11*b* standard. Therefore, wireless devices adhering to 802.11*b* will not communicate with devices using 802.11*a*. Another standard, 802.11*g*, is compatible with 802.11*b*, and transfers data at 54 Mbps, using OFDM on the 2.4 GHz frequency band. Two other flavors of WiFi, 802.11*h* and 802.11*i*, have yet to be accepted. However, because these standards deal with issues pertaining to wireless security, look for these specifications to become accepted standards in 2003. Security is a major concern with wireless networks, and healthcare administrators implementing

802.11*a,b,c* must pay careful attention to the privacy and security of data being transmitted over a wireless network.

WiFi Security

Because wireless devices communicate over the same frequencies, a person within range of a wireless signal can use their wireless device to pick up and decipher data as they are being transmitted across the network. This means anyone, whether premeditated or not, can walk by a wireless network and get instantaneous access to e-mail, medical records, and files stored on a healthcare facilities server. The art of detecting and breaking into a wireless network is called war driving, and war drivers, using a WiFi-enabled device and software programs such as AIRSNORT, WEPCRACK, and NETSTUMBLER cruise through city streets and residential neighborhoods looking for wireless networks. One method of securing a wireless network is to enable the wired equivalent privacy (WEP) security protocol that comes with the software shipped with WiFi equipment. WEP encrypts data on a wireless network, making it hard for war drivers to access information. The problem with WEP is that it is not a very strong encryption protocol, and it can be broken into by experienced war drivers. To fully secure a wireless network, health administrators should implement a virtual private network (VPN) application. VPNs provide advanced encryption and security that makes it extremely hard for war drivers to crack.

Bluetooth

Another standard used to connect wireless devices is Bluetooth (802.15). Bluetooth is good for allowing wireless devices to communicate over short distances, roughly 33 feet, with throughput of 750 kbps, and limited power consumption. Bluetooth-enabled devices can automatically connect to create a personal area network (PAN). When a new device comes within range of a PAN, it will automatically join in, provided it has the proper security authorization [22]. The key to Bluetooth is that many companies are developing products that can have immediate impact on the healthcare industry. For example, products such as toilet seats, smart shirts, beds, and digital stethoscopes are being designed to collect individual vital signs, which can then be relayed directly to a healthcare provider. For example, a patient with heart problems can be outfitted with a smart shirt. The smart shirt monitors blood pressure, heart rate, respiration, temperature, and can even perform an EKG. Coupled with a Bluetooth-enabled laptop connected to the Internet, or handset, the information can then be directly transferred to the patient's doctor. To communicate, a device must have built-in Bluetooth capability, or a Bluetooth card installed. Bluetooth is secure because it constantly alters the frequencies used to transmit data. This makes it hard for a war driver to intercept messages because frequencies used to transmit data change with each transmission. Moreover, because Bluetooth is used to communicate over short distances, it would be hard not to notice someone hacking into your wireless PAN. Bluetooth supports 128-bit encryption, which is a more secure method of transferring data across a network.

Fixed wireless networks using WiFi and Bluetooth should become the norm in both the home and healthcare facility within the next 5 years. Competition for the wireless market share is being generated by a set of standards falling under the rubric of mobile computing. At the center of the mobile computing movement are handset devices connected to public phone companies, which claim to offer voice, data, and Web-enabled access to information. Access to services such as voice, data, e-mail, and the Internet for handset devices is provided by a set of standards known as 1 G, 2 G, 2.5 G, and 3 G. Each standard has its own set of protocols (modulation techniques), which provides a different and not always comparable set of services. Public services, such as Palm.Net and GoAmerican.Net, provide PDAs made by Palm and Blackberry access to e-mail and other news services. The problem with the mobile computing industry is that there is no uniformity of acceptance in North America, let alone the rest of the world. What that means is that physicians using their handsets may get great voice and Web access in their local areas, only to have poor quality voice and no Web access if they travel to another part of the U.S. This makes selecting a mobile computing service hard, because uniformity of service across the country, let alone the same city, is hard to guarantee. In what follows, each of the mobile computing standards will be discussed, along with the role they play in providing wireless access to health-related information.

The Gold Standard

To take wireless service to the next level, end users will need more bandwidth, security, and reliability, which will provide them with access to video on demand, mobile e-commerce, online multimedia, and wireless Web surfing [23]. However, many industry analysts are not sure how these services will be provided [24,25]. For example, early mobile computing handsets used the 1G communication standard. This provided end users with analog, circuit-based, narrowband, voice-only communication. This was followed by the growth of the 2G standard. This standard was digitally based and provided voice and very limited data communications. It was also very slow. The 2G standard used TDMA (USA), GSM (Europe/Asia), and CDMA (USA) to modulate the data. Because 2G modulation techniques did not provide end users with the services they needed, two other standards, 2.5G and 3G, have been offered as viable alternatives.

2.5G is appealing because it is an upgrade to 2G, so there are no technology infrastructure replacement costs. It also provides more bandwidth than 2G while still using the same frequency spectrum. 2.5G offers three different modulation techniques, which include iDEN (North and South America, China, Japan, with throughput of 64 Kbits), GPRS (China, Europe, USA, with throughput of 171 Kbits), and EDGE (USA with throughput of 384 Kbits). One of the major drawbacks with the 2.5G standard is that is was not designed to optimally handle voice and data simultaneously [23].

This leaves 3G, which is supported by three similar, but not fully compatible, modulation techniques. These techniques include W-CDMA (Europe and Japan), CDMA2000 (Korea), and TD-CDMA (China). The U.S. is experimenting with all three; however, it appears that W-CDMA is the technique that will gain overall support. To implement 3G on a wide scale, changes will need to be made to the communications infrastructure. 3G uses high-end radiofrequencies and different modulation techniques, which require cell towers to be closer together. Furthermore, the federal government controls much of the spectrum needed to enable 3G communications, and it seems unlikely that it will relinquish that control in the near future. In theory, 3G can provide up to 2.05 Mbps of throughput for a stationary device, this changes to 384 kbps (slow moving), and 128 kbps (user in a vehicle). For 3G to take wireless access to the next level it must provide a reliable enough medium for accessing content other than voice communication. Finally, the service will need to be made available in a large number of areas throughout the world.

In the future, mobile computing may face competition from WiFi as the standard for public access to wireless information. For example, in many American cities such as

Aspen, New York, Portland, San Francisco, and Seattle, Internet service customers are using wireless technology to give neighbors free access to online connections, creating neighborhood area networks (NANs). Some cities are even exploring the idea of installing wireless access points in bus stops, subway stations, and local thoroughfares. This will let anyone with a 802.11 wireless device or laptop access to the Internet. If this trend continues to grow, individuals could walk through cities and neighborhoods continuously connected to the Internet, without having to have a mobile computing service provider [26,27].

Providing Content on a Wireless Device

Because of its ubiquitous nature, the World Wide Web allows access to its services to all types of devices. However, just because PDAs and wireless handsets can access Web content does not mean the content will appear the same on all devices. In fact, to take full advantage of the way a wireless device such as a PDA or handset displays Web-based information, content must be tailored to the device. This can lead to innumerable problems when physicians want to view information from a CPOE system, medical Web page, or electronic medical record. Therefore, healthcare administrators need to consider several technologies and techniques to prepare Web-based content for display on small screen wireless devices. Content development can be accomplished using one of the following: hypertext markup language, extensible markup language (xml)/extensible stylesheet language (xsl), screen scrapping or transducing, voice-enabled interfaces, and wireless services providers (WISP)/Web enablers. Explanations of how these technologies work are beyond the scope of this chapter. For a more detailed discussion see Bergeron [20] and Schilit et al. [28]. The point is that for Web content to be displayed on a small screen wireless device, some form of content preparation is required. At this point, the types of wireless devices available and their methods of communicating have been discussed. In what follows, examples of how wireless devices have been used to access, retrieve, and acquire healthcare information will be explored. Within that discussion, several factors healthcare administrators must consider when adopting wireless technology will be introduced.

Miami Children's Hospital Project

Dr. Redmond Burke, chief of cardiac surgery at Miami Children's Hospital, wanted to begin tracking information about cardiac surgery performed within the facility and find a method that would allow his staff to review this information at the bedside of the patient. To that end, Dr. Burke and several programmers developed an Access 97 database. This database tracked detailed information about each surgery, including the type of equipment and the procedures used, mortality, and length of stay. Also included in the database were the progress notes [SOAP] that doctors used to record patient outcomes. One of the major goals for developing the database was to help physicians better manage postoperative care, which can make up between 80 and 85 percent of the care a patient receives in the hospital. Most pediatric patients can spend several weeks to months in the hospital's intensive care unit. The database would be the perfect means of tracking how a patient responded to the type of postoperative care they received.

About 2 years ago, a set of Palm Pilots was purchased, and with help from Jeffrey White, a member of the hospital's Information Technology staff, a form was developed that allowed physicians to enter information into the Palm Pilot to record progress notes. The form contained more than 250 different fields; most of them used checkboxes to record information because entering large amounts of text in a Palm can be very difficult. To get the information from the Palm Pilot to the Access database, a physical connection or hot synchronization unit was used. White developed a specialized hot synchronization conduit using Pendragon Forms software to make sure that data were processed directly into the database during the synchronization phase. As White explains, "the process of updating a patient record became a nightmare. Information had to be entered into the Palm, hot synchronized with the desktop, and then updated on the database server."

After the system had been up and running, White conducted a survey among the physicians using the pediatric database, by asking the question: "Which device is being used most: palm or desktop? After 2 months, 80 percent of the physicians used the Palm. After 8 months, 20 percent used the Palm. More of the physicians were using the desktop to enter information.

Why Did More Physicians Prefer the Desktop? What Are the Issues?

The fact that physicians had to use the hot synchronization process turned them off because it took too much time to perform. It disrupted their normal workflow. Furthermore, using the desktop was faster because it allowed physicians to enter information about patient care events and plans for treatment, both full-text fields, more rapidly than on the Palm. However, as White explains, the straw that broke the camel's back was the fact that "the MIS department needed to make sure that hospital applications, databases, and information collection devices conformed to HIPAA. Many of the physicians owned their own Palm Pilots, which contained data about patients. Most physicians took their devices home at night, and if the device was lost or stolen—this would became both a privacy and security issue."

Solution

Another problem with which White had to contend is the fact that referring physicians generate much of health care. A physician refers a patient to another doctor or a healthcare facility. The problem is that after the referral is made the referring physician is left out of the loop and the decision-making process. Moreover, when the patient goes home, the primary contact is the referring physician. To provide a successful level of care, he or she needs to know all the issues with the patient, what went on in the hospital, what medications the patient might need, and what are the symptoms of upcoming complications. Therefore, White needed to find a method to keep the referring physician in the loop and part of the decision-making process. His solution also needed to take into consideration the desire of parents or caregivers to monitor patient progress, especially if they were living some distance from the hospital.

White decided to use a Web-based system, because most computers and institutions are using the World Wide Web. The solution that White and the pediatric surgeons at MCH choose was I-ROUNDS™. I-ROUNDS was developed by TEGES and is described by Bergeron as a Web enabler, or a company that can take information from a healthcare facility's data sources and create Web pages that caregivers can use to provide real-time patient care [20]. The beauty of I-ROUNDS is that it takes information from 15 MCH data sources, including bedside monitors, using 802.11b, up-to-date pictures of the patient, patient's vital statistics, X-rays, laboratory results, progress notes, and EKG heart traces, and place them on a set of Web pages that all healthcare providers can assess together simultaneously, whether they are using the hospital local area network or using a wireless device at home. The system also provides healthcare providers with one seamless interface and one system log-on, making it easier for the healthcare provider to get the needed information as quickly as possible. White explains that most of the physicians are using a Web pad to access the I-ROUNDS system. A Web pad is a wireless device similar to the new tablet, but half the price. In the final analysis, White thinks that one of the major problems with PDAs and handsets is screen size. "The patient record is huge. How can you play chess when you only see part of the screen? How do you know what your opponent is doing? For the Palm or iPAQ to be successful, applications need to be developed that deliver the most vital information as compactly as possible. Screen real estate is important. You only have 11 lines of screen space with which to work on most PDAs. Also, screen resolution can be a problem. Physicians want full-color, high-resolution images to make accurate diagnoses."

The Miami Children's Hospital Project shows how wireless devices can be meshed with other wired devices, along with the World Wide Web, to provide instant access to patient information. As the use of PDAs becomes more pervasive, companies that make CPOE products need to make sure their applications support the use of handheld devices to view, update, and track patient information [29]. Without the support of major CPOE and healthcare application vendors, handheld devices and handsets will be used strictly for scheduling, address book functions, prescription writing, and voice communication applications [30]. Use of wireless networking will not be restricted to healthcare facilities such as hospitals and outpatient clinics. As the healthcare industry looks at methods to reduce cost and utilization of services, wireless and pervasive computing will become more prevalent in assisted living facilities and in the home. One example is Oatfield Estates, an assisted living facility located in Milwaukie, Oregon [31–34]. What sets Oatfield Estates apart from other facilities is the ingenious use of wireless technology to provide residents with a more independent lifestyle. Each room in the facility is equipped with infrared/radiofrequency sensors that can track residents' comings and goings. To make this possible, each resident wears a transponder around his or her neck, which also gives off infrared and radiofrequency signals. This allows staff to quickly locate a resident when the resident signals for help using a button on the transponder. Distress signals that go unanswered for more than 5 minutes are followed up by an e-mail message sent directly to a supervisor's handset. The transponder also gathers residents' vitals statistics and monitors their changing cognitive and physical conditions; using wireless technology (802.11b); it then uploads the information into a database. Outside, a set of cameras and tripped beam sensors alert staff members if a resident strays too far from the facility. Moreover, beds that residents sleep on have a set of "load cells" controlled by electromechanical transducers. These load cells can be used to track changes in a resident's weight, to monitor sleeping patterns, and, if a resident follows the same pattern every night, to turn on the light in the bathroom. This pervasive technology can also be used to protect residents from harming themselves. For instance, if a patient with Alzheimer's wanders into the kitchen, the system can issue an e-mail alert to a supervisor. If that resident has a caregiver present, the system acknowledges this with the quiet reserve of a 21st-century Jeeves.

The most compelling feature of the Oatfield Estates experience is the capability it provides family caregivers and other healthcare providers. For example, if a resident of Oatfield Estates has a daughter living in Pittsburgh, Pennsylvania, that daughter has the capability to log-on securely to the facility's database and view her mother's daily activities. The daughter can see that her mother went outside for a walk with three of her friends, or that she took a nap at four in the afternoon, and that over the past week she has been sleeping normally. This type of technology can not only allay family caregivers fears, but it can allow family members to ask more provocative questions of their relatives ("Why didn't you eat breakfast?") or of the caregivers themselves ("My mother has lost 5 pounds in the last 2 weeks, do you think this is a problem?"). With this type of pervasive technology coming into place, distance in the foreseeable future will not be a concern, as caregivers, both familial and medical, are able to track the health of an individual over great distances.

In a more familiar surrounding—the home—researchers, like those at the Rochester Center for Future Health are looking at ways to help individuals prevent the need for prolonged medical care [35]. One device, known as the "Smart Bandage," is equipped with a miniature sensor that can detect when a wound contains contaminant bacteria [36]. In the near future, a wireless device can be used with the "Smart Bandage" to determine the type of contaminating bacteria present (*Escherichia coli, Salmonella, Pseudomonas aeruginosa*), then, using a wireless network, to alert the individual and his or her physician as to the best antibacterial agent to use to kill the contaminant. Other devices, such as the "Smart Shirt" (Sensatex) and the "Life Shirt" (VivoMetrics) can record information about an individual's respiratory, cardiology, and sleep patterns over a specific period, store the information into a wireless PDA, which then transfers the results to a laptop or handset with a wireless network connection to a healthcare provider for review.

As the acquisition and storage of data becomes more pervasive, and healthcare facilities grapple with the new HIPAA security and privacy laws, healthcare providers must seek out new methods for securing data and ensuring that only authorized individuals gain access to confidential patient information. In the movie *The Fugitive*, Richard Kimble (Harrison Ford) impersonates a staff member of a large Chicago hospital, thereby gaining access to patient records. Under HIPAA regulations a violation of this nature would result in the hospital having to pay a hefty fine for allowing a breach in patient privacy. Although the example is fictionalized, it is not so far-fetched. As healthcare providers, family caregivers, and patients access information using wired and wireless devices, better methods are needed to ensure that individuals submitting and accessing health-related information are really the persons they claim to be, especially with "war driving" growing in prevalence.

Biometrics

One technology that is being hailed as the vanguard in securing healthcare information is biometrics. Biometrics uses individual physiological or behavioral characteristics to determine or verify identify [37]. The most commonly used biometrics falls into two categories: physiological, which are a direct measurement of a part of the human body; and behavioral, which are "derived from an action and indirectly measure characteristics of the human body" [37]. The most common physiological biometrics includes finger-scan, iris scan, hand-scan, and retina-scan. Behavioral biometrics is typified by voice and signature scans. Before biometrics is widely accepted by healthcare administrators, the best methods for securing health information need to be identified, and it must be "demonstrated that their benefits of deployment outweigh the risks and costs" [37]. Moreover, for a biometric solution to be successful, it cannot disrupt the healthcare professional's daily routine. For instance, if use of biometric verification requires physicians to wait 1 minute and 30 seconds before it is verified, their willingness to use the system will be greatly reduced. They may even find ways to circumvent the system. Also, huge time delays could force physicians to batch process orders in CPOE all at once, rather than one at a time. This batch process routine could lead to errors as physicians mix up patients and orders.

To shed light on this concern, the following discussion focuses on why biometrics is the ideal solution to the security problem. Next, it will explore how biometrics works. Finally, it will discuss identification of those technologies most likely to find a niche in securing a healthcare information system.

Deployment of biometrics is advantageous by the way it provides added security, convenience, reduction in fraud, and increased accountability. Biometrics provides a higher level of security by providing access to health information to authorized individuals and locking out those with nefarious intent.

Security

Because biometric security is based on a unique feature of an individual's body, for instance, a fingerprint, it is very difficult to copy, steal, or replicate this information. On the other hand, passwords, personal identification numbers (PIN), and smart cards can be easily obtained or even shared. Biometrics also reduces the need to remember complicated passwords or go through the process of changing a password after a specified period of time.

Convenience

Unlike passwords and smart cards, biometrics cannot be forgotten. Furthermore, biometrics allows a healthcare facility to manage access better to different data sources. For years, healthcare providers have complained that to get information about a patient they had to log-on to separate databases. With biometric security, physicians only have to log-on once, and then they have access to laboratory results, CPOE, and the radiology database. Furthermore, a hospital network can be biometrically protected, thereby protecting sensitive information from attacks by "war drivers" and other hackers.

Fraud Reduction

Some hospital services, especially those designed for seniors, the poor, and the indigent, require registration. In some cases, individuals can register several times, using different aliases. Use of biometrics makes sure that an individual's information does not already exist in the hospital database. Biometrics can also deter fraud, because individuals who know that such a system is in place will be less likely to try and register more than once.

Increased Accountability

With HIPAA regulations looming over their heads, health administrators must be able to verify who has accessed specific files, at a given time, on a specific computer. Biometrics, combined with a computer operating system, provides administrators with more pronounced auditing and reporting capabilities.

To understand how a biometric system works, it is important to know that a distinction exists between verification and identification. Verification tries to answer the question: "Am I who I claim to be?" An individual presents a user name, ID number, and then their biometric information. The system searches a database and determines whether the username and biometric information match the same information stored in the database. If a match is found, the user has been authenticated. Authentication is referred to as 1:1 (one-to-one) matching. Identification attempts to answer the question: "Who am I?" With the identification process, a user not does provide an identity, just their biometric information. The system then compares this information with biometrics stored in the database. This is called 1:N (one-to-many) matching. It is obvious that one-to-many matching can be more time intensive and computational processing intensive. Because a one-to-many database contains many individuals, it will be necessary for the system to compare the data provided with the data in the database until a match is found or a decision of nonmatch is rendered. On the other hand, one problem with verification is that it cannot determine whether a person is in the database more than once.

The Biometric Process

The biometric process begins with enrollment. Depending on the type of biometric being used, physiological or behavioral data are acquired and then stored in the system as a template. One of the misconceptions regarding biometrics is that the system stores all the information, whether it is a fingerprint or scan of an individual's face. In reality, depending on the system and the type of algorithms used, certain key features are extracted during enrollment and used to create a template. Each biometric vendor has its own enrollment algorithms, and some are better than others. A template can be stored locally on a PC or a network server.

To verify or identify a person, an individual must present his or her biometric information to the system. As in the enrollment phase, not all the raw biometric data collected during presentation are used. A template is created and then compared to the biometric stored within the system. The act of comparing a presentation template with an enrollment template is called matching. When a presentation template is matched with an enrollment template, a score is generated. The score is then compared against a threshold that can be set by a system administrator. The score is generated, based on the degree of similarity between a comparison of the two templates.

How a biometric system generates a score is a very important process and should be carefully evaluated when considering various biometric applications. A threshold is a number set by the system administrator that establishes the degree of correlation necessary for a comparison between an enrollment template and a presentation template to be considered a match. Depending on the level of security desired, the threshold can be set very high or very low. To understand the impact that a threshold can have on a system, it is important to understand the concepts of "false match rate," "false nonmatch rate," and "failure to enroll rate." False match rate is the probability that a user's template will be incorrectly judged to be a match for a different user's template. Basically, this means that an impostor is trying to log-on to the system, and he or she succeeds, but the biometric information is similar to an individual already in the system. To lower false match, system administrators can set the biometric application so it has a very high threshold. The problem is that setting the threshold level high increased the false nonmatch rate, which is the probability that a user's template will be incorrectly judged to not match his or her enrollment template. This means that a valid user of the system has been denied access because a strong correlation does not exist between their verification and enrollment template. Why does this happen? Because no two presentations are ever the same. Changes in a user's biometric data can occur.

A person may get a cut or scratch on a finger. In facial recognition, a change in hairstyle or glasses can affect nonmatch rate. Therefore, no two presentation templates are the same. By raising the threshold, the system will require that a presentation template contain more biometric features than a lower threshold setting.

Related to false match rate and false nonmatch rate is the failure to enroll rate. This is the level of probability that a person's biometric data cannot be used to enroll him or her in the system. Again, the threshold level will determine how much information is needed to create an enrollment template. Together, these three indicators can affect system effectiveness and should be discussed with the vendor of a biometric product being considered. Vendors who understand the ramifications of how these concepts affect each other will openly discuss how their system provides a balanced approach to counteracting the effects of these concepts on each other to make their system work efficiently. No biometric system can guarantee 0 percent false matches or 0 percent false nonmatches. Somewhere in the system, a balance must be struck. From the discussion above, when comparing and contrasting different biometric systems, health administrators need to carefully examine how a specific application acquires a biometric image, how it processes that image, the distinctive features it captures, how it creates templates, and how it matches enrollment and presentation templates to determine an appropriate decision: match or nonmatch. Robust systems that address these specified areas will be worthy of consideration for purchase.

Biometrics in Health Care

The most promising biometric technology for adoption by the healthcare industry is the finger-scan. Finger-scan can be used to provide access to personal computers and healthcare networks. Also, many devices, keyboards, mice, and PDAs, already have finger-scan technology built in. The strengths of finger-scan are that it is already a proven technology that provides high levels of accuracy; it can be deployed in a wide range of environments (desktop, laptop, provides physical access to an information storage facility), it is easy to use, and users can enroll multiple fingers for verification and authentication. Problems with finger-scan appear to be that not all user populations can be enrolled in the system, such as the elderly and individuals who do a lot of manual labor. Another drawback to finger-scan is that devices used to collect presentation data can malfunction with wear and tear. This necessitates constant upkeep and replacement.

The New York State Office of Mental Health was an early implementor of finger-scan. Initially, this healthcare institution purchased more than 6000 finger-scan units to enhance network security and protect the confidentiality of patient information.

Another biometric, iris-scan, is also suitable for use by healthcare institutions. Iris-scan can verify or identify a person, based on the unique characteristics of the human iris. The strengths of iris-scan include its high resistance to false matching, the stability of the iris over time, and the ability to use this biometric to provide access to healthcare information or entry into a physically secure location, such as a medical record keeping or information technology department. Drawbacks to the system include its difficulty in use. During enrollment and presentation, individuals must remain perfectly still, or the system will not be able to scan the iris, therefore causing false nonmatching and failure-to-enroll anomalies to occur. Finally, users are sensitive to any device the shines a light into their eyes.

The final biometric that could gain wide use in the healthcare sector is the hand-scan. This biometric uses the unique aspects of the human hand, especially the height and width of the back of the hand, to verify and identify an individual [37]. The hand-scan can be used to provide physical access to highly secure areas and monitor when an individual arrives and leaves the workplace. The strengths of this technology include its ability to be used in different environments, reliability, and convenience. Drawbacks are price and limited applicability. In terms of future use, look for the finger-scan to be the most widely accepted biometric by the healthcare industry.

Putting It All Together: Customer Relations Management

Meanwhile, back on the *Enterprise*, Captain Kirk had a wealth of information at his disposal using the ship's computer system. If he needed information about the ship's WARP drive, it was readily available via the computer. If he needed personal information about a crew member, the status of an officer in sick bay, or a detailed report on earth's history dating back to the 20th century, all Kirk had to do was make a request. Within seconds, the computer provided the information. How was this possible? Because all the *Enterprise*'s major systems were tied directly into the ship's computer. Engineering, sick bay, hangar deck, and personnel files were all tied together to ensure that the ship functioned in a smooth and efficient manner.

Most healthcare delivery organizations (HCOs) can be likened to a ship, much like the *Enterprise*. However, a major problem with these HCOs is that many of the major systems that allow the organization to operate are tied to disparate legacy information systems. For example, radiology may be running on a VAX, while accounting is using COBOL. Human resources and the medical records department are still using paper to track employee and patient comings and goings. The medical records department is working to adopt a new coding software program that may or may not work with the proposed CPOE system being installed next year. And down in pharmacy, an automated drug-ordering system running on Windows 2000 Professional will be available next month. From this brief description, it is easy to see that many HCOs do not provide their administrators, physicians, and even their patients with the same seamless access that the *Enterprise* computing systems afforded Captain Kirk. If physicians need an MRI report "stat," they either have to call down to the radiology department, send one of their staff to retrieve the records, or try accessing the information through that department's somewhat Byzantine computing system. This example shows that as an HCO grows, either through mergers or through the installation of fragmented and disparate information systems, "choke points" begin to appear in the immediate delivery of information [38]. These choke points not only affect the delivery of care, but they can affect the bottom line and the HCO's most important benefactor, the healthcare consumer, who can decide to take his or her business elsewhere.

Rise of a New Type of User

Phillips and Panchal report that in the past HCOs interested in the bottom line would go after the physician [39]. The thinking was that if they were able to attract the physician to the organzation, the patients would follow. With the rise of the Internet, more and more individuals are using the World Wide Web to locate health-related information and are beginning to demand greater control over "the access to and delivery of care" [39]. The new healthcare consumers want "personalized and customized health service." They want to have the distinct feeling that the HCO is keeping track of their interactions with the organization and its physicians, and that it is doing everything possible to help the consumers manage their health. Consumers become frustrated when they can log-on to their bank's Web site, get a detailed list of activity in their checking and savings accounts, or find out how much they owe on a loan, but when they call their HCO to check on laboratory results, schedule an appointments, or try to determine if a specific procedure is covered, they are placed on hold and required to wait an unnecessarily long time.

Because of this fact alone, Phillips and Panchal point out, "HCOs need to build and manage personalized relationships with both patients and physicians," to develop longitudinal histories of the customers' interactions and track their interests. To build and manage these relationships, an HCO needs to embrace the concept of customer relationship management (CRM). At the core of CRM is the use of software and technology to integrate an HCO's disparate systems—payer, EMR, and scheduling—to create various touch points such as Web portals, telephone services, PDA messaging services, and kiosks, which enable both the patient and the physician to give and receive more personal, customized care [39]. Many out-of-the-box CRM applications require a great deal of configuration and preinstallation planning. Health administrators must work closely with CRM vendors to make sure their implementation meets the demands of their customers. When evaluating a CRM system, administrators should look for a system that provides a functionality that includes customer profiles, relationships, case structure, workflow and automation, scripts and frequently asked questions, and business intelligence [39]. Each of these functions will be briefly discussed.

Customer Profiles

A CRM system should provide the capability to gather important patient demographics, insurance coverage, and preferences. This information can be shared throughout the HCO and used to make interactions, whether online or in person, more intimate.

Relationships

Does the customer have a spouse, children, multiple physicians, and health plans? All this information needs to be recorded, so that all interactions with the HCO can be tracked and monitored to provide premium service.

Case Structure

Service requests can be assigned to one or more HCO representations. This will provide for more accountability on the part of the HCO, and more satisfaction for the customer.

Workflow and Automation

This function sets the ground rules for how business is done. If a case has not been resolved after a number of days, it is sent to a department administrator for resolution. For patients with e-mail, appointment reminders can be sent. For patients new to the HCO, a set of maps and parking information can be delivered either by e-mail or through the regular postal service.

Scripts and Frequently Asked Questions

This is a support service that guarantees that service requests are handled in a consistent and professional manner. It also provides insurance that specific business processes and policies are followed to the letter.

Business Intelligence

This provides the capability of gathering information about customers, both physicians and patients. It is used to inform and make intelligent business decisions. It also can be used to help the customer make important decisions. For example, many patients want to know the type and number of operations a physician performs on a yearly basis. This information can be made available to patients to help allay their fears and to assure them that they are in good hands.

The goal of CRM is tie together the disparate systems that operate within an HCO and to provide customers with greater access to information through a set of touch points. Again, these touch points can be traditional: phone, television, fax, radio, and prints. Or they can be nontraditional and make use of new wireless technologies: handsets, PDAs, and laptops. Furthermore, through the use of CRM, HCOs can develop Web portals that allow patients who have the proper security clearance access to their medical records, laboratory results, and information about their physicians, such as the types of services they provide and their educational background. In deciding whether to implement CRM, HCOs should consider how this application can set them apart from their competition. With profit margins getting increasingly narrow, and reimbursements for specific treatments getting lower and lower, CRM is one way that HCOs can garner and retain more of their customers and gain a greater market share in their region.

References

1. Kohn LT, Corrigan JM, Donaldson MS, editors. To err is human: building a safer health system. Committee on Quality Health Case in America, Institute of Medicine. Washington, DC: National Academy Press; 2000.
2. Lang RD. An interview with Joanne E. Turnbull, PhD, Executive Director, National Patient Safety Foundation. J Healthcare Inform Manag 2002;16(1):25–26.
3. Wennberg JE. Dealing with medical practice variations: a proposal for action. Health Affairs 1984;3(2):7–32.
4. Dartmouth Atlas of Health Care 2001. Available at: http://www.dartmouthatlas.org/. Accessed November 20, 2002.
5. Vergano D. Operations often depend on where you live. USA Today 2000; September 19; Sect. A:1.
6. McConnell T. Safer, cheaper, smarter. Health Manag Technol 2001;22(3):16–18.
7. Ash JS, Gorman PN, Hersh WR. Physician order entry in U.S. hospitals. Proc AMIA Annu Symp 1998;235–239.
8. Meadows G, Caiken BP. Computerized physician order entry: a prescription for patient safety. Nurs Econ 2002;20(2):76–77, 87.
9. Eisenberg F, Barbell AS. Computerized physician order entry: eight steps to optimize physician workflow. J Healthcare Inform Manag 2002;16(1):16–18.
10. Kilbridge P, Welebob E, Classen D, and First Consulting Group. Overview of the Leapfrog group evaluation tool for computerized physician order entry. Available at http://www.fcg.com. Accessed November 20, 2002.
11. Teich JM. Inpatient order management. J Healthcare Inform Manag 1999;13(2):97–110.
12. Eskew A, Geisler M, O'Conner L, Saunders G, Vinci R. Enhancing patient safety: clinician order entry with a pharmacy interface. J Healthcare Inform Manag 2002;16(1):52–57.
13. Mekhjian HS, Kumar RR, Kuehn L, et al. Immediate benefits realized following implementation of physician order entry at an academic medical center. J Am Med Inform Assoc 2002;9(5):529–539.

14. Scalise D. CPOE (computerized physician order entry). An executive's guide. Hosp Health Netw 2002;76(6):41–46.
15. Armstrong C. AHA guide to computerized physician order entry system. American Hospital Association. Available at: http://www.aha.org/medicationsafety/poe-execsumA3115.asp.
16. Cook RI. Safety technology: solutions or experiments. Nurs Econ 2002;20(2):80–82.
17. Ahmad A, Teater P, Bentley TD, et al. Key attributes of a successful physician order entry system implementation in a multi-hospital environment. J Am Med Inform Assoc 2002; 9(1):16–24.
18. Sittig DF, Stead WW. Computer-based physician order entry: the state of the art. J Am Med Informatics Assoc 1994;1(2):108–123.
19. Chan W. Increasing the success of physician order entry through human factors engineering. J Healthcare Inform Manag 2002;16(1):71–79.
20. Bergeron B. The wireless Web and healthcare. Chicago, IL: Healthcare Information and Management Systems Society; 2002.
21. Comer DE, Droms RE. Computer networks and Internets, with Internet applications. 3rd ed. Englewood Cliffs: Prentice Hall; 2001.
22. Ferenczi PM. Personal area networking. Computer Buyer's Guide and Handbook 2002; 21(10):36–40.
23. Garber L. Will 3G really be the next big wireless technology? Computer 2002;35(1):26–32.
24. Dreazen Y. Space wars: the future of wireless depends on companies getting more room on the spectrum. But who is going to give it up? Wall Street Journal 2002 Sept. 23; R9.
25. Chittum R. Calls in question: why are wireless networks still plagued by dropped signals, bad reception and 'dead zones'? Wall Street Journal 2002 Sept. 23; R:8.
26. Paulson LD. Users create underground wireless networks. Computer 2002;35(1):25.
27. Drucker J, Angwin J. Unleashed: new way to surf the Web is giving cell carriers static. Wall Street Journal 2002 Nov. 29; A:1.
28. Schilit BN, Trevor J, Koh TK. Web interaction using very small Internet devices. Computer 2002;35(10):37–45.
29. Holmes BJ, Brown EG, Twist AE. Doctors connect with handhelds. Forrester Research, Inc.; 2001.
30. Criswell DF, Parchman ML. Handheld computer use in U.S. family practice residency programs. J Am Med Inform Assoc 2002;9(1):80–86.
31. Shellenbarger S. The brave new world of eldercare: gadgets track loved ones' every move. Wall Street Journal 2002 July 18.
32. Shellenbarger S. Technology holds promise for easing families' worries over the elderly. Wall Street Journal 2002 July 25.
33. Fox C. Technogenarians: the pioneers of pervasive computing aren't getting any younger. Wired 2001;9(11):1–8.
34. Donahue B. Byte, byte, against the dying of the light. Atlantic Monthly 2001 May.
35. Rochester Center for Future Health. Available at http://www.futurehealth.rochester.edu/news/index.cfm. Accessed November 21, 2002.
36. Chan S, Horner SR, Fauchet PM, Miller BL. Smart Bandage. J Am Chem Soc. 2001;123:11797–11798.
37. Nanavati S, Thieme M, Nanavanti R. Biometrics: identity verification in a networked world. New York: Wiley; 2002.
38. Frazier G. Chokepoints as a source of system inefficiency. Personal communication; 2002 November 12.
39. Phillips J, Panchal S. Meeting the needs of customers with health CRM. J Healthcare Inform Manag 2002;16(3):35–39.

34
Evidence-Based Medicine: Enabling Physicians to Make Better Decisions

Velma L. Payne

The solution is not to remove the decision-making power from the physician, but to improve the physician's capacity to make better decisions.

Healthcare Challenges

There was a day when physicians, armed with a degree and a mission, had the confidence that based on their knowledge they could see patients, hear their complaints, and determine the best course of action to cure or ease their pain. Physicians were trusted and left to rely on their expertise to determine what was in the best interest of each patient. The medical profession, like every avenue of life, has gone and continues to go through a profound transition. The days when physicians were trusted to make the proper decision to heal the sick are gone. The basic assumption of the past, that what a physician decides by definition is correct, is being challenged. The root of the challenge is a concern for quality health care. According to David Eddy, "The plain fact is that many decisions made by physicians appear to be arbitrary—highly variable, with no obvious explanation. The very disturbing implication is that this arbitrariness represents, for at least some patients, suboptimal or even harmful care" [1]. Eddy states "substantial variations in what physicians see have been reported in virtually every aspect of the diagnostic process, from taking a history, to doing a physical examination, reading laboratory tests, performing a pathological diagnosis, and recommending a treatment" [1, p. 2]. These variations are centered on observations, perceptions, reasoning, conclusions, and practices [1, p. 2]. Statistics provided indicate that observers looking at the same thing will disagree with each other or even with themselves from 10 percent to 50 percent of the time [1, p. 2]. Eddy also feels that even though there is variability in medicine, it is not randomly practiced. Physician decisions might be variable, but they are not flippant or whimsical decisions. Variability in decisions occurs due to the complexity of problems occurring under difficult circumstances. Physicians are in the impossible position of not knowing outcomes of different actions, but having to act on them anyway. Physicians are in a position where they not only must deal with the mysteries of human biology and disease and con-

Velma L. Payne, MS, MBA, is Chief Information Officer at OB/GYN Partner, LLC, in Pittsburgh, PA.

tinually expanding technologies, but a montage of other forces such as the expectations of patients and their families, personal, professional and financial goals, changing reimbursement systems, competition, malpractice, peer pressure, and politics, as well as incomplete information.

So how can physicians make better decisions? What is required to ensure that health-care providers are making the best decision possible? There are two main ingredients needed for accurate decisions regardless of the profession—evidence and the ability to analyze the evidence [1, p. 5]. Without such formal evidence, healthcare providers have no alternative but to turn to their own personal experiences and knowledge. However, oftentimes such personal experience does not include a large number of observations, there are no controls, and follow-up is usually short term and incomplete. For optimal health care, the ability to analyze the evidence is required. However, even if physicians were provided with extensive evidence, they could not possibly sort through it all in their heads in an instant when seeing a patient. Physicians must have access to solid information about the outcomes, consequences, risks and benefits of different choices. Physicians must also be able to process this information quickly and accurately. The solution to today's problem in the healthcare profession is not to remove the decision-making power from the physician, but to improve the capacity for the physician to make better decisions. Physicians must be given the information required; the skills to utilize that information must be institutionalized; and the process to support, not dictate, decisions must be built.

Evidence-Based Medicine Philosophy

Formally, evidence-based medicine (EBM) is "the conscientious, explicit, and judicious use of current best evidence in making decisions about the care of individual patients" [2]. "The practice of evidence-based medicine requires integration of individual clinical expertise and patient preferences with the best available external clinical evidence from systematic research" [2]. The objective of evidence-based medicine is to make efficient use of published literature to help with patient care. Simply put, the goal of evidence-based medicine is to be aware of the evidence that exists on various ailments, diseases and sicknesses; to be able to question the evidence and determine its soundness; determine its applicability to the patient; and finally to determine how to apply the evidence to the patient in need with a perfect balance of risk and benefit.

Before the adoption of evidence-based medicine, clinical decisions were based on intuition, unsystematic clinical experiences, and pathophysiological rationale. Evidence-based medicine relies on evidence from clinical research and on a formal set of rules to effectively interpret the research results, all of which are used to complement the clinician's common sense and medical training. Initially, the focus of evidence-based medicine centered on applying the best research evidence relevant to a clinical problem for a resolution of the problem. Modern-day versions of the evidence-based model emphasize that research evidence alone is not an adequate guide to the application of the evidence. The modified model is based on patients' circumstances, preferences, and actions, along with the best research evidence, with a central role for clinical expertise to integrate these components [3]. This modified model extends the original model to say that clinicians must apply their expertise to evidence as well as the patient's preferences and values before making a management recommendation [3]. The new model, depicted in Figure 34.1, has recently been defined as "the integration of best research evidence with clinical expertise and patient values" [3].

FIGURE 34.1. The updated model for evidence-based clinical decisions.

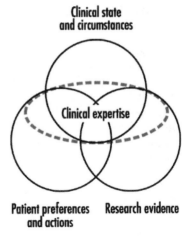

Clinical state and circumstances

Clinical expertise

Patient preferences and actions   Research evidence

Clinical state and circumstances is described as the dominant factors that affect clinical decisions, which include patients' clinical state, the clinical setting, and the clinical circumstances that patients find themselves in when they seek medical attention. For example, patients with retrosternal chest pain when in a remote location may be forced to settle for aspirin, whereas those living close to a tertiary care medical center will have more options, assuming they recognize the symptoms and act promptly [3]. Evidence-based decisions vary from patient to patient according to their individual clinical circumstances.

The model also includes *patient preferences and actions*. Without regard to a patient's preferences, physicians may find that the patient may resent the prescribed treatment, its adverse effects, or its costs, thus resulting in the patient not following the prescribed course of action. It has been determined that "clinicians' estimates of their patients' adherence to prescribed treatments have accuracy no better than chance" [3]. The integration of patient preferences and actions within the evidence-based model is an indication that physicians must accurately access the probability that the patient will follow the prescribed treatment.

The *research evidence* reflected in the evidence-based model provides detailed guides to the determination of the ultimate and pertinent evidence for specific clinical decisions. Research evidence is a key component and plays an imperative part in the personalization of the evidence to the patient's specific circumstances. Finally, the role of *clinical expertise* encompasses all three of the other components of the modified evidence-based model. Clinical expertise must not only encompass but also balance the patient's clinical state and circumstances, relevant research evidence, and the patient's preferences and actions for a successful and satisfying result.

Evidence-based models do not come without limitations, however. The major limitation of the evidence-based models is the lack of depiction of all the elements involved, including the extremely important role that society and healthcare organizations play in providing and/or limiting health services resources [3]. Another limitation is the impossibility of accurately predicting the patient's likelihood of following the treatment program [3]. Due to these limitations, the model is conceptual rather than practical and continuously remains under development.

The Evolution of Evidence-Based Medicine

A number of determined individuals became the first pioneers in the discovery of variations in clinical practice. Paul M. Ellwood, Jr., MD, a national leader in the efforts to make the health system accountable to consumers for delivering high-quality care, and who now recognizes individuals who have devoted lifetime efforts toward this goal with "The Ellwood Award," is only one of these individuals. John E. Wennberg, MD, MPH, who trained at Johns Hopkins University in internal medicine and is currently the director of the Center for Evaluative Clinical Sciences and a professor at Dartmouth Medical School, is another pioneer on variants within practice. Wennberg's research on variations in health care revealed large differences in allocation of hospital resources, physician supply, and the use of high-risk procedures. According to Wennberg, "most people view the medical care they receive as a necessity provided by doctors who adhere to scientific norms based on previously tested and proven treatments" [4]. However, Wennberg feels that the type of medical service provided is often found to be as strongly influenced by subjective factors related to the attitudes of individual physicians as by science [4]. Wennberg's work culminated in the production of the Dartmouth Atlas, the most comprehensive report on variations in health services throughout the United States. He has continued to conduct research, bringing to light questions never posed to the healthcare system. The basis of Wennberg's theories of practice variations is primarily scientific. A shift to an evidence-based style of practice, it is believed, would narrow this variation [2].

Such a shift to an evidence-based style of practice began in the late 1970s with a group of clinical epidemiologists at McMaster University in Canada who began working on a series of articles, later published in the *Canadian Medical Association Journal* in 1981, that would advise clinicians on how to read clinical journals. After several years, the group, consisting of David Sackett, Brian Haynes, Peter Tugwell, and Victor Neufeld, began to realize the necessity of motivating clinicians to move beyond what they termed "critical appraisal," or browsing literature, to actually utilizing the information in solving patient problems or "practical application of evidence from the medical literature to patient care" [5]. In the spring of 1990, Gordon Guyatt, MD, Residency Director of the internal medicine program at McMaster, approached the Department of Medicine with the mission of training physicians to practice this new brand of medicine. This medicine, which he entitled "scientific medicine," is based on knowledge and understanding of the medical literature supporting each clinical decision. He proposed this "bringing critical appraisal to the bedside" as a philosophy of medical practice.

The philosophy, later termed evidence-based medicine, first appeared in the autumn of 1990 in an informational document intended for residents entering or considering application to the residency program at McMaster. In 1991, the term appeared in print in the *ACP Journal Club*. In 1992 the McMaster Group, allied with a group of academic physicians primarily from the U.S., who later become the first international evidence-based medicine working group, published an article that expanded on the existing description of evidence-based medicine labeling it a "paradigm shift" [5]. This group later produced a new set of articles to present a much more practical approach to applying the medical literature to clinical practice in a 25-part series called "The User's Guides to the Medical Literature," which was published in *JAMA* between 1993 and 2000 [5].

The term evidence-based medicine did not stop there. Healthcare practitioners realized the principles of evidence-based medicine were applicable to allied healthcare workers such as nurses, dentists, orthodontists, physical therapists, occupational thera-pists, chiropractors, and podiatrists, which resulted in the creation of terms such as evidence-based health care and evidence-based practice.

The Evidence-Based Medicine Process

The practice of evidence-based medicine involves five steps [6]:

- *Formulate the question:* convert the need for information about diagnosis, prognosis, therapy, causation, and prevention into a question that can be answered.
- *Find the evidence:* conduct research on the best evidence that will answer the pro-posed question.
- *Analyze the evidence:* critically appraise and summarize the evidence for validity and determine its impact and applicability in clinical practice.
- *Apply the results:* integrate the critical appraisal, clinical expertise, and the patient's values and circumstances.
- *Assess the outcome:* evaluate the effectiveness and efficiency of the evidence research and the patient response to the treatment.

Formulating the Question

Applying evidence-based medicine to practice involves defining the patient's problem and searching for literature to resolve that problem. Defining the patient's problem involves framing the question in the proper form. There are four elements of a well-built clinical question, commonly referred to as *"PICO,"* which include determin-ing the appropriate patient *population*, determining the *intervention* that should be used, *comparing* various strategies available, and determining the clinical *outcome* of interest [7]. Establishing each of these factors for a case under consideration is crucial.

Determining the proper question is only one aspect of question formulation. Another pertinent step to evidence research is determining the type of study commonly used to answer the question at hand. Different studies are used during a clinical process to resolve different types of questions. There are four types of clinical questions, includ-ing therapy, harm, diagnosis, and prognosis, each with a preferred study design used as the base of evidence [5].

Therapy is the process of determining the effect of different treatments on the improvement of a patient's function and/or if the treatment avoids adverse events. A randomized controlled trial (RCT) is commonly used to answer questions on thera-peutic issues. A process comparable to flipping a coin is used to determine if the participant will receive an experimental treatment or a control treatment. Once par-ticipants are allocated to the designated treatment or control group, the participant is monitored to determine the existence or absence of the outcome of interest.

Harm studies ascertain the effects of potentially harmful agents on patient function, morbidity, and mortality. Observational studies are used to determine harm. In such studies, patients with and without the exposure are observed to determine if the outcome of interest occurs.

Diagnosis-based questions establish the power of an intervention to differentiate between those with and without a target condition or disease. Diagnostic test studies, commonly used to determine a diagnosis, involve investigators identifying a group of patients who may or may not have the disease or condition of interest, which is called the target condition. After determination of the collection of patients who may have the target condition, the patients undergo both a diagnostic test and a "gold standard," or a test considered to be the diagnostic standard for a particular condition. The investigator evaluates the diagnostic test by comparing its classification of patients with that of the gold standard.

Prognosis is the estimation of the future course of a patient's disease and is assessed using observational studies. Investigators identify patients that belong to a particular group with or without factors that may modify their prognosis. Over time investigators follow the patients to determine if they experience the target outcome.

Before searching for evidence, the clinician must determine the proper question. If the proper question is not being addressed, the search for evidence will not be beneficial. Determining the proper question involves specifying the type of question being considered along with the type of study commonly used to answer that question. These steps are critical before beginning the search for evidence.

Find the Evidence

Even if clinicians have determined the proper question and study method to search for, one of the most oppressive obstacles they face is a limitation of time to conduct research. With such diminished time, clinicians must maximize their research efforts for evidence relating to patient issues. The rapid evolution of resources to support evidence-based healthcare decisions, as well as the swift pace of innovation and technology, enable the clinician to gather, summarize, and apply critical evidence in an expeditious manner.

Major Providers of Evidence

With today's state-of-the-art technology, many evidence providers have provided their content over the Internet. These online databases make it more efficient for clinicians to search for evidence. Some of the major providers of evidence-based medicine databases are listed in Table 34.1. This list is by no means a complete list; many sources are available.

Searching for evidence includes determining the optimal medical information based on the question being researched. The researcher should match the question to the

TABLE 34.1. Major providers of online evidence-based databases.

Resource	Internet address
ACP Journal Club	http://www.acpjc.org
Cochrane Library	http://www.update-software.com/cochrane/
UpToDate/ MEDLINE	http://www.uptodate.com
OVID Reviews	http://www.ovid.com
Scientific American Medicine	http://www.samed.com
Clinical Evidence	http://www.clinicalevidence.com
Best Evidence	Available via the ACP Journal Club and OVID EBMD Review

source of information that will most likely provide the appropriate answer. Textbooks are best for clinical use; however, keeping textbooks up to date proves a continual challenge [7]. Investing in evidence databases, evidence-based journals, and online services such as the Cochrane Library, Clinical Evidence, UpToDate, or Best Evidence and accessing computerized clinical decision support systems are a means of obtaining critical evidence [7]. Detailed information of some of the more prevalent sources follows.

Cochrane Library, disseminated by an international organization, The Cochrane Collaboration, focuses primarily on systematic reviews of controlled trials of therapeutic interventions. This source does not address other aspects of medical care such as diagnostic tests or prognosis. There are three sections of the Cochrane Library, updated quarterly, including the Cochrane Database of Systematic Reviews (CDSR), which is a complete report for all the systematic reviews that have been prepared by members of the Cochran Collaboration; the Database of Reviews of Effectiveness (DARE), which includes systematic reviews published outside the collaboration; and Cochrane Controlled Trials Registry (CCTR), which contains a list of over 268,000 references to clinical trials that Cochrane investigators have found by searching a wide range of sources including Medline and Excerpta Medica (EMBASE) bibliographic databases, hand searches, and reference lists of relevant original studies and reviews that refer to randomized trials and observational studies.

UpToDate is an online textbook that references many high-quality studies chosen by its section authors. A measure of explicit methodologically quality criteria is not utilized for this source.

MEDLINE, maintained by the U.S. National Library of Medicine, is a bibliographic database that includes over 11,000,000 citations of both clinical and preclinical studies. This source is an extremely comprehensive database covering numerous medical journals.

Clinical Evidence, published by BMJ Publishing Group and the American College of Physicians/American Society of Internal Medicine, focuses on providing a concise account of the current state of knowledge, ignorance, and uncertainty about the prevention of treatment regarding common and important clinical conditions.

Best Evidence is the cumulative electronic version of *ACP Journal Club* and the international evidence-based medicine secondary journals. Its focus is on systematic reviews and original studies of clinical questions. These journals present the review or study, along with an accompanying commentary by an expert who offers a clinical perspective on the study results and other notable articles.

Internet and Wireless Device Evidence-Based Tools

With the state-of-the-art technology dominating today's society, almost all evidence-based tools available today are Internet based, with many tools being available for wireless handheld devices. Numerous companies have jumped on the bandwagon hoping to gain the majority of market share in offering such tools. The well-known *Clinical Evidence*, previously only offered in print and on CD-ROM, is now offered in its entirety on the Internet as well as in a handheld/PDA version.

McKesson Information Solutions: In their attempt to review and research the current healthcare system, McKesson determined that a variability of care was occurring due to physicians deviating from conventional standard care by slightly altering patient treatment. This variability cost U.S. healthcare organizations $250 billion every year [8]. McKesson states the automation of evidence-based medicine can reduce this variability of care, ultimately reducing costs. McKesson developed a Clinical Decision Support Order Entry System to resolve this problem. One aspect of their system, Horizon Expert Orders, is a system that automates evidence-based medicine by integrating current best practices, protocols, knowledge bases, and patient data, which will allow the physician to make the best care decisions at the point of care due to the access of valuable information.

POEMs: The evidence tools discussed thus far have been "disease-oriented" evidence tools that represent outcomes without verifiable positive outcomes to patients. POEMs, or "patient-oriented evidence that matters," are tools that reflect outcomes based on demonstrated positive outcomes important to patients [2]. The POEM information selection process consists of monthly reviews of numerous journals for valid and clinically applicable new evidence that measures outcomes important to patients and addresses the issues faced by patients and physicians. The use of POEMs can significantly increase the efficiency of a physician's practice by providing new evidence that not only is medically sound but is patient oriented. InfoPOEMs is offered on various platforms including a desktop computer, the Internet, as well as handheld computers. The diversity of InfoPOEM's availability provides clinicians with a tool that will reach them with the most convenient means and at a time that will be most beneficial to them. With the push technology option, clinicians are not even required to perform a search to become aware of the latest research evidence. The data are pushed to the clinicians' designated devices, including wireless devices, based on categories they designate are of interest. Such a technology exemplifies not only the growth, but also extreme benefits, of information technology in the healthcare industry. Such information, available at a clinician's fingertips, will increase the quality of care tremendously.

Analyze the Evidence

Once assembled, the evidence must be analyzed for quality and applicability. Analyzing the evidence involves critically appraising and summarizing the evidence for validity and assessing the impact of the effect in clinical practice. For each category of therapy, harm, diagnosis, and prognosis, the researcher should assess the study by asking three major questions:

- Did the study produce valid results?
- What are the results?
- Can the results be applied to my patient?

For each category the specific questions that are used to assess the study are slightly different, as detailed in Table 34.2. Even though there are some differences across the categories in the administration of the study, the concepts of reviewing the study and determining its impact on the patient are very similar.

Did the Study Produce Valid Results: Was it Administered Properly?

Researchers analyzing the validity of studies should consider three major categories, which include prognostic factors, patient follow-up, and group analysis.

TABLE 34.2. Common questions for validation and use of studies in clinical practice.

Study	Are the results valid?	What are the results?	Can the results be applied to our patient?
Therapy	Was the assignment of patients to treatment randomized? Was randomization concealed? Were all patients analyzed in the groups they were randomized? Were groups similar at the start of the trial? Were patients and clinicians kept blind to treatment? Were groups treated equally, apart from the experimental therapy? Was follow-up of patients sufficiently long and complete?	What is the magnitude of the treatment effect? How precise is the estimate of the treatment effect?	Is our patient significantly different from those in the study that the results cannot apply? Is the treatment feasible in our setting? What are our patient's potential benefits and harms of the therapy? What are our patient's values and expectations for the outcome we are trying to prevent and the treatment we are offering?
Harm	Were there clearly defined patient groups similar in important ways? Were the treatments/exposures and clinical outcomes measured in the same way in the groups being compared? Was follow-up of the study patients complete and sufficiently long enough for the outcome to occur?	What is the magnitude and precision of the association between the exposure and outcome?	Is our patient so different from those included in the study that its results do not apply? What is our patient's potential benefit from the therapy?
Diagnosis	Was there an independent and blind comparison with a reference standard of diagnosis? Was the diagnostic test evaluated in an appropriate spectrum of patients? Was the test validated in a second, independent group of patients?	What were the diagnoses?	Are the study patients similar to the patient being considered? Is it unlikely that the disease possibilities or probabilities have changed since this evidence was gathered?
Prognosis	Was a defined and representative sample of patients assembled at a common point in the course of their disease? Was patient follow-up sufficiently long and complete? Were objective outcome criteria applied in a blind fashion?	How likely are the outcomes over time? How precise are the prognostic estimates?	Are the study patients similar to our own? Will this evidence make a clinically important impact on our conclusions about what to offer or tell our patient?

Source: Refs. [5,7].

Determinants of an outcome, called prognostic factors, are items such as a patient's age, severity of illness, and the presence of comorbid conditions. If these prognostic factors are unbalanced within the study population, the outcome of the study will be biased to under- or overestimate the effect of the treatment. Clinicians must review prognostic features of the study's population at commencement and establish a baseline. The inclusion of all patients with the clinical problem from a defined geographical area, or the inclusion of a consecutive series of all patients with the clinical problem that receive care at the investigators' institutions, are two of the most commonly used methods for ensuring representation [5]. The wider the spectrum of patients in the sample, the more representative the sample will be of the whole population, resulting in exceptionally valid results. If the magnitude of prognostic factor differences is large, the validity of the study may be compromised. If the magnitude of the factors is vast, statistical techniques permit the adjustment of the study result for baseline differences; however, both unadjusted and adjusted analyses must generate the same conclusion for readers to gain confidence in the study's validity [5].

Proper follow-up is essential to the success and validity of the study. Once the treatment is administered, patient follow-up must be long enough to accurately determine the outcome. Short follow-up periods will not provide clinicians with accurate results. Ideally, at the conclusion of a trial, investigators will know the outcome of each patient that was entered into the study. The greater the number of patients whose outcome is unknown, or "lost to follow-up," the greater a study's validity is compromised. With long follow-up periods, there is the potential for patient dropouts. A high patient dropout rate threatens the validity of a study. When patients drop out, the reason for the loss may be crucial and must be considered. If patients dropped out due to adverse outcome, this absence from the analysis would lead to an overestimation of the efficacy of the treatment [7]. For studies of diagnosis, 1 to 6 months for acute and self-limited symptoms and 1 to 5 years for chronically recurring or progressive symptoms is the recommended follow-up period [5].

When reviewing a study for validity, it is important that the evidence reveal that the investigators analyzed the groups properly. Group analysis differs slightly for each category. For therapy studies, the patient population is randomized. In this type of study, randomization of patients must exist and be concealed from those making the decision of patient eligibility for the study to yield valid results. Unblinded or unmasked randomization could lead to the enrollment of sicker, or less sick, patients to the treatment or control group, resulting in biased results. Concealing randomization can be accomplished in ways, such as the preparation of blinded medication in a pharmacy, or remote randomization in which the individual recruiting the patient can access a specified Internet site to discover the arm of the study to which to allocate the patient. For therapy studies, all patients must be analyzed within the groups to which they were randomized. An "intention-to-treat analysis," which is the analysis of outcomes based on the treatment arm to which the patient was randomized, rather than the treatment they received, will preserve the value of randomization and ensure the resulting effect was only from the treatment assigned [7].

For harm studies, observational study designs are used when administering the study. There are three main observational study designs including cohort studies, case-control studies, and case reports [7]. In a cohort study, the investigator identifies exposed and nonexposed groups of patients, each a cohort, and then follows them forward in time, monitoring the occurrence of the predicted outcome [5]. Cohort studies have many advantages; however, it takes an extensive amount of time to develop rare outcomes, which threatens the feasibility of such studies. An alternative to cohort studies is case-control studies in which investigators identify patients that have already developed the target outcome, then choose controls, or a group who are reasonably similar to the cases with respect to important determinants of outcome such as age, sex, and medical conditions but who have not suffered the target outcome [7]. Once both groups are determined, the investigators assess the relative frequency of exposure to the alleged harmful agent on each group while adjusting for differences in the known predictive variables [7]. Case-control studies permit the assessment of cause–effect relationships without extending the study over years required to determine if an outcome will be present on one patient.

The third study, case reports, or case series, are sometimes used to answer questions of harm. These types of studies lack comparison groups and are usually only sufficient for hypothesis generation, and therefore investigators often rely on other studies [7]. For harm studies, it must be assured that information is not biased by either recall bias due to increased patient motivation or due to interviewer bias resulting from probing by the interviewer. Clinicians must ensure that bias-minimizing strategies were used by making sure patients and interviewers were blind to the hypothesis of the study.

For diagnosis studies, valid evidence will only occur if the investigators arrive at a correct final diagnosis; this requires the application of explicit criteria when assigning the final diagnosis to each patient [5]. Each diagnosis study should include the findings needed to confirm each diagnosis, as well as the findings useful for rejecting the diagnosis. The search for these criteria should be comprehensive enough to detect all the important causes of the clinical problem to reduce the chances of invalid conclusions. Once determined, the explicit diagnostic criteria must be applied consistently, otherwise they will be useless. Even with the consistent application of the criteria, some patients' problems may remain and be left unexplained. The higher the number of undiagnosed patients, the greater the chance of error in the estimates of disease probabilities [5]. For prognosis studies, individuals determining the outcomes must be blinded to the presence of prognostic factors; otherwise, the study will be biased.

Information technology can greatly enhance each study category. The use of computerized databases of claims, medical records, etc., provides a way for investigators to obtain valuable information without an introduction of recall or interviewer bias. Given specific parameters such as patient age, illness severity, presence or absence of comorbid conditions, geographical region, sex, and race, database search utilities can quickly and accurately derive an acceptable patient population for the study. As previously noted, for studies requiring randomization of treatment between experimental and control groups, randomization can easily be performed by computer programs that will assign an equal number of patients to each group. For harm studies in particular, a source of information in case-control studies is often computer-based record keeping.

Linking computer-based health insurance databases with drug plan sources can provide the case and control groups required for such studies. For example, these sources can assist investigators in the determination of the use of various drugs by patients with a certain condition. As with cohort studies, information technology has provided an expedient manner of obtaining the case and control groups without extensive and laborious resources. Computerized medical, pharmaceutical, healthcare, and patient records are providing an extremely valuable source of information for researchers and clinicians to determine what works, what does not work, what will cause a patient to overcome an illness, and what will harm patients. Computer systems can also accurately track each individual's response to the treatment as well as their diagnosis, prognosis, adverse affects, etc. No matter what the study type, each patient can be directed to visit a Web site to enter his or her health progress or decline and signs and symptoms on a daily, weekly, bimonthly, or monthly basis. If the patient does not enter his or her status for a specific check-in period, push technology can be used to send an e-mail reminder to the patient. If the patient still does not respond, alerts can be sent to the study administrator's e-mail, cell phone, or handheld device to follow up with the patient. Once the study has been completed, information technology will prove extremely valuable in the analysis of data entered by the participants. A researcher will easily be able to determine if the study has produced valid results, and can be assured of the results, all due to enhanced, sophisticated, and accurate information and decision support systems.

What Are the Study Results?

Once the validity of the study is determined, the actual results of the study should be determined. Without an accurate assessment of the results of the study, obviously the study will not be of value to a clinician. An understanding of the various statistical measures used to reveal outcomes is essential to this phase of the evidence-based medicine process. The manner in which study results are determined varies for each study category.

Therapy studies utilize randomized clinical trials that produce dichotomous outcomes and involve monitoring how often patients experience an adverse event or outcome. Patients either suffer an event or do not. There are several ways to disclose the proportion of patients who develop such events. An absolute risk reduction, relative risk, and relative risk reduction are the most common ways to summarize the conclusions of a study [7]. The absolute risk reduction is the absolute difference between the proportion that had the target outcome in the control group and the proportion that had the target outcome in the treatment group [7]. The relative risk is the risk of events among patients on the new treatment, relative to that risk among patients in the control group [5]. The most commonly reported measure of dichotomous treatment effects is the relative risk reduction, or the complement of the relative risk expressed as a percent [5]. When determining if a therapy study can be applied to a patient, each figure should be assessed for preciseness and relevance.

For harm studies, the clinician must determine the strength of the association between exposure and outcome and the precision of the estimate of risk. Without a precise and accurate result, a clinician should not consider administering the study to the patient. For diagnoses studies, the actual diagnoses and the associated probabilities must be understood by the researcher. Without this understanding, the clinician runs the risk of causing harm to the patient.

Not only is validity a concern for the clinician researching prognostic studies, the actual results are just as important. Quantitatively, the results are represented as the number of events that occur over time. Oftentimes, the results of a prognostic study are represented in the form of a survival curve, which is a graph of the number of events over time, or conversely, the chance of being free from these events over time. To adequately graph study results, the events must be discrete and the time at which they occur must be precisely known [7].

As with each stage of the evidence-based medicine process, information management systems prove to be an irreplaceable entity in the determination of the study results. Many information systems exist on the market, based on various technologies and platforms, which provide the ability to analyze a tremendous amount of data in a short time frame, to calculate various statistical measures such as absolute risk reduction, relative risk reduction, relative risk, and survival analysis. Manual calculations of such figures would not only take an excessive amount of time, but would result in a greater potential for error, ultimately with a greater potential of harm to the patient. There are times when a physician needs to obtain information on what evidence has proven effective in an extremely short time frame because a patient is faced with a life-threatening disease. Information management systems are expedient, efficient, and relentless and have become an integral part of the clinician's process. With the explosion of technology to platforms never thought possible, such as wireless handheld personal digital assistants and cell phones, coupled with the delivery of data in an automated fashion without any intervention to pull the data from various heterogeneous data sources, the possibilities of healthcare information management systems are endless.

Can the Results Be Applied to Our Patient?

Once the validity of the study, the magnitude of the precision of the treatment, and the results of the study are known, the final consideration of the clinician is how this evidence can be applied to the patients in their clinical practice. Four considerations must be weighed during this phase of the evidence-based medicine process: similarity of patients in the study to the patient at hand, feasibility of the treatment or process, benefit and harm analysis, and, most importantly, the values, preferences, and expectations of the patient must be considered.

To apply the procedure to a patient, the study patients should be similar to the clinician's patient. To demand a complete fit of every inclusion criterion would not be sensible. There may be a difference in age, social class, or responsiveness to the procedure. Rather than try to "fit" our patient into the criteria of the study, a more appropriate approach may be to determine if there is a compelling reason why the results should not be applied.

Along with the study fitting the patient, the feasibility of the treatment at the institution and by the patient must be assessed. If the treatment is not feasible to the patient, clinician, and the healthcare system in terms of not only administration, but also monitoring and the required follow-up, there is no reason to further consider the study's evidence [7].

The magnitude of the risk to the patient is of enormous concern for the practicing physician. Physician's must ensure they do not inflict unnecessary harm to their patients. Not only must the potential benefits and harms to the patient be determined, but the benefits outweighing the risk also need to be contemplated. Even if a study produces favorable effects of treatment on a clinically important outcome, one must also consider the possible deleterious, or unexpectedly harmful, effects on outcomes. How likely, or unlikely, it is that the disease probabilities have changed since the evidence was gathered is another crucial assessment that is not optional during this stage. As time passes, disease frequency can be altered by more stringent controls, or even elimination, of a disease. Along with the analysis of the risks and benefits, another key element of a decision to start treatment is to deliberate the patient's risk of the adverse event if the patient is left untreated [7]. What will happen if the patient is not treated at all? Will this be more of a risk or will it ultimately be a benefit? Such questions are difficult to answer and are specific to each case being considered.

By far the most important consideration before applying the treatment to the individual is does it fall within the patient's values, preferences, and expectations? The patient should be asked to make value judgments about the severity of the bad outcome that is hoped to be prevented, as well as the adverse events or side effects that might be a result of the treatment [7]. The patient needs to determine how severe they consider one relative to the other on a scale of death to full health. Once determined, the patient's values for these outcomes need to be integrated with the probability of their occurrence. The ultimate goal of the implementation of any treatment is to provide the patient with the outcome they most desire. Without patient satisfaction, no therapy is worth the execution.

Healthcare information management systems and information technology is also valuable at this stage of the process. Computer systems can determine the similarity of the patients, perform a risk analysis on benefits and harms, as well as determine the feasibility of a procedure provided at a certain facility, and determine if the procedure is within the limits set by the patient's healthcare insurance. When assessing if the procedure coincides with the patient's values and preferences, however, the patient will ultimately have to make this critical decision.

Apply the Results

A major part of every clinician's day is making patient management decisions, some of which are minor, others of extremely great consequence, and some are a matter of life and death. Every decision involves weighing the benefits, risks, gains, and losses, as well as recommending and implementing a course of action that is in the best interest of the patient. Applying the results or putting evidence into practice involves the integration of the critical appraisal of evidence, clinical expertise, and the values and circumstances of the patient. Recommendation development required by clinicians, commonly labeled clinical decision making, is to specify the alternative courses of action and the possible outcomes, or target outcomes. During this process all reasonable alternatives are considered, and all beneficial and adverse outcomes are identified. Once the options and outcomes are identified, the links between the two are evaluated. In evaluating these links, questions such as "How are potential benefits and risks likely to vary in different groups of patients?" and "What benefits and harms will the alternative management strategies bring to a patient?" must be answered. Based on the answers to these questions, treatment recommendations are made about the relative desirability, or undesirability, of possible outcomes. These outcomes are the basis of moving from evidence to action. Decision analysis and clinical practice guidelines are used by clinical investigators and experts when putting evidence into action [6].

Decision Analysis

According to the Evidence-Based Medicine Working Group, decision analysis "provides a formal structure for integrating the evidence about the beneficial and harmful effects of treatment options with the values or preferences associated with those beneficial and harmful effects." [6]. Clinical decision analyses are studies that use formal mathematical approaches to analyze decisions in patient care to decide whether to screen for a condition, choose a test strategy, or select a type of treatment. The first step to clinical decision analysis is to build a decision tree, which is a graphical representation of the decision to analyze, strategies to compare, and clinical outcomes of each strategy [6]. The second step in decision analysis is to generate probabilities of the likelihood of events ranging from zero for impossible to one of absolute certainty

[6]. The third and final step of decision analysis is to calculate the total value associated with each possible course of action by multiplying the probability by the utility. The branch with the highest total value, the more preferable is that clinical strategy. The lower the total value, the less desirable the clinical strategy will be [6]. These decision analysis methods can be performed using software programs that model what might happen to a hypothetical cohort of patients over a series of time cycles. These models are called multistate transition models or Markov models and permit a more sophisticated and true-to-life depiction and ultimately a more accurate decision analysis.

Clinical Practice Guidelines

Practice guidelines are "systematically developed statements to assist practitioner and patient decisions about appropriate health care for specific clinical circumstances" [6]. These guidelines provide an alternative edifice for integrating evidence into practice and utilize values to reach treatment recommendations. Practice guidelines rely on the consensus of a group of decision makers such as experts, frontline clinicians, and patients who carefully consider the evidence and decide the implications. Typically, these guidelines may be used to provide recommendations for a country, region, city, hospital, or clinic. The guidelines based on the evidence are dependent on who uses them. Clinicians practicing in rural areas of less industrialized countries without resources to monitor its intensity may provide different guidelines from an urban large institution serving an affluent community.

Assessing Recommendations

Recommendations pertain to decisions that involve particular groups of patients, the choices that will affect those patients, and the consequences of the choices. These recommendations must consider all patients who are relevant, or they will not be valid and will not be applicable. Along with the proper consideration of patient groups, and management options, the consequences of the options must also be measured. The clinician must determine all the outcomes that may result from a particular treatment to adequately prepare, counsel, and treat the patient. Clinicians recommending screening must identify all potential outcomes of the treatment to maximize the probability of the target outcome becoming reality. Once the clinician is sure the recommendation is based on all relevant patient groups, management options, and possible outcomes, and has detailed the options and outcomes, they must estimate the likelihood that each outcome will actually occur. This involves reviewing all the recommendations, consolidating and combining the relevant evidence that is detailed in systematic reviews, all without bias that will distort the results. Even considering all the right patient groups and options and ensuring there are systematic reviews of evidence linking options to outcomes is not enough. There also has to be an appropriate specification of values and preferences associated with the outcomes. The skill of linking treatment options with outcomes is a matter of science; the assignment of preferences to outcomes, however, is a matter of values.

A critical part of the application of evidence is patient safety. The evidence, guidelines, and treatment selected must be applied in a manner that will not harm the patient. Medical errors are a leading cause of death in the U.S. [7]. There are more deaths in hospitals each year from preventable medical mistakes than there are from vehicle accidents, breast cancer, or AIDS [7]. Up to 98,000 Americans die each year from preventable medical mistakes they experience during hospitalizations, according to the Institute of Medicine [7]. Because American health care remains very far below obtainable levels of error prevention and customer value, consumers are not appropriately educated about the extent of preventable healthcare mistakes, providers have not been given the rewards and incentives necessary to sustain a continual improvement process that will lead to a reduction of medical mistakes, and purchasing strategies needed to incorporate innovative ways to reduce mistakes. Organizations such as The Leapfrog Group are needed to assist in this error reduction process [7]. The Leapfrog Group was created to help save lives and reduce preventable medical mistakes by mobilizing employer purchasing power to initiate breakthrough improvements in the safety of health care and giving consumers information to make more informed hospital choices [7]. This group is a coalition of more than 100 public and private organizations that provide healthcare benefits. They work with medical experts throughout the U.S. to identify problems and propose solutions that it believes will improve hospital systems that could break down and harm patients. The Leapfrog Group, which represents approximately 32 million healthcare consumers in all 50 states, provides important information and solutions for consumers and healthcare providers. Some will view this type of organization as just another layer of bureaucracy to contend with; however, when it comes to patient safety, there should not be any action that should constitute a "burden" on our healthcare industry and health providers.

This stage of the evidence-based medicine process is largely a matter of judgment and values. However, information technology can be used to derive decision trees and Markov models. The complexity of such models that includes the calculation of probabilities is best suited for computer crunching rather than human calculation. The key consideration at this stage is the values, beliefs, and preferences of the patient; no computer system can decide for the patient what their values and expectations are and if a procedure is right for them. If the evidence-based medicine process has proven that a study is valid and feasible and the study population is similar to the patient at hand, at a minimum, the study results will provide a base for clinicians to determine what steps to take next. If nothing else, it will provide the clinician with a starting point for a discussion with the patient and the family, and, if necessary, lead to counseling about recovery, pain reduction, or end-of-life concerns.

Assess the Outcome

Assessing the outcome is the evaluation of the effectiveness and efficiency of the evidence research with the patient response to the treatment. Once a patient has been treated, and the outcome of the treatment has been determined, the clinician should go back and conduct some self-evaluation of how they performed during the evidence-based medicine process. During this self-evaluation, the clinician should evaluate his or her performance in asking the right questions, questions that resulted in the proper evidence. It should be determined if one asked well-formulated questions that included questions about background knowledge as well as those to determine the proper diagnosis. Clinicians should ask themselves if the questions being asked resulted in finding the proper evidence that matched the patient's population, symptoms, and preferences. The clinician should determine if they were able to narrow the search to the best source when searching for the evidence. Questions should be asked such as: Did I achieve access to the hardware and software required to obtain the best evidence for my clinical discipline? Do I have the right tools in the proper locations to be able to conduct a search quickly—at "just the right time"—when the patient is available to discuss the potential treatment? Did I access the proper sources and determine the proper study that would result in the evidence that fit my patient's situation? Was the evidence search efficient? If I was unable to find the proper evidence immediately, what methods were required to find the proper evidence? Clinicians should also determine if the level of critical appraisal skills they possess are sufficient to adequately determine if the evidence found is valid and fits the situation at hand. Physicians must determine if they are becoming more accurate and efficient in applying the critical appraisal measures.

One of the most import aspects of the self-evaluation process is for clinicians to determine if they have acquired the skills necessary to integrate evidence and the patient's values. A physician needs to become efficient in adjusting critical appraisal measures to fit the individual patient. Without a successful application of the evidence to the patient's situation, and within the patient's values and preferences, the treatment will ultimately fail. It is imperative for clinicians to conduct such an evaluation of their skill throughout the evidence-based medicine process. For without such an evaluation of these items, physicians will not develop the proper skills to adequately find and apply the proper evidence, and their patients will not receive the ultimate level of diagnosis and treatment necessary to bring them to optimal health.

Barriers to Evidence-Based Medicine

The application of evidence-based medicine in everyday clinical practice is not an easy task. Sources indicate there are at least four major barriers to application including (1) the difficulty in finding sound evidence, (2) the lack of clarity of standards of evidence and interpretation, (3) the mismatch between existing evidence and the clinical situation at hand, and (4) the increasing time pressures and constraints on clinicians that make it extremely challenging to find, synthesize, and interpret evidence that is relevant to a patient's problem [2]. There are also many social, organizational, or institutional barriers that inhibit the incorporation of research-based evidence into clinical practice. It is often difficult to locate and access patient-relevant information at the point of patient care. These barriers, however, can be overcome. Many naturally occurring as well as planned experiments and actions are under way that will in time overcome these barriers. Physician assistants, information specialists, and other healthcare professionals are increasingly becoming a part of physician practices and are integral in identifying evidence and recommending courses of action for implementation of such evidence.

Conclusion

Evidence-based medicine is not a cure-all or panacea whose practice will result in the best solution for each patient's problem. It is the integration of clinical expertise with the best available clinical evidence derived from systematic research, patient preferences, and choices. It is not intended to replace clinical expertise and judgment but rather is intended to enhance it. The practice of evidence-based medicine is a process of self-directed learning in which caring for patients creates the need for clinically important information about diagnoses, prognoses, treatment, harm, and many other aspects of health care. Evidence-based medicine provides a way for clinicians to keep up with the rapidly growing body of medical literature and to sharpen their skills of critically appraising evidence with clinical expertise and each patient's circumstances, all with the ultimate goal of providing the best care possible.

This new paradigm of medicine, combined with the remarkable advances in information technology, are the key components that are required to reach this ultimate goal. Information technology will virtually ensure the accessibility of a vast amount of reliable evidence to use for informed decisions, provide the means of analyzing the evidence, and applying the evidence, all within real-time patient care. Once the evidence has been obtained, analyzed, and applied, information technology will also prove instrumental in assessing the outcome of the application to the patient. Information technology touches all aspects of the evidence-based medicine process. Without the coupling of evidence-based medicine and information technology, two very important aspects of our healthcare industry, the patient will not receive the optimal care available. Information systems used within the healthcare industry, and in every stage of the evidence-based medicine process, have proven to be beneficial and will continue to influence the future and advancement of this field beyond what anyone ever imagined.

References

1. Eddy D. The challenge, clinical decision making from theory to practice. Sudbury: Jones and Bartlett; 1996. p. 2, 5.
2. Geyman J, Deyo R, Ramsey S. Evidence-based clinical practice concepts and approaches. Kidlington, Oxford: Butterworth-Heinemann; 2000.
3. Haynes B, Devereaux, PJ, Guyatt G. Clinical expertise in the era of evidence-based medicine and patient choice. ACP Journal Club 2002; Mar.–Apr.;136:A11.
4. Wennberg J. Dealing with medical practice variations: a proposal for action. Health Affairs 1984;3(2):6–32.
5. The Evidence-Based Medicine Working Group. In: Guyatt G, Rennie D, editors. User's guides to the medical literature essentials of evidence-based clinical practice. Chicago: AMA Press; 2002.
6. Gray G, Gray L. Evidence-based medicine: applications in dietetic practice. Perspect Practice Mag 2002;102(9):1263–1272.
7. Sackett D, Straus S, Richardson S, Rosenberg W, Haynes B. Evidence-based medicine: how to practice and teach EBM. 2nd ed. Edinburgh: Leith Walk; 2000.
8. McKesson Information Solutions Web site. http://infosolutions.mckesson.com/products/sets/clinical2.asp.
9. The Evidence-Based Medicine Working Group. In: Guyatt G, Rennie D, editors. User's guides to the medical literature: a manual for evidence-based clinical practice. Chicago: AMA Press; 2001.
10. Leapfrog Organization Web Site. http://www.leapfroggroup.org. The Leapfrog Group for Patient Safety Rewarding Higher Standards.

35
Aligning Process and Technology: Balancing Capability with Reality-Based Processes

KAREN L. KNECHT, MARION J. BALL, and NHORA CORTES-COMERER

Healthcare organizations need to place greater emphasis on optimizing workflow and on new automation tools that focus on how work is carried out.

The pressures on the healthcare industry continue to escalate. In addition to concerns about improving financial performance, the industry is also beleaguered by the effects of reduced reimbursements, severe staff shortages in critical areas such as nursing and pharmacy, and the ever-increasing burden of regulatory compliance. More recently, the release of two reports by the Institute of Medicine (IOM) on the state of health care in the United States cast a further pall. In 2000, the IOM's Committee on Health Care Quality in America released dramatic figures connected to the numbers of deaths attributed annually to medical errors [1]. A second report followed suit in 2001 calling for the creation of a new health system that would help bridge what the Institute characterized as a quality chasm in the delivery of health care. Among the imperatives cited by the report to help the industry arrive at such a system were the effective application of information technologies and the reengineering of care processes [2].

The criticism exhibited by these reports is not intended to suggest that health care in the U.S. is a technological wasteland. To the contrary, U.S. medical research and technology is world renowned. Yet the system of healthcare delivery is such that it is stifling the application of that knowledge for the benefit of patient care. Critics point out that the healthcare industry in the U.S. has been among the least progressive in terms of adopting information technologies and innovative management practices. In fact, the hospital industry is the only remaining one whose mainline core processes are not yet automated. While other industries, such as manufacturing, long ago declared war on quality—guided by principles of total quality control, Six Sigma standards, and business process reengineering—the healthcare industry lags far behind. A comparison of healthcare quality's statistics with other industries indicates that to compete in world-class markets, manufacturing and service industry quality systems should operate in the range of five to six Sigma, or between 230 and 3.4 defects per million opportunities

Karen L. Knecht, RN, BSN, is Vice President of Advisory/Benefits Realization at Healthlink Incorporated in Houston, TX. Marion J. Ball, EdD, is Vice President for Clinical Informatics Strategies at Healthlink Incorporated in Baltimore, MD. Nhora Cortes-Comerer, BA, is a former Independent Consultant in healthcare informatics based in New York.

[3,4]. This same report claims that health care today operates in the range of two to four Sigma, or between 308,000 and 6210 defects per million [5].

To its credit, health care has been making serious strides in its efforts to adopt enabling technologies for the betterment of patient care. Critics maintain, however, that most of these innovations have focused on cost reduction, staffing, and improvement of function, and that these efforts are not sufficient. If the industry is to gain the greatest benefits from investments in technology, then process redesign needs to be a significant part of the equation. In essence, healthcare organizations need to place greater emphasis on aligning process and technology—on optimizing processes with new automation tools to transform the delivery of health care.

Origins of Process Redesign

The idea of aligning process and technology is not new. There have been references to this concept at least since the introduction of Michael Hammer and James Champy's revolutionary book *Reengineering the Corporation* in 1993 [6]. Other pioneers of redesign have also noted characteristics of processes that are especially relevant to health care. In 1990, Davenport and Short defined process redesign as "the analysis and design of workflows and processes within and between organizations" [7]. They further characterized processes as having customers, internal or external, and being based on three dimensions:

- *Entities*. Processes take place between organizational entities. They can be interorganizational or cross-functional.
- *Objects*. Processes result in the manipulation of objects. These objects an be physical or informational.
- *Activities*. Processes can involve two types of activities: managerial (e.g., developing a budget) and operational (e.g., filling a customer order).

In 1994, Teng et al. introduced the concept of metrics when they defined business process reengineering as "the critical analysis and radical redesign of existing business processes to achieve breakthrough improvements in performance measures" [8].

Process Redesign in Health Care

So how well do these concepts relate to health care? The healthcare enterprise, with its interchange of participants and entities, is host to myriad processes that cross organizational lines. Chief among the players is the patient, who is seen as the ultimate customer. Information is manipulated and managed continuously in both managerial and operational frameworks. And measurable process improvement is the rule of the day. Obvious complexities are involved in tying healthcare processes across an enterprise. The introduction of automation to streamline and reduce these complexities is critical to making significant improvements in the delivery of health care today.

Some of the challenges involved in automating health care have been attributed to the complexities of integrating disparate solutions in clinical and financial areas. The trend among healthcare information technology vendors has been to minimize these complexities by providing solutions on more common architectures. In addition, the introduction of workflow-based applications has increased. But none of these solutions is a "silver bullet." Applying automation, even the newer, more sophisticated solutions, without focused, intentional process redesign can increase the very complexities intended to be streamlined.

Most organizations considering process redesign as part of their implementation strategy have the best intentions at the start of large complex technology projects; however, too often, the following can occur:

1. There is a lack of a clearly defined organizational strategy and goals that are

a. Focused.
b. Understandable.
c. Achievable.
d. Measurable.

2. There is often executive sponsorship but lack of executive guidance on how to achieve these goals. This includes making the executive-level decisions required to guide the implementation teams in their efforts.
3. These is a lack of a focused and dedicated process redesign effort that is tightly linked with the system implementation effort and that can be carried forward postimplementation. Too many times, the same resources responsible for system implementation are also responsible for process redesign associated with system implementation.

Typical system implementation often begins with planning efforts focused on getting project teams defined and trained, conducting environmental assessments, and installing hardware. There is often a project kickoff with a few words by the executive sponsors and then . . . the design teams are off and running. Design sessions are held that use focus groups made up of systems analysts and subject matter experts who understand the specifics of how detailed work in their areas is carried out. These design teams are focused on making decisions that relate to system configuration, and the discussions are generally technology driven: What screen should come next? What fields should appear on this screen? What data should populate system tables? These sessions are an appropriate context for decisions related to system design, but the sessions do not take process implications and process redesign opportunities into consideration. When a significant decision arises during the course of a design session where a system configuration may impact operational processes, these groups will react in either of two ways: they will answer the question in such a way that they recreate their current world, or they will not feel empowered to make significant changes and will halt the design process while a more appropriate group considers the question. This results in a system design that is less likely to move the organization toward its goals and objectives and almost always includes delay, confusion, and lost time.

Alignment of process and technology calls for balancing the technology capabilities of commercially available products with reality-based process changes. It requires an approach that streamlines the system implementation, does not slow it down, ensures that new processes are put in place with the new systems, and provides a foundation for continuous optimization postimplementation. An important first step in that direction is the establishment of a project governance structure framed by a well-defined strategy, goals, and objectives.

Governance

The governance structure should follow a model that represents all aspects of the stakeholder community and provides a clear path for decision making (Figure 35.1). This may call for the refinement of existing committees and organizational structures or it may require the creation of a new structure from the ground up. It is important to

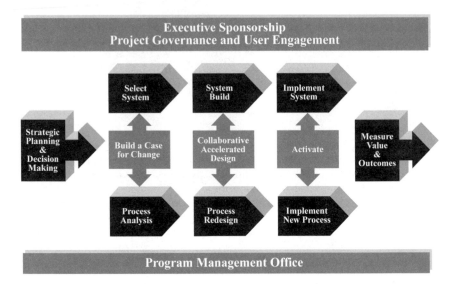

FIGURE 35.1. The governance structure for a process redesign project should represent all aspects of the stakeholder community and provide a clear path for decision making and accountability for these decisions.

ensure success from the beginning by having representation from the top tier of the organization, including the CEO, CFO, CIO, CNO, and physician leadership.

The senior executive leadership is responsible for more than just project sponsorship. It is responsible for providing ongoing executive guidance through timely and focused decision making as well as by establishing clear accountability for these decisions. It is also critical that ownership of the process redesign effort be driven by operational leadership, not by the technology side of the organization.

Another critical component of the project management structure is the process redesign team itself. The ability to carry out an analysis of the enterprise and develop a plan for the successful implementation of technology-supported process redesign requires an experienced team with the right balance of a unique set of skills including knowledge of vendors and their respective products, knowledge of available technologies, operations and processes, management of organizational change, project management, and group facilitation (Figure 35.2). In addition, the importance of user participation, particularly physician engagement, cannot be overemphasized. It is not enough to elicit physician buy-in after decisions have been made. Physicians must be fully engaged as participants in the analysis, selection, and decision-making process. The process redesign team works in collaboration with the executive team, organizational operations, as well as the systems team. Its broad responsibilities include:

1. Developing a thorough understanding of the enterprise operation.
2. Evaluating vendor potential and limitations.
3. Ensuring that system design decisions are balanced with the intended process redesign goals and objectives.
4. Determining performance metrics.
5. Developing change management strategies.

An often-overlooked role in the project governance structure is that of a skilled facilitator. The needs of various stakeholders, including organizational operations, the vendor, as well as the information technology team can often be in conflict. A skilled facilitator is responsible for:

1. Ensuring that effective work is carried out during the analysis and design phases of the project.
2. Identifying areas of opportunities, determining working solutions, and gaining consensus on decisions in a time-sensitive manner.
3. Facilitating decision making through tools such as nominal rankings and pros and cons analysis.
4. Developing and coordinating presentations of pertinent data (background, problem statement, findings, alternatives).
5. Capturing and managing decisions, issues, and next steps.
6. Maintaining meeting discipline.
7. Identifying cross-departmental, multidisciplinary, and cross-product interdependencies.

Finally, while engagement of the user community and the composition of the project teams are critical, a clear alignment of the decision-making process is required to

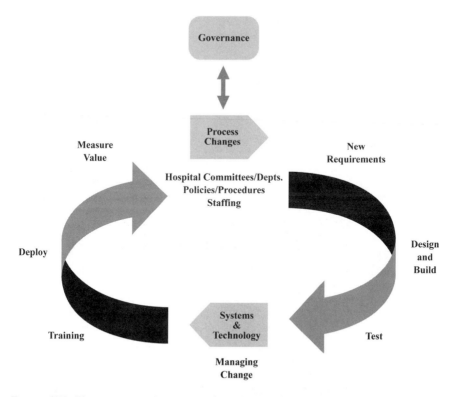

FIGURE 35.2. The process requires an experienced team with the right balance of skills including knowledge of vendors and their respective products, knowledge of available technologies, operations and processes, management of organizational change, project management, and group facilitation.

provide the directional framework within which the teams can operate successfully. A key component of the governance model is aligning decision making at the appropriate level of the organization so that those key business decisions that support the organization's goals and objectives are made at the top levels of the organization and communicated to the project teams.

Process and Workflow Analysis

Analysis of operations is one of the most important functions in process design. When well executed, it leads to a broad understanding of the enterprise and will usually show what processes currently in place are not effective. A map of the enterprise is a valuable tool in demonstrating how work is transmitted across the organization by function, geography, institution, system, and business unit (Figure 35.3).

In conducting the analysis of operations and of individual business units, the project team should keep in mind that information technology solutions are best applied to automate key processes where documents, information, or tasks are passed from one participant or department to another for action (whether human or machine), according to a set of rules or business logic. It is also important to align the organization's redesign strategy with the organization's business goals. The majority of these goals fall into one of seven broad categories: reducing operating expenses, increasing revenues,

Enterprise Map

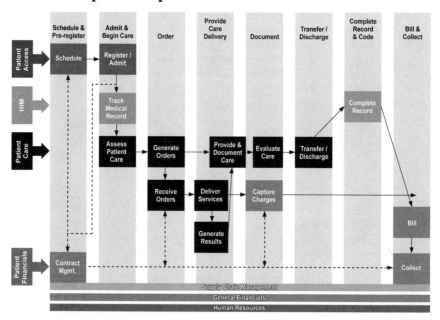

FIGURE 35.3. A map of the enterprise is valuable in demonstrating how work is transmitted across the organization by function, geography, institution, system, and business unit. A complementary process map diagrams the work path for each process and subprocess.

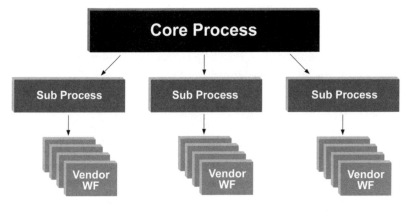

35.4

Process Levels - Example

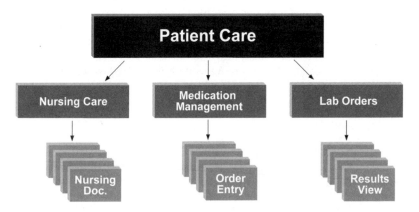

35.5

FIGURE 35.4, 35.5. Process redesign solutions are best applied to those automated key processes where documents, information, or tasks are passed from one participant or department to another for action. Within the healthcare organization's business structure, several operational processes can be identified either as core processes or subprocesses. Examples shown include Patient Care as a core process with Nursing Care, Medication Management, etc., as corresponding subprocesses, and additional subprocesses under each of these categories. Specific, detailed system workflows that apply to these processes and subprocesses can be identified.

complying with regulations, improving the quality of care, retaining staff, enhancing physician satisfaction, and/or enhancing patient satisfaction. Within these categories, a number of operational processes, both core processes and subprocesses, can be identified (Figures 35.4, 35.5).

Analysis of operations sets the stage for carrying out process analysis in conjunction with system design. Process analysis illuminates people and information flow issues and enables participants to understand where handoffs occur and the impact of specific design decisions on the overall process. Areas of impact include roles and responsibilities, policies and procedures, and organization culture as well as the facility.

Process tools such as process mapping and workflow diagrams are critical to under-standing and communicating these effects. Process mapping provides a means of illus-trating how work is carried out. Process maps provide a big-picture outlook for specific design decisions around workflow. This helps ensure that decisions are made in a way that benefits the organization as a whole, not just a specific department or group of users. The key to successful process analysis is a focused analysis that demonstrates immediate benefits around key system functions and provides a foundation for ongoing process optimization after initial system implementation.

A New Paradigm

Successful process redesign also requires the adoption of a new paradigm that calls for the analysis of individual operations within a framework of process and workflow, along with system function, and from the business unit level to the individual users (Figure 35.6). Less emphasis is placed on current state analysis with more emphasis on devel-oping the future state model and on operational impact analysis around the features and functions provided by vendor solutions. In the past, much effort was put on detailed current state analysis and building a future state that did not reflect the realities of the vendor solutions or organization strategies and timelines.

Designing a future state that incorporates both an understanding of the vendor's capabilities and supports the organizational business objectives becomes the basis for

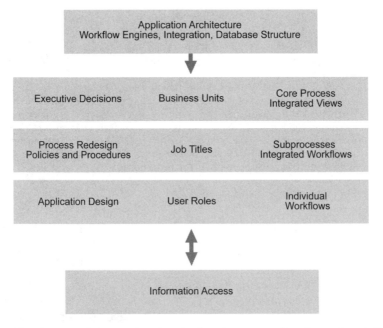

FIGURE 35.6. Process redesign requires the adoption of a new paradigm that analyzes individual operations within a framework of operational workflows, along with system functions, and from the business unit level to the individual user.

understanding the key business decisions required to design new processes and systems. Executive-level decisions are made, documented, and communicated at the start of the effort.

This new paradigm allows design sessions to be conducted within a framework of clearly defined goals and in the context of critical business decisions that were made by the executive and physician leadership. These decisions support the process decisions that are then made by the people who understand how the work is done on a day-by-day basis. When system design sessions are conducted within a framework of clearly defined goals and critical business decisions that have been made by senior management and physician leadership, these sessions can then focus on "How will we carry out the work that we've agreed to do?"

Process maps provide the big picture context for specific design decisions and support the redesign efforts related to policies and procedures as well as roles and responsibilities. Detailed workflows, on the other hand, illustrate individual roles within a process and how that role interacts with the system as defined by a set of business rules set out by the executive decisions. These workflows provide a context within which to make system design and configuration decisions in the context of how work is carried out.

Process redesign efforts continue throughout the entire implementation life cycle. Training is focused on how the system supports new processes, not just instructions on what buttons to select, which screens to use, and how to sign on to the system. Process maps can be used as a foundational tool during testing activities so that new processes along with the new technology are tested. Finally, in preparation for deployment, facility preparation is carried out to ensure that users understand the decisions made during the early design process and are prepared to make the organizational and operational changes needed to ensure success working under the new business model. Two essential principles to keep in mind are:

1. There needs to be an organized systematic approach to implementation.
2. Focus on changing those practices that represent the greatest effect on the patient experience and organizational efficiency.

Some Thoughts About Return on Investment

Regardless of the process being redesigned, metrics are typically cast in the form of expected benefits or results and include such factors as customer wait times, number of claims denials, etc. While these examples provide one way to measure the success of redesign efforts, how do they relate to the inevitable question of return on investment (ROI)? According to a study by Chapin, Forrer, and Timur, the vast, but hard-to-measure intangible benefits of information technology (IT) make it difficult to measure ROI using traditional methods and creates a unique challenge for managers [3].

Traditional ROI models assume that costs and benefits are known and expressed in a common metric, such as money [3,9]. This is not always the case when measuring ROI for IT in health care. One major reason is the close interaction between structure, process, and outcome that makes the tracking of specific benefits to IT so complex. As Chapin et al. state, clinical process improvement through the use of technology cannot be considered IT projects in themselves, but projects targeted at developing new or improved processes or activities. According to Chapin et al. and also Axson, the best method to measure ROI is to take the three areas of people, process, and technology and then translate these into quantifiable returns related to utility of the products and services offered and the cost of delivering them [3,10]. Isolating a single input and attempting to measure its impact, they maintain, is akin to assessing the direct contribution of cheese to a pizza [3,10].

The IT–ROI debate will undoubtedly continue fo some time to come. Meanwhile, the best approach for managers is to continue articulating objectives in terms of business goals, for example, to evaluate and modify processes in terms of the best applicable technology that will lead to increased productivity, less paperwork, increased employee morale, and customer satisfaction.

References

1. Kohn LT, Corrigan JM, Donaldson MS, editors. Committee on Quality Health Care in America, Institute of Medicine. To err is human: building a safer health system. Washington, DC: National Academy Press; 2000.
2. Committee on Quality of Healthcare in America, Institute of Medicine. Crossing the quality chasm: a new health system for the 21st century. Washington, DC: National Academy Press; 2001.
3. Chapin MA, Forrer DA, Timur A. The examination on return on investment for information technology in healthcare (hospital) industry to achieve quality of care. International College (unpublished).
4. Swinney Z. Should you calculate your process sigma?—with examples. Retrieved December 5, 2001 by Chapin, Forrer, and Timur from http://www.isixsigma.com/library/content/c010730b.asp.
5. Merry MD, Crago MG. The past, present and future of health care quality. The Physician Executive 2001 Sept–Oct. Retrieved November 20, 2001, by Chapin, Forrer, and Timur from informatics-review.com/benefits.html Web site: http://www.informatics-review.com/benefits.html.
6. Hammer M, Champy J. Reengineering the corporation. New York: Harper Business; 1993.
7. Davenport TH, Short J. The new industrial engineering: information technology and business process redesign. Sloan Manag Rev 1990; 31(4):11–27.
8. Teng J, Grover V, Fiedler K. From business process reengineering to organizational transformation: charting a strategic path for the information age. Cal Manag Rev 1994;36(3):9–31.
9. Laudon KC, Laudon JP. Management information systems: organization and technology in the networked enterprise. Englewood Cliffs: Prentice Hall; 2000.
10. Axson D, CEO perspectives: calculating return on IT investment: a pointless effort? Review 2001; 1–4. Retrieved December 5, 2001 by Chapin, Forrer, and Timur, from http://www.dmreview.com/master.cfm?NavID=55&EdID=3015.

36
Clinical Decision Support Systems: Impacting the Future of Clinical Decision Making

Eta S. Berner and Tonya La Lande

If used properly, Clinical Decision Support Systems have the potential to change the way medicine has been taught and practiced.

With the increased focus on the prevention of medical errors that has occurred since the publication of the landmark Institute of Medicine report, *To Err Is Human*, computer-based physician order entry (CPOE) systems have been proposed as a key element of systems approaches to improving patient safety [1–4]. While CPOE systems alone can eliminate several types of errors, their major impact will be when they are linked to clinical decision support systems. Clinical decision support systems (CDSS) are computer systems designed to influence clinician decision making about individual patients when these decisions are made. If used properly, they have the potential to change the way medicine has been taught and practiced. This chapter will illustrate several types of CDSS, summarize current data on the use and effect of CDSS in practice, and will provide guidelines for users to consider as these systems begin to be incorporated in commercial systems and implemented outside the research and development settings.

Types of CDSS

There are a variety of systems that can potentially support clinical decisions. Even Medline and similar healthcare literature databases can support clinical decisions. Decision support systems have been incorporated in healthcare information systems for a long time, but these systems usually have supported retrospective analyses of financial and administrative data [5]. Recently, sophisticated data mining approaches have been proposed for similar retrospective analyses of both administrative and clinical data [6]. Although these retrospective approaches can be used to develop

Eta S. Berner, EdD, is Professor of Health Informatics in the Department of Health Services Administration at the School of Health Related Professions at the University of Alabama at Birmingham. Tonya La Lande is a graduate assistant in the Health Informatics Program of the Department of Health Services Administration at the School of Health Related Professions at the University of Alabama at Birmingham.

guidelines, critical pathways, or protocols to guide decision making at the point of care, such retrospective analyses are not usually considered to be CDSS. These distinctions are important because vendors often will advertise that their product includes decision support capabilities, but that may refer to the retrospective type of systems, not the kind that are designed to assist clinicians at the point of care. Metzger and her colleagues [7,8] have described CDSS using several dimensions. According to their framework, CDSS differ in the *timing* at which they provide support (before, during, or after the clinical decision making), how active or passive the support is, that is, whether the CDSS actively provides alerts or passively responds to physician input or queries. CDSS also differ in whether the information provided is general or clearly based on patient-specific information. Finally CDSS vary in how easy they are for busy clinicians to access [7]. Although CDSS have been developed over the past 30 years, many of them have been standalone systems or part of noncommercial computer-based patient record systems. In recent years, some of the originally noncommercial systems are now being more widely marketed and other vendors are beginning to incorporate CDSS with their computer-based patient records and physician order entry systems.

Another way that CDSS have been categorized is whether they are knowledge-based systems or nonknowledge-based systems that employ machine learning and other statistical pattern recognition approaches. We will focus on the knowledge-based systems, but will also discuss some examples of other approaches as well.

Knowledge-Based Decision Support Systems

Many of today's knowledge-based CDSS arose out of earlier expert systems research, where the aim was to build a computer program that could simulate human thinking [9,10]. Medicine was considered a good domain to which these concepts could be applied. In the past 15 years the developers of these systems began to adapt them so that they could be used more easily to support real-life patient care processes [11]. The intent of these decision support systems was no longer to simulate an expert's decision making, but to assist the clinician in his or her own decision making. The system was expected to provide information for the user, rather than to come up with "the answer," as was the goal of earlier expert systems [12]. The user was expected to filter that information and to discard erroneous or useless information. The user was expected to be active and to interact with the system, rather than just be a passive recipient of the output. This focus on the interaction of the user with the system is important in setting appropriate expectations for the way the system will be used.

There are three parts to most CDSS. These parts are the knowledge base, the inference or reasoning engine, and a mechanism to communicate with the user [13]. The knowledge base consists of compiled information, often, but not always, in the form of IF-THEN rules. An example of an IF-THEN rule might be, for instance, IF a new order is placed for a particular blood test that tends to change very slowly AND IF that blood test was ordered within the previous 48 hours, THEN alert the physician. In this case, the rule is designed to prevent duplicate test ordering. Other types of knowledge bases might include probabilistic associations of signs and symptoms with diagnoses or known drug–drug or drug–food interactions.

The second part of the CDSS is called the inference engine or reasoning mechanism, which contains the formulas for combining the rules or associations in the knowledge base with actual patient data.

Finally, there has to be a communication mechanism, a way of getting the patient data into the system and getting the output of the system to the user who will make the actual decision. In some standalone systems, the patient data need to be entered directly by the user. In most of the CDSS incorporated into electronic medical record (EMR) systems, the data are already in electronic form and come from the computer-based patient record, where they were originally entered by the clinician or may have come from laboratory, pharmacy, or other systems. Output to the clinician may come in the form of a recommendation or alert at the time of order entry, or, if the alert was triggered after the initial order was entered, systems of e-mail and wireless notification have been employed [14,15].

CDSS have been developed to assist with a variety of decisions. The example above described a system designed to provide support for laboratory test ordering. Diagnostic decision support systems have been developed to provide a suggested list of potential diagnoses to the users. The system might start with the patient's signs and symptoms, entered either by the clinician directly or imported from the EMR. The decision support system's knowledge base contains information about diseases and their signs and symptoms. The inference engine maps the patient signs and symptoms to those diseases and might suggest some diagnoses for the clinicians to consider. These systems generally do not generate only a single diagnosis, but usually generate a set of diagnoses based on the available information. Because the clinician often knows more about the patient than can be put into the computer, the clinician will be able to eliminate some of the choices. Most of the diagnostic systems have been standalone systems, but the Wizorder system developed at Vanderbilt University has a diagnostic system that runs in the background, taking its information from the data already in the EMR [16]. This system has been incorporated into the McKesson Horizon Clinicals™ system.

Other systems can provide support for medication orders, a major cause of medical errors [1,17]. The input for the system might be the patient's laboratory test results for the blood level of a prescribed medication. The knowledge base might contain values for therapeutic and toxic blood concentrations of the medication and rules on what to do when a toxic level of the medication is reached. If the medication level were too high, the output might be an alert to the physician [17,18]. There are CDSS that are part of physician order entry systems that take a new medication order and the patient's current medications as input, the knowledge base might include a drug database, and the output would be an alert about drug interactions so the physician could change the order. Similarly, input might be a physician's therapy plan, the knowledge base would contain local protocols or nationally accepted treatment guidelines, and the output might be a critique of the plan compared to the guidelines [18]. Some hospitals that have implemented these systems allow the user to override the critique or suggestions, but often the users are required to justify why they are overriding it.

Nonknowledge-Based CDSS

Unlike knowledge-based decision support systems, some of the nonknowledge-based CDSS use a form of artificial intelligence called machine learning, which allows the computer to learn from past experiences and/or to recognize patterns in the clinical data [19]. Artificial neural networks and genetic algorithms are two types of nonknowledge-based systems [19].

Artificial Neural Networks

Research in neural networks has been going on since the 1940s [20]. Artificial neural networks (ANN) simulate human thinking and learn from examples [19]. An ANN consists of nodes called neurodes (which correspond to neurons) and weighted connections (which correspond to nerve synapses) that transmit signals between the neurodes in a unidirectional manner [19,21]. An ANN contains three layers, which include the input layer, output layer, and hidden layer [19]. The input layer is the data receiver and the output layer communicates the results, while the hidden layer processes the incoming data and determines the results [19].

This structure bears some similarities to the knowledge-based decision support systems, but rather than having a knowledge base derived from the medical literature or from an expert clinician's knowledge, the ANN analyzes the patterns in the patient data to derive the associations between the patient's signs and symptoms and a diagnosis. Many of the knowledge-based CDSS cover a wide range of diseases. For instance, the input may be the signs and symptoms exhibited by a patient and the output may be the possible diseases the patient may have. Neural networks often focus on a more narrow range of signs and symptoms, such as those associated with a single disease, such as myocardial infarction [22].

These systems can learn from examples by supplying them with known results for a large amount of data [21]. The system will study this information, make guesses for the correct output, compare the guesses to the given results, find patterns that match the input to the correct output, and adjust the weights of the connections between the neurodes accordingly to produce the correct results [21]. This iterative process is known as training the artificial network [21]. In the example with myocardial infarction, for instance, the data including a variety of signs and symptoms from large numbers of patients who are known to either have or not have a myocardial infarction can be used to train the neural network. Once the network is trained, that is, once the weighted associations of signs and symptoms with the diagnosis are determined, the system can be used on new cases to determine if the patient has a myocardial infarction.

There are many advantages and disadvantages to using artificial neural networks. Advantages include eliminating the need to program IF-THEN rules and eliminating the need for direct input from experts [19]. ANNs also can process incomplete data by inferring what the data should be and can improve every time they are used because of their dynamic nature [19]. ANNs also do not require a large database to make predictions about outcomes, but the more comprehensive the training data set is, the more accurate the ANN is likely to be [21]. Even though all these advantages exist, there are some disadvantages. The training process involved can be time consuming [19]. ANNs follow a statistical pattern recognition approach to derive their formulas for weighting and combining data. The resulting formulas and weights are often not easily interpretable, and the system cannot explain or justify why it infers certain data the way it does, which can make the reliability and accountability of these systems a concern [19].

Despite the above concerns, artificial neural networks have many applications in the medical field. In a review article of the use of neural networks in health care, Baxt provides a chart that shows various applications of ANNs, which include diagnosis of appendicitis, back pain, dementia, myocardial infarction, psychiatric emergencies, sexually transmitted diseases, skin disorders, and temporal arteritis [23]. Study results have shown that ANN's diagnostic predictions for pulmonary embolisms were as good or better than physicians' predictions [24]. Another study also showed that neural networks did a better job than two experienced cardiologists in detecting acute myocardial infarction in electrocardiograms with concomitant left bundle branch block [25]. Studies have also shown that ANNs can predict which patients are at high risk for cancers such as oral cancer [26]. The studies described in Baxt's chart illustrate other applications of ANNs, including predicting outcomes for things such as surgery recovery, liver transplants, cardiopulmonary resuscitation, and heart valve surgery as well as the analysis of waveforms of ECGs and EEG [23].

Genetic Algorithms

Another nonknowledge-based method used to create CDSS is with a genetic algorithm (GA). GAs were developed in the 1940s by John Holland at MIT and are based on the evolutionary theories by Darwin that dealt with natural selection and survival of the fittest [19]. Just as species change to adapt to their environment, "GAs 'reproduce' themselves in various recombinations in an effort to find a new recombinant that is better adapted than its predecessors" [19]. In other words, without any domain-specific knowledge, components of random sets of solutions to a problem are evaluated, the best ones are kept and are then recombined and mutated to form the next set of possible solutions to be evaluated, and this continues until the proper solution is discovered [27]. The fitness function is used to determine which solutions are good and which should be eliminated [19]. GAs are similar to neural networks in that they derive their knowledge from patient data.

Genetic algorithms have also been applied in health care, but there are fewer examples of this type of CDSS than those based on neural networks. For example, GAs have proved to be a helpful aid in the diagnosis of female urinary incontinence [28].

Although research has shown that CDSS based on pattern recognition and machine learning approaches may be more accurate than the average clinician in diagnosing the targeted diseases, many physicians are hesitant to use these CDSS in their practice because the reasoning behind them is not transparent [24]. Most of the systems that are available today involve knowledge-based systems with rules, guidelines, or other compiled knowledge derived from the medical literature. The research on the effectiveness of CDSS has come largely from a few institutions where these systems were developed.

Effectiveness of CDSS

Clinical decision support systems have been shown to improve both patient outcomes as well as the cost of care. While many of the published studies have come out of Brigham and Women's Hospital, LDS in Utah, and the Regenstrief Medical Institute, which have had these systems for a long time, there are an increasing number of studies from other places that have shown positive impact [4,17,29–33]. The systems can minimize errors by alerting the physician to potentially dangerous drug interactions, and the diagnostic programs have also been shown to improve physician diagnoses [33–35]. The reminder and alerting programs can potentially minimize problem severity and prevent complications. For instance, in the past few years there have been articles in *JAMA* and the *New England Journal of Medicine* that have shown how programs that warn of early adverse drug events have had an impact on both cost and quality of care [4,29,32,36]. These data have prompted the Leapfrog Group and others to advocate their use in promoting patient safety [3]. However, most of the studies that have shown the strongest effect on reducing medication errors have been done at institutions with very sophisticated, internally developed systems and where use of an EMR, CPOE, and CDSS are a routine and accepted part of the work environment. Without that cultural milieu, and an understanding of the strengths and limitations of the systems, integration of these systems may prove more difficult [37].

Several published reviews of CDSS have emphasized the dearth of evidence of similar effectiveness on a broader scale and have called for more research and especially qualitative research that elucidates the factors which lead to success outside the development environment [38,39]. Studies of the Leeds abdominal pain system, an early CDSS for diagnosis of the acute abdomen, showed success in the original environment and much more limited success when the system was implemented more broadly [40,41]. Not only is there a lack of studies on the impact of the diffusion of successful systems, but also there are still few places utilizing the systems themselves [36]. The KLAS research and consulting firm conducted an extensive survey of the sites that had implemented CPOE systems [42]. As KLAS defines these systems, CPOE systems usually include CDSS that were defined as, ". . . alerting, decision logic and knowledge tools to help eliminate errors during the ordering process." [42]. Although most of the CPOE systems provide for complex decision support, the results of the KLAS survey showed that most sites did not use more than 10 alerts and many sites did not use any of the alerting mechanisms at order entry. These data on system use outside the research and development sites underscore that despite evidence that CDSS has many benefits, as the KLAS report states, "The use of active complex alerts is in its infancy" [42].

Metzger and McDonald report anecdotal case studies of successful implementation of CDSS in ambulatory practices [8]. While such descriptions can motivate others to adopt CDSS, they are not a substitute for systematic evaluation of implementation in a wide range of settings. Unfortunately, when such evaluations are done, the results have sometimes been disappointing. A recent study incorporating guideline-based decision support systems in 31 general practice settings in England found that although care was not optimal before implementing the computer-based guidelines, there was little change in health outcomes after the system was implemented. Further examination showed that although the guideline was triggered appropriately, clinicians did not go past the first page and essentially did not use it [18].

There is a body of research that has shown that physicians have many unanswered questions during the typical clinical encounter [43,44]. This should provide an optimal opportunity for the use of CDSS, yet a study tracking the use of a diagnostic system by medical residents indicated very little use [45]. This is unusual given that this group of physicians in training should have even more "unanswered questions" than more experienced practitioners, but may partially be explained by the fact that the system was a standalone system not directly integrated into the workflow. Also, Teich et al. suggest that reminder systems and alerts usually work, but systems that challenge the physicians' judgment or require them to change their care plans are much more difficult to implement [46]. A case study of a CDSS for notification of adverse drug events supports this contention. The study showed that despite warnings of a dangerous drug level, the clinician in charge repeatedly ignored the advice. The article describes a mechanism of alerting a variety of clinicians, not just the patient's primary physician, to assure that the alerts receive proper attention [17].

Thus, although these systems can potentially influence the process of care, if they are not used, they obviously cannot have an impact. Integration into both the culture and the process of care is going to be necessary for these systems to be optimally used.

Wong et al., in an article published in 2000, suggest that the incentives for use are not yet aligned to promote wide-scale adoption of CDSS [37]. Those incentives may be changing, but these systems are not equally attractive to all stakeholders. As Doolan and Bates [36] illustrate, hospital administrators are beginning to see advantages to adoption of CDSS and other clinical computing applications, but the perceived disadvantages for physicians loom larger than the advantages. There are several reasons why implementation of CDSS is challenging.

Some of the problems include issues of how the data are entered. Other issues include the development and maintenance of the knowledge base and issues around the vocabulary and user interface. Finally, since these systems may represent a change in the usual way patient care is conducted, there is a question of what will motivate their use, which also relates to how the systems are evaluated.

Implementation Challenges

The first issue concerns data entry, or how the data will actually get into the system. Some systems require the user to query the systems and/or enter patient data manually. Not only is this "double data entry" disruptive to the patient care process, it is also time consuming, and especially in the ambulatory setting, time is scarce. It is even more time consuming if the system is not mobile and/or requires lengthy log-on. Much of this disruption can be mitigated by integrating the CDSS with the hospital information system and EMR. As mentioned above, several commercial products have integrated decision support capabilities. What that means is if the data are already entered into the medical record, the data are there for the decision support system to act upon, and, in fact, many systems are potentially capable of drawing from multiple ancillary systems as well. This is a strength, but not all clinical decision support systems are integrated, and without technical standards assuring integration of ancillary systems, such linkages may be difficult. There are also a number of standalone systems, some of the diagnostic systems and some drug interaction systems, for example. This means that patient data have to be entered twice, once into the medical record system and again into the decision support system. For many physicians, this double data entry can limit the usefulness of such systems.

A related question is who should enter the data in a standalone system or even in the integrated hospital systems. Physicians are usually the key decision makers, but they are not always the person who interacts with the hospital systems. One of the reasons for linking CDSS with physician order entry is that it is much more efficient for the physician to receive the alerts and reminders from decision support systems. The issue is not just order entry, but also mechanisms of notification. The case study mentioned earlier described a situation where the physician who received the alert ignored it [17]. These systems can be useful, but their full benefits cannot be gained without collaboration between the information technology professionals and the clinicians.

Although it might not seem that vocabularies should be such a difficult issue, it is often only when clinicians actually try to use a system, either a decision support system or computer-based patient record or some other system with a controlled vocabulary, that they realize either the system cannot understand what they are trying to say or, worse yet, it uses the same words for totally different concepts or different words for the same concept. The problem is that there are no standards that are universally agreed upon for clinical vocabulary and, since most of the decision support systems have a controlled vocabulary, errors can have a major impact.

Future Uses of CDSS

Despite the challenges in integrating CDSS, when properly used, they have the potential to make significant improvements in the quality of patient care. While more research still needs to be done evaluating the impact of CDSS outside the development settings and the factors that promote or impede integration, it is likely that increased commercialization will continue. There is increasing interest in clinical computing and, as handheld and mobile computing become more widely adopted, better integration into the process of care may be easier [47]. In addition, the concerns over medical errors and patient safety are prompting a variety of initiatives that will lead to increased incorporation of CDSS. Physicians are legally obligated to practice in accordance with the standard of care, which at this time does not mandate the use of CDSS. However, that may be changing. The issue of the use of information technology in general, and clinical decision support systems in particular, to improve patient safety has received a great deal of attention recently [1,2,48]. Healthcare administrators, payers, and patients are concerned now more than ever before that clinicians use the available technology to reduce medical errors. The Leapfrog Group [3] has advocated physician order entry (with an implicit coupling of CDSS to provide alerts to reduce medication errors) as one of their three main quality criteria.

Even if the standard of care does not yet require the use of such systems, there are some legal and ethical issues that have not yet been well addressed. One interesting legal case that has been mentioned in relation to the use of technology in health care is the Hooper decision. This case involved two tugboats (the T.J. Hooper and its sister ship) that were pulling barges in the 1930s when radios (receiving sets) were available, but not widely used on tugboats. Because the boats did not have a radio, they missed storm warnings and their cargo sank. The barge owners sued the tugboat company, even though the tugboat captains were highly skilled and did the best they could under the circumstances to salvage their cargo. They were found liable for not having the radio, even though it was still not routinely used in boats. Parts of the following excerpt from the Hooper decision have been cited in other discussions of CDSS [49].

> ... whole calling may have unduly lagged in the adoption of new and available devices. It never may set its own tests, however persuasive be its usages. Courts must in the end say what is required; there are precautions so imperative that even their universal disregard will not excuse their omission. But here there was no custom at all as to receiving sets; some had them, some did not; the most that can be urged is that they had not yet become general. Certainly in such a case we need not pause; when some have thought a device necessary, at least we may say that they were right, and the others too slack [50].

It has been suggested that as CDSS and other advanced computer systems become more available, not only may the Hooper case provide legal precedent for liability for failure to use available technology, but the legal standard of care may also change to include using available CDSS [51]. Since this area is still new, it is not clear what type of legal precedents will be invoked for hospitals that choose to adopt, or avoid adopting, CDSS. One legal scholar suggests that while the use of CDSS may lower a hospital's risk of medical errors, healthcare systems may incur new risks if the systems either cause harm or are not implemented properly [52]. In any case, there are some guidelines that users can follow that may help to ensure more appropriate use of CDSS.

Guidelines for Selecting and Implementing CDSS[1]

Assuring That Users Understand the Limitations

In 1986, Brannigan and Dayhoff highlighted the often different philosophies of physicians and software developers [53]. Brannigan and Dayhoff mention that physicians and software developers differ in regard to how "perfect" they expect their "product" to be when it is released to the public [53]. Physicians expect perfection from themselves and those around them. Physicians undergo rigorous training, have to pass multiple licensing examinations, and are held in high esteem by society for their knowledge and skills. In contrast, software developers often assume that initial products will be "buggy" and that eventually most errors will be fixed, often as a result of user feedback and bug reports. There is usually a version 1.01 of almost any system almost as soon as version 1.0 has reached most users. Because a CDSS is software that in some ways functions like a clinician consultant, these differing expectations can present problems, especially when the knowledge base and/or reasoning mechanism of the CDSS is not transparent to the user. The vendors of these systems have an obligation to learn from the developers and to inform the clinicians using the CDSS of its strengths and limitations.

Assuring That the Knowledge Is from Reputable Sources

Users of CDSS need to know the source of the knowledge if they purchase a knowledge-based system. What rules are actually included in the system and what is the evidence behind the rules? How was the system tested before implementation? This validation process should extend not just to testing whether the rules fire appropriately in the face of specific patient data (a programming issue), but whether the rules themselves are appropriate (a knowledge-engineering issue). Sim et al. advocate the use of CDSS to promote evidence-based medical practice, but this can only occur if the knowledge base contains high qualify information [54].

Assuring That the System Is Appropriate for the Local Site

Vendors need to alert the client about idiosyncrasies that are either built into the system or need to be added by the user. Does the clinical vocabulary in the system match that in the EMR? What are the normal values assumed by a system alerting to abnormal laboratory tests and do they match those at the client site? In fact, does the client have to define the normal values as well as the thresholds for the alerts?

The answers to the questions on what exactly the user is getting are not always easy to obtain. We conducted a survey of the nine vendors listed in the top 100 companies of the annual vendor revenue survey of *Healthcare Informatics*, who also indicated that their CPR systems contained decision support functionality [55,56]. We began by reviewing the vendor Web sites to see how much information about the CDSS they contained. If we could not find answers to our questions on the Web site, we telephoned the vendors to find an appropriate person to answer our questions.

---

[1] Significant parts of this section and smaller parts of other sections were reprinted with permission from Berner ES. Ethical and legal issues in the use of clinical decision support systems. J Healthcare Inform Manag, 2002;16(4):34–37.

The survey asked vendors whether they provided a knowledge base/medical logic model to their customers. If they answered yes, they were asked what the knowledge source was, if the knowledge base was updated, how often the knowledge base was updated, and if there was an additional charge for the updates. If they answered no to providing a knowledge base, they were asked if they provided templates for the user to develop rules, if there was an additional charge for these templates, how much effort was involved for the customer to build these rules, and whether they provided mechanisms to obtain/buy rules from somewhere else, and if there was a charge.

None of the vendor Web sites contained answers to all the questions on the survey. The knowledge source was given on one of the nine vendor Web sites, and two of the nine vendor Web sites indicated that they provided templates to develop the rules. All nine of the vendors needed to be contacted to obtain additional information. Obtaining this information turned out to be a more challenging task than expected.

Three of the vendor representatives with whom we spoke were very helpful and open to answering the questions. The other six did not know the answers to some or all of the questions and said they would refer our questions to someone else who would call us back. After waiting a month with no response from the vendors, we utilized our personal contacts with users of five of the remaining systems to request either answers or a referral to another vendor contact. Two of those contacts returned answers to most of our questions, leaving us with four companies for whom we could not obtain answers to most of our questions.

The results of our survey are based on the full answers to the questionnaire from four of the nine clinical decision support vendors as well as the information that was obtained from the Web sites and the partial answers from one of the five remaining vendors. The results show that five of the nine vendors provide a knowledge base/medical logic models. Two of the five vendors said their knowledge base comes from rules they developed based on experience with their customer base in the past. One uses a physician order entry system and knowledge source that was developed and is currently used by a well-known academic medical center, and one of the five vendors did not know the source of their knowledge base. Three of the five vendors said they update their knowledge base, one does not perform updates, and two vendor representatives did not know if their knowledge base was regularly updated. Two of the vendors who said they provided updates were not sure how often these occurred.

The results also show that seven of the nine vendors provide templates to develop the rules. Three of these seven vendors did not have an answer to the question about the amount of effort that is involved for the customer in building these rules. Four of the seven vendors said it did not take much effort to build the rules with the templates. In fact, one vendor pointed out that the time-consuming part was researching, validating, and approving new rules. Also, one vendor said they provide a community Web site for their customers so they can post and share rules on the Web. Four vendors said they did not provide mechanisms to obtain/buy rules from somewhere else, one vendor said clients could obtain rules from professional committees and organizations, and four vendors did not have an answer to this question.

When users ask questions like those in our survey, they may find, as we did, that the decision support system provided is really just an expert system shell and that local clinicians need to provide the "knowledge" that determines the rules. For some systems, an effort has been made to use standards that can be shared among different sites, for example, the Arden syntax for medical logic modules [57], but local clinicians must still review the logic in shared rules to assure that they are appropriate for the local situation. Using in-house clinicians to determine the rules in the CDSS can assure its applicability to the local environment, but that means that extensive development and testing must be done locally to assure the CDSS operates appropriately. Often a considerable amount of physician time is needed. Without adequate involvement by clinicians, there is a risk that the CDSS may include rules that are inappropriate for the local situation, or if there are no built-in rules, that the CDSS may only have limited functionality. On the other hand, local development of the logic behind the rules may also mean that caution should be exercised if the rules are used in different sites. The important thing is for the user to learn at the outset what roles the vendor and the client will have to play in the development and maintenance of the systems. Based on our experience, and despite the fact that many of the vendors did make an effort to provide the answers for us, there were still many important questions for which we could not easily obtain the information. These results can help to explain the findings from the KLAS survey of CPOE users, which involved users of systems of many of the same vendors we surveyed. Although these systems have decision support capabilities, the effort involved in customizing the CDSS for the local site may be considerable and the result may be that these capabilities are underutilized [42].

Assuring That Users Are Properly Trained

Just as the vendor should inform the client how much work is needed to get the CDSS operational, the vendor also should inform the client how much technical support and/or clinician training is needed for physicians to use the system appropriately and/or understand the systems' recommendations. It is not known whether the users of some CDSS need special clinical expertise to be able to use it properly, in addition to the mechanics of training on the use of the CDSS. For instance, systems that base their recommendations on what the user enters directly or on what was entered into the medical record by clinicians may reach faulty conclusions or make inappropriate recommendations if the data on which the CDSS bases its recommendations are incomplete or inaccurate. Also, part of the reason for integrating CDSS with physician order entry is that it is assumed that the physician has the expertise to understand, react to, and determine whether to override the CDSS recommendation. Diagnostic systems, for instance, may make an appropriate diagnostic suggestion that the user fails to recognize [35,58]. Thus, vendors of CDSS need to be clear about what expertise is assumed in using the system and those who implement the systems need to assure that only the appropriate users are allowed to respond to the CDSS advice.

As these systems mature and are more regularly integrated into the healthcare environment, another possible concern about user expertise arises. Will users lose their ability to determine when it is appropriate to override the CDSS? This "de-skilling" concern is similar to that reported to happen when calculators became commonplace in elementary and secondary education, and children who made errors in using the calculator could not tell that the answers were obviously wrong. The solution to the problem is not to remove the technology but to remain alert to both the positive and negative potential impact on clinician decision making.

Monitoring Proper Utilization of the Installed CDSS

Simply having a CDSS installed and working does not guarantee that it will be used. Systems that are available for users if they need them, such as online guidelines or protocols, may not be used if the user has to choose to consult the system and especially if the user has to enter additional data into the system. Automated alerting or reminder systems that prompt the user automatically can address the issue of the user not recognizing the need for the system, but another set of problems arises with the more automated systems. They must be calibrated to alert the user often enough to prevent serious errors, but not so frequently that they will be ignored eventually. As mentioned earlier, there have been reports of CDSS triggering an alert that the patient's physician ignored [17]. What this means is that testing the system with the users and monitoring its use is essential for the CDSS to operate effectively in practice as well as in theory.

Assuring the Knowledge Base Is Monitored and Maintained

Once the CDSS is operational at the client site, a very important issue involves the responsibility for updating the knowledge base in a timely manner. New diseases are discovered, new medications come on the market, and issues like the threat of bioterrorist actions prompt a need for new information to be added to the CDSS. Does the vendor have an obligation to provide regular knowledge updates? Such maintenance can be an expensive proposition given both rapidly changing knowledge and systems with complex rule sets. Who is at fault if the end user makes a decision based on outdated knowledge, or, conversely, if updating one set of rules inadvertently affects others, causing them to function improperly? Such questions have been raised for more than 15 years [59], but because CDSS are still not in widespread use, the legal issues have not really been tested or clarified.

The Food and Drug Administration (FDA) is charged with device regulation and has recently begun to reevaluate its previous policy on software regulation. Up to now, many standalone CDSS have been exempt from FDA device regulation because they required "competent human intervention" between the CDSS advice and anything being done to the patient [60]. Even if the rules change and CDSS are required to pass a premarket approval process, monitoring would need to be ongoing to assure that the knowledge does not get out of date and that what functioned well in the development process still functions properly at the client site. For this reason, local software review committees, who would have the responsibility to monitor local software installations for problems, obsolete knowledge, and harm as a result of use, have been advocated [61].

Conclusion

With the increasing interest and availability of CDSS, the likelihood is that more vendors will begin to incorporate them. As skepticism about the usefulness of computers for clinical practice decreases, the wariness about accepting the CDSS advice that many clinicians currently exhibit is likely to decrease. As research has shown, if CDSS are available and convenient, and if they provide what appears to be good information, they are likely to be heeded by clinicians [29,48,62, p. 953]. Finally, as CDSS become widespread, we must continue to remember that the role of the computer should be to enhance and support the human who is ultimately responsible for the clinical decisions.

References

1. Kohn LT, Corrigan JM, Donaldson MS, editors. To err is human: building a safer health system. Committee on Quality Health Care in America, Institute of Medicine. Washington, DC: National Academy Press; 2000.

2. Institute of Medicine. Crossing the quality chasm: a new health system for the 21st century. Washington, DC: National Academy Press; 2001.
3. The Leapfrog Group. www.leapfroggroup.org.
4. Bates DW, Leape LL, Cullen DJ, et al. Effect of computerized physician order entry and a team intervention of prevention of serious medical errors. JAMA 1998;28:1311–1316.
5. Oliveira, JO. A shotgun wedding: business decision support meets clinical decision support. J Healthcare Inform Manag 2002;16(4):28–33.
6. DeGruy KB. Healthcare applications of knowledge discovery in databases. J Healthcare Inform Manag 2000;14(2):59–69.
7. Perreault LE, Metzger JB. A pragmatic framework for understanding clinical decision support. In: Middleton B, editor. Clinical decision support systems. J Healthcare Inform Manag 1999;13(2):5–21.
8. Metzger J, MacDonald, K. Clinical decision support for the independent physician practice. California Healthcare Foundation; 2002.
9. Shortliffe EH, Axline SG, Buchanan BG, Merigan TC, Cohen SN. An artificial intelligence program to advise physicians regarding antimicrobial therapy. Comput Biomed Res 1973; 6(6):544–560.
10. Miller RA, Pople HE Jr, Myers JD. Internist-I, an experimental computer-based diagnostic consultant for general internal medicine. N Engl J Med 1982;307:468–476.
11. Miller R, McNeil M, Challinor S, Masarie F, Myers J. The Internist-1/Quick Medical Reference project: status report. West J Med 1986;145:816–822.
12. Miller RA, Masarie FE Jr. The demise of the "Greek Oracle" model for medical diagnostic systems. Methods Inform Med 1990;29:1–2.
13. Tan JKH, Sheps S. Health decision support systems. Gaithersburg: Aspen; 1998.
14. Kuperman GJ, Teich JM, Bates DW, et al. Detecting alerts, notifying the physician, and offering action items: a comprehensive alerting system. Proc AMIA Symp 1996;704–708.
15. Shabot MM, LoBue M, Chen J. Wireless clinical alerts for physiologic, laboratory and medication data. Proc AMIA Symp 2000;789–793.
16. Geissbuhler A, Miller RA. Clinical application of the UMLS in a computerized order entry and decision-support system. Proc AMIA Symp 1998;320–324.
17. Galanter WL, DiDomenico RJ, Polikaitis A. Preventing exacerbation of an ADE with automated decision support. J Healthcare Inform Manag 2002;16(4):44–49.
18. Eccles M, McColl E, Steen N, et al. Effect of computerised evidence based guidelines on management of asthma and angina in adults in primary care: cluster randomised controlled trial. BMJ.com 2002.
19. Marakas GM. Decision support systems in the 21st century. Upper Saddle River, NJ: Prentice Hall; 1999.
20. Devillers J, editor. Neural networks in QSAR and drug design. London: Academic Press; 1996.
21. Hirshberg A, Adar R. Artificial neural networks in medicine. Isr J Med Sci 1997; 33(10):700–702.
22. Cross S, Harrison R, Kennedy RL. Introduction to neural networks. Lancet 1995;346: 1075–1079.
23. Baxt WG. Application of artificial neural networks to clinical medicine. Lancet 1995;346: 1135–1138.
24. Holst H, Astrom K, Jarund A, et al. Automated interpretation of ventilation-perfusion lung scintigrams for the diagnosis of pulmonary embolism using artificial neural networks. Eur J Nuclear Med 2000;27(4):400–406.
25. Olsson SE, Ohlsson M, Ohlin H, Edenbrandt L. Neural networks—a diagnostic tool in acute myocardial infarction with concomitant left bundle branch block. Clin Physiol Funct Imaging 2002;22(4);295–299.
26. Naguib RNG, Sherbet GV, editors. Artificial neural networks in cancer diagnosis, prognosis, and patient management. Boca Raton: CRC Press; 2001.
27. Levin M. Use of genetic algorithms to solve biomedical problems. MD Comput 1995; 12(3):193–199.

28. Laurikkala J, Juhola M, Lammi S, Viikki K. Comparison of genetic algorithms and other classifications methods in the diagnosis of female urinary incontinence. Methods Inform Med 1999;38:125–131.
29. Evans RS, Pestotnik SL, Classen DC, et al. A computer-assisted management program for antibiotics and other antiinfective agents. N Engl J Med 1998;338:232–238.
30. Teich JM, Merchia PR, Schimz JL, et al. Effects of computerized physician order entry on prescribing practices. Arch Intern Med 2000;160:2741–2747.
31. Tierney WM, Miller ME, McDonald CJ. The effect on test ordering of informing physicians on the charges for outpatient diagnostic tests. N Engl J Med 1990;322:1499–1504.
32. Doolan DF, Bates DW, James BC. The use of computers for clinical care: a case series of advanced U.S. sites. J Am Med Inform Assoc 2003;10:94–107.
33. Berner ES, Maisiak RS, Cobbs CG, Taunton OD. Effects of a decision support system on physician diagnostic performance. J Am Med Inform Assoc 1999;6:420–427.
34. Berner ES, Maisiak RS. Influence of case and physician characteristics on perceptions of decision support systems. J Am Med Inform Assoc 1999;6:428–434.
35. Friedman CP, Elstein AE, Wolf FM, et al. Enhancement of clinicians' diagnostic reasoning by computer-based consultation. A multisite study of 2 systems. JAMA 1999;282:1851–1856.
36. Doolan DF, Bates DW. Computerized physician order entry systems in hospitals: mandates and incentives. Health Affairs 2002;21(4):180–188.
37. Wong HJ, Legnini MW, Whitmore HH. The diffusion of decision support systems in healthcare: are we there yet? J Healthcare Manag 2000;45(4):240–249; discussion 249–253.
38. Hunt D, Haynes R, Hanna S, Smith K. Effects of computer-based clinical decision support systems on physician performance and patient outcomes: a systematic review. JAMA 1998; 280(15):1339–1346.
39. Kaplan B. Evaluating informatics applications: clinical decision support systems literature review. Int J Med Inform 2001;64:15–37.
40. de Dombal FT. The diagnosis of acute abdominal pain with computer assistance: worldwide perspective. Ann Chir 1991;45:273–277.
41. Adams ID, Chan M, Clifford PC, et al. Computer aided diagnosis of acute abdominal pain: a multicentre study. Br Med J 1986;293:800–804.
42. KLAS Research and Consulting Firm. CPOE digest (computerized physician order entry). KLAS Enterprises, LLC; 2003.
43. Covell DG, Uman GC, Manning PR. Information needs in office practice: are they being met? Ann Intern Med 1985;103:596–599.
44. Gorman PN, Helfand M. Information seeking in primary care: how physicians choose which clinical questions to pursue and which to leave unanswered. Med Decision Making 1995; 15:113–119.
45. Berner ES, Maisiak RS, Phelan ST, et al. Use of a diagnostic decision support system by internal medicine residents. Unpublished study.
46. Teich JM, Merchia PR, Schmiz JL, Kuperman GJ, Spurr CD, Bates DW. Effects of computerized physician order entry on prescribing practices Arch Intern Med 2000; 160(18):2741–2747.
47. Turisco F, Case J. Wireless and mobile computing. California Healthcare Foundation; 2001.
48. Morris AH. Decision support and safety of clinical environments. Qual Saf Health Care 2002; 11(1):69–75.
49. Weed LL, Weed L. Opening the black box of clinical judgment—an overview. BMJ 1999;319:1279. Data supplement—complete version. http://www.bmj.org/cgi/content/full/319/7220/1279/DC1.
50. The T.J. Hooper. 60 F.2d 737 (2d Cir. 1932).
51. Osler, Harkins & Harcourt Law Firm. Ten commandments of computerization. Reprinted by permission by the Canadian Information Processing Society; 1992. http://www.cips.ca/it/resources/default.asp?load=practices.
52. Terry NP. When the machine that goes "ping" causes harm: default torts rules and technologically-mediated health care injuries. St. Louis U Law 2002;46:37.
53. Brannigan VM, Dayhoff RE. Medical informatics. The revolution in law, technology and medicine. J Legal Med 1986;7(1):53.

54. Sim I, Gorman P, Greenes RA, et al. Clinical decision support for the practice of evidence-based medicine. J Am Med Inform Assoc 2001;8:527–534.
55. Kittelson B. Spotlight: CPR systems. Healthcare Inform 2002;18(5):41–47.
56. The 2002 Healthcare Informatics 100. Healthcare Inform 2002;18(6):33–64.
57. Poikonen J. Arden syntax: the emerging standard language for representing medical knowledge in computer systems. Am J Health Syst Pharm 1997;54(3):281–284.
58. Berner ES, Maisiak RS, Heudebert GR, Young KR Jr. Clinician performance and prominence of diagnoses displayed by a clinical diagnostic decision support system. Proceedings, AMIA Symposium; 2003.
59. Miller RA, Schaffner KF, Meisel A. Ethical and legal issues related to the use of computer programs in clinical medicine. Ann Intern Med 1985;102:529–536.
60. Fried BM, Zuckerman JM. FDA regulation of medical software. J Health Law 2000; 33(1):129–140.
61. Miller RA, Gardner RM. Recommendations for responsible monitoring and regulation of clinical software systems. American Medical Informatics Association, Computer-based Patient Record Institute, Medical Library Association, Association of Academic Health Science Libraries, American Health Information Management Association, American Nurses Association. J Am Med Inform Assoc 1997;4(6):442–457.
62. Berner ES, Kennedy JI, Blackwell G, et al. Use of computer-generated ECG reports by residents and faculty. Proceedings of the Nineteenth Annual Symposium of Computer Applications in Medical Care. Philadelphia: Hanley & Belfus; 1995. p. 953.

37
Web-Enabled Medicine: The Challenge of Ensuring Quality Information and Care

GEORGE D. LUNDBERG and PATRICIA L. LUNDBERG

What started out as a medium for the delivery of content now has the potential to enhance the art and practice of medicine for both patients and physicians.

The Internet changes everything! Well, not exactly everything. The earth still gets its energy from the sun; Avogadro's number is still 6.023×10 to the 23rd; the Red Sox and Cubs will never meet in a World Series. But access to information has never realized such potential before the Internet. It speeds to our monitor screens—a potentially bewildering array of formal speeches, barroom conversation, music, newspapers, television and radio programs, telegraph messages, magazines, movies, medical journals, esoteric research publications, and other assorted items. John Seely Brown has called it "an entirely new medium, likely to change nearly every aspect of how we live, work and learn" [1]. The medical Internet encompasses eContent, eCommerce, eCommunity, eConnectivity, and now, even eCare and eCME (continuing education). The Internet knows neither geographic nor legal boundaries. Still, it is only a medium, not the message. As we move from a medium that delivers copious health information (eContent) to one that can transact eCommerce worldwide to one that will actually enhance the art and practice of medicine for patients and physicians alike (eConnectivity, eCare, and eCME), the challenge is to ensure the trustworthiness of information and care delivered as Web-enabled medicine on the Internet.

Trusting the Internet

Daniel Masys has termed the Internet the "flag bearer" of the societal trend of information technologies influencing the healthcare workforce. Because of access to every level of health information on the Internet, hundreds of millions of people worldwide will be able to participate in the knowledge economy, and, at the least, put new stress on their medical caregivers, and, at the most, replace them as irrelevant. As long ago

George D. Lundberg, MD, ScD, is Editor of Medscape General Medicine, www.medgenmed.com, and Special HealthCare Advisor to the Chair and CEO of WebMD. Patricia L. Lundberg, PhD, is Associate Professor and Executive Director of the Center for Cultural Discovery and Learning at Indiana University Northwest.

as 1996, Masys reported, former Speaker of the U.S. House of Representatives Newt Gingrich predicted (correctly) that motivated patients with chronic conditions would use information on the Internet to become more knowledgeable than some of their doctors about the management of their diseases [2].

A central concern about this powerful medium is that people may value too highly the information they receive on the Internet. People might be persuaded to think that, if it is on the Internet, it must be true, especially if the site is glitzy. The quality of the technology, however, is much greater than the quality of much of the information it conveys. Some people don't believe anything they read on the Internet because there is so much junk there, but neither can we believe everything we read on paper. How do we go about separating the truly beneficial elements of the medical Internet from the useless and the dangerous? And how do we transmit knowledge efficiently given that only 1 percent of the world's population owns a computer and only 30 percent of the world's population is literate? Similarly, not everyone in the United States owns a computer. The great potential to improve world health is thus limited by both the quality of Internet information and the ability of poor, third-world countries to retrieve it [3].

The Internet represents the most significant advance in human communication since the printing press. It is more important than the telephone, radio, or television, although Internet technology obviously draws from these technologies as well as others. Although it is still new, evolving, and difficult to understand, it represents a giant step to fast-forward. Anyone with an Internet-ready computer and a telephone line can communicate with anyone else, anywhere else in the world, almost instantly. Furthermore, we can communicate without government restrictions in most countries and few to no economic restrictions. The click of a mouse transmits words, ideas, sounds, and video images. The Internet enhances the exercise of freedom of the press, freedom of speech, and the free flow of information at very low cost.

The expansion of the Internet for medical use that occurred since 1995 defines a bona fide technological revolution in the delivery of medical care. In 1997, only 27 percent of U.S. consumers used the Internet for medical or health purposes. That number grew to 44 percent by 2002; of that number, 50 percent of consumers used the Internet to explore treatment options, 37 percent to seek information on disease prevention, 37 percent to investigate risk factors, 34 percent to obtain information about drugs, and 21 percent to research clinical trials. In 1995, only 3 percent of U.S. physicians were able to access the Web. In 1996 physician usage increased to 15 percent. In 1997, 20 percent of U.S. physicians used the Internet for medical purposes. In 2000 the number increased to 90 percent. In 2002 about 61 percent use it regularly; and of that number, 90 percent looked for clinical information, 74 percent read medical journals online, 63 percent conversed with their peers, 58 percent participated in online continuing medical education, and 42 percent attended conferences online. Rarely has physicians' use of any technology that they have not been paid to adopt taken off so rapidly. Once they understood the potential of such technology for their practice, they embraced it as readily as the general public has [4].

The Internet has become the primary means by which consumers access healthcare information. In 2002, 55 percent of consumers seeking health information go to the Web to find it. When asked in 2002 which Web sites they have used for health information over the previous 12 months, U.S. consumers answer: WebMD Network (includes WebMD, AOL Health, MSN Health, and Medscape), 72 percent; MayoClinic, 22 percent; Discovery Health, 19 percent; NIH, 16 percent; and CDC, 13 percent. The Internet is followed by TV news, 44 percent; health magazines, 37 percent; magazine advertisements, 19 percent; and TV ads, 18 percent. Of the total time spent accessing health information, consumers spent 32 percent on the Internet, followed by 23 percent on magazines, 22 percent on TV programs, 8 percent on TV ads, and 7 percent on magazine ads [5].

One of the megatrends of the 1990s was the drive toward patient autonomy. Patients began to increase the degree to which they took charge of their health. And why shouldn't they? It is their health, after all. The Internet did not create the movement toward patient autonomy, but it did enhance it. By functioning as the world's greatest medical library, at a fingertip and generally free of charge to anyone with a computer, modem, and line connector, the Internet provided the opportunity for patients to quickly access virtually the same information as the doctor on virtually any disease or condition, significantly, to any depth. Often, the motivated e-savvy patient may now know substantially more about a given condition than the physician, although not necessarily with the perspective and judgment brought by a full medical education. In 2002, 92 percent of U.S. physicians report that patients have talked to them about information that they have seen on the Internet about a medical condition or drug. This compares favorably with the 95 percent of physicians who report that patients have spoken to them about information they have seen on a TV commercial about a medical condition or drug [5].

No one knows exactly how many eHealth sites are available to the public. The number may be in the thousands or the millions, ranging in quality from excellent to abominable, with potential effects ranging from the very helpful to the dangerous. Anyone who knows how to navigate the Internet can be the author, editor, publisher, and owner of the information on a Web site. How valid is the information flooding across our monitor screens? This is a critical question for the 98 million Americans who use the Internet for health information.

Many sites are misinformed, some sites convey excellent health information, and a lot are in between. Many eHealth sites are managed without the traditional checks and balances of the medical journal world, where scientific articles are reviewed by peer scientists before publication, or even the fact-checking and confirmation of sources routine among newspapers, magazines, radio, and television. There is always some level of editorial control in the traditional public media: someone is identified as owning the publication or broadcast station, and someone, usually an editor or producer, is accountable for the information. On the other hand, on the Internet there may be no quality control beyond that exercised by the person who puts the information on the site, and no way to judge a site's timeliness or applicability. We used to say *caveat emptor* (let the buyer beware), but with the Internet, it is *caveat lector et viewor* (let the reader and viewer beware) [6].

Governing eContent, eCare, and eCME in America's Health

The governance of the medical Internet has been worked out well for some functions and not so well for others. eContent, eConnectivity, eCommerce, eCommunity, and eCare are all related but different. eContent and eCommunity are covered under the rubrics of the International Committee of Medical Journal Editors (ICMJE), Health on the Net (HON), HiEthics, and the Internet Health Care Coalition (IHC) eHealth Code of Ethics. eCommerce in the U.S. falls under the Federal Trade Commission. eConnectivity is largely governed by the Health Insurance Portability and Accountability Act (HIPAA), with particular attention to privacy and security. eCare in the U.S.

falls under the Council on Ethical and Judicial Affairs of the American Medical Association (CEJA), and the state licensing boards.

Because the Internet is the medium and not the message, all the various laws, regulations, rules, and ethics that apply to human discourse and intercourse also apply here. However, the historical silliness of some of our existing laws is magnified on the Internet. The U.S. licenses physicians state by state. But how is it sensible that a physician licensed in Pennsylvania can practice in eastern Pennsylvania but cannot practice across the Delaware River in western New Jersey? Geographic boundaries become even more artificial in cyberspace. Patients know this. Medscape asked readers in December 2000 to respond to a survey about whether responders would support new Internet medical licenses, the current system of medical licensing by states, or a national medical license. Respondents totaled more than 3000. The results demonstrated a desire for change: 66 percent favored a national medical license, 16 percent medical licensing by state, 11 percent a special Internet license, and 4 percent were uncertain [7].

T.E. Miller and A.R. Derse in *Health Affairs* in July 2002 argue that online care requires a "new regulatory paradigm" and that the distinction between providing health information and practicing medicine online needs to be more clearly delineated. They recommend a hybrid system that combines state and federal oversight to address interstate care [8]. Alan Green in a personal communication has proposed another approach, modeled along the lines of drivers' licenses, to maintain one in the state in which one lives and be subject to discipline there, but be allowed to drive (and practice) in all 50 states. Without a change in the current licensing system, it is illegal for physicians to practice across state or national boundaries. But medicine is already practiced across state or national boundaries through doctor-to-doctor consultations. It is both ethical and legal. Think of the patient in Kuwait with a complicated heart condition. The patient's Kuwaiti physician can transmit the EKG or cardiac catherization data electronically to Brigham and Women's Hospital in Boston over the Internet. A cardiologist there can interpret the data and consult by Internet immediately with the Kuwaiti physician, who then makes the decision and implements the therapy, following information that comes from this second opinion. This is now done through a company in Cambridge, Massachusetts, called World Care [3].

When the medical Internet emerged in the mid-1990s, its forerunners recognized that the medical Internet needed standards; as in all good medicine, the essence of professionalism is self-governance based on high ethical principles. The medical Internet can draw from at least five other major sources of intellectual and ethical development as historically tested springs of important thought: the ethics of the medical Internet is informed by the ethics of medicine and journalism, medical education, good business practices, and medical journals. One of the really good reasons the American Medical Association was founded in 1846 was to create a code of medical ethics. It did so, and over the ensuing 158 years, its Council of Ethical and Judicial Affairs (CEJA) has published updates of medical ethics based on nine principles that now fill more than 200 pages. The simplest explication of medical ethics is doing the right thing for patients and for populations of patients.

Primary source, peer-reviewed medical and science journals began simultaneously in France and England about 300 years ago [9]. This new system tested the validity of new information through expert scrutiny from others in the field. Peer review established limits on the publication of scientific articles and led to the medical science editorial enterprise as we know it today. We view this development, the erection of barriers to publishing bad stuff, as one of the most important events in the history of science. But it was not until 1978 that this enterprise was formalized. Editors from the *New England Journal of Medicine* (*NEJM*), the *Journal of the American Medical Association* (*JAMA*), the *British Medical Journal* (*BMJ*), and the *Annals of Internal Medicine* founded the so-called Vancouver Group, the International Committee of Medical Journal Editors (ICMJE), which began to delineate rules of behavior for medical journal authors, editors, publishers, peer reviewers, and advertisers [10]. It took 300 years to elaborate an internationally accepted code of ethics, the "Uniform Requirements," thereby adding assurance of the trustworthiness of published information for physicians, health reports, and the public at large. We could call that "Gutenberg time." And by the year 2000—6 short years after the founding of the medical Internet—we had at least six well-developed sets of rules, policies, or standards available to guide authors, editors, publishers, owners, peer reviewers, advertisers, sponsors of Internet medical and health information; we call that "Internet time." The time warp created by the Internet has sped us from Gutenberg—print heavy—time to Internet—speed of light—time [11].

Just as one of the functions of the ICMJE has been to guide professional self-governance in the medical literature, with the desirable result of precluding governments from enacting laws to govern how medical journals work, so too, successful self-governance of the medical Internet community has so far dissuaded governments from enacting laws to legislate or regulate how the medical Internet works. Key to this achievement were early regular meetings of staff from the American Medical Association (AMA) and the United States Food and Drug Administration (FDA), which planned cooperatively how the medical Internet should develop. This effort involved the World Health Organization (WHO) as well.

Patients and professionals alike may now consult the codes of the ICMJE itself, the American Medical Association, the HI Ethics (implemented by the American Accreditation Health Care Commission [URAC]), the Health on the Net Foundation (HON), or the Internet Healthcare Coalition (IHC). This cornucopia of ethical leadership benefits readers who can test sites against these high standards and bookmark those they can most likely trust for the best health and medical information.

Five simple process rules, first published in *JAMA* for anyone seeking health information from the Internet, can put every health site to the test: [6]

1. Who wrote what is on the screen? Without a name, the information cannot be trusted because the "author" cannot be queried.
2. If the author's name appears, where does that person work? Can he or she be e-mailed or visited? Is there an address, an institutional connection, a reputable place?
3. Where does the information come from? If it was not written originally for the site—and a great deal of information on sites does not originate there—where did the information first appear? Look for attribution, and consider the source.
4. Who owns the site? Who funds it? Whether the site is sponsored by advertising, subscription, or an owner's underwriting, disclosure should be easily determined.
5. When was the information posted? Newer information can invalidate older information or put another angle on it or balance it. Information on the Internet may be changed over time, making proper dating crucial.

A recent study from the *Consumers Union*, reported on October 29, 2002 in the *Wall Street Journal* [12], found that while professionals evaluating the qualities and credibility of a health Web site may well follow these rules, especially valuing authorship, consumers may still be more persuaded by the "look and feel" of a site, in other words, pretty packaging or functionality, rather than content. Site users must be diligent in valuing the quality of the message over a glitzy presentation or packaging.

Finding Trustworthy Internet Sites

If a site satisfies these five questions, users know that those running the site are reasonably competent. They at least understand the principles of journalism, the principles of medical ethics, and good business practices. But having such knowledge does not necessarily make their information valid.

Site users need to go further. The next step after answering the five questions is to find "brand-name" identification. If the information comes from prestigious institutions such as Harvard Medical School, the Mayo Clinic, Johns Hopkins Hospital, the Centers for Disease Control and Prevention (CDC), or the National Cancer Institute (NCI), chances are good that the information is valid. Such institutions put their reputations on the line whenever they put information on the Internet. For-profit sites such as Medscape, where George Lundberg served as Editor in Chief from 1999, earn trust through the reputations and credentials of the people who work there. In the new fast-forward Internet time, Medscape, launched in May 1995 and now part of the WebMD family, is one of the older medical information sites. Medscape seeks authorities for all its information, and the peer-review and editing process is virtually as rigorous as that of *JAMA*. Authors are trusted names in their fields from the best institutions, which vouch for their work.

Internet users enter through an access point, or portal, with a variety of search engines from which investors make money. Users are at the mercy of whoever put the search engine together because they can retrieve only what the search engine provides. So where does one begin for reliable information? One good way to start is with the National Library of Medicine at PubMed, www.pubmed.gov or www.pubmed.com, or with www.healthfinder.gov. These sites offer a mass of government information that is easy to navigate and free of charge. An excellent source of peer-reviewed information is offered by Medline, produced by the National Library of Medicine, available as a link through many eHealth sites. Medline has online 4000 of the best medical journals of the world in various languages dating from 1967. One can enter the database, search with key words, and bring up dozens, hundreds, or thousands of articles from the journals. Only abstracts are published on the site, not full text. Although some 30,000 medical journals are published worldwide, the vast majority of the best, most frequently cited new information in medical literature comes from fewer than 500 of the 4000 journals carried by Medline.

Few people seek such in-depth information. Medscape, strategizing that people are searching not for huge volumes of information, but rather for the best information they can obtain quickly and easily, identified the "best" 269 journals of the 4000. The result, Medscape Select at www.medscape.com, provides the "best" answers to the most frequently asked questions of medical literature [13].

U.S. physicians reported in 2002 that they used many sources of information to inform their medical practices. Dominant are medical journals, 99 percent; communication with peers, 98 percent; conferences, 97 percent; pharmaceutical detail representatives, 89 percent; dinner seminar meetings, 89 percent; and the Internet, 87 percent. When asked which Web sites physicians have gone to in the past 12 months for medical information related to their practice, they report: WebMD Medscape, 67 percent;

Medline/National Library of Medicine, 55 percent; NIH, 32 percent; CDC, 29 percent; Physicians On Line (POL), 25 percent. The same studies show usage of *The New England Journal of Medicine* at 67 percent and *JAMA* at 61 percent. Forty-five percent of U.S. physicians report that they visit WebMD Medscape at least once a month. Comparable figures for Medline/NLM are 33 percent; for NIH, 17 percent; CDC, 15 percent; and POL, 13 percent [5].

When asked about their satisfaction level with health information in various forms of media, U.S. consumers in 2002 answered yes to "extremely or very satisfied": 51 percent, Internet; 46 percent, TV news; 46 percent, health magazines; 24 percent, TV ads; 20 percent, magazine ads.

U.S. physicians in 2002 were asked to rate four sources of information—medical journals, the Internet, pharma symposia, and detail representatives—as credible, comprehensive, timely, and up to date on treatments. Physicians rating each as good or excellent were Internet, 85 percent; journals, 83 percent; symposia, 65 percent; and detail reps, 56 percent. Journals scored highest on credibility, with the Internet second; the Internet scored highest on comprehensiveness, with journals second; the Internet scored tops on both timeliness and latest therapy, followed by journals and symposia. The question of whether drug or disease information first seen on the Internet, and driving patients to see doctors thereafter, is a good thing is an open question, awaiting definitive research. The most obvious negative effect would be that some consumers might convince some doctors to prescribe a drug that is unnecessary, expensive, and thus wasteful or even potentially harmful. The most obvious positive effect would be for a patient to receive proper pharmaceutical treatment for a disease or condition that they would otherwise not have received without the information as stimulant via the Internet, and from which they benefited. Be that as it may, we know that online activities drive offline actions by both consumers and physicians. For consumers, WebMD has demonstrated numbers like 36 percent of readers talking to their doctors about a condition after visiting WebMD or 16 percent asking their doctors for a specific brand name. Forty percent of physicians who are regular monthly users of Internet medical sources report that it has influenced their medical practice and 38 percent say it has improved their communication with patients [5].

The Long, Slow Path to Medical Cyberspace

Medicine is both an art and a science. Much of the practice of medicine devolves into two major categories. The first involves the "high-touch" activity of caring, which includes intense interpersonal relational feelings. The second involves information: the seeking, observing, gathering, assimilating, interpreting, dispensing, feeding back, and monitoring of information. In what ways, then, might the Internet be applicable to transmitting high-quality medical information? The answers are many: it can be used as a medical library; it can replace functions served by the telephone or fax machine; it can replace hand-delivered notes, letters, brochures, or certificates; it can be used to place orders for diagnostic tests or for medications, to report laboratory or X-ray results, and to record verbal communications; and it can be used whenever distance separates people and copies are needed quickly. In short, the Internet provides virtual stat service. In 2000, through sampling techniques, Cyberdialog, a Web research company now called Manhattan Research, reported that 34 million Americans wished to communicate with their physicians electronically but only 3 million had actually done so [5]. This is a terrific opportunity gap for physicians to fill. Harris Interactive polls reported that 84 percent of U.S. consumers want electronic alerts from physicians; 83 percent wanted lab results online; 80 percent wanted personalized medical information; 69 percent desired online charts to monitor their chronic conditions; and 43 percent said that they would select a physician based at least in part on the availability of Internet services.

Why haven't a greater number of physicians responded to these patient requests and market demands? Many doctors feel that they are already overly busy and that e-mail will tie up their time even more. So far there are few ways for them to get paid for e-mail medicine (a problem that also applies to telephone consultations). Some doctors believe that the Internet will cause them to lose close contact with patients; they prefer to maintain the "high-touch" factor essential to the art and practice of medicine. Others fear the misuse of specific documentation that e-mail establishes, preferring telephone interaction as less of a potential liability.

But physicians and patients in actuality will save, not lose, time by using e-mail, since wasted minutes playing "telephone tag" can be eliminated. Like all professionals, physicians need to be compensated fairly for their time. Experimental methods of payment for e-mail use are now under way. The physician, given the economic informed consent of the patient, can charge directly for e-mail interaction without bothering with an insurance carrier. An electronic communication between two people who know each other can be meaningful, clear, and succinct—in many instances, an even better outcome for both patient and physician than "high-touch" care. Physicians need to experiment with the use of an e-mail triage nurse or physician's assistant in cases where time worries persist. Also, the clear permanent record of an e-mail interaction provides excellent documentation of exactly what transpired between physician and patient, with little room for misinterpretation in case something does go amiss and there is a need to investigate. So the Internet, far from posing a threat, has the potential to become a positive opportunity for better medical practice.

At last we are positioned to make "mouse calls" in lieu of house calls [4]. When we started using computers in clinical labs in the 1960s, one of our main purposes was to connect the lab result with the physician at the bedside. With information in hand, the physician could quickly make the proper judgment and treat the patient appropriately. Today that system is routine.

The path to medical cyberspace is clearly mapped. eConnectivity is here. We might have a lab test done in Austin, Texas, for a patient in Johnson City, a big geographic gap now bridged instantaneously by the computer. Because we now have the technology that ensures this kind of eConnectivity, information transfers like this are already happening. In another scenario a patient can enter a symptom into the computer and transmit the information to a physician who interprets it, orders the appropriate test, and sends the patient to a laboratory. The test results are quickly transmitted to the physician by e-mail or telephone, or through a handheld personal digital assistant (PDA) device. The physician then e-mails the patient directly with instructions to change the dosage of a drug, stop taking the drug, go directly to a hospital emergency room for immediate care, or to the physician's office as appropriate. In another scenario, a patient might do a glucose test at home and transmit the results via computer to the physician. The physician would get a printout or a graph on the office computer screen and e-mail the patient to recommend a change in insulin dosage. The patient would never have to come in for a visit.

Such connectivity between physician and patient is advisable only for patients and doctors who know one another; skipping an initial office visit for those who have never met would breach current ethical principles. The seemingly mundane practices of medicine, such as carefully observing the patient, noting reactions to queries, listening for voice inflections, and feeling the pulse can be critically important. Clinicians develop a sixth sense from observing patients directly, an experience no one can get solely from the Internet. However, once a relationship is established, significant benefits can be derived from e-mail exchanges between patients and physicians. No more telephone tag. That kind of connectivity cuts through voice mail frustration and documents the interaction.

The Internet also can be an antidote to managed care. In strictly managed care, administrators with MBAs determine the amount of time a physician is allowed to spend with any one patient, especially in an office setting. However, once a patient and physician have established a therapeutic relationship, they can expand contact time through the Internet, which is outside the reach of bean counters. A lot of information can flow back and forth with the click of a mouse, and it can be more thoughtful and better managed, to the greater satisfaction of both patients and physicians.

Sometimes too much information seems to be floating about. A number of physicians have complained about patients who come in with reams of computer printouts. They are good patients; they want to do the right thing, but it is frustrating for the physician because a lot of the printed-out information could be garbage, and a lot of time can be wasted sorting through the data to determine what is trustworthy and what is not. Explaining everything could take an inordinate amount of time, a rare commodity for those in managed care networks. Some physicians say they wish they could pull the plug on their patients' computers.

But no one should stop patients from accessing the Internet, and no one can censor what they receive. Physicians need to direct patients to trusted sites. Patients will self-select their own level of sophistication, from newsbyte for public consumption to cursory abstract to abstruse journal article for medical professionals. We learned our lessons on how patients access information some years back, early in the development of the American Medical Association's Web site in 1995–1996. Bill Silberg and George Lundberg, with pharmaceutical company grant money, developed a sophisticated section on HIV-AIDS. It was intended to provide state-of-the-art clinical practice and practical research information for physicians caring for HIV-AIDS patients. They were surprised to discover that the principal users of this site turned out to be patients and their friends and families, not physicians. These profoundly interested consumers became extremely sophisticated readers. That observation quickly caused us to espouse the view and the practice that medical and health information should be freely available to any and all, and that the reader should decide what level of sophistication was appropriate for them. That insight shaped Medscape and similar models.

Internet Privacy Concerns

Few things are of more concern to patients than the privacy of their medical information. People generally do not want other people talking about their medical problems, but privacy is difficult to maintain. Unfortunately, there are no secrets in hospitals. The issue of invasion of privacy antedates the Internet, the computer, and the telephone. People tend to find it "interesting" if you have cancer, syphilis, or HIV. Some can be trusted with this information, and some cannot. Publicly sharing private information is unfortunately prevalent in such places as hospital elevators. Events that occur in the patient–physician relationship are themselves private, the business only of the patient and the physician. But they also become the business of the closest family members, and then to some extent they become the business of the insurance carrier or the managed care organization, if the contract allows access to information for billing and payment purposes. Psychiatrists and other mental health caregivers often have patients who pay for care out of pocket because they do not want any insurance records of their therapy, given the unfortunate cultural bias against patients seeking mental health care. Of course, pharmacy information is also available to many.

Private information on the Internet presents a heightened but not insurmountable problem. There is a dramatic difference between the old hospital system, in which there were no or few secrets, and the new era, with its technical capability of distributing mass information at the touch of a finger. What one person tells another in the elevator or cafeteria pales in comparison with what can happen to computerized information. In approaching the Internet as a therapeutic information transfer device, patients should be aware that private information could become public and be wary of what they confide about themselves over cyberspace. This delicate issue has to be addressed with great sensitivity. Yet the established rules must apply to both paper and electronic recording. HIPAA, a giant new federal law long in gestation, is being implemented in 2002–2003; one part is intended to "solve" the privacy and security problems. Of course it will not succeed fully, but it will be interesting to observe what effects it actually has.

Generally, information generated from the patient–physician relationship should be kept private. Exceptions to this privacy practice are certain celebrities whose health is in the public interest, especially those running for high public office and mentally ill patients who pose a threat to others. By now it is fairly well accepted that someone running for president of the United States has to surrender much of his or her medical file to the public, especially given older revelations about Franklin D. Roosevelt and Woodrow Wilson and very recent revelations about just how ill John F. Kennedy was while President. The power of the office is so great that the health of those who seek it is a legitimate and public point of concern. In the second instance, a psychiatrist is obliged by law to break patient confidentiality, if a patient says, for example, that he plans to kill his wife. The threatened person has to be warned. Protecting life is a principle that overrides the principle of privacy.

eCare Today

eCare is now a reality. Large numbers of physicians are willing to provide it. Fair methods of payment for services are being developed. Professional liability insurance carriers have participated in establishing practice standards tolerable to them. Privacy and security concerns have been assuaged to a realistic level by encryption when needed. Agencies that license physicians have adopted acceptable rules of practice behavior. Some elements of industry with investor funding have entered the field. And many branches of organized medicine have invested in its creation and growth.

Two prototype eCare organizations have led the way: Medem in San Francisco and HealinX (now Relay Health) in the East Bay area of California. While they share similar goals, connecting doctors and patients electronically to promote rapid, efficient, effective, documented medical practice decisions, they have sharply different business models. Leaders of Medem believe that the speed and convenience of eCare will be so great that patients will be happy to pay personally for care by credit card without involving insurance or managed care companies. CEO Ed Fotsch points out that payment for a visit to the physician office is only a small part of the burden of going to see the doctor. Often, the patient may have to drive and pay for parking, take a taxi or bus many miles, lose half a day of work, and hire a babysitter in addition to paying the doctor. Insurance only reimburses part of the cost of the doctor. In eCare, all transactions take place electronically from the comfort of home or office at no cost to the patient, other than the direct charge of the physician. Medem believes that patients will pay $20 to $35 by credit card out of pocket for an eVisit and that many doctors will be comfortable with eCare for patients whom they know already. Medem takes a small percentage from each such encounter. Relay Health, on the other hand, believes that patients expect much of their medical care to be paid by insurance.

This model anticipates that the ease and efficiency of eCare will control costs and justify payment from insurance and managed care carriers, with a high level of satisfaction from a healthy and pleased patient. As of this writing (December 2002), Medem is launched and growing smartly, demonstrating support for the concept. Relay Health is also, and has positive customer satisfaction ratings to support its approach. Both companies may be right, as may others who enter this young field that is destined for success.

The Internet not only provides physicians with new tools to improve patient care; it also gives patients an unprecedented opportunity to take charge of their health care with the best medical information. More than 100 million computer users in the United States have accessed the Internet for health information so far—especially information regarding specific disease, diagnosis, and treatments. Online health users are more typically women than men; they also tend to be older, Caucasian, married, and college educated. They tend to arrive at the doctor's office with a printout of options and too often leave with a lower opinion of a practitioner who seems less informed than they. Unfortunately, data show that only 15 percent of U.S. physicians recommend any specific medical Internet site to their patients. But we suggest that all physicians should encourage patients to become Internet savvy—specifically, by recommending two or three general health information Web sites with demonstrated high standards of quality and two or three condition-specific sites on which they rely for whatever ails them. In this way, patients can be armed with information that the physicians themselves trust, and they can study this information on their own time, away from the stopwatches of the managed care bean counters.

Electronic medical records provide a useful tool both for achieving high-quality efficient medical care and for preventing medical errors. To a greater degree than almost any other force, consumer activism in medical care—including careful Internet searches for reliable medical information—can drive doctors and hospitals to use electronic tools more rapidly. Informed patients can protect themselves by insisting that both doctors and hospitals automate their information handling for the patient's benefit and safety and freely share access to the patient's medical records with the patient who, after all, owns them. Of course, health insurance claims should also be electronic. In the U.S., approximately 2 billion insurance claims are filed from physician offices each year. About one half are still on paper. It costs about $3.50 to process one such claim on paper but only $0.35 electronically. It seems that making that switch is a complete "no brainer." WebMD's Envoy provides such services to offices of more than 300,000 U.S. physicians.

Understand that changing physician behavior, like any human behavior, can be very difficult. Methods for change include education, feedback, administrative changes, and financial rewards and penalties. According to Forrester Research [14], a doctor is more likely to use an electronic or Internet tool if it saves time, works as advertised, has a trusted quality stamp, strengthens the doctor's power position, helps meet a mandate or requirement, and is free of charge. Healthtech 2001 [15] has reported that physicians consider the following to be "essential" Internet applications: clinical diagnostic reporting, medical records, administrative claims processing, eligibility and referral authorizations, and information technology systems support.

In theory, the Internet could virtually eliminate the health insurance industry in America. With Internet technology, people—individually or collectively—can negotiate directly with physician groups or other providers for their care. They would have to assume some risk, but the banding together of patients or providers can spread that risk. In addition, secondary insurers may be able to cover procedures with huge price tags, such as organ transplants. But the money that could be saved by eliminating or greatly downsizing the health insurance industry (which has only marginally higher public approval ratings than the for-profit managed care companies) could be as much as $200 billion a year in administrative overhead and profit. This newfound money could help cover the uninsured and fund preventive medicine/public health initiatives as well [4].

eCME

We believe that continuing education will be one of the most useful applications of Internet medicine. Since the science of medicine is constantly changing, all medical professionals know that they must be committed to lifelong learning. Sources for accredited continuing education, be it for physicians, nurses, pharmacists, dentists, or various others, have traditionally been videotapes, reading of medical journals, or courses taken in person at society conventions, meetings, or at educational institutions. Learning from teaching materials delivered on the Internet has burgeoned in the past few years. The ACCME states that eCME programs accounted for 7 percent of all CME activities in 2001, doubling since the 2000 figures of 3.4 percent and more than tripling the 1999 2.1 percent [16]. The actual number of credit hours awarded is a difficult national number to find. We do know that Medscape was the source of about 100 credit hours in February 1999. In 2000 it was approximately 100,000 credit hours; 2001 was 200,000; and 2002 300,000. So, growth is extraordinary. These numbers do aggregate nurses, pharmacists, and physicians. The benefits of Internet CME/CE are many: it is usually free of charge to the viewer, it is funded by sponsorships, and the educational experience can be in the home or office of the professional at any time of day or night. All proper Accreditation Council for CME (ACCME), IEMJE, IHC, AMA, FDA, HON and HiEthics rules must be followed. The very best authorities and evidence-based medicine are the teachers, and a certificate awarding credit can be printed out immediately upon completion of the course requirement. Thus, it is not hard to agree that this modality has a great future and could turn out to be the dominant form of CE/CME.

Web-Based Medicine and Quality of Care

Crossing the Quality Chasm, published by the Institute of Medicine, has become widely recognized as the standard for healthcare quality in America that we should all strive toward [17]. It lists 10 rules or goals for day-to-day practice needed to "cross the chasm": care based on continuous healing relationships; customization based on patient needs and values; the patient as the source of control; shared knowledge and the free flow of information; evidence-based decision making; safety as a system property; the need for transparency; anticipation of needs; continuous decrease of waste; and cooperation among clinicians. Virtually all are based on information flow or need. The Internet is part of the mechanism that should be used to follow all 10 rules. In 2002, the California Healthcare Foundation performed a wonderful service by contracting with the First Consulting Group to issue an iHealth report detailing the ways information and communication technology can be used to achieve these 10 aims [18].

Organizing the 10 IOM rules into four general principles of care, this report details 12 IT applications that can be used to realize patient empowerment; reliability and safety; care relationship beyond the encounter; and public accountability for quality. The report describes multiple actual information technology (IT) applications from medical facilities in multiple states. Most have a Web-based core or component to help achieve one or more of these four general principles of quality of care.

The large and well-established field of medical informatics has benefited from distinguished academic leadership for many decades. The creation of complex and comprehensive hospital information systems has become robust and nearly ubiquitous in and around academic medical centers, stemming from the fledgling systems of the late 1960s. Individual laboratories, radiology, billing, admissions, pharmacy, and other systems have become integrated, but often with home-grown solutions requiring substantial on-site dedicated staff thus lacking the capability of communicating seamlessly with other home-grown systems.

Most American physicians are self-employed and in small practices with few funds to invest in complex computer equipment and information technology expertise. So the newer systems based on personal computers, the Internet, and Application Service Provider (ASP) models allow use in smaller physician office practices with lower start-up costs. Small physician office practices did begin to use billing systems fairly early, but the implementation of clinical components has been quite slow, and many would say retarded, compared to many Northern European countries, the U.S. military, and the Veterans Health Administration. This situation has changed abruptly due in large part to the dominant emergence of the Internet and Web-based technologies that allow the use of remotely hosted applications. Expensive mainframe computers or complex personal computer networks are not required in the small offices of physicians. Vendors offer information technology services to physicians merging the ASP model, spreading costs over use time rather than as large start-up costs.

The advent of personal digital assistants (PDAs) as wireless handheld devices is another great technological advance that can prevent the requirement of equipping each room where a doctor sees a patient with an actual wired computer terminal. With the emergence of these new technological capabilities, handheld devices, wireless networks, ASP, and Web-based technology, many vendors who previously bypassed the clinical information needs of the small physician office practice have now entered it, recognizing that between 30 and 40 percent of all clinically active U.S. physicians engage in solo or small-office practices—a substantial market.

The California Healthcare Foundation has published two other very helpful monographs in 2002 that report on the uses of information technologies in a wide range of specific physician office settings [19,20]. Many use the Web. Handheld devices can access the Web to download the most up-to-date electronic drug reference information for real-time application with patients. Physicians can now "write" prescriptions online with Web-based direct transmission to participating pharmacies for all but controlled substances, eliminating the pervasive problem of physicians' illegible handwriting, speeding up the process greatly, and essentially eliminating the need for pharmacist call-backs.

Many vendors provide a wide range of coverage of Web-based applications and tools for the physician office. Such tools include Web-based ASP; handheld PDAs; electronic coding, charge capture and payer connectivity; electronic information transcription transmission and documentation; electronic laboratory test order entry and routing of test results; e-prescribing with prescription transmission, refills, drug alerts, checking of formularies, and drug references; clinical decision support tools with point-of-care practice analysis and patient registries; and many other electronic medical record features.

In studying which physician offices chose to automate, the California Health Care Foundation (CHCF) reported that there were four common themes. All practices that chose to automate recognized that they had specific problems not being solved in their manual modes, and they sought specific IT solutions. While some technological fixes that physicians employ address only single functions, many available products offer multiple solutions. Physicians themselves must be the catalyst for IT implementation, often as the leader. Tangible and intangible, but nonetheless real, benefits have been achieved in many settings, as judged by cost-effectiveness, greater efficiencies, fewer delays and errors, and happier patients and staff.

Yet another way in which the Web can enable better medicine is by making clinical decision support available far away from the academic medical center. Decision support tools can identify patients who are due for specific interventions or follow-up of prior work; alert the physician to dangers that might accompany a planned clinical action; make easily available current knowledge applicable to a specific clinical situation to the physician at the time and place needed; and identify and call to the attention of the physician patient information that should activate intervention.

A substantial number of vendors and some medical associations have entered this market providing knowledge tools. The American College of Physicians/American Society of Internal Medicine is leading medical associations by introducing in 2002 the PIER (Physicians Information and Education Resource) free to members. It is a Web-based, standalone tool, organized by disease topic, and capable of being integrated into electronic medical records (EMRs) and handheld products. Another pioneer in this field is Massachusetts-based Up to Date, which has grown from paper through CD-ROM to an online offering. This is a knowledge tool easily accessible for rapid searching in the office. Medscape is one of the oldest and by far the largest and most used knowledge tools. Offered free since 1995, Medscape information is tailored for many medical specialties as well as medical students, nurses, and pharmacists. www.medscape.com enjoys more than 4 million registered users in 237 countries, who record nearly 1 million page views daily, entirely over the Internet.

The Medical Manager system of physicians' office information was born in the mid-1980s in Florida and has garnered the largest market share of physician office practice (about 185,000 U.S. physicians in 2002). The success of Medical Manager, in addition to early mover advantage and high-quality products and support services, stems from it being modularized. Different physicians possess different levels of interest and sophistication in computer applications. The Medical Manager system provides a range of options, from the simplest office scheduling to a complex EMR within its Intergy product as well as a Web-based handheld called Ultia [21]. For claims processing, Medical Manager and other such office management systems interface electronically with Envoy and smaller vendors.

Important New Initiatives

Davidoff and Florance in 2000 [22] proposed that a new health professional, the "informationist," be developed in the ranks of clinical librarians and that such workers, in constant touch with the Internet, would provide rapid information retrieval for "just-in-time," "up-to-date" clinical answers at the "point-of-care."

Don Kemper, CEO of Healthwise, champions the idea of information therapy, as "prescription-strength" health information from physicians through secure online messaging. In an interview in the CHCF's *iHealthBeat*, Kemper describes information therapy as "the prescription of specific, evidence-based medical information to a specific patient, caregiver, or consumer at just the right time to help them make a specific health decision or behavior change." This is different from the usual consumer search for health information on the Internet because it removes most of the chance or luck factor of the usual search, it is efficient, it comes from a trusted source (the regular physician), and there is a record that documents the event. As with everything else in our society, there is a cost created by this process, and to make it fly, there needs to be a way to pay for it [23].

Of the several organizations that have been very helpful in getting Internet medicine off to a flying start, the eHealthInitiative stands out as a leader. This Washington D.C.-based, not-for-profit organization is dedicated to improving the cost-effectiveness, quality, and safety of American health care by appropriate use of IT. Janet Marchibroda, the CEO, envisions that the offices of all healthcare providers will create and maintain EMRs, interconnected as appropriate between providers, patients, payers, purchasers, and public health agencies [24].

This group promulgates the standardization of data methodologies so as to allow this interconnectivity in practice. The tragic events of September 11, 2001, followed by the anthrax bioterrorism attacks, focused national attention on the sad state of our medical IT infrastructure, both for medical diagnosis and care and for early recognition and public health interventions. Fresh federal money was quickly appropriated in 2001 and pumped into the public health system beginning in 2002. This obvious national need and the infusion of fresh funding motivated many national and state public health leaders to respond in a variety of ways, including the building of new IT interconnected infrastructure. The eHealthInitiative has been one key in crafting a public–private collaboration to include public health officials, laboratories, standard setters, and healthcare providers to work together to create such an information structure. The task is a large one. Technology exists; standards have been set; the public health community is on board. The principal problem is the small penetration of routine clinical practices in the U.S. by EMRs, estimated by some as low as 5 percent. In a recent Washington, D.C. group brainstorming session sponsored by the National Comprehensive Cancer Center Coalition, widespread agreement was reached that the entire national cancer care program was impeded by the paucity of available shared data on all aspects of cancer care. There David Hopkins, PhD, of the Pacific Business Group on Health proposed that our country needed a "Hill-Burton" type of legislation to fund and implement the available and needed healthcare information technology nationwide at all levels. An organization like the eHealthInitiative, because of its 501C3 and 501C6 tax law structures, could help lead the way to make such change happen.

Although most Internet health information is free to the user, there are some services available for fees. These include medical search services. For several hundred dollars, companies such as www.canhelp.com, www.findcure.com, www.thehealthresource.com, and www.canceradvisors.org will provide comprehensive targeted, screened searches for specific medical problems or treatments. Of course, broad-based free automated search engines like www.google.com of Mountain View, California, provide searches of more than 1 billion Web pages in less than 1 second and are revolutionizing the total world information business. In contrast, the human discretion, judgment, and focus added for these fee-based specialized search products may be worth the money for some users [25].

Conclusion

With the announcement in November 2002 that the U.S. Department of Defense has approved its integrated information system for patient medical records around the world—the Composite Health Care System II—for beginning implementation in 2003, we see at long last the realization of the dream so many have had for so long [26].

Finally, the Institute of Medicine is at it again. Within a blockbuster report issued on November 19, 2002, are 12 pages proposing that the federal government and the main private sector healthcare players declare a goal of creating a "paperless" healthcare system in 5 years by creating multiple pilot projects that would virtually eliminate paper-based processes through three implementation phases. This IOM report requires uniform data standards with the federal government providing most of the initial funding comparable to federal government funding of interstate highways. Payers are urged to compensate for e-mail consultations, remote consultations, and care delivered by information and communication technologies [27].

With all these actual activities, in addition to the extraordinary information and communication technology available to us, we are finally on a roll. The long-standing inertia to resist change appears to have been converted into inertia to power change. There is still nothing more powerful than an idea whose time has come.

References

1. Brown JS. Learning in the digital age. In: Devlin M, Larson R, Meyerson J. The internet and the university: Forum 2001. Cambridge, MA, and Boulder, CO: Forum for the Future of Higher Education and EDUCAUSE; 2002. p. 65–91.
2. Masys DR. Effects of current and future information technologies in the health care work-force. Health Affairs 2002;21:33–41.
3. Lundberg GD with Stacey J. Severed trust: why American medicine hasn't been fixed. New York: Basic Books; 2001.
4. Lundberg GD, Stacey J, Waters T, Lundberg PL. Patient-focused control: fixing our broken health system. In: Lundberg GD with Stacey J. Severed trust. Revised and updated with comprehensive solutions to the health care dilemma. New York: Basic Books; 2002.
5. WebMD Proprietary Information. Market Facts Consumer Health Media Study, July 2002; BCG Harris Interactive eHealth Physicians Study, June 2002; Manhattan Research Physician Health Media Study, July 2002; Fulcrum Analytics, CyberCitizen Health, 2001; AMA Physicians and the Internet Study, 1997; Jupiter Media Metrix, 1997.
6. Silberg W, Lundberg GD, Musacchio RA. Assessing, controlling and assuring the quality of medical information on the internet. JAMA 1997;277:1244–1245.
7. http://www.medscape.com/px/instantpollservlet/view?ActiveFlag=1&BackURL=/px/instantpollservlet/result?PollID=560.
8. Miller TE, Derse AR. Between strangers: the practice of medicine online. Health Affairs 2002;21:168–180.
9. Kronick DA. Peer review in eighteenth century scientific journalism. JAMA 1990;263:1321–1322.

10. http://www.icmje.org/.
11. Lundberg GD. The ethics of the medical internet. MedGenMed September 10, 1999. vol 1, number 2. http://www.medscape.com/viewarticle/408003.
12. How do people evaluate a Web site's credibility? Consumer Web Watch News. Research report. November 2002. http://www.consumerwebwatch.org/news/report3.
13. Lundberg GD, Anderson SM, Goodhue, J, DuBois DD, O'Malley K, Smith SE. A virtual core collection: Medscape Select. http://www.medscape.com/pjsp/public/help/search/medline/medscape/medscapeselect.html.
14. Barrett M. Why doctors hate the net. Forrester Research Report, March 2000. http://www.forbes.com/asap/2000/1127/248_2.html.
15. http://www.newswise.com/articles/2001/3/HTECH.TFC.html.
16. http://www.accme.org/incoming/119_2001_annual_report_data.pdf.
17. Committee on Quality of Health Care in America. Crossing the quality chasm: a new health system for the 21st century. Washington, DC: National Academy Press; 2001.
18. Kilbridge P. Crossing the chasm with information technology: bridging the quality gap in health care. Oakland, CA: California Health Care Foundation; 2002.
19. Metzger J, MacDonald K. Clinical decision support for the independent physician practice. Oakland, CA: California Health Care Foundation; 2002.
20. MacDonald K, Metzger J. Achieving tangible IT benefits in small physician practices. Oakland, CA: California Health Care Foundation; 2002.
21. Integrated practice management, clinical and e-health solutions. Santa Clara, CA: The Medical Manager Health Systems; 2002.
22. Davidoff F, Florance V. The informationist: a new health professional? Ann Intern Med 2000; 132:996–998.
23. Commentary. Q&A with Don Kemper, Healthwise CEO. iHealthBeat. The Advisory Board Company. August 5, 2002.
24. Commentary. Q&A with Janet Marchibroda, CEO, eHealthInitiative. iHealthBeat. The Advisory Board Company. September 9, 2002.
25. Parker-Pope T. Firms help patients find latest cures for illnesses. The Wall Street Journal Online, November 26, 2002.
26. Caterinicchia D. DOD approved medical system. FCW.com. Federal Computer Week, November 7, 2002.
27. Committee on rapid advance demonstration projects: health care finance and delivery systems. Corrigan JM, Greiner A, Erickson SM, editors. Information and communications technology infrastructure: a "paperless" health care system. In: Fostering rapid advances in health care: learning from system demonstrations. Washington, DC: Institute of Medicine; 2002.

38
Combating Terrorism: A New Role for Health Information Systems

JOHN S. SILVA and EDWARD N. BARTHELL

This chapter addresses the issue of global terrorism and proposes how health systems need to be integrated within a homeland security response network.

Global terrorists have declared a "holy" war on the American homeland. The destruction they have caused and could cause in the future exceeds the capacity of our existing health systems to respond and treat casualties. This chapter addresses this issue and proposes how health systems need to be integrated within a homeland security response network.

Life in the United States changed forever the morning of September 11, 2001. Suicidal terrorists declared war on the American Homeland by slamming airplanes into the World Trade Towers in New York City and the Pentagon in Washington, D.C., killing nearly 3000 Americans. The subsequent "anthrax letter" attacks paralyzed the federal government, disrupting the operations of the Senate, the Supreme Court, and post office facilities, as well as affecting private enterprises. The economic consequences of these attacks to the country were just as devastating: multiple business sectors lost many billions of dollars in revenue and the Stock Market suffered the single largest loss in its history. Cleaning up and restoring after both these attacks cost additional billions. Most important, our sense of security has been shattered, becoming perhaps the first casualty in the new war.

As catastrophic as these initial attacks were, subsequent ones could be much worse. A chemical or biological weapon attack could result in tens of thousands of Americans dead or severely injured—millions in the case of smallpox. "We are simply not prepared to respond to a biological or chemical attack," states Dr. Steven Morse of Columbia University in a recent interview with *Newsweek* [1]. In an example of how unprepared we may be, Oklahoma Governor Frank Keating and former senator Sam Nunn failed to control or manage a smallpox attack in a recent bioterrorist war game called Dark Winter. "No central authority collected information from hospitals so the extent, speed and even the existence of the epidemic was unknown . . . Hospitals were overwhelmed [1].

The anthrax-tainted letters discovered in Florida, Washington, D.C., and New Jersey killed 5 people, infected 18, and put more than 30,000 Americans on antibiotics. These

---

John S. Silva, MD, is the Chief Architect with Silva Consulting Services in Eldersburg, MD. Edward N. Barthell is Vice President with Infinity Healthcare in Mequon, WI.

letters were the first significant biological attack within the U.S. Serious deficiencies were exposed, particularly in America's health system and in its ability to detect and manage a biological terrorist attack. The anthrax letters showed the government that even a relatively unsophisticated, small-scale attack could cause human casualties and enormous economic disruption. The fragmented, disconnected, and stove-piped health systems were not capable of detecting the attack, nor did they respond with sufficient alacrity to protect our citizens.

These two attacks demonstrate the spectrum of terrorist activities:

- Overt attacks that are obvious and cause significant local destruction and loss of life, such as planes flying into the World Trade Towers or sarin gas released in the Tokyo subways.
- Covert attacks that are not obvious until individuals become sick, like the postal workers who became ill after exposure to anthrax that was released from letters in mail-handling facilities.

Both types of attacks may result in overwhelming numbers of casualties and deaths and cause significant disruption of "business as usual."

Problems Associated with Terrorist Attacks

While there are certainly many problems that must be identified and managed during and responding to an attack, the information-related ones that are particularly relevant to health workers are:

- Too many things to do right now—Detect, Protect, DECON, Triage & Treat.
- Deal with casualties that may overload hospitals.
- Need to know what is actually going on—and where.
- Data needed to manage situation hard to get, hard to disseminate.

These information needs result in requirements placed on the health system, at a time when all participants will be under extremely stressful conditions. City, state, and federal agencies and officials must have accurate and up-to-date information so they can manage the overall incident, allocate resources appropriately, and ensure that response activities are effective. Much of this information must come from the incident scene, first responders, and hospitals that will treat casualties. All these tasks must be done while maintaining some level of care for the "daily" illnesses that will continue to occur. To compound the situation, there is a good likelihood that multiple incidents will occur at or near the same time, some of which may be targeted directly at our response capabilities.

The following example will give the reader a sense of the urgency and magnitude of these problems. A set of tools was developed to estimate the number of casualties that could occur following an airborne release of various toxins and biological weapons [2]. Figure 38.1 illustrates the effect of an airborne release of 1 kg *Staphylococcus entero-toxin* B (SEB). The innermost clear ellipse in Figure 38.1 represents a greater than 95% probability that persons within that area would become sufficiently ill to require medical attention. The relative hourly casualty presentation rate estimates the number of individuals per hour that would need treatment for SEB intoxication. The vertical axis shows the number of hours after release of the agent and the horizontal axis depicts the number of casualties, where each tick mark represents 10,000 casualties. The estimated number of persons who would need to be treated within the first 8 hours was well in

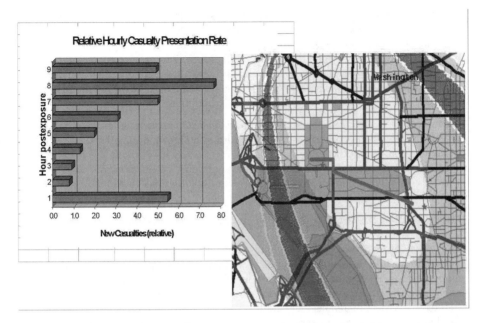

FIGURE 38.1. Estimated casualties following airborne release of 1 kg *Staphylococcus enterotoxin* B (SEB).

excess of 150,000. Clearly, that number would overwhelm existing response and casualty management approaches for any city. The estimates did not include individuals exposed without intoxication or individuals who believed they might have been exposed. Data from the Tokyo sarin attack estimated that for every 1 person exposed to sarin, there were at least 10 "worried well" who were seen by the health system.

Imagine, for a minute, what the Emergency Operations Center in the city might look like as it responds to this incident. The phone lines become immediately overwhelmed; cell phones will be so overloaded that they are not useful. To which hospital do casualties get sent? How many beds are available? How do ambulances get to the incident scene? How many people are sick? What are their symptoms? The scene at hospitals will be just as difficult. Emergency departments would become quickly filled to capacity. And where would the overflow go? These were the earliest problems identified in three major casualty simulations described below.

All health systems, even those not engaged at the incident scene, become "first responders" in scenarios where the number of casualties exceeds the carrying capacity of a city. These systems will need to be integrated into the citywide command and control system so that decision makers can have accurate and timely information from the incident and treatment locations. Integrated command and control systems for response must:

- Provide correct *"What to Do"* to who needs it, where it is needed.
- Display up-to-the-minute picture for all.
- Manage coordination across ALL responding agencies.

In these settings, logistics and supply of critical health resources and personnel to the locations where they are needed are the key determinants of successful response.

There will be no time to create or bring in new systems to manage the problem; they must be in place *before* an incident of this magnitude occurs. There will be no time to train on any disaster-only system. These systems must be used daily to manage current incidents and already be integrated with all the responding organizations. As a result of analyzing a number of existing response systems and many discussions with first responder and health system users, the following overarching system requirements are offered:

- Must adapt to user's environment—no specialty hardware or software requirements.
- Must NOT disrupt workflow—no added burden on responders.
- No additional manpower required—will not get any.
- Data must be captured "real-time"—As a by-product of users doing their job.

Integrated Homeland Security Response Network

The threat of terrorism spans bombings, chemical or hazardous materials releases, nuclear or dirty bombs, and biological agent attacks. Their potential for unthinkable numbers of casualties and fatalities require the healthcare sector to rethink how it approaches preparing for and managing patients during disasters. The all-hazard nature of today's disasters mandates that health systems be fully integrated into all the efforts for detecting, identifying, responding to, and recovering from catastrophic events. The magnitude of these terrifying events suggests that the public safety sector, including health systems, must organize itself to optimize all its resources to successfully mitigate an attack of any kind.

The U.S. military has recognized that information superiority, coupled with precision weaponry, wins wars. The response to terrorist attacks has to be similar. Local, regional, and federal responders and agencies need to know what is the agent, what is its extent, how many casualties are likely and where they will be located, what medical resources are required to treat, and what is currently available. That information, coupled with field response, transportation, and traffic control assets, will support movement of casualties to treatment locations, which may include temporary "field" hospitals. Working with command and control centers, health systems need to provide data on its resources, know the number and type of casualties it must treat, and identify shortfalls. Each of these types of information will be changing dynamically as the incident evolves and the health systems receive and treat casualties.

Response managers will be continuously optimizing resource allocations, identifying critical resource deficits, and developing contingency plans as the incident(s) evolve. Without data interoperability across the public safety sector and responding agencies, it will be nearly impossible to manage an effective response. Poorly managed incidents have a real potential to exacerbate the loss of lives. Response managers will also be in constant contact with other decision makers—mayors, governors, and federal agencies—all of whom need to know what the current "operational picture" is.

The conceptual framework shown in Figure 38.2 presents a schematic of how the various members of the public safety and response communities could exchange information and provide their data to a coordinating city or county emergency operations center (EOC). The collection of systems becomes the "local node" in a homeland security response network. Software systems in the EOC would aggregate multiple data feeds, provide analysis, and generate products, like a common operational picture, that

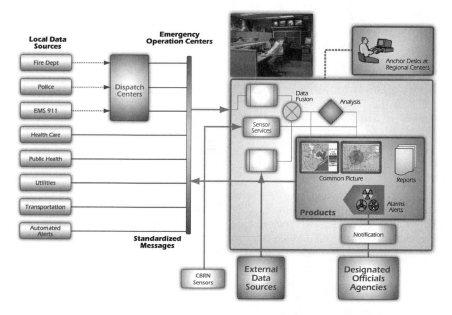

FIGURE 38.2. Framework for data interoperability. (By permission of Silva Consulting Services.)

all the entities could use. The key element to this framework is that individual responder information systems must be able to share and receive data from other responder systems. Thus, this framework does not suggest a traditional systems integration effort in which all local systems are integrated into one gigantic system. Rather, the framework specifies data interoperability via a defined set of common data elements that will be exchanged using standardized messages, most likely via standard XML messages [3].

Currently, fire, police, and EMS receive emergency calls from a 911 service. These messages flow into separate computer-aided dispatch (CAD) systems and appropriate response units are dispatched to the incident scene. While the dispatchers may share a common building, few jurisdictions share data among their CAD systems. Developing a common operational picture for a city, state, or region will require each CAD system to share a common set of data about the incidents it is supporting. The National Institutes of Justice is working with the law enforcement community to develop a set of standard critical incident messages. The ComCARE Alliance is working with the fire and EMS communities to accomplish the same for their incidents. Clearly, these messages must be harmonized.

Health care, public health, transportation, utility, weather, and sensor systems do not generally share information outside their own community. As described above, emergency managers and decision makers need a comprehensive picture of the current state of an incident. Without real-time data provided by each of the responding or treating entities, it will be impossible to effectively mitigate the effects of terrorist attacks.

The city or county EOC is a key "node" of a new system of systems—the homeland security response network. The EOC system needs to collect automatic data feeds from local systems including:

- Critical incidents.
- 911 dispatches.
- Health system status, such as emergency department (ED) diversion and number of beds available.
- Public health surveillance system reports.
- Sensor networks (environmental, weather, and chemical/biological sensors).
- Public works.
- Transportation, such as the Intelligent Traffic System.

Data fusion functions within the EOC system will aggregate data feeds and provide integrated view(s) of the day's incidents within jurisdiction and locations of police, fire, and EMS resources using a map-based graphical information system (GIS). In the event of a critical incident, the same system generates an up-to-the-minute common picture of the situation including incidents, hazards, resource and unit locations, and other critical information. Reporting functions will generate the reports required by responders, local, state, and federal agencies, and government officials. A notification function will send alert and alarm messages to designated officials, agencies, and responders.

Hazardous Material Release

Several of the capabilities outlined above exist today. The following scenario shows how various systems can exchange messages and interact to orchestrate the response to a hypothetical release of chlorine gas in the Orlando, Florida area.

- A driver of a semitrailer truck loses consciousness and his truck rolls off the freeway, close to the intersection of Routes 417 and 408, hitting a tree and causing chlorine to leak.
- Qualcomm sensors on the truck note the sudden deceleration and forward an Automated Crash Notification (ACN) message [4] (an XML standard document from ComCARE Alliance; www.Comcare.org) to an Intelligent Message Broker (IMB) (developed by Orillion; www.orillion.com).
- The IMB takes the coordinates of the crash scene from the ACN message. It then matches the crash location against the regions specified by agencies and systems stored within the EPAD geo-database (Electronic Provider Access Directory; ComCARE). During the registration process, an agency is required to specify its region of interest on a map, the coordinates of which are stored in EPAD (Figure 38.3).
- The Incident command center at the EOC, using the Homeland Incident Reporting and Tracking System (HIRTS; DynCorp, www.dyncorp.com), is registered in EPAD and receives the ACN XML message containing the crash location and type and amount of hazardous material (Figure 38.4).
- HIRTS extracts the location and HAZMAT information from the XML document, plots the incident and, following approval, forwards a HIRTS ALERT message to EMSystem (Figure 38.5).
- The incident command center staff reviews the crash site, and, noting that one hospital is within the path of the chlorine plume, closes the ED. Using EMSystem (www.EMSystem.com), the staff issue a "RED BAR" alert requesting that local EDs

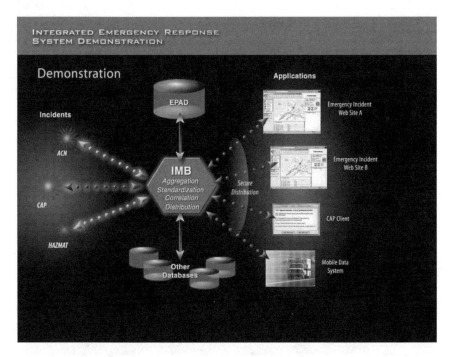

FIGURE 38.3. Integrated Response System forwards telematics data from HAZMAT trucks and sends it to organizations registered in EPAD using standardized XML document messages. (Courtesy of David Aylward, ComCARE Alliance.)

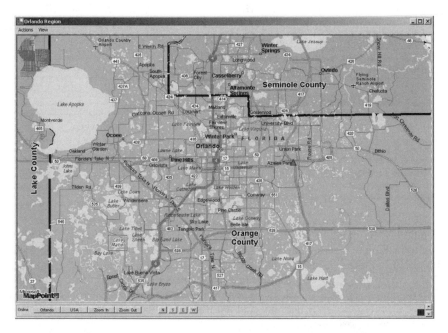

FIGURE 38.4. Homeland Incident Reporting and Tracking System (HIRTS) displays the location of the HAZMAT incident scene. (Courtesy of William McCeney, DynCorp.)

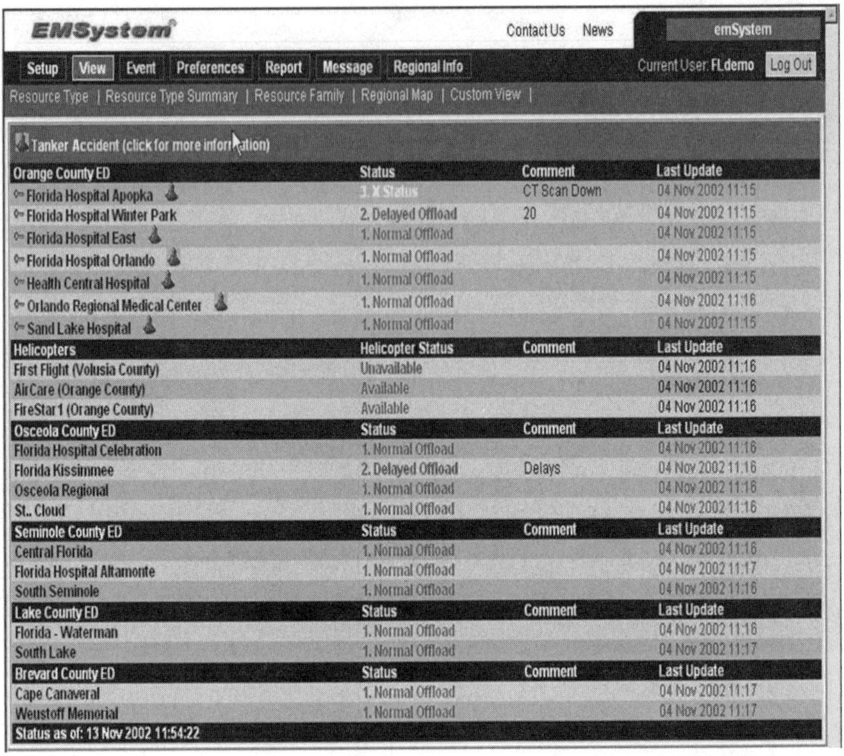

FIGURE 38.5. EMSystem displays the HAZMAT alert message to affected hospitals (*cone icons* next to their name) and dispatch centers.

initiate mass casualty procedures and mark their resource availability and capability to receive victims from the incident using EMSystem (Figure 38.6).

- In addition, the staff attach the Material Safety Data Sheet for chlorine to the alert so that all hospitals and first responders will have immediate access information about chlorine and how to manage casualties (Figure 38.7).
- EMS dispatch systems use EMSystem display to route ambulances to hospitals based on real-time availability (Figure 38.8).

This short scenario demonstrates how disparate systems that communicate via standard XML messages through an EOC can dramatically improve a city or region's ability to mount a coordinated and appropriate response to a large-scale incident. Importantly, these systems exist today and use XML documents to exchange information securely and easily. Before the complexity, extent, and number of terrorist situations increase, regional homeland security response networks must be fashioned to interconnect the currently disconnected entities and agencies within cities and states and the federal government.

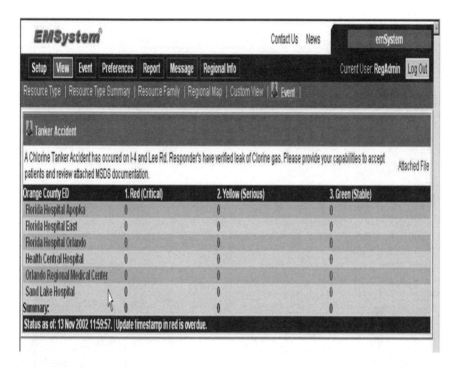

FIGURE 38.6. Hospitals that will receive victims are requested to identify bed availability online.

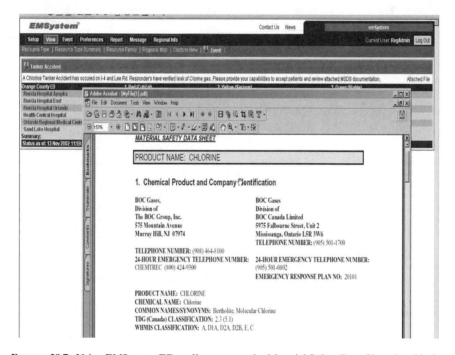

FIGURE 38.7. Using EMSystem, ED staff can access the Material Safety Data Sheet for chlorine and have immediate access to treatment information.

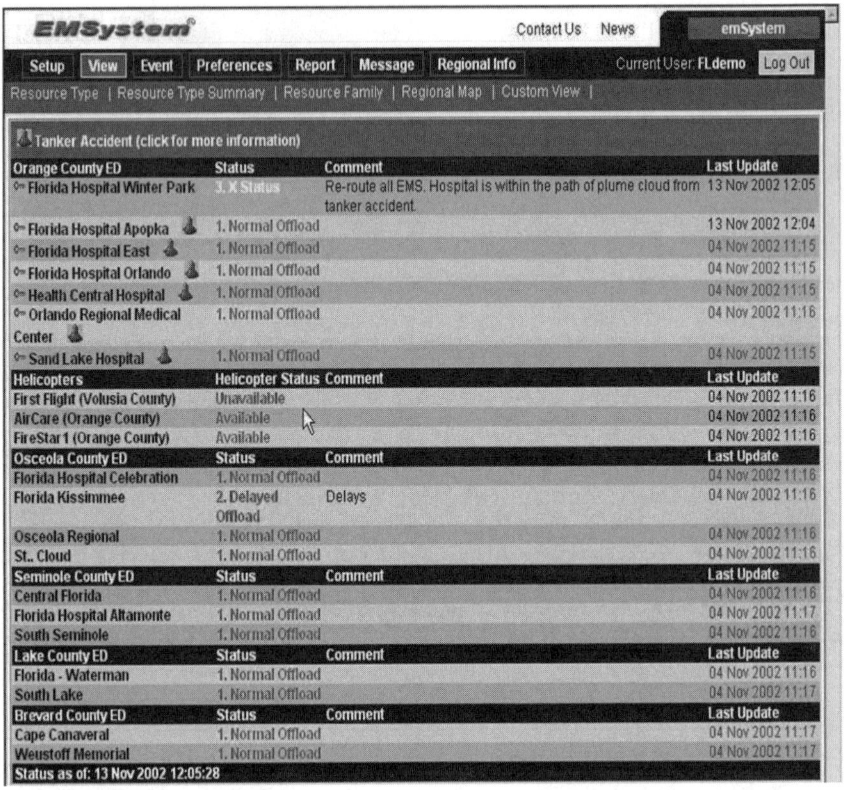

FIGURE 38.8. Dispatch center and Emergency Operations staff use EMSystem displays to monitor bed and ED availability.

Bioterrorism

The threat of bioterrorist attack has grown substantially since the "anthrax letters" of October 2001 and the war with Iraq. Two national exercises, TOPOFF in May 2000 and Dark Winter in June 2001, have graphically described this potential. In the TOPOFF simulation, a covert release of plague occurred in Denver. Within 4 days after plague had been identified, Denver was overwhelmed, the disease had spread to other states, and local jurisdictions were competing for scarce medical resources. The Dark Winter simulation had similar problems, including spread to 25 states and 15 other countries. Lessons learned from this exercise were summarized and included the findings that existing organizations are not structured to manage such an incident, there is no surge capacity within the health system to provide treatment, and containing such an incident will pose unique logistic, medical, and legal challenges [5]. The Medical Disaster Conference held at Dartmouth in June 2001 attempted to quantify the number and type of resources that would be needed to respond to and manage a biological attack [6]. Their simulation was a tularemia attack in the Dartmouth area resulting in 5000 casualties. Using resource estimation tools, they predicted that 1000 responders would be needed by day four of the outbreak and nearly 6000 by day six.

The predicted human resource needs were well beyond those available locally, leading the conference attendees to postulate a system of "Cybercare" to support large-scale disasters [7].

Early detection of a bioterrorist attack is the most important lesson learned from these exercises and simulations. Detecting the disease while the number of seriously ill individuals is low provides a short interval to initiate aggressive treatment and prophylaxis measures that, if effective, would substantially reduce the mortality, morbidity, and resource requirements following an attack. Kaufman et al. analyzed the effect of delaying effective treatment on mortality and cost [8]. Not surprisingly, starting treatment within the first 72 hours was most effective for both anthrax and tularemia attacks. Starting treatments after 5 days did not substantially reduce the overall mortality or cost.

The need to detect a potential bioterrorist attack has led to the introduction of numerous "biosurveillance" systems. The primary focus of these systems is to detect the onset of nonspecific disease prodrome symptoms as early as possible *before* the patients present with classic disease syndromes or die of disease. Teich et al. have summarized the epidemic curve and detection strategies for anthrax and described general aspects of biosurveillance and bioagent detection [9]. Syndromic surveillance systems are classified into those that collect surveillance data continuously or those that collect data for specific events. To the extent possible, surveillance data for detection of a potential outbreak or attack should be collected continuously and not require hospital, ED, or clinic resources to input any information. The Real-Time Outbreak and Disease Surveillance System (RODS) is one such system and is described in a separate chapter (Chapter 39) in this book. Event-based surveillance systems usually collect a small amount of syndromic data from specific settings within a city or region, most often EDs. It does require additional work on the part of health providers and additional personnel to enter the syndromic data into a Web-based collection form. The advantage of event-based surveillance is that it requires a health provider to assign a specific patient to a syndrome or describe signs and symptoms. The Web forms are often tailored for the specific event and can collect more "targeted" information such as demographic data, presence or absence of specific diseases, signs or symptoms, and epidemiological data from the patient.

Green used retrospective data on clinic and ED visits to create threshold curves, and then superimposed a simulated anthrax attack based on the Svredlovsk data [10]. Figure 38.9 demonstrates their theoretical model and characterizes the shift from prodrome symptoms that appear first in clinic settings to disease-specific ones that appear in EDs. It should be noted that syndromic surveillance systems are focused on early detection of unusual occurrences or anomalies in the number of persons with some indicator that "things are not right." They are not diagnostic systems that provide the identification of the pathogen. For more details concerning surveillance systems, the reader is referred to description of CDC's early system [11]. Lober et al. report on a Roundtable on Bioterrorism Detection that summarizes the features of a number of different surveillance systems [12] and a recent National Syndromic Surveillance Conference held by the New York Academy of Medicine [13].

Coming back to the theme of this chapter, let us look at what could happen once a surveillance system has detected an anomaly or an astute clinician has observed a sentinel patient. Following detection of an anomaly or report of a sentinel case, public health organizations begin the process of outbreak investigation. They need to know as soon as possible if the anomaly is a false positive and the observed variations are just more "flu" cases. They also need to identify the offending agent, assess the extent of the problem, and monitor the number of new cases. If it appears to be a serious health problem, they need to activate appropriate intervention strategies including treatment, prophylaxis, isolation vaccination, and the like.

City and state decision makers need to be aware of the status of all active anomaly investigations and be notified early if the outbreak is a potential bioterrorist incident. This highlights the need for information sharing across health systems, public health networks, and local and state command and control systems. The messages that will be sent among the various systems need to be defined before an incident, as do the response and recovery plans, in such a way that each member of the community knows what the message means to them, what portion of the plan they must perform, and how they will update or notify appropriate entities about the status of their area of responsibility. Figure 38.10 depicts how surveillance systems cooperate during various phases of an anomaly assessment and send messages between the health systems, public health, and EOC.

Continuous surveillance systems monitor the health of a target population—city, state, or region—by collecting and analyzing data feeds from the community. When an anomaly is detected, the specifics of the anomaly are fed to the appropriate public health officials who proceed expeditiously to investigate the anomaly. Event-based surveillance may be used by public health to request specific information from health providers within the community to help determine the geographic extent of the potential outbreak and develop an accurate epidemic curve. Messages sent to the EOC will notify staff that an anomaly workup is in progress and keep them informed of its status. Messages could be sent to other local or state EOCs, or to the state and federal public health agencies in the event that this problem may be regional or national in nature. If an outbreak or bioterrorist attack is confirmed, both continuous and event-based surveillance systems would monitor the efficacy of treatment and prophylaxis measures. The rate of new cases and morbidity and mortality of existing cases should be positively affected by the introduction of appropriate therapy. Failure to achieve reduction in any of the above case rates would imply that treatments may not be effective and suggest a strain that was modified to resist standard therapy. In addition, accu-

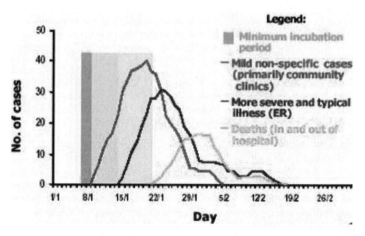

FIGURE 38.9. Theoretical model for a terrorist attack: sudden exposure during a short period to aerosolized anthrax. (Courtesy of Dr. Manfred Green, Israel Center for Disease Control.)

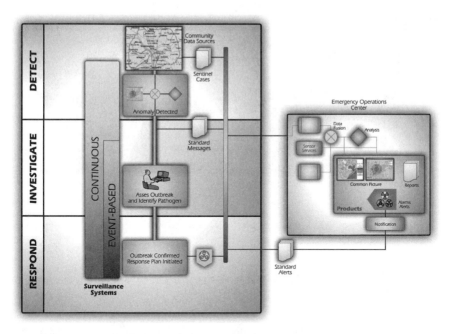

FIGURE 38.10. Interoperable data sharing among surveillance and response systems is essential for successful response. (By permission of Silva Consulting Services.)

rate and timely information regarding numbers of new cases will be critical to optimize resource allocations and logistics necessary to maintain an effective distribution across the community.

Bioterrorist Attack

The following hypothetical scenario involving a bioterrorism attack in the Orlando region is provided to demonstrate how surveillance systems need to interact with a regional EOC to provide the "homeland security response network."

The U.S. has invaded a foreign country in response to its weapons of mass destruction program and a number of militant Islamic organizations have threatened retaliation. Intelligence reports indicate that a terrorist cell in the southeastern U.S. may be preparing to release a biological agent in the next 2 to 3 weeks. One week later, an astute clinician in a Miami suburb reports a critically ill Arab immigrant with buboes and sepsis from what appears to be a possible case of plague. The patient is intubated and on a respirator and cannot be questioned. Samples sent to a CDC-approved laboratory confirm plague.

- The Orlando regional EOC and local public health department activate syndromic surveillance using the in-place EMSystem for all Orlando hospitals. Each facility reports daily total numbers of patients seen in the ED and the number of patients with a temperature above 100.6°F every shift (Figure 38.11).
- A message is sent to each Orlando area ED every 8 hours requesting they fill in the form shown in Figure 38.12.

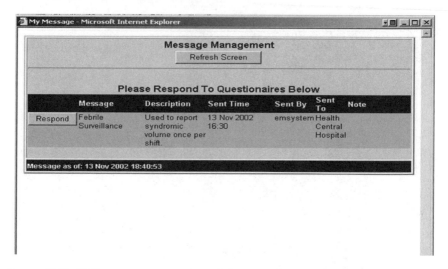

FIGURE 38.11. EMSystem message sent to each Emergency Department per shift to enter temperature data.

- This questionnaire is automatically delivered every shift; audio prompts alert department personnel to fill it out. Once posted, data from the completed questionnaire are sent securely to the Orlando Public Health Department via a standard XML message.
- On the fifth day of collecting fever information, the public health office observes an anomaly in two hospitals (Figure 38.13).

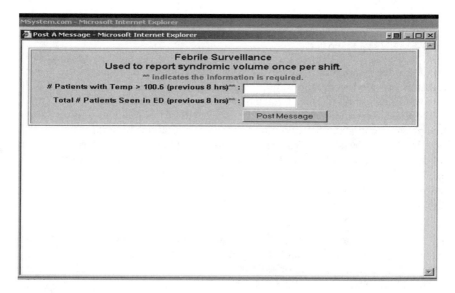

FIGURE 38.12. Temperature data form that each ED is requested to fill in with the number of patients with fever over the past 8 hours.

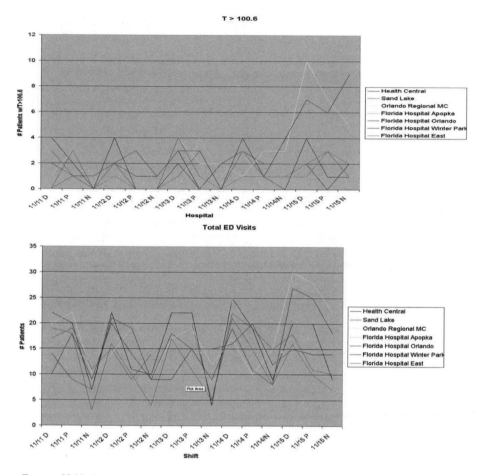

FIGURE 38.13. Excessive number of patients with fever detected by surveillance software in two hospitals on day five.

- EMSystem, reporting through HIRTS, notify public health staff that the number of fever cases from two geographically adjacent hospitals significantly exceed the expected number of fever cases reported for the past 24 hours. HIRTS notifies the regional EOC and, with public health staff, initiate an aggressive investigation of the outbreak.
- To assess the extent of the outbreak and determine more accurately the epidemic curve, public health staff develops a questionnaire specific to plague and will request that Orlando physicians begin immediately to fill out an emergency surveillance questionnaire (ESQ).
- Public health staff issue a RED BAR ALERT via EMSystems to area EDs to begin using ESQ for all patients with fever. Hospitals with the Red icon all receive the alert and those with message icons (the envelope) will automatically receive the questionnaire. The RED BAR also contains additional information that ED staff can access with a simple mouse click (Figure 38.14).

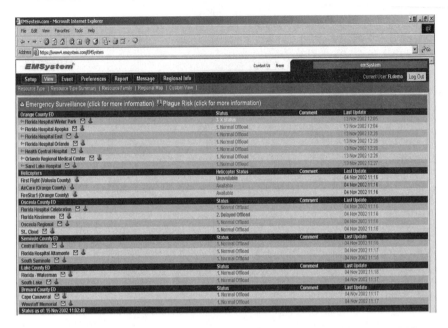

FIGURE 38.14. "RED BAR" alert is sent from Public Health via EMSystem to all EDs.

- The plague ESQ is very short and requires minimal data entry. It does provide additional information to the public health and EOC staff to rapidly construct epidemic curves and identify the extent of the outbreak. If public health or EOC need additional information, the form can be modified very quickly and posted immediately to all the hospitals.
- Data entered into the forms are sent in a secure fashion to the public health and/or EOC system via a standard XML message for analysis and reporting (Figure 38.15).
- The public health and EOC staff post information about plague and the detailed medical response plan to the RED BAR so that ED staff can retrieve it immediately at the point of care (Figure 38.16).

In this particular scenario, the region did not have a continuous surveillance system in place. After being alerted to a potential threat, they were able to activate event-based surveillance via a Web form to give them insight into the number of fever cases reported every 8 hours. Following the detection of an excess number of fever cases, they collected additional information to help determine extent and number of potential plague cases. The medical response plan would contain details regarding management of suspected plague cases, how to confirm the diagnosis, and appropriate prophylaxis and treatment regimens. In addition, the same EMSystem could have been used to monitor bed availability and other critical resources within the ED and hospital, thus providing the EOC, public health, and government officials with a comprehensive and timely picture of the outbreak status. Secure, standard message exchanges using XML is the keystone to sharing information between HIRTS and EMSystem and the ability to deliver "just the right" information to EOC and public health systems.

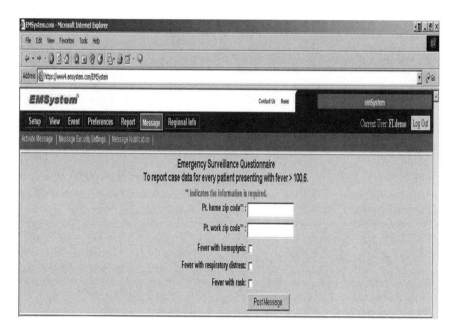

FIGURE 38.15. Specific signs and symptoms data form that each ED is requested to fill out for each patient meeting the criteria.

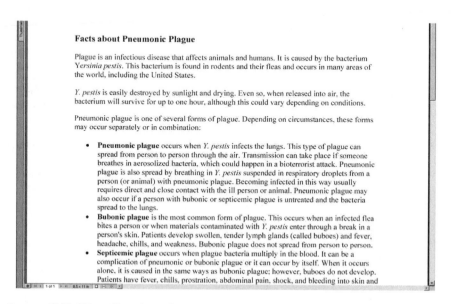

FIGURE 38.16. ED staff can immediately access information from Public Health regarding the outbreak and obtain details on what types of diagnostic tests and therapeutic procedures and treatments are recommended.

Summary

The need for a homeland security response network is clear. Terrorist threats are no longer academic exercises. Today's health systems must be fully prepared to support effective and efficient responses to all hazards, even those with overwhelming casualties. This chapter has identified the information problems, has proposed a standard message framework to share information, and provided two "visionary" scenarios of how health systems, public health, and public safety systems could come together in the very near future to handle an initial version of a homeland security response network. Perhaps in the near future mayors and governors and public health officials will be telling CNN what is happening rather than watching CNN to find out.

References

1. Newsweek 2001 Oct 8.
2. Silva JS. This tool was developed under a DARPA program called ENCOMPASS. Dr. Gene McClellan from Veridian was the principal investigator.
3. Silva JS. Fighting cancer in the information age. An architecture for national scale clinical trials. MD Comput 1999;16(3):43–44.
4. ComCARE Alliance ACN Data Set Working Group. www.comcare.org/research/news/releases/011205acnstandard.html.
5. ANSER. Dark Winter: Summary; 2001. www.homelandsecurity.org/darkwinter/index.cfm.
6. Rosen J, Gougelet R, Mughal M, Hutchinson R. Conference report of the Medical Disaster Conference, June 13–15, 2001. Hanover, NH: Dartmouth College; http://thayer.dartmouth.edu/~engg005/MedDisaster/.
7. Rosen J, Koop EC, Grigg EB. Cybercare 2002 July. www.homelandsecurity.org/journal/Articles/cybercare.html.
8. Kaufman AF, Meltzer ML, Schmid, GP. The economic impact of a bioterrorist attack: are prevention and postattack intervention programs justifiable? Emerg Infect Dis 1997;3:83–94.
9. Teich JM, Wagner MM, Mackenzie CF, et al. The informatics response in disaster, terrorism and war. J Am Med Inform Assoc 2002;9:97–104.
10. Green MS, Cohen D, Kaufman Z, et al. Use of simulated bioterrorist attacks to evaluate syndromic surveillance systems based on multiple data sources. Presented at National Syndromic Surveillance Conference, September 2002. New York Academy of Medicine, New York, NY.
11. Silva JS. Global Expeditionary Medical Surveillance (GEMS) support of domestic preparedness. In: Ramsaroop P, Ball MJ, Beaulieu D, Douglas JV, editors. Advancing federal sector health care: a model for technology transfer. New York: Springer-Verlag; 2001. p. 316–324.
12. Lober W, Bryant T, Wagner M, et al. Roundtable on bioterrorism detection. J Am Med Inform Assoc 2002;9:105–115
13. National Syndromic Surveillance Conference, September 2002, New York, NY. www.nyam.org/events/syndromicconference/.

39
Public Health Surveillance: The Role of Clinical Information Systems

MICHAEL M. WAGNER, JEREMY U. ESPINO, FU-CHIANG TSUI, and RON M. ARYEL

This primer on public health surveillance and clinical information systems draws on actual experiences in exploring the synergy between both systems.

Health departments across the United States have begun collecting new types of surveillance data from hospitals in near real time. In New York City, Boston, and Washington, D.C., for example, hospitals send daily reports of patient visits to emergency departments to the respective health departments [1–3]. Hospitals in Utah and the Commonwealth of Pennsylvania send such data in real time via health level seven (HL7) interfaces [1]. Similar projects are under way in other states [4].

This new trend is driven by the need for early detection of surreptitious biological attacks. The trend is likely to accelerate because evidence is accumulating that these new approaches work—that they can detect outbreaks earlier than existing methods and even identify outbreaks that have previously gone unnoticed [5–8]. This trend has important implications for researchers and developers in clinical informatics because it is creating new design requirements for clinical information systems.

This chapter is written for the public health reader as well as researchers and developers in clinical informatics. For clinical informaticians, it provides a primer on public health surveillance, drawing on examples from our experience with the RODS (real-time outbreak and disease surveillance) system, which is an example of a public health surveillance system that collects and processes these new types of data. For public health workers, it provides a primer on clinical information systems, also drawing on examples from our experience with the Health System Resident Component (HSRC), a hospital-based system similar to a clinical event monitor.

This chapter begins with a scenario depicting a future in which tight coupling between public health surveillance systems and clinical information systems enables earlier detection of disease outbreaks.

Michael M. Wagner, MD, PhD, is an Associate Professor of Medicine and Intelligent Systems and Director of the RODS Laboratory at the Center for Biomedical Informatics at the University of Pittsburgh. Jeremy U. Espino, MD, is a National Library of Medicine Postdoctoral Fellow at the RODS Laboratory at the Center for Biomedical Informatics at the University of Pittsburgh. Fu-Chiang Tsui, PhD, is an Assistant Research Professor of Medicine and Associate Director of the RODS Laboratory at the Center for Biomedical Informatics at the University of Pittsburgh. Ron M. Aryel, MD, MBA, is a Consultant at Del Rey Technologies in Santa Monica, CA.

It is noon, January 1, 2006, and a bioterrorist has just introduced *Bacillus anthracis* by aerosol route into a sporting event in Pittsburgh. Anthrax is treatable, thus early detection of this attack is imperative so that resources can be mobilized to respond to the needs of the exposed population.

At the time of the release, the real-time outbreak and disease surveillance (RODS) system computes a probability of anthrax outbreak in Pittsburgh—absent intelligence data indicating a heightened threat level and health surveillance data showing patterns normal for that time of year—of less than 0.0001, well below its threshold for recommending action. Since biosensors for *B. anthracis* are not yet installed at the stadium due to cost and public relations concerns, the attack itself is not detected and therefore does not produce an update in RODS's probability.

Thirty-six hours postrelease, RODS updates its probability of anthrax attack to 0.01, which results in a notification to public health authorities that an investigation of the possibility of anthrax attack be initiated. RODS computes this probability based on algorithmic analysis of data collected automatically and in real time from clinical information systems and other existing information systems about employee and school absenteeism, requests for appointments, triage calls, visits to healthcare systems, orders for tests, and purchases of over-the-counter flu remedies. These algorithms detect activity that is increasing steeply and has just exceeded seasonal baselines by 3 standard deviations. The public health authorities log-in to existing Web-based electronic medical records to gather additional information about patients with respiratory symptoms in emergency departments. RODS automatically updates decision support logic in point-of-care systems in hospital and clinics. These systems begin to prompt clinicians to collect additional information about patients with respiratory symptoms and to order rapid diagnostic tests for anthrax. RODS also recommends that the National Pharmaceutical Stockpile (a military-style distribution system with palletized stockpiles of antibiotics and vaccine stored at airports, as well as a command and control structure) be called to standby status.

Forty hours postrelease, RODS updates its probability of anthrax attack to 0.5. RODS computes this probability from routinely collected data and from new data collected by point-of-care systems. The new analysis in particular reflects two cases of patients admitted to ICUs with gram-positive *Bacillus* bacteremia, anthrax-like symptoms, and mediastinal widening on chest radiograph. Immediate review of these cases by infectious disease experts, prompted and facilitated by RODS, confirms that they fit the definition of probable anthrax, and treatment is initiated. One of these cases is from San Francisco, but the infectious disease expert review reveals that the affected patient had just returned from a weekend in Pittsburgh. At about this time, automatic spatial analysis of the data by BARD (Bayesian aerosol release detector) helps characterize the attack as a 1-kg release north of the football stadium on January 1. Based on cost–benefit criteria, including the high probability of anthrax attack and estimates of the numbers of exposed individuals, RODS recommends immediate movement of supplies and troops to Pittsburgh and passes detailed case data to the command and control computers of the Bioterrorism Emergency Response System.

Forty-two hours postrelease, supplies and personnel have begun to arrive. RODS updates its probability of anthrax attack to 0.95 based on increasing trends in the data, especially the appearance of four additional anthrax-like syndromes. RODS reminds public authorities that at this level of confidence, the mayor should appear on local and national media to instruct attendees of the sporting event to take specific actions.

Fifty-two hours postrelease, the first positive culture for *Bacillis anthracis* is confirmed by a clinical laboratory.

Relationship Between Public Health and Health Care

As in the foregoing scenario, the practices of public health and health care should in an ideal world be tightly coupled. Information such as laboratory test results collected by health care is essential to the practice of public health. Information collected by public health, for example, about the prevalence of disease, is essential to practice of health care. Medical schools in fact teach doctors to consider the prior probability (prevalence) of disease in their diagnostic and management decision making for individual patients. Students are instructed to consider the most likely etiologies first, invoking the classic metaphor "upon hearing hoof beats, think of horses, not zebras." They are taught Bayes theorem as the basis of rational decision making.

For a variety of pragmatic reasons, however, the practices of public health and health care are loosely coupled, at best, and information sharing is limited and oftentimes slow. The barriers to better information sharing include the cost and effort to develop technical means. These barriers have not been addressed because doctors and public health officers could perform their jobs acceptably well with manual systems (which is not to say that all preventable morbidity and mortality was prevented).

Primer I: What Health Care Should Know About Public Health Surveillance Systems

Immediately following the October 4, 2001, anthrax cases in Boca Raton, Florida, the limitations of current approaches became very apparent. Public health needed immediate information about whether other suspected anthrax cases were being seen in hospitals throughout the United States. Physicians in every hospital and clinic needed to know the scope of the problem, what risk factors (such as postal employment) indicated potential exposure, and what treatments were proving effective. The data exchanges necessary to satisfy these information needs had to occur in real time. They did not occur and will not occur effectively until information systems are built to support such exchanges. This section is about public health surveillance systems being developed to meet those needs, and the following section is about clinical information systems that can collect needed information and that can be extended to collect additional information and coordinate response.

The Infectious Disease Threats

There are scores of infectious diseases of interest to public health, and they are discussed and enumerated in both reportable disease lists [9] and threat lists [10–12]. Our prior research suggests that outbreaks of such diseases fall into two key patterns that have very different implications for information technology, which we label *Anthrax* and *Smallpox* [13].

Anthrax Pattern

At one extreme are abrupt outbreaks that result from near simultaneous exposure of a cohort of individuals to contaminated air, food, or water. A terrorist release of anthrax (Figure 39.1), is one example. The figure shows the speed at which mortality would accumulate following a hypothetical attack with aerosolized *B. anthracis*. The shape (not height) of the curve is based on the outbreak in 1979 in the city of

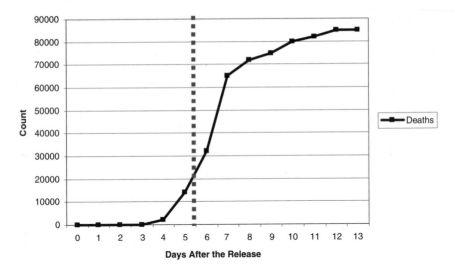

FIGURE 39.1. Anthrax cumulative mortality curve. The shape of the anthrax curve is based on the Sverdlovsk curve, as reported by Meselson. The absolute numbers are projections to a very large-scale release.

Sverdlovsk, Russia. Anthrax is a treatable disease; there is a window of opportunity lasting approximately 4 days within which it is possible to mitigate the effects of the attack [14].

The relative narrowness of this window of opportunity is a key characteristic of this pattern. Within that window, not only must public health detect an attack, but it also must respond, which may involve administration of treatment or quarantine of thousands of individuals. Delays of just hours may translate into significant morbidity and mortality.

Smallpox Pattern

At the other extreme are disease outbreaks, such as smallpox or severe acute respiratory syndrome (SARS), which start with one or a few cases and then grow in number due to communicability [15]. In such outbreaks, the first patient will become very ill and present for medical care even before the secondary cases become symptomatic. The earliest opportunity for detection of these kinds of outbreaks requires an astute clinician who when presented with a fully declared example of the disease performs the appropriate workup, formulates a correct differential diagnosis, and takes the necessary actions such as notification and quarantine. Even very late detection of the case (e.g., at autopsy) could still be of considerable value if it leads to prevention of other cases. The kind of information technology most suited for this is decision support at the point of care, as described below under Primer II: Clinical Event Monitors.

Early Warning Systems for Public Health Surveillance

Public health surveillance systems have been defined as networks of people and activities that may function at a range of levels from local to international [16]. In the U.S., surveillance is provided by more than 50 systems that are themselves loosely coupled and undergoing constant change. They are collectively the product of an evolutionary process rather than the result of implementation from a single set of prespecified functional requirements [13].

Current public health surveillance systems are based largely on reporting by laboratories of reportable diseases (that have been diagnosed by microbiological and other testing) and by astute clinicians and lay people who notice individuals or groups of individuals with problems of public health importance. These methods are manual and are known to suffer from delays in reporting and underreporting.

Mitigating an *Anthrax pattern* outbreak will require vast improvements in the rapidity of detection and of response decision making in public health. Improvements of even an hour over current capabilities may reduce economic impact by hundreds of millions of dollars [17].

A promising new approach being pursued by research groups, including our own, is real-time analysis of secondary data, which are data being collected routinely for other purposes (for example, clinical data collected by electronic medical record systems) [17,18]. The RODS system is an example of this class of systems. RODS has been deployed since 1999 in Pennsylvania and since the 2002 Winter Olympics in the state of Utah. We make RODS available free for noncommercial use (available by click download from www.health.pitt.edu/rods/sw).

Figure 39.2 illustrates some of the functions of RODS. Data from a large region are collected in real time and stored in a database. The data are diverse, including microbiology cultures, chief complaints, and over-the-counter (OTC) sales of health products. Algorithms periodically analyze the data for anomalous densities of cases and bring those cases to the attention of public health officials by e-mail or pager notification. Investigators can analyze the spatial and temporal distributions of cases, or can use a look-back capability to access electronic medical records (also discussed in Primer II, below).

Figure 39.2A is the main screen from RODS that displays the temporal pattern of seven prodromes in emergency department visits in a region. In particular, it shows the daily numbers of patients registering with respiratory, diarrheal, rash, constitutional, neurological, botulinic, and encephalitic chief complaints.

Figure 39.2B shows a general query facility, called EpiPlot, for examining temporal distribution of cases. The user can select the data to be plotted, for what time frame and from what geographic region. Figure 39.2C shows a general query facility called MapPlot for examining spatial distribution of cases. Figure 39.2D is an interface that allows a user such as a public health officer with proper access rights to review the details of individual cases in a suspicious "spike" of cases. This service is provided through automatic linkage with the results-review functions of a health systems electronic medical record system. A user must present a valid user ID and password to the native system to gain access.

In summary, our research and that of others is beginning to identify functional requirements for public health surveillance systems that have implications for clinical information systems. These requirements include the ability to quickly create and apply new case definitions; the ability to collect data in real time needed to test case definitions for a wide range of diseases; and the ability to collect and analyze other data including host characteristics, spatial data, food consumption, water consumption, personal contacts, veterinary and zoonotic data, and preclinical data such as biosensor data and OTC drug sales.

The research has also identified types of clinical data that are of importance in public health surveillance [19].

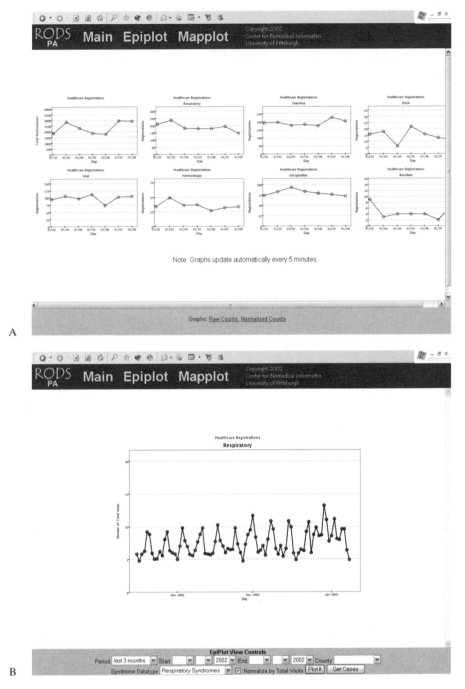

FIGURE 39.2. RODS (real-time outbreak and disease surveillance system) interfaces. (A) Main screen. Each graph plots daily counts of reasons for visits to eight emergency departments. The first graph (reading *left to right*) plots both the total number of visits (all cause) and the total number of visits for problems conceivably related to infectious disease. The other graphs plot counts of viral illness, respiratory illness, diarrhea, rash, and encephalitis. (B) A standard epidemic plot. The controls at the bottom of the page allow configuration of the time frame and the syndrome type data for the plot.

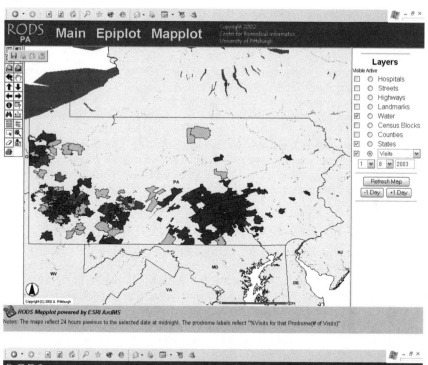

C

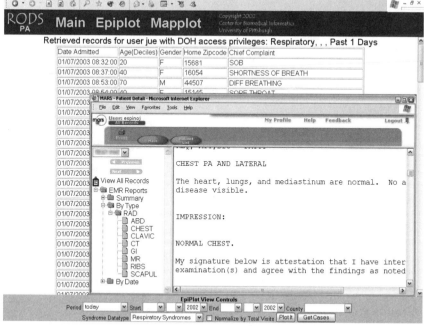

D

FIGURE 39.2. (C) A commercial off-the-shelf mapping function. Maps may be zoomed, moved, and detailed to the street level. *Darker areas* indicate increased activity. (D) Electronic medical record review. This screen displays a subset of patients derived from a query executed earlier in a session. With appropriate access privileges, a user can query the electronic medical record of a particular patient for dictated reports, images, laboratory tests, and cultures, as shown in the *inset*.

- *Nonspecific syndromes:* Examples of data needed for detection of patients with early stages of disease are data about symptoms of colds or diarrhea and ICD-9 coded diagnoses of upper respiratory illnesses. Other examples include questions asked by patients to clinicians (via health Web sites or call centers).
- *Specific syndrome:* Examples of data needed include histories of exposures, vital signs, physical findings, laboratory results, radiology results, and preliminary results from microbiology laboratories (e.g., Gram stains).
- *Definitive agent:* Examples of data include microbiology cultures or autopsy reports.
- *Clinical epidemiology:* Examples include clinical data, plus information on the whereabouts of patients prior to onset of disease, food and water consumption, contacts with affected individuals, work and home addresses. We discuss the clinical information systems that may provide these data in the Primer II section below.

Privacy and the Architecture of Early Warning Systems

For reportable diseases, public health departments are entitled by law to receive identifying information from clinicians about the affected individuals for the purposes of treatment and investigation of the cause of the outbreak. However, for other types of data needed for early warning public health surveillance, the legal basis for hospitals to provide identifiable information is much less firmly established. *This relatively firm constraint dictates a distributed detection system design in which some detection functions, such as linking of clinical data about a single patient to determine whether a patient satisfies a case definition, must reside within healthcare institutions.*

A distributed design is illustrated in Figure 39.3, in which elements of detection logic are located within each healthcare institution in a component that we call a *health-system-resident component* (HSRC). With this design, healthcare institutions do not have to pass detailed data about all patients to an external public health surveillance system. Instead, they pass only those cases that satisfy case definitions. The HSRC is discussed below as an example of a potential new component in healthcare information architectures.

CDC's National Electronic Disease Surveillance System

The CDC's National Electronic Disease Surveillance System (NEDSS) Project will influence the evolution of public health surveillance. NEDSS is a combination of reference architecture for public health surveillance systems, standards for data encoding and messaging, a process of funding, and actual components for system builders. At the time of this writing, the NEDSS-guided development of electronic public health surveillance systems in state and county health departments has a focus on automation of health department functions. The link to clinical data focuses on Web-based interfaces that clinicians and laboratorians can use to report notifiable diseases [20].

Primer II: What Public Health Should Know about Clinical Computing

A modern healthcare enterprise operates scores of computer systems for scheduling, registration, billing, radiology, laboratory, pharmacy services, dictation, ordering of tests, recording of clinical observations, emergency room management, and intensive

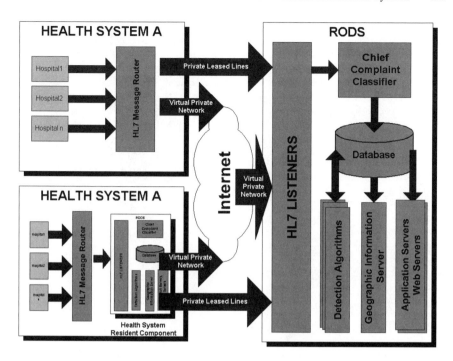

FIGURE 39.3. RODS and health system resident component (HSRC). Located in the University of Pittsburgh Medical Center Health System (UPMC-HS) is a health-system-resident component. Other health systems that do not have an HSRC interact with RODS directly using HL7 to transmit data. RODS maintains the connections from the HSRC(s) and message router(s), accepts and parses data, calls the inference engines, applies outbreak detection algorithms, and handles notifications. The HSRC provides the ability to apply additional case definitions and infection control functions. It consists of the same components as RODS (a database, epidemic detection logic, a Web application server, access control, and modules that generate spatial and temporal displays), albeit in smaller scale.

care unit operations. It is therefore surprising that, although public health practice is highly dependent on data from healthcare systems for surveillance, there are few if any direct links between clinical information systems and public health. Instead, data are typically transferred back and forth by fax, mail, or phone between the two domains of practice. The untapped potential of data collected by existing computer systems (and the untapped potential of point-of-care systems to support real-time, decision-supported interactions between healthcare providers and public health) is enormous. This section summarizes the types of clinical systems, the data they collect relevant to public health surveillance, and market penetration (Table 39.1).

HL7 Message Routers

Figure 39.4 illustrates typical health system information architecture. Health Level Seven (HL7) is a dominant messaging standard in healthcare computing that allows systems built by different vendors to more readily exchange data. Although we do not know the exact national market penetration of HL7 as a deployed standard, in our

TABLE 39.1. Clinical systems, data, and market penetration (estimated).

Clinical system	Data	Hospital/health system	ED	Office/home health	LTCF	Potential uses
Registration	Chief complaints, addresses, age, gender	High	High	?	—	Syndrome-based detection strategies
Scheduling	Appointments and reasons	High	High	?	—	Syndrome-based detection strategies
Billing	CPT-4 codes	High	High	High	—	Indirect evidence
Laboratory	Cultures, tests	High	High	High	High	Culture- and test-based detection strategies
Radiology	Chest radiographs	High	High	High		Test-based strategies
Pathology	Biopsies, autopsies	Mod.	Mod.	Mod.		Diagnosis-based strategies
Dictation	Symptoms and signs	High	High			Symptom and sign data
Pharmacy						Indirect evidence
Orders	Tests, drugs ordered	Low	Low	Low	Low	Indirect evidence
Data warehouse	All clinical data	Low	—	—	—	All the above
Event monitor	—	Low	—	—	—	—
Point-of-care systems	Coded symptoms, vital signs, signs, diagnoses, orders, epidemiological data	Low	Low	Low	—	Data needed to satisfy case definitions; potential for decision support for physicians
Patient Web portals and call centers	Symptoms, referrals appts.	Low	—	—	—	Collect early symptom information, potential for decision support for patients and doctors

ED, emergency department; LTCF, long-term care facility; —, not applicable; ?, unknown.

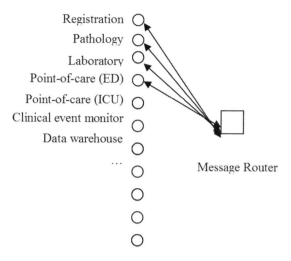

Registration
Pathology
Laboratory
Point-of-care (ED)
Point-of-care (ICU)
Clinical event monitor
Data warehouse
...

Message Router

FIGURE 39.4. Representative information technology (IT) architecture of a modern health-care system. Various clinical systems feed HL7 message data to an HL7 message router to be distributed.

work in Pennsylvania and Utah we found it to be nearly ubiquitous. HL7 message routers are recognized as a key leverage point for bidirectional, real-time communications among existing clinical systems described in this chapter and public health surveillance systems.

Registration, Scheduling, and Billing Systems

Most healthcare systems handle patient registration, scheduling, and billing automatically. There are a few vendors that supply the systems and most provide HL7 outbound interfaces. Data useful for public health surveillance include chief complaints and reasons for a health visit, patient age, gender, and home address. Many research groups in bioterrorism detection are investigating the use of such systems and data to provide an earlier signal than current methods [1,5,17,21].

Electronic registration is almost ubiquitous in emergency departments and hospital-based or associated practices as well as large HMOs. Smaller practices may not utilize electronic systems to as great an extent, however. Billing, scheduling, and registration data are collected at the health system level; thus, to achieve regional surveillance, multiple health systems data must be integrated. There is heterogeneity in coding practices and schemes used that represent moderate obstacles to data integration.

Clinical Laboratory Systems

The data supplied by laboratories are important to surveillance of virtually every public health threat. Happily, the vast majority of clinical laboratories in the U.S. are highly automated, utilizing computers to run tests, store results, and communicate results. Clinical laboratories perform tests on a variety of human tissues and fluids: blood, urine, stool, cerebrospinal fluid (CSF), saliva, mucus, semen, and fluid aspirated from joints. Laboratory test results are often important in establishing diagnoses and are generally available online very soon after they are run, making the laboratory's time lag among the shortest of all data systems. Results are available not only directly from the laboratory systems, but, where deployed, also through the laboratory reporting interfaces of point-of-care systems. Thus, because of ubiquitous availability, public health authorities are justified in closely examining methods of integrating laboratory data into an early warning system for threats to public health, as they have been doing [22,23].

Radiology Systems

Radiology departments were also relatively early conversions in health care to computer processing. Most healthcare systems today handle radiology scheduling and resulting automatically. There are a few vendors that supply the systems and most provide HL7 outbound interfaces. Data useful for public health surveillance include results of imaging, especially of chest and lungs. Many research groups in medical informatics have investigated methods for processing radiology imaging reports to recover information about patient characteristics, such as presence or absence of pneumonia on chest radiograph [24–29]. Technical advances have made the digital storage and presentation of images at the point-of-care feasible, although the market penetration of this functionality is low at present. Such functionality would be of limited use for public health and is mainly reserved for detailed investigation of new disease outbreaks that are eluding characterization and requiring expert analysis of source materials.

Pathology

Pathology information systems are more recent additions to healthcare computing because of the image-intensive nature of pathology practice (gross and microscopic examinations). Thus, penetration into the market is less than for laboratory or radiology systems. Data useful for public health surveillance include orders for tests and results. Data accuracy would be expected to be very high. Timeliness and availability are not as good as for laboratory systems due to the nature of pathology practice and the fact that these systems in many places are free-standing (used to generate printed reports), and integration has not been as critical a design factor as in laboratory or radiology resulting.

Dictation

Dictation systems are a mainstay of clinical data recording in the hospital, emergency department (ED), and outpatient settings. Dictation services can range from single part-time transcribers working with word processing software to transcription pools producing reports in dedicated systems manufactured by companies such as Lanier. Although dictations are rich in clinical detail, including the patient's presenting complaint, the history of the illness, exposure information, vaccinations, vitals signs and physical findings, and diagnostic impressions, the data are in English and difficult to process computationally. There is also a time delay due to transcription that further limits data utility. Nevertheless, the value of the information is sufficiently high that many researchers in medical informatics have developed approaches to processing these data. The accessibility of these data is lower than that of laboratory systems because dictations are less frequently routed through a message router.

Pharmacy

Pharmacy information systems receive and process orders for medications. These orders may include antibiotics and antidotes for toxins that provide indirect evidence of a patient's symptoms or diagnosis. In most implementations, the orders are received on paper and transcribed by the pharmacist into the pharmacy information system; thus, there is a delay from the time the physician expresses his or her understanding of the clinical problem in the form of orders to the time that information is available electronically. The reliability of the information is extremely good, however, since pharmacists use expert knowledge and contextual information (available in the orders themselves, the pharmacy information system, and sometimes from review of the patient chart or contact with the physician) to validate the order before dispensing a medication. Pharmacy data are not highly accessible to other computer systems in most health systems; however, the importance of pharmacy data for prevention of medication errors has created a strong motivation for hospitals to upgrade their pharmacy systems

Orders

Many healthcare systems have computer applications that allow ward clerks to communicate physician orders to the laboratory and other departments in the healthcare system. Orders, similar to pharmacy orders, contain indirect information about a patient's condition. For example, if a CSF examination or blood cultures are ordered, this action suggests that the patient may have an infectious condition. If respiratory isolation is ordered, this action may indicate that the patient should be seen by hospital infection control. In a very small number of healthcare institutions, physicians enter orders directly into computers, eliminating the time delay and creating an opportunity for direct interaction and decision support of the clinician [30–33]. The potential of this type of data and activity is discussed under point-of-care systems below.

Data Warehouses and Results Review

Healthcare systems often operate data warehouses to integrate data from multiple information systems and multiple hospitals. Data warehouses have become increasingly prevalent as a result of the mergers and acquisitions that occurred in health care in the 1990s. Although data warehouses do not represent a primary source of data like systems previously discussed, they represent a point of integration of data that can be considered as a leverage point for public health surveillance. Data warehouses are not always real time, although if they are being used by a healthcare system to achieve a useful consolidated view of data for clinical purposes (referred to as "results review") they will have the real-time characteristic. The availability of real-time data warehouses in health care is moderate at present.

Results review has potential value for accelerating the conduct of public health investigations. With appropriate permissions, public health investigators will read electronic charts rather than traveling to all locations at which affected individuals have received care.

Clinical Event Monitors

A clinical event monitor is a type of clinical information system with considerable potential to contribute to public health surveillance. Clinical event monitors first appeared in the 1970s. They have been referred to variously as reminder systems [34–42] and alerting systems [43–45]. Clinical event monitors perform real-time collection and analysis of clinical data for the purpose of improving the care, both preventive and acute, of *individual patients* [46].

The potential for public health surveillance has been partly explored by empirical research on detection of cases of tuberculosis [28,47] and in the related field of hospital infection control [29,48–51].

The relevance of clinical event monitors to public health surveillance is suggested by their feed-forward, data-driven architectures and their core capabilities, which include (1) access to relevant data collected routinely by other clinical information systems, and (2) facilities for operators to define logical patterns that can be compared to incoming patient data. In particular, they are well suited for implementing case-detection logic and for supporting real-time interactions with clinicians to influence clinicians' actions.

Point-of-Care Systems and Decision Support

Point-of-care systems refer to systems that are used by clinicians to record directly details of patient encounters, to review information, and to order tests and other services. Vendors sell point-of-care systems specialized for diverse settings including ED, office, hospital, intensive care units (ICU), long-term care facilities, and home health care. Point-of-care systems can be of use even in prehospital care settings. "Ruggedized" handheld computers have been deployed in the field to aid emergency medical units in the delivery of care to patients.

Rapid detection and response depend on tight coupling between the activities of public health workers and the activities of individual clinicians. This coupling can be accomplished best through embedding of decision support and disease-reporting capability within clinical information systems. The importance of point-of-care systems is the ability to embed decision support that can interact with the physician at the time the patient is being seen and thereby influence decision making about testing and treatment. Such an infrastructure will help clinicians adhere to rapidly changing population-based guidelines needed to optimally manage individual cases, and it will provide public health officials with aggregate information about disease activity needed for public health surveillance.

Unfortunately, in the U.S., point-of-care systems are deployed in fewer than a quarter of hospitals nationwide and in even fewer physicians' offices; even this number can overstate the extent of their actual availability, since, for example, in this statistic, a point-of-care system present in one department within a hospital is sufficient to be counted. A small minority of agencies responsible for prehospital care, such as fire and emergency medical services, utilize point-of-care systems. The Surgeons General's offices of the nation's military services, when interviewed, were not aware of widespread use of point-of-care systems in military facilities; if they are deployed, such deployments may be scattered in specific facilities. On the other hand, the Veterans Administration has a high level of deployment of point-of-care systems.

In the United Kingdom, by contrast, point-of-care systems are ubiquitous. The value of these systems for public health surveillance is illustrated by the rapidity with which the U.K. will be able to implement an anthrax surveillance strategy. By changing the decision support logic only once in a central location, the ability will exist to detect postal workers presenting with influenza symptoms at the time of phone or physical presentation to any primary care physician. Moreover, the ability to provide advice at that very moment to the physician seeing the patient will also exist.

Patient Web Portals and Call Centers

Two additional types of information systems are now appearing in healthcare settings. Patient Web portals are designed to provide scheduling and triage information for patients. Call centers are designed to provide similar functionality for those patients who do not have access to, or the inclination to use, Web services. Call centers also support communication among physicians, as in the case of physician-to-physician consultation. The types of data collected by these systems justify their inclusion in this discussion, despite their very low market presence. Patient Web portals have the potential to collect symptom-level data as early as the day of onset of illness. Call centers have similar potential, but only if patients can be persuaded to use them early, rather than waiting for illness to progress. The reliability and availability of such data have the potential to be very high, especially if such services are designed from the ground up with the needs of regional integration of data for public health surveillance purposes in mind.

Health System Resident Component

An example of a new component in health system architectures is the Health System Resident Component (HSRC). It is similar in function and architecture to a clinical event monitor, and, in fact, we initially developed HSRC from an existing clinical event monitor that was developed and maintained by two of the authors (FCT, MMW). That system, called CLEM (CLinical Event Monitor), currently operates within the University of Pittsburgh Medical Center Health System in Western Pennsylvania (Figure 39.4) [52]. Like other event monitors, CLEM analyzes data routinely collected by other computer systems (e.g., laboratory information systems, radiology systems, and the registration system). These systems transmit data in the form of HL7 messages over a network to an HL7 message router and then via the message router to CLEM. The transmissions occur without delay unless there is a problem with an interface, in which case messages are stored temporarily in the sending system or the message router. Clinical event monitors often include communication subsystems that convey results of analyses directly to responsible physicians. In CLEM, the notification subsystems use databases that map between patients and responsible physicians and communication channels such as pagers and e-mail [53–55].

With the HSRC, a healthcare information system can detect and automatically transmit to the health department reportable cases of disease based on microbiology data, provide deidentified clinical data to public health surveillance systems such as RODS, and detect cases using specific case definitions (e.g., define a possible anthrax case as a patient with a wide mediastinum on a chest X-ray and gram-positive rods in their blood). The HSRC provides additional services beyond the support of public health surveillance activities. In particular, the HSRC provides infection control support through immediate detection of high-risk infectious diseases such as tuberculosis; detection of nosocomial infections; and detection of hospital-based outbreaks and computer-assisted outbreak investigations. In addition, the HSRC provides a specialized user interface for infection control practice consisting of line listings of patients with positive cultures, reports of any anomalies in the microbiology data that might signify an outbreak, and maps of the floors of the hospital on which infectious disease data can be plotted. In the HSRC, the user can toggle between hospital and community views. In hospital view, only data for hospitalized patients are counted and plotted, and the list of cultures and case definitions of potential interest available for plotting changes to reflect diseases of interest for hospital infection control (e.g., Vancomycin-resistant enterococcus). In community view, similar to RODS, only data for emergency visits are counted and plotted based on patients' free-text triage chief complaints.

Summary

Clinical data are highly relevant to public health surveillance. Clinicians and health systems are a primary point of data collection about the sick, including data about demographics, risk factors, symptoms, signs, special testing, and diagnoses. Clinical data in the U.S. at present, however, are not highly available to public health. Part of the reason is data availability; the use of computers to record clinical information has lagged behind administrative use, and market penetration is variable depending on the type of system. Clinical information systems are widely deployed in clinical laboratories, radiology departments, and for registration; less so in pathology departments; and least used as point-of-care systems. Some administrative systems such as registration, scheduling, and billing have data that are of value for public health surveillance, and developers of new strategies for early detection of disease outbreaks are using them. Examples of data that are highly available include chief complaints, demographic information, and laboratory results. Data that are needed but not available include symptom and sign data, which are often recorded using English in dictated notes, not computer encoding.

Point-of-care systems represent an important resource for detection of *smallpox pattern* outbreaks. The reason is that point-of-care systems can embed decision support that can assist a clinician in the recognition of rare diseases. Point-of-care systems also afford public health an opportunity to interact directly with front-line clinicians in real time. Thus, if a patient is identified by public health surveillance to require special treatment or data collection, a point-of-care system provides a channel into the process of care to effect those goals. In addition, point-of-care systems are capable of collecting additional types of data such as symptom and sign data needed for public health surveillance.

Barriers to integration of clinical systems into public health include legal, administrative, and technical barriers. At present, health systems typically provide detailed information to public health only about patients with notifiable diseases. Although public health has a legal basis to access any data needed for public health purposes, routine access of data needed for early detection is a new area without established precedents and practices. There are few models for how such use would be supervised or supported financially. The technical barriers include differences in how data are coded and represented that can involve expensive interface development. A bright note is that the clinical computing industry has been working on the problem of interfacing and data integration for several decades, so there is a large body of work already completed toward solutions that can be applied directly to the problem of integrating clinical data into public health practice.

Acknowledgments. We are indebted to the programmers who assisted in the creation of RODS and HSRC: Hoah-Der Su, Zhen Liu, and Xiaoming Zeng. This work was supported in part by grants GO8 LM06625-01 and T15 LM/DE07059 from the National Library of Medicine; contract no. 290-00-0009 from the Agency for Healthcare Research and Quality; contract F30602-01-2-0550 sponsored by the Defense Advanced Research Projects Agency and managed by Rome Laboratory; and by Cooperative Agreement Number U90/CCU318753-01 from the Centers for Disease Control and Prevention (CDC). The views and conclusions contained in this document are those of the authors and should not be interpreted as necessarily representing the official policies, either expressed or implied, of the Defense Advanced Research Projects Agency, Rome Laboratory, or the United States government, and its contents are solely the responsibility of the authors and do not necessarily represent the official views of CDC.

References

1. Lober WB, Thomas Karras B, Wagner MM, et al. Roundtable on bioterrorism detection: information system-based surveillance. J Am Med Inform Assoc 2002;9(2):105–115.
2. Anonymous. Syndromic surveillance for bioterrorism following the attacks on the World Trade Center—New York City, 2001. MMWR (Morb Mortal WKLY Rep) 2002;51:13–15.
3. Green MS, Kaufman Z. Surveillance systems for early detection and mapping of the spread of morbidity caused by bioterrorism. Harefuah 2002;141:31–33.
4. Tsui F-C, Espino JU, Wagner MM, et al. Data, network, and application: technical description of the Utah RODS Winter Olympic Biosurveillance System. Proc AMIA Symp 2002.
5. Tsui F-C, Wagner MM, Dato V, Chang C-CH. Value of ICD-9-coded chief complaints for detection of epidemics. Proc AMIA Symp 2001;711–715.
6. Quenel P, Dab W, Hannoun C, Cohen JM. Sensitivity, specificity and predictive values of health service based indicators for the surveillance of influenza A epidemics. Int J Epidemiol 1994;23(4):849–855.
7. Brinsfield K, Gunn J. Using volume-based surveillance for an outbreak early warning system. Acad Emerg Med 2001;8(5):492.
8. Welliver RC, Cherry JD, Boyer KM, et al. Sales of nonprescription cold remedies: a unique method of influenza surveillance. Pediatr Res 1979;13(9):1015–1017.
9. Roush S, Birkhead G, Koo D, Cobb A, Fleming D. Mandatory reporting of diseases and conditions by health care professionals and laboratories. JAMA 2001;282(2):164–170.
10. Department of Defense. Chemical and Biological Defense Program: annual report to Congress. 2000.
11. NATO handbook on the medical aspects of NBC defensive operations AMedP-6(B). NATO; 1996. [Army Field Manual 8–9; Navy Medical Publication 5059; Air Force Joint Manual 44–151.]
12. Anonymous. Biological Diseases/Agents List (online) 2002 (cited 2002; 12/20). Available from: http://www.bt.cdc.gov/Agent/agentlist.asp.
13. Dato V, Wagner M, Allswede M, Aryel R, Fapohunda A. The nation's current capacity for the early detection of public health threats including bioterrorism. Washington, DC: Agency for Healthcare Research and Quality; 2001.
14. Meselson M, Guillemin J, Hugh-Jones M, et al. The Sverdlovsk anthrax outbreak of 1979. Science 1994;266(5188):1202–1208.
15. O'Toole T. Smallpox: an attack scenario. Emerg Infect Dis 1999;5(4):540–546.

16. Buehler J. Surveillance. In: Rothman K, Greenland S, editors. Modern epidemiology, 2nd ed. Philadelphia: Lippincott-Raven; 1998.
17. Wagner M, Tsui F-C, Espino J, et al. The emerging science of very early detection of disease outbreaks. J Public Health Manag Pract 2001;6(6):50–58.
18. Centers for Disease Control and Prevention. Preventing emerging infectious diseases: a strategy for the 21st century (online) 2000 (cited 2001 April 30). Available from: http://www.cdc.gov/ncidod/emergplan/.
19. Wagner MM, Aryel R, Dato V. Availability and comparative value of data elements required for an effective bioterrorism detection system. Washington, DC: Agency for Healthcare Research and Quality; 2001 (11/28/01).
20. National Electronic Disease Surveillance System (NEDSS): a standards-based approach to connect public health and clinical medicine. J Public Health Manag Pract 2001;7(6):43–50.
21. Espino J, Wagner M. The accuracy of ICD-9 coded chief complaints for detection of acute respiratory illness. Proc AMIA Symp 2001;164–168.
22. Effler P, Ching-Lee M, Bogard A, Man-Cheng L, Nekomoto T, Jernigan D. Statewide system of electronic notifiable disease reporting from clinical laboratories: comparing automated reporting with conventional methods. JAMA 1999;282(19):1845–1850.
23. Panackal AA, M'ikanatha NM, Tsui F-C, et al. Automatic electronic laboratory-based reporting of notifiable infectious diseases. Emerg Infect Dis 2001;8(7):685–691.
24. Jain NL, Knirsch CA, Friedman C, Hripcsak G. Identification of suspected tuberculosis patients based on natural language processing of chest radiograph reports. Proc AMIA Ann Fall Symp 1996;542–546.
25. Fiszman M, Chapman WW, Aronsky D, Evans RS, Haug PJ. Automatic detection of acute bacterial pneumonia from chest X-ray reports. J Am Med Inform Assoc 2000;7(6):593–604.
26. Chapman W, Haug P. Comparing expert systems for identifying chest x-ray reports that support pneumonia. Proc AMIA Symp 1999;216–220.
27. Chapman WW, Fizman M, Chapman BE, Haug PJ. A comparison of classification algorithms to automatically identify chest X-ray reports that support pneumonia. J Biomed Inform 2001; 34(1):4–14.
28. Hripcsak G, Knirsch C, Jain N, Stazesky RJ, Pablos-Mendez A, Fulmer T. A health information network for managing innercity tuberculosis: bridging clinical care, public health, and home care. Comput Biomed Res 1999;32(1):67–76.
29. Knirsch C, Jain N, Pablos-Mendez A, Friedman C, Hripcsak G. Respiratory isolation of tuberculosis patients using clinical guidelines and an automated clinical decision support system. Infect Control Hosp Epidemiol 1998;19(2):94–100.
30. Sittig DF, Stead WW. Computer-based physician order entry: the state of the art. J Am Med Inform Assoc 1994;1(2):108–123.
31. Bates DW, Boyle DL, Teich JM. Impact of computerized physician order entry on physician time. In: Proceedings of the annual symposium on computer applications in medical care. 1994. p. 996.
32. McDonald CJ, Tierney WM, Overhage JM, et al. The Regenstrief Medical Record System—experience with MD order entry and community-wide extensions. Proceedings of the annual symposium on computer applications in medical care 1994. p. 1059.
33. Tierney WM, Miller ME, Overhage JM, McDonald CJ. Physician inpatient order writing on microcomputer workstations: effects on resource utilization. JAMA 1993;269(3):379–383.
34. McDonald CJ. Protocol-based computer reminders, the quality of care and the non-perfectibility of man. N Engl J Med 1976;295:1351–1355.
35. McDonald CJ, Hui SL, Smith DM, et al. Reminders to physicians from an introspective computer medical record. Ann Intern Med 1984;100(1):130–138.
36. Frame P. Can computerized reminder systems have an impact on preventive services in practice? J Gen Intern Med 1990;5(suppl 5):S112–S115.
37. Winickoff R, Coltin K, Fleishman S, Barnett G. Semiautomated reminder system for improving syphilis management. J Gen Intern Med 1986;1(2):78–84.

38. Ornstein SM, Garr DR, Jenkins RG, Rust PF, Arnon A. Computer-generated physician and patient reminders. Tools to improve population adherence to selected preventive services. J Fam Pract 1991;32:82–90.
39. Rind DM, Safran C, Russell SP, et al. The effect of computer-based reminders on the management of hospitalized patients with worsening renal function. In: Clayton PD, editor. Proceedings of the fifteenth annual symposium on computer applications in medical care. Washington, DC: McGraw-Hill; 1993. p. 28–32.
40. McDonald CJ, Hui SL, Tierney WM. Effects of computer reminders for influenza vaccination on morbidity during influenza epidemics. MD Comput 1992;9(5):304–312.
41. McDonald C. Action-oriented decisions in ambulatory medicine. Chicago: Year Book Medical; 1981.
42. McDonald CJ. Use of a computer to detect and respond to clinical events: its effect on clinician behavior. Ann Intern Med 1976;84(2):162–167.
43. Bradshaw KE. A computerized laboratory alerting system to warn of life threatening events. PhD dissertation, University of Utah, Department of Medical Informatics. 1988.
44. Kuperman GJ, Gardner RM, Pryor AT. HELP: a dynamic hospital information system. New York: Springer-Verlag; 1991.
45. Rind DM, Safran C, Russell SP, et al. Effect of computer-based alerts on the treatment and outcomes of hospitalized patients. Arch Intern Med 1994;154:1511–1517.
46. Hripcsak G, Clayton P, Jenders R, Cimino J, Johnson S. Design of a clinical event monitor. Comput Biomed Res 1996;29:194–221.
47. Hripcsak G, Knirsch C, Jain N, Pablos-Mendez A. Automated tuberculosis detection. J Am Med Inform Assoc 1997;4(5):376–381.
48. Classen D, Pestotnik S, Evans R, Burke J. Description of a computerized adverse drug event monitor using a hospital information system. Hosp Pharm 1992;27(9):776–779.
49. Evans R, Larsen R, Burke J, et al. Computer surveillance of hospital acquired infections and antibiotic use. JAMA 1986;265:1007–1011.
50. Kahn M, Steib S, Fraser V, Dunagan W. An expert system for culture-based infection control surveillance. In: Proceedings of the annual symposium on computer applications in medical care. 1993. p. 171–175.
51. Larsen RA, Evans RS, Burke JP, Pestotnik SL, Gardner RM, Classen DC. Improved perioperative antibiotic use and reduced surgical wound infections through the use of computer decision analysis. Infect Control Hosp Epidemiol 1989;10:316–320.
52. Wagner M, Pankaskie M, Hogan W, Tsui F, Vries J. Clinical event monitoring at the University of Pittsburgh. Proc AMIA Symp 1997;188–192.
53. Wagner M, Tsui F, Pike J, Pike L. Design of a clinical notification system. Proc AMIA Symp 1999;989–994.
54. Wagner M, Eisenstadt S, Hogan W, Pankaskie M. Preferences of interns and residents among e-mail, paging, and traditional methods for the delivery of different types of clinical information. Proc AMIA Symp 1998;140–144.
55. Tsui F-C, Wagner M, Wilbright W. A feasibility study of two methods for end-user configuration of a clinical event monitor. Proc AMIA Symp 1999;975–978.

40
Leveraging Patient Data to Support Clinical Practice

CRAIG S. LEDBETTER

To truly promote best practice, access to accurate and complete patient data at the point of care is required.

Sources of Data

To manage appropriately the clinical care of their patients, clinicians must simultaneously consider information from a number of sources:

a. The health history of the patient and the patient's family.
b. The current health problems of the patient.
c. The clinical status of the patient including laboratory and other physiological results.
d. The current treatment regimen and the patient's individual response to selected treatment options.
e. A body of knowledge concerning diagnostic possibilities and their treatment recommendations.
f. Evidence about the efficacy and risks of the various treatment options.
g. The expected outcomes and prognosis of patients with similar health problems, clinical status, and treatment regimen.
h. A large body of general scientific and medical knowledge that facilitates the understanding and interpretation of all this information.

Some of this information comes from data in the individual patient's record. Some of it comes from studies of population-based aggregations of patient data. Some comes from the general study of science, medicine, and other related disciplines. This listing of information required for clinical management suggests that the patient record is a most important source of data for clinical decision making.

Applications developed to provide support for clinical practice must be able to access information from both patient-specific and population-based perspectives, as well as relevant information from specialized knowledge bases. Without access to patient-specific clinical data, a system cannot provide patient-specific recommendations. Although there may be value in a system that simply provides easy access to sets of standard practice guidelines, order templates, or searchable knowledge bases, such applications can provide only general support for clinical practice.

Craig S. Ledbetter, RN, BSIS, is Manager of Product Development for Misys Healthcare Systems.

Patient Data and Clinical Decision Support

Clinical decision support system (CDSS) refers to a wide range of functionality in clinical software systems. This includes clinical alerting capabilities, knowledge base access, dosage computation and other clinical calculations, context-driven documentation templates, diagnostic algorithms, predefined treatment protocols and order sets, and other computer-based facilities that can support clinical decision making to some degree. These may be implemented as standalone systems or integrated into a computer-based patient record system.

There are many examples of the successful application of specific CDSS functionality within a healthcare information systems environment [1]. This is good; the need for comprehensive CDSS is becoming critical. The healthcare industry is currently being driven by unprecedented economic, social, and political forces to improve healthcare quality, patient safety, and access to care while still decreasing costs [2–6]. If the benefits of a CDSS are to be fully realized, it seems clear that a comprehensive set of CDSS tools will need to be integrated into a computer-based patient record (CPR) system to support clinical decision making at every point along the clinical care management process. Access to the patient-specific data available in the CPR makes possible patient-specific recommendations in the form of alerts, practice guidelines, clinical pathways, or other mechanisms that encourage appropriate care [1]. Particularly critical is the integration of CDSS facilities with computerized physician order entry, when clinicians are actually creating the plan of care [7].

Due to the complexity of this task, it is likely that such a comprehensive point-of-care CDSS will have to be constructed incrementally. But building software systems using an iterative software development model requires a well-defined set of prioritized business requirements to be successful. Many have contributed to such a set of requirements for CDSS [8–11], and additional requirements will continue to be identified as the industry gains experience with these systems. The identification of business requirements and conversion into an appropriate system design is the goal of systems analysis and design. Examining the business and system requirements for a comprehensive CDSS is an interesting exercise that may provide insight for healthcare organizations that are seeking to meet the business imperatives they face today by implementing one or more applications that support clinical decision making.

Business Requirements for Comprehensive CDSS

Clinical Process

The clinical process, as it is taught to physicians, nurses, and other allied health professionals, is an adaptation of the scientific method. By examining the process that clinicians follow as they manage the clinical care of their patients, the operational scope of a comprehensive CDSS can be understood. Clinical decision support capabilities are useful in all phases of the clinical process: (a) assessment, (b) planning, (c) intervention, and (d) evaluation. The clinical process is a continuous cycle in which clinicians constantly integrate new clinical patient information, refine assessments and diagnoses, and revise the plan of care. The kinds of decision making performed by clinicians in each of these phases might be targeted with specific applications of CDSS technology.

A model for business requirements discovery for CDSS can be developed by asking, "Where in the process of care would clinicians benefit from access to specific information or other decision support services?" Once this model has been developed, the analysis can be further refined by determining the type(s) of information and services that could be helpful at each point in the clinical process, and how that support would best be presented. This process would help define the functional scope of a comprehensive CDSS (Table 40.1).

TABLE 40.1. Business requirements for clinical decision support systems.

Clinical process	Patient focus (point-of-care): Transactional Analysis	Population focus (retrospective): Aggregate Analysis
Assessment		
Intellectual support	• Clinical documentation templates • Relevant knowledge base access • Clinical group membership • Differential diagnosis generation	• Clinical group identification • Analysis of disease processes • Community health analysis • Epidemiological analysis
Error prevention	• Result field range checking • Criteria-based result fields	• Clinical risk factor analysis
Clinical environment	• Relevant patient data display • Risk factor flags • Critical value alerts • Reminders • Calculations/conversions	• Case-mix analysis • Disease prevalence studies • Study group identification • Outlier case identification
Planning/intervention		
Intellectual support	• Order templates • Protocol order sets • Relevant knowledge base access • Evidence citation access • Expert drug dosing • Treatment option generation	• Clinical pathway development • Evidence-based practice guideline development • Protocol development • Care standards development • Antibiotic sensitivity report
Error prevention	• Allergy warnings • Drug interaction check (vs. drug, procedure, diet, disease/problem) • Procedure interaction check • Criteria-based orders/referrals • Duplicate order checks • Corollary orders • Dose calculation checking	• Protocol/pathway variance analysis • Adverse drug reaction analysis • Advisory override analysis • Drug dispensing error analysis • Drug administration error analysis
Clinical environment	• Drug cost warnings • Procedure cost warnings • Procedure availability information • Clinical reminders (scheduled and criteria-based) • Relevant patient data display • Patient education templates • Interdisciplinary order display	• Resource availability analysis • Service turnaround time analysis • Acuity staffing analysis • Service volume analysis • Service delay analysis
Evaluation		
Intellectual support	• Variance indicators • Relevant knowledge base access	• Benchmarking • Outcomes measures • Process quality indicators • Wellness management analysis • Disease management analysis
Error prevention	• Critical value alerts • Criteria-based alerts • Abnormal result highlighting	• Sentinel event investigation
Clinical environment	• Relevant patient data display • Reference range display • Result verification processing	• Clinical risk adjustment • Utilization review analysis • Patient satisfaction results

Source: Adapted with permission from CS Ledbetter and MW Morgan, Journal of HIMSS 2001; 15(2): 119–131.

Clinical Decision Making

This approach sounds deceptively easy—just two steps to a set of business requirements for a comprehensive CDSS. Our understanding of the clinical process is fairly complete, as it is a man-made model for approaching the clinical management of patients that is taught almost universally to clinical professionals in schools of medicine, nursing, and the allied health disciplines. Developing an understanding of how care providers make clinical decisions is much more complex, however.

There is very interesting work being done to further our understanding of clinical reasoning and decision psychology [12] from which we may glean some insight about the kinds of information and services that might facilitate clinical decisions. A number of models have been proposed to help understand how clinical reasoning occurs [13]. Such models must be simplifications of the cognitive organization and processing of knowledge, as no single model seems to explain all aspects of clinical decision making [14]. However, the models are useful for thinking about how and when a CDSS could be helpful to practicing clinicians, or for categorizing the reasons for failures of clinical judgment [12].

Patient Safety and Medical Errors

An increasing level of concern about patient safety in the United States was brought into focus by the Institute of Medicine's (IOM) 2000 report *To Err is Human: Building a Safer Health System* [3]. This report gave estimates for the number of deaths and other adverse clinical events related to medical errors that were surprisingly high to most readers (adverse events occur in 2.9 to 3.7 percent of hospitalizations, resulting in 44,000 to 98,000 deaths annually). The IOM estimated annual healthcare costs of *preventable* adverse events to be $9 to $15 billion. In addition to the high economic costs and patient suffering associated with preventable adverse medical events, a new focus on patient safety from federal and state policy makers [4,5] has placed increasing pressure on healthcare organizations to take action to report and reduce medical errors.

In this environment, an analysis of the business requirements for a CDSS must include the identification of those activities in the clinical care process that are most frequently associated with medical errors and/or adverse patient outcomes. As a starting point, providing targeted decision support facilities at points along the process of care where errors are more likely to occur is a reasonable design approach.

Clinical Errors

Diagnostic and other clinical errors might be divided into "no-fault" errors, "system" errors, or "cognitive" errors [15]. "No-fault" errors occur because it is not always possible to be certain of a diagnosis or treatment choice. This type of error may be reduced through the introduction of new knowledge from scientific study and the evidence-based practice of medicine. "System" errors occur due to latent imperfections in the healthcare delivery system. This type of error is perhaps the most easily addressed by CDSS and other forms of care process automation (workflow queues, reminders, communication facilities, etc.) provided by CPR systems.

"Cognitive" errors reflect failures in clinical judgment, from misdiagnosis to faulty data collection (omissions included), flawed reasoning, or lack of knowledge. Diagnostic error is more challenging to address in the design of a CDSS. The dependence on patient-specific data is greater, the knowledge bases and algorithms required are extremely complex, and the system must more directly interact with the clinician to provide help here. Although there are computer-based programs that can support diagnostic decisions by providing extensive differential diagnoses based on the patient's clinical information [1], a clinician still must determine the appropriateness of the suggested diagnoses. Initially, CDSS may help avoid cognitive errors by providing context-specific information, documentation templates, and other indirect means of supporting the clinician's diagnostic decision-making efforts.

Preventing Errors

Failures in clinical judgment might never occur if the intellectual demands of medicine did not exceed human intellect, if clinicians always diligently checked for errors, or if the clinical process or system itself provided sufficient safeguards [16]. If CDSS can intervene by supporting the clinician's intellect, checking for and guarding against errors, and in general, making the clinical operational environment more efficient and effective, clinical errors may be decreased. As a starting point, these goals can add an additional dimension to the analysis of requirements for a comprehensive decision support system (see Table 40.1).

Patient Data and the Computer-Based Record

To truly promote best practice, access to accurate and complete patient data at the point of care is required. Providing relevant patient-specific data as well as evidence to support a particular clinical pathway can mean the difference between a pathway that is followed or one that is ignored by clinicians [9]. The effective scope of a CDSS is extremely limited in the context of a paper-based medical record—only niche CDSS applications can be implemented. Any patient data that a standalone application requires must be redundantly entered. Such standalone systems have not been widely adopted by clinicians, which limits their influence in eliminating unwanted practice variation or improving outcomes [9]. It can be argued that a prerequisite to a truly comprehensive CDSS is a CPR that supports the entire clinical care process. Only if clinicians use the computer during every patient care management activity can CDSS provide support throughout the entire scope of the clinical care process.

An examination of the existing patient record can be used to determine the degree to which CDSS will be able to support a specific clinical environment. Each instance of handwritten clinical documentation or orders in the patient record represents a point in the clinical process where only niche, standalone CDSS applications are feasible. Even in those areas of the enterprise where CDSS is integrated into a CPR, the patient data on the handwritten portions of the record are unavailable to the system. Access to patient-specific data is incomplete, and this affects the scope and functionality of the CDSS. Handwritten clinical notes and orders in the patient record represent holes in the ability of an integrated CDSS to help prevent errors, facilitate clinical operations, and otherwise provide intellectual support to clinicians.

Computerized Physician Order Entry

Few points along the clinical process of care provide more opportunity for effective CDSS applications than when the clinician is creating the plan of care—the point of order entry [7]. Direct order entry by clinicians is the ideal. Even if nurses or clerks enter handwritten physician orders into the CPR, most of the advantage gained from real-time, interactive CDSS facilities (alerts, relevant knowledge base access, and other context-driven CDSS features) is forfeited.

Medication Orders

A lot of attention has been given recently to medication orders and the impact of medication errors and adverse drug events (ADEs) on patient safety. Drug interaction checking, drug dosing calculations, drug allergy checking, drug laboratory value checks, corollary order prompting, and other interactive CDSS at the point of order entry may reduce medication-related errors [7]. Access to drug guidelines at the time of administration and access to drug information and patient instructions at the time of dispensing could also enhance the safety of drug therapy at those important points in the clinical process.

Mechanism to Implement Best Practice

Clinician orders include more than medications—they represent the entire plan of care. CDSS applications at the point of order entry provide a mechanism for implementing changes in clinical practice by presenting best practice recommendations and evidence to support those recommendations at the appropriate time. Access to patient data allows the system to avoid unnecessary "nuisance" prompting of the physician with irrelevant alerts and recommendations. When properly integrated into order entry in a CPR, CDSS applications can improve compliance with protocols, practice guidelines, clinical pathways, and other best-practice tools [1].

Transactional Analysis

At the point of care, clinical interventions are transactional in the sense that they are ordered, scheduled, performed, and documented within fairly well-defined clinical operational processes. From a patient-specific perspective, information analysis must be supported at the level of an individual point-of-care transaction in the CPR system.

A number of CDSS applications can be triggered by an individual clinical transaction (e.g., the entry of an individual test result or treatment order) to provide interactive alerts, context-specific protocol orders, or other rules-based support. Data from a single clinical transaction can be evaluated, or the evaluation can also include data within other transactions from the same patient encounter, or data within transactions from other encounters. These data can be tested against one or more predefined rules that may access independent knowledge bases and apply specialized algorithms to determine system response. CDSS applications implemented at the transaction level can be interactive and context specific, and provide support for decisions about a particular patient at a particular point along the clinical process—the point of care.

Aggregate Analysis

Clinicians, administrators, and researchers also require aggregate analysis of clinical data for retrospective, population-based studies. Aggregate analysis of appropriate data can help make the difference between medicine as an art, where anecdotal evidence and individual experience influence clinical decisions, and medicine as a science, where statistically valid evidence about clinical and process outcomes drives clinical decisions [17].

Transactional patient data from the CPR can be grouped and aggregated to provide the evidence required to guide improvements in clinical practice, establish protocols, design clinical pathways, and develop quality indicators. CDSS applications implemented at the aggregate level should be able to provide statistically valid information to support decisions about a particular patient population across the entire clinical process, supporting evidence-based practice.

Published journal articles can provide evidence on which to base clinical decisions, but for any given clinical case, the applicability of the published study to the specific patient or population of patients being cared for must still be determined by the clinician. Aggregate analysis of a local patient population can facilitate comparisons to the study population to help determine if a published study is germane.

The clinical decision support requirements listed in Table 40.1 have been separated into patient-focused, point-of-care requirements that require transactional analysis of patient-specific data and population-focused, retrospective requirements which require aggregate analysis of population-specific data.

Knowledge Bases

Access to relevant, up-to-date knowledge resources (drug information databases, disease databases, journal articles, etc.) is also necessary to provide the full scope of information needed for clinical decision making. To achieve widespread use by clinicians, CDSS facilities must be easily accessible and readily available at the time of clinical decision making [9]. These requirements go beyond the simple model of knowledge base "libraries" that can be accessed by clinicians through search engine functionality. Simply providing easy access to relevant knowledge resources at appropriate points in the clinical care process does provide a basic infrastructure that supports the need for reference information. However, the ability of a system to deliver relevant reference information to the clinician at the point of care based on specific patient data from the current transaction and from within the current patient record goes beyond simple library functionality and enables context-specific knowledge base access.

This review of the business requirements for a CDSS is meant to be representative, not comprehensive. We will undoubtedly be analyzing clinical practice and discovering new ways to support clinical decision making for a long time to come. CDSS applications in actual practice are relatively new, and their impact on clinical practice and patient outcomes is just beginning to be studied. Not all the assumptions made here regarding the potential benefits of any particular application of CDSS technology are theory free. However, this requirements set is large enough to provide a sense of the scope of a comprehensive CDSS and to begin to define the system infrastructure and functionality that could support CDSS across the entire clinical care process. The goal of providing insight for healthcare organizations that are seeking to implement CDSS applications can be met by providing this glimpse of the system requirements for a comprehensive CDSS.

System Requirements for a Comprehensive CDSS

Processing Patient Data

As an overriding goal, CDSS should support patient-specific clinical decision making at the point of care. This implies that CDSS applications are created from a set of knowledge-based tools fully integrated into the clinical workflow and with access to a repository of complete, accurate patient-specific clinical data [8]. The best way to achieve this from a systems perspective is to integrate the CDSS functionality into a CPR that supports the full clinical care process. Patient data and clinical workflow support are provided by the CPR, and this represents an enabling infrastructure for CDSS.

This does not necessarily mean that, as an intermediate step, a CDSS application cannot be implemented as a standalone system. It does imply that the ultimate goal would be to integrate that application into a CPR to avoid redundant data entry, share patient-specific clinical data with other systems, and make the application accessible to all appropriate clinical users.

Transactional Processing

A CPR system stores and retrieves discrete clinical transactions at a very high rate to support real-time patient data entry and patient data review across a large healthcare enterprise. The CPR accesses patient data from the repository in a longitudinal, patient-centric manner. To support the real-time clinical care process, any data from any encounter for a particular patient must be retrievable for display or processing with subsecond response time. Online transactional processing (OLTP) is the term used to describe this type of data processing.

In many cases, CDSS applications must analyze patient data at the transactional level in context with other patient data or with data from specialized knowledge bases. Algorithms designed to produce information useful for clinical decision making can be applied in this type of real-time, online transactional analysis (OLTA). Many transactional systems support the integration of functionality during transactional processing through filing triggers or other application programming interfaces (APIs) that expose the patient data from within a clinical transaction to other computer processes. These triggers can supply transactional data to CDSS applications that provide alerts, messaging, and other criteria-based actions that depend on the data in the current transaction.

The analysis rules for each CDSS application could be coded into the application at the time of development, but this produces a system that is difficult and costly to modify and maintain. A better design is the integration of a rules engine, with facilities for defining and modifying rules without the need for additional programming. Each CDSS application would then query this OLTA "rules engine" by passing patient data from individual transactions for specific analysis. Based on a Boolean response from the rules engine, the CDSS application would either perform or not perform the specific action it was programmed to do.

The definition of the rules to be applied by the OLTA rules engine should be stored in a configuration database, to facilitate frequent additions or modifications as required by the decisions and recommendations of the Medical Staff, clinical quality improvement committees, or other organizational best practice development activities. This provides an architecture that is flexible enough to support the iterative improvement process typical of continuous quality improvement (CQI) and evidence-based medicine (EBM) methodologies.

When a large amount of specialized knowledge is required to support the evaluation of rules, a knowledge database should be integrated with the system in such a way that the rules engine can make use of the specialized data for comparison or other required analysis. A drug information database is an example of such a specialized knowledge base, which is typically provided by a commercial vendor who retains responsibility for updating the information regularly. This relieves the CDSS application and the rules engine of the large maintenance responsibility for the drug information in the database.

Aggregate Processing

Even in this era of gigahertz processors, the sheer volume of transactions encountered by CPR systems requires that they be specifically designed and tuned to handle OLTP. Database architecture, indexing, disk caching, and other parameters are optimally configured for rapid transactional processing and access to the longitudinal patient record. System performance may suffer if the system is used for other types of processing (e.g., aggregate, population-based analysis or multidimensional reporting), thus affecting system response at the user interface.

Clearly, many of the CDSS requirements described depend on information produced from retrospective, population-based aggregations of patient data, or, to coin a new term, online aggregate analysis (OLAA). The type of data processing required to support such aggregate analysis can tax a CPR system designed primarily for OLTP. The architectural design that enables efficient OLTP is fairly inefficient for aggregate analysis and multidimensional reporting, causing competition for available processing resources, and leading to unacceptable delays at the point of care.

It is possible to design a database system to support the complex set operations and high-volume disk reads required for the retrospective, aggregate analysis of large volumes of patient data. A clinical data warehouse (CDW) is an example of such a system. Extraction of patient data from the OLTP system and reorganization of the data within the CDW enable efficient population-based and multidimensional analysis and avoid the impact of inefficient aggregate processing on the real-time transactional system.

Attributes of a Clinical Data Warehouse

Nussbaum and Ault described fairly thoroughly the attributes of a CDW, making the distinction that it is not just a large collection of clinical data [18]. A CDW includes patient data from the CPR and (potentially) data from other enterprise systems, stored on a separate system and reorganized to support retrospective analysis. The data are filtered and manipulated to provide an integrated data set with common units and conforming dimensions. Specialized data structures (e.g., the fact and dimension tables of star-schema architecture) are created to support multidimensional analysis, and the data may be stored redundantly at various levels of aggregation to support ease of reporting and enhance performance. The data are often organized into subject-oriented domains (data marts) to support various user populations and simplify security. Database architecture and system configuration are adjusted to optimize the CDW system for aggregate analysis.

The CDW does not contain a mirror image of the patient data in the transactional system, but rather a subset of data useful for retrospective aggregate analysis. Data needed only for real-time clinical process management are not needed in the CDW. For example, the OLTP system may contain data required to determine proper work queue flow and resolve other real-time processing questions. The CDW does not need these data, but rather contains the results of the clinical processes that occurred—orders, results, and clinical documentation from the patient record.

The CDW is not a real-time system. Real-time processing should be done on the OLTP system to make the data from those transactions available to the OLTA rules engine. There are "best-of-breed" clinical systems that integrate patient data from multiple departmental systems using real-time interfaces. This architecture can consolidate all patient data into a single repository, but the repository itself must handle a high volume of update and read transactions as well as support any real-time clinical rules analysis. Because the system requirements for transactional processing must be considered in their design, these systems poorly support the need for aggregate or multidimensional analysis [19]. A separate CDW specifically tuned for retrospective, population-based aggregate analysis of patient data seems to be a system requirement for comprehensive CDSS.

System Design

The system requirements outlined here suggest a number of application components that appear to be necessary for a comprehensive CDSS. Figure 40.1 is a high-level diagram of a comprehensive decision support model. From this model it is clear to see what would be lost without the feedback mechanism provided by the CDW and the aggregate processing that it supports. Information obtained from the CDW should be integrated back into the clinical process in several ways. Rules-based clinical alert criteria evaluated during transactional processing can be based on information obtained through aggregate analysis using the CDW. In this way, real-time alerts and reminders will address specific opportunities for improvement discovered in the clinical data. The effectiveness of those rules can be monitored in the same way. Clinical pathways, protocol order sets, and other standards of care utilized during the clinical care process

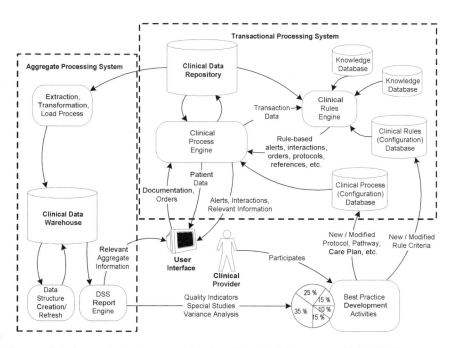

FIGURE 40.1. System design for comprehensive clinical decision support (CCDSS). The system requirements outlined here suggest a number of application components that appear to be necessary for a comprehensive CDSS. (Adapted with permission from CS Ledbetter and MW Morgan, Journal of HIMSS 2001;15(2):119–131.)

can be developed and monitored using aggregate information from the CDW. This represents an evidence-based, iterative approach to achieving best practice. Relevant aggregate information (pathway variance reports, special study results, etc.) from the CDW can be presented to the clinician at the point of care to support treatment decisions for populations of patients. Slowly changing community health factors, such as the prevalence of certain diseases or the recent antibiotic resistance patterns for locally cultured pathogens, can be constantly updated and available to the clinicians.

Management Information

The types of information needs that can be supported through aggregate analysis with a CDW can be categorized based on the type of reporting tool required to produce them. Management reporting meets predictable information needs using basic reporting applications that allow the generation of predefined or "canned" reports. Most if not all commercially available reporting tools support predefined report generation, and they can manage and maintain large libraries of these reports. The typical management report that provides monthly departmental statistics is an example of a report that meets a predictable information need in the healthcare organization.

Ad Hoc Information

Unpredictable information needs are met by reporting applications that allow the user to produce ad hoc queries or that support "drill down" into the data. This allows users to answer questions that arise unpredictably and that are not answered by the available management reports. Most multidimensional reporting tools provide this type of reporting environment, although the performance of these tools can depend on the specialized architecture of the underlying data structures in the CDW. These tools produce the type of retrospective, population-based analysis required for many CQI, EBM, and CDSS development initiatives.

Data Mining

Discovery and predictive modeling information needs are met by reporting applications that analyze targeted data sets using traditional statistical methods or artificial intelligence techniques to determine the significance of findings (confirmatory analysis) or to discover significant patterns and correlations within the data that were previously unknown (exploratory analysis). Data mining is a rapidly growing area of business intelligence that uses specialized decision support tools to go beyond traditional analysis by query.

Data mining tools that support discovery can find patterns in patient data without the need for the user to provide a specific hypothesis to test, and they can produce graphs or other visualizations to display the discovered patterns to the user.

Data mining tools that support predictive modeling can supply values for unknown variables based on previously discovered patterns and correlations. A pertinent example of predictive modeling would be the assignment of a clinical risk adjustment value based on documented physical assessment and diagnostic test results contained in the patient record. This would allow a CDSS system to alert the clinician if a particular patient was at high risk for morbidity, mortality, or even excessive resource utilization while there was still time to intervene.

Data mining tools that support forensic analysis can find statistically unexpected values in a target data set. This allows the identification of opportunities for improvement, where variation in clinical practice or some other special cause has produced outlier results. Such outliers can be easily detected at the time that they happen if a particular process of care is being measured and monitored regularly. This type of data mining tool allows the system to discover these unexpected results in care processes that are not being monitored with performance indicators.

Examples of Comprehensive CDSS

Studies of the impact of widespread implementation of CDSS within the framework of a full-featured CPR and supporting CDW do not yet exist, but studies of smaller implementations of CDSS functionality indicate that the potential to impact clinical care and patient safety is great [1]. Advanced CDSS implementations that depend on sophisticated integration into the CPR infrastructure are beginning to be cited in the literature, and these examples provide additional lessons that will have implications beyond the design phase of the software system development life cycle.

The implementation methodology and change management approach utilized for any specific CDSS application can affect the impact the application will have on actual clinical practice after go-live. Installing a comprehensive set of CDSS tools is not enough. Integrating those tools into the CPR and providing a CDW, knowledge bases, and other supporting infrastructure is not enough. If the goal of CDSS is to positively impact clinical practice, then the implementation of a comprehensive CDSS must be considered as part of a larger plan to support the evidence-based practice of medicine and promote best practices. An actual case study from the recent literature can illustrate this [9].

Case Study from University Health Networks

University Health Networks (UHN) in Toronto, Canada, is a large, 1000-bed, integrated healthcare delivery network that includes Princess Margaret Hospital, Toronto Western Hospital, and Toronto Medical Laboratories. UHN has implemented the Misys CPR(TM) system developed by Tucson based Misys Healthcare Systems (www.misyshealthcare.com). The Misys CPR system is a high-availability transactional system that provides a patient data repository with integrated clinical operational workflow management, a criteria-evaluation engine (OLTA rules engine), and integrated knowledge bases. It supports all phases of the clinical care process. In Figure 40.1, Misys CPR functionality is represented by those processes within the area labeled "Transactional Processing System." Misys CPR at UHN is accessible to authorized clinicians from more than 5000 desktops across the enterprise and contains data for more than 3 million patients and 12 million visits over the past decade.

The CDW at UHN is Misys Data Warehouse(TM), also developed by Misys Healthcare Systems. Extracted patient data from Misys CPR populates the Misys Data Warehouse, which is implemented on the Oracle® Enterprise Edition relational database management system (www.oracle.com). In Figure 40.1, Misys Data Warehouse functionality is represented by the area labeled "Aggregate Processing System."

Organizational Environment

Two years ago UHN established a Clinical Advisory Committee to oversee all CDSS initiatives. This committee is chaired by a practicing physician and includes representatives from both clinical and administrative areas. Their goal is to provide clinicians with CDSS tools that can improve the quality and efficiency of clinical care.

This committee approved an initiative that sought to reduce inappropriate utilization of the erythrocyte sedimentation rate (ESR) laboratory test. Aggregate analysis identified this opportunity for improvement when it was discovered that 12,000 ESR tests were being performed annually. A clinical working group evaluated the available evidence and developed a guideline that would limit the indications for the use of ESR tests to cases in which temporal arteritis was suspected or when monitoring connective tissue disease activity. This guideline was based on evidence (studies) from the literature, not anecdotal examples or individual clinician experience, an important distinction to note for this best practice development activity. Physician involvement in the prioritization, development, testing, and implementation of the CDSS application was seen as a critical factor in the success of the initiative [9].

Application Design

The guideline was approved by the Clinical Advisory Committee, and the Shared Information Management Team (SIMS) at UHN became responsible for the development, testing, deployment, and evaluation of the CDSS application to implement this new practice guideline. From the comprehensive set of CDSS tools provided by the Misys CPR system, the team developed a rule-based alert that triggered at the time of clinician order entry. Rather than simply implement an alert describing the new protocol, the SIMS team provided an option for the clinician to see the evidence on which the new guideline was based. This was accomplished through services provided by Ovid Technologies (www.ovid.com), a leading provider of Web-based EBM content. Misys partnered with Ovid to streamline access to Ovid content, avoiding the need for any additional sign-on process or content searching. Selecting the option to see the evidence from the order entry screen in Misys CPR directly produced the specific reference document desired.

Application Impact

Immediately after implementation of this CDSS application, the utilization of ESR tests at UHN dropped nearly 50 percent. This reduction has continued in the intervening 2-year period. The design of the alert took a number of factors into account:

1. There was good evidence that allowed the clinical working group to define specific indications for the appropriate use of the ESR test.
2. The alert was implemented at precisely the point in the process of care where clinicians were making the decision to order the test.
3. The evidence that supported the new clinical protocol was directly available at the point of decision, without any undue overhead required to retrieve it.
4. The size of the improvement opportunity was known before the decision to implement the alert.

Additional Experience

UHN has implemented a number of similar alerts since the ESR utilization initiative but with mixed success [9]. The variation in effectiveness of similar CDSS applications might be explained by one or more of the design factors mentioned above. This is most dramatic where some of these design factors were not specifically addressed in the CDSS implementation.

Standard duplicate alerts for laboratory and other tests can easily be configured in the Misys system. These duplicate alerts can be defined to inform the clinician if a previous order for the same test has been placed within a certain time period (e.g., the last 24, 36, or 48 hours). The clinician can then decide whether to place the order anyway. No clinical protocol is displayed that describes specific indications for repeating the test, and no links to evidence in support of the alert are provided. However, these standard duplicate alerts do occur at the point of clinician order entry, addressing that important design factor, and the number and rate of duplicate orders for any given test can be determined through aggregate analysis before a decision to implement an alert.

UHN implemented a standard duplicate alert for chest radiograph (X-ray) orders. If a chest X-ray had previously been ordered within the past 24 hours, the system displayed an alert when a clinician ordered an additional chest X-ray. The clinician could choose to override the alert and order the duplicate test. Chest X-rays ordered for patients in the intensive care units were not included in this alert. (In a very unstable patient, multiple chest X-rays within a 24-hour period might be indicated.) This was a general clinical alert that was not associated with an evidence-based guideline or supporting references. This alert had no impact on the utilization of chest X-rays.

UHN also enabled standard duplicate alerts for the top 27 (by volume) laboratory tests. Simply enabling these alerts alone, without specific ordering guidelines or references to applicable evidence, produced no significant impact on test utilization for approximately 50 percent of the laboratory tests.

Changing the practice behavior of clinicians appears to require more than unsupported prompts or alerts during order entry. At UHN, the CDSS alerts that offered relevant evidence through an educational approach tended to be more effective in guiding the clinician toward best practice than those which were less specific regarding the basis for the alert [9]. This finding highlights the importance of a comprehensive approach to designing and implementing CDSS applications to ensure best practice is achieved.

Conclusions

Access to patient data is a critical design consideration for CDSS applications. CDSS can be beneficial throughout the entire clinical care process, particularly during clinician order entry. Integration of CDSS applications into the CPR may be the best way to achieve the goal of comprehensive clinical decision support.

As a first step, CDSS applications can be deployed where it is likely that they can prevent or reduce clinical errors. CDSS can provide intellectual support, error checking, and general environmental support to help prevent errors. Although some clinical decisions (e.g., diagnosis) are inherently complex and the cognitive process used during clinical reasoning is not yet well understood, CDSS with full access to patient data can enable patient-specific or context-based information and alerts that can indirectly support such complex clinical decisions.

Experience with CPR systems that have integrated, comprehensive CDSS tools available is currently limited. Early examples suggest that there are design factors that may influence the effectiveness of individual applications of CDSS technology which are not necessarily related to gaps in system functionality. Valid evidence, developed through the analysis of patient data and scientific study, may be a critical prerequisite to changing clinician behavior in many cases. Although this means that even a comprehensive CDSS is not necessarily a silver bullet that will end unwanted practice variation and usher in an era of best practice in health care, it does suggest that one of the most powerful uses of CDSS is to further the use of evidence-based medicine in the clinical environment.

References

1. Trowbridge R, Weingarten S. Clinical decision support systems. In: Shojania KG, Duncan BW, McDonald KM, et al., editors. Making health care safer: a critical analysis of patient safety practices. Evidence Report/Technology Assessment No. 43 (prepared by the University of California at San Francisco–Stanford Evidence-based Practice Center under contract no. 290-97-0013); AHRQ Publication No. 01-E058. Rockville, MD: Agency for Healthcare Research and Quality; 2001. p. 589–594.
2. Committee on Quality of Health Care in America, Institute of Medicine. Crossing the quality chasm: a new health system for the 21st century. Washington, DC: National Academy Press; 2001.
3. Committee on Quality of Health Care in America, Institute of Medicine. Kohn LT, Corrigan JM, Donaldson MS, editors. To err is human: building a safer health system. Washington, DC: National Academy Press; 2000.
4. Medical errors—congressional and federal agency activity on errors. JHITA Advocacy Paper. Joint Healthcare Information Technology Alliance. November 2000. Available on-line: http://www.jhita.org/mederrors.htm.
5. Booth M, Riley T, Rosenthal J. Medical errors and adverse events: a report of a 50-state survey. NASHP Publication No. GNL31. Portland, ME: National Academy for State Health Policy; 2000.
6. Forum for State Health Policy Leadership. Frequently asked questions . . . access and the uninsured. Washington DC: National Conference of State Legislatures. 2002. Available on-line: http://www.ncsl.org/programs/health/forum/faqaccess.htm.
7. Kaushal R, Bates D. Computerized physician order entry (CPOE) with clinical decision support systems (CDSS). In: Shojania KG, Duncan BW, McDonald KM, et al., editors. Making health care safer: a critical analysis of patient safety practices. Evidence Report/Technology Assessment No. 43 (prepared by the University of California at San Francisco–Stanford Evidence-based Practice Center under contract no. 290-97-0013); AHRQ Publication No. 01-E058. Rockville, MD: Agency for Healthcare Research and Quality; 2001. p. 589–594.
8. Perreault LE, Metzger JB. A pragmatic framework for understanding clinical decision support. J HIMSS 1999;13(2).
9. Wu R, Peters W, Morgan MW. The next generation of clinical decision support: linking evidence to best practice. J HIMSS 2002;16(4):50–55.
10. Metzger J, Stablein D, Turisco F. Clinical decision support: finding the right path. First reports series. Long Beach, CA: First Consulting Group; 2002.
11. Raiford R. The power and value of embedded clinical decision support. CARING Newsletter. Columbia, MD: The Capital Area Roundtable on Informatics in Nursing; 2002.
12. Elstein AS, Schwarz A. Clinical problem solving and diagnostic decision making: selective review of the cognitive literature. BMJ 2002;324:729–732.
13. Elstein AS. Clinical problem solving and decision psychology: comment on "the epistemology of clinical reasoning." Acad Med 2000;75:S134–S136.
14. Norman GR. The epistemology of clinical reasoning: perspectives from philosophy, psychology, and neuroscience. Acad Med 2000;75(suppl 10):S127–S133.
15. Graber M, Gordon R, Franklin N. Reducing diagnostic errors in medicine: what's the goal? Acad Med 2002;77:981–992.
16. Redelmeier DA, Ferris LE, Tu JV, et al. Problems for clinical judgement: introducing cognitive psychology as one more basic science. CMAJ (Can Med Assoc J) 2001;164(3):358–360.
17. Framework for improving performance. Oakbrook Terrace, IL: Joint Commission on Accreditation of Healthcare Organizations; 1994.
18. Nussbaum GM, Ault SP. The best little data warehouse. J HIMSS 1998;12(4):79–93.
19. Amatayakul M. The state of the computer-based patient record. J AHIMA 1998;69(9):34–40.

41
Winona Health Online: Connecting the Community for Better Health

GARY EVANS and KATHRYN BINGMAN

> *In Winona, Minnesota, a bucolic, but progressive, community*
> *becomes the test bed for a visionary project that catapults*
> *healthcare delivery into the future.*

Strong Community, Big Vision

To the first-time visitor, Winona, Minnesota, may appear somewhat typical of a small Midwestern town: neat and clean, a collection of small houses and businesses that are nestled between the bluffs and the Mississippi River. To be sure, the area is beautiful. Its residents are friendly and hard working. Many of them are descendants of the German and Polish immigrants who arrived in the mid-1800s to operate the lumber mills that sprawled along the riverbanks and to develop the railroad system that was moving West.

The community, today, also seems largely untouched by the bustle of modern-day life ... peaceful, maybe even sleepy. In fact, the quiet pace of life and natural beauty caused Paul Harvey, a popular syndicated radio commentator, to call it one of the "best-kept secrets of the upper river," a phrase adopted by the local Chamber of Commerce to attract visitors.

But those first impressions mask other attributes of the city that was started 150 years ago by the early travelers of the great Mississippi River, on a sandbar, just 50 miles north of the point where Minnesota, Iowa, and Wisconsin connect. Analysts say that, during all of its 150 years, the community has been blessed to have people of great vision among its residents. The quiet, natural beauty almost hides a bustling and progressive community that, from its earliest moments, embraced the concept of education as important to its growth and development. The early visionaries stepped up, money in hand, to create the first teacher training institute west of the Mississippi River and funded Minnesota's first public high school. Their never-waning love for education led to the development of expansive public and private elementary and secondary systems, two universities, and a technical college.

Gary Evans is President and CEO of Hiawatha Broadband Communications, Inc. Kathryn Bingman is Vice President and General Manager of the Cerner Corporation and President of Cerner IQHealth.

Modern-day visionaries sensed the power of technology as the Internet took its fledgling steps. Community leaders first established an educational network dedicated to extending the reach of teaching and learning. They also ensured that Winona would have a prominent presence on the information superhighway by building a community fiberoptic telecommunications network that would provide Winona residents with high-speed connectivity through a company called Hiawatha Broadband Communications.

As an adjunct to education, the roots of the community's healthcare system were established in 1894, growing into a modern complex called Winona Health. Today, Winona Health consists of one acute care hospital, three extended care facilities, one assisted living facility, one clinic, one pharmacy, and one ambulance service. This system is dedicated to improving the health of the regional community through initiatives that are aided and advanced by leading-edge technologies.

Advancing Community Health Care

In Kansas City, Missouri, Cerner Corporation has been pioneering healthcare automation since 1979 by providing software, services, and content to healthcare organizations. These solutions are designed to address the needs of the entire healthcare continuum—from the ICU to the living room. Cerner's unique architecture places each person at the center of his or her own care by extending solutions and empowering the individual to manage his or her own health in better ways.

Then, Neal Patterson, Cerner's founder, chairman, and CEO, had a vision that involved searching for an ideal community to test a unique proposition: To use integrated technology solutions to connect citizens and healthcare providers, and, ultimately to improve the health status of a community. The combination of Winona's health system and community attributes attracted Patterson to choose Winona as the test bed for his vision. "To pioneer this type of shift, to a more involved consumer," says Patterson, "we searched for a city with a strong healthcare community, a population that valued knowledge and innovation, and a leadership that embraced technology as a means of establishing meaningful, ongoing relationships with its citizens."

A partnership between Winona Health, Hiawatha Broadband Communications, and the Cerner Corporation was formed, and Winona Health Online (WHOL) was christened on June 9, 2000. The underlying premise of WHOL is that health improves with more efficient, timely communication between health professionals and consumers who have access to appropriate, accurate, and individualized health information.

WHOL's goal was to provide the following services to the citizens of Winona:

- *A personal health system.* WHOL envisioned offering residents a secure place on the Internet where they could keep and control access to their own personal health information. A personal health record (PHR) is provided, enabling consumers to store and track their personal medical data. This information includes the results of laboratory tests, allergies, medications, conditions, and other pertinent medical history.
- *Quality health information.* WHOL wanted to provide a setting where health information from trusted sources could be made available to the Winona community via the Internet. WHOL chose information suppliers who would provide quality health, drug, and drug-interaction information. This has served to arm residents with the resources needed to make intelligent healthcare choices consistent with the opinions of their physicians.

- *Enhanced communication.* To extend care beyond the four walls of the hospital and enhance the patient–physician relationship, WHOL sought to encourage secure and private communications between consumers and their healthcare providers. WHOL accomplished this by providing consumers with the capability to schedule appointments, refill prescriptions, receive lab results, and ask follow-up questions to office visits.
- *Improved patient satisfaction.* Like other health organizations, WHOL sought a solution to the elusive "perfect patient" experience. By supporting consumers as they manage their own care at home, providing them with easy access to pertinent, reliable health information, and by making available additional communication with healthcare providers, WHOL offers a relationship management mechanism that surpasses traditional methods.
- *Improved community health.* Ultimately, WHOL set out to validate the premise that an innovative approach to healthcare practices—providing a framework for relevant prevention strategies, enhanced communications, and engaging empowered consumers—would result in better patient compliance, more appropriate treatment, and, ultimately, improved health outcomes.

Technology Considerations

Personal Health Records

WHOL sought to provide each resident in the community with his or her own personal health record (PHR). The PHR differs from an electronic medical record in that the information is owned and maintained by the consumer. Although there are many different approaches to the ideal PHR, the one taken by WHOL is based on the concept that a PHR should be:

- Populated by both consumer-entered information and clinical data collected across the continuum of care.
- Accessible by healthcare professionals at the appropriate time.
- Controlled by the consumer.
- Portable.

A recent Gartner report predicted that in 2002 and beyond, PHR models that rely primarily on patient-entered information are doomed to failure (0.9 probability) [1]. WHOL's vision, however, is to supply residents with a PHR that contains both their self-entered information and information that is supplied by their physicians or caregivers.

Security

Security continues to be vitally important in the development and use of consumer-driven healthcare management. The system used requires a unique user name and password and employs Secure Socket Layer 3.0 (SSL) and 128-bit encryption. A Personal Digital Certificate (PDC) was initially installed to offer the highest level of security possible for consumers, but this also presented a significant barrier to adoption. The PDC was removed after several months, which resulted in increased ease of registration. Individuals are also required to provide authentication by picture identification before sharing any clinical information. All communications are encrypted messages rather than simple e-mail messages.

Adoption Efforts

Given the broad goals of WHOL, physician acceptance and support was considered critical for its ultimate success. Physicians were involved in the planning and development process from the beginning. A medical advisory board was established to engage community physician leaders and healthcare professionals in guiding project development and implementation. Initially several meetings were held with physicians and their staff to explain how the system worked, how they could use it, and how patients would use it.

Simultaneously, WHOL began an extensive marketing campaign to inform consumers throughout the community. Marketing techniques included direct mail, presentations at local health fairs, newspaper and billboard advertisements, on-site employer presentations, and the use of student interns to promote WHOL. Computer kiosks were set up in highly visible, high-traffic areas to make it easy for individuals and families to sign up and access WHOL. Last, a $50 credit (equal to 3 months of Internet service) was offered to all users who signed up and took a health risk assessment on WHOL.

Status

Currently, 40 (of 50) physicians, the hospital (including lab and radiology), long-term care facilities, and four (of seven) pharmacies are participating in the project. As of December 2002, nearly 3600 consumer accounts are active. Currently, WHOL members can:

- Create and control a portable, online PHR.
- Take an online health risk assessment to share with their healthcare team.
- Receive lab results from their physicians and store them in their PHR.
- Participate in disease management programs and trigger alerts to their providers based on consumer-entered values.
- Ask questions of their providers, request and confirm appointments day or night.
- Access health information Web sites (including those recommended by their own providers), and receive information about prescriptions and over-the-counter drugs and their potential interactions.

Added Community Connections

WHOL provides value to many individuals outside the "four walls" of the traditional healthcare organization. For example, Home and Community Options is a not-for-profit organization that provides nearly 200 clients with complex healthcare and behavioral needs with residential and support services. They use WHOL to coordinate and update medical information. This is a unique value that provides a technologically accessible (24/7 with Internet access) single point of information and communication for multiple service providers from vastly different disciplines.

Other community organizations that rely upon WHOL include:

- Winona Health Services.
- Development Achievement Centers.
- Winona Workforce Centers.
- Public Health Department.
- Hiawatha Valley Mental Health.

Movement Toward Self-Care

Healthcare delivery organizations are seeking methods to provide their patients with better support while they are at home and managing their own care. Currently there are many different agencies, health systems, and providers that recommend self-care standards by disease state. The standards can be used by PHR systems to send reminders, provide information in the context of the individual's health state, and alert patients and their providers if their measurements are not within the normal and expected clinical ranges. Self-care needs also should include the integration of home monitoring devices. Providing guided self-care ultimately extends patient safety to the home.

WHOL sought to improve self-care within the community and initiated a diabetes-specific program. In October 2002, WHOL introduced the Diabetes Center as part of the Winona Diabetes Study. The Diabetes Study is being conducted through a partnership between Winona Health, Winona Family Medicine, Cerner, and a consultant affiliated with the University of Wisconsin. The study is designed to demonstrate the impact of online communications on the health outcomes of patients with diabetes versus nonparticipants with diabetes. Through the Diabetes Center, the study provides:

- A Diabetes Diary to track and communicate blood glucose levels and related diabetic information with members of each participant's diabetes care team (nutritionist, educators, physicians and other healthcare professionals).
- Templated and free-text messages that allow the diabetes care team to respond quickly and easily to the data that are communicated through participants' diaries and secure messages.
- The ability to securely send and receive messages among the care team.
- The ability for the care team to send discrete clinical lab results to participants.
- Participants with the tools to review and accept discrete clinical data that can be automatically stored in their PHR.
- Accurate information on diabetes, diabetes management, and related conditions.

This program helps patients feel more safe and supported in the management of their diabetes, but also works to improve workflow for clinicians and reduce paperwork and faxes. The diabetes program will be the foundation from which other disease-specific programs will grow.

Vision for the Future

Increased value for consumers will become evident as WHOL physicians forward medical visit summaries, laboratory test results, interpretation of radiological and other examinations, and medication data for inclusion in the PHR. As Gartner indicates, even motivated patients tend to lose interest over time or cannot accurately recall what has been done for them or discussed with them [1]. To create "sticky" Web-based community models, data must be autopopulated into the PHR from clinical systems. Centralized discrete data that the consumer owns and shares as they see appropriate presents a strong value proposition. Solving the broader challenges around the cross-organizational sharing of clinical information will yield the benefit of having personal health records be truly all-inclusive and connected. This is uniquely possible in Winona.

One of the key lessons learned in the WHOL project is that involving physicians in recruiting participants greatly influences adoption. By the end of 2003, all physicians in Winona will have the ability to connect to consumers within their normal workflow. Adoption rates will improve with ease in workflow for all those involved in the care process—physicians, nurses, office staff, and the patient.

The immediate focus is to provide solutions for people who have an ongoing, highly interactive relationship with the health system. Projects will be initiated to support women and children's health and additional disease focused programs such as congestive heart failure and asthma. Additionally, the ability to automatically add medical device data, such as glucometer readouts, directly to the PHR will serve to reduce significantly the barriers that patients face in keeping their PHR information current. Once data such as glucometer readouts can be incorporated automatically into the PHR, rules-based logic will then be used to notify healthcare providers when a patient's glucose levels are no longer in a predetermined range.

As more information is collected on an individual, the personal health system will be tailored to meet the individual's needs and help them better manage not only their own health but also that of others they care about. A wide variety of community organizations will have the ability to use blinded data to send targeted messages announcing classes, educational activities, or community testing that might directly address an individual's health issues. Clinicians will have the ability to recommend self-care guidelines and provide meaningful content to those whom they are treating.

WHOL also seeks to improve value for members through the inclusion of other entities that influence overall health. Other areas that are being explored include local employers, schools, and public health authorities.

WHOL has already demonstrated great vision and strides in connecting various entities within the Winona community. Early successes include the collaboration of local health organizations, businesses, and the support of Cerner to engage members of the community on the improvement of their own health. The future of the effort will, no doubt, be marked as other community programs from Winona have been—by a strong vision, success and strength of community involvement.

Reference

1. Healthcare predictions for providers: 2002 and beyond. The Gartner Group; 2001; Dec. 28.

42
INTERNATIONAL PERSPECTIVE
Global Outlook for Health Information and Communication Technologies

KLAUS A. KUHN

The status of health information systems worldwide is highly dependent on the sociotechnical and socioeconomic context of each country.

A Digital Divide

In April 2002, the Working Group on Health Information Systems of the International Medical Informatics Association (IMIA WG 10/HIS) held a Working Conference in Heidelberg, Germany, where international experts discussed the problems, challenges, and solutions currently confronting the development and deployment of healthcare information systems worldwide [1,2]. The perspective outlined in this chapter will comprise an overview of the results elaborated during this conference. While the Heidelberg conference was focusing primarily on the status of health care in highly industrialized nations, an overview of the situation in developing countries will be added as well.

The global state of healthcare information systems is characterized by a digital divide. Expenditures on information and communication technologies (ICTs) differ drastically among high-, low-, or middle-income economies, according to figures presented in the World Development Reports of the World Bank [3]. For the year 2000, the number of PCs per 1000 people—an important development indicator—was 20.1 in low- and middle-income economies, while it was 392.7 in high-income economies.

In the sections that follow, the status of and perspectives on developing countries and industrialized nations are described separately. Then, a section on global outlook will explore the challenges they have in common.

Klaus A. Kuhn, Professor, Dr. Med., is Professor and Director of the Institute of Medical Informatics and Chief Information Officer of the Philipps-University Marburg Medical Center in Marburg, Germany. Dr. Kuhn is also Chair of the IMIA Working Group on Health Information Systems.

Health ICT in Developing Countries

The IMIA Working Group on Health Informatics for developing countries (IMIA WG 9) has pointed out that political, economic, and social frameworks, as well as technological advances, are critical to the use and effectiveness of information and communication technologies, and that there are differences between developing countries and industrialized nations in these respects [4]. These frameworks also differ among developing countries. The role of information technology (IT), however, is directly dependent on the context of each country, the country itself, and its health system [5].

Relevance of Socioeconomic and Sociotechnical Issues

Several problems have been identified in the deployment and use of information and communication technologies in developing countries. Among the major ones are an inadequate communications infrastructure and a lack of human resources. Better access to hardware and to the Internet is needed and anticipated, but a lack of prerequisite skills for introducing, operating, and maintaining IT systems may be a serious limiting factor [6,7]. Insufficient programming capacity is also a problem because there are not enough companies that can write the required necessary applications software [8].

It is generally true that health information systems need to be adapted to the socioeconomic and technological context of each country, and this is particularly relevant in developing countries. Reports from Africa indicate that software to support healthcare processes cannot routinely be found off the shelf, so local development and end-user participation are necessary [9–11].

Although equipment may be inadequate, technology as such is similar worldwide. Differences exist, however, in the socioeconomic environment between developing and highly industrialized countries, and these differences have an impact on the design and use of health information systems in respective areas of the world. In a situation where financial and human resources are limited, goals and objectives need to be clearly identified and defined to develop effective IT support for healthcare processes. This is true in industrialized countries, and it is also of significant importance in developing countries. To optimize IT support of healthcare processes, organizational restructuring may be necessary; that is, instead of concentrating resources on major hospitals and focusing on upward reporting, local information management could be strengthened, thus supporting primary health care and prevention [12,13]. The development of the healthcare sector needs to be conceptualized and planned within the context of the broader infrastructure of the country. To establish the necessary skills, human resource development and educational programs are required [14,15].

These concrete areas in which information and communication technologies can bring improvements for developing countries have been identified [16]:

- Providing tools for continuing education.
- Delivering health and disaster management services to poor and remote locations.
- Increasing the transparency and efficiency of governance.

The necessity to take into account socioeconomic context has implications on the software engineering process and on the information system development process, both of which will benefit from a methodology that is fast and calls for optimal adaptation to organizational purposes. For example, the following has been suggested for Africa:

a software life cycle with an iterative process, including rapid application development, use cases as a simple and robust subset of UML for the overall design, and risk analysis [17].

The Role of the Internet

There have been predictions that the Internet will significantly help to bridge the digital divide between industrialized and developing countries [18]. In terms of health care, it is believed that telecommunications and the Internet may contribute significantly to improving global health systems performance and to reducing the inequities that separate the industrialized nations from the developing world. By means of the Internet, global access to information and knowledge, to education, and to healthcare services can become possible. A high number of factual databases and knowledge bases from around the world are already accessible via the Internet.

Access to the Internet, however, may also be limited. Estimates of Internet users worldwide [19] are about 1 in 30 on average worldwide, about 1 in 3 for Europe and North America, 1 in 125 for Latin America and the Caribbean, 1 in 200 for Southeast Asia and the Pacific, 1 in 200 for Sub-Saharan Africa, and 1 in 250 in East Asia. These figures are growing rapidly, but bottlenecks, such as telephone infrastructure problems and shortages of technical staff and of skilled personnel, may slow down progress in developing countries. It has been discussed that ICTs diffuse more slowly in developing countries and that they might bring fewer benefits and greater costs in comparison to industrialized nations, while alternative ICT solutions might fit better in a local context [20]; for example, tools such as CD-ROMS may be a good alternative for education and training. In industrialized nations, the Internet is expected to be a driving force toward the creation of collaborative information systems. In developing countries, it could also play a role in the collection of statistical and epidemiological data with the goal of improving strategies at the organizational and community levels [21]. In any case, the Internet is presenting an opportunity for global empowerment and for improved access to medical information and knowledge.

Health ICT in Industrialized Countries

The General Situation

In contrast to the situation in many developing countries, a highly developed health IT industry exists in industrialized countries. The IMIA WG HIS Heidelberg conference has provided an overview of the efforts and successes of this industry. Motivated by the need for keeping healthcare quality high in spite of massive cost pressures, care providers are demanding more comprehensive health information systems that provide clinical functionality and support work practice. Vendors have invested significantly, and the functionality discussed in Heidelberg shows their successes. Features like order entry, scheduling, and result reporting are becoming more prevalent and better adapted to the care providers' work practice. As academic centers increasingly replace their self-developed systems with commercial modules, cooperation between academic institutions and the health information systems industry has been established, often resulting in new and optimized solutions [22–27].

The Internet is having a massive impact on access to medical information and knowledge, on education, and on health care in general. Collaborative information systems are being created, which combine existing concepts, functionality, and roles [28]. Their potential for empowering patients and supporting communication, consultation, and collaboration among institutions, healthcare professionals, patients, and their families have been shown [29]. As one consequence, in industrialized nations, underserved, disadvantaged, and vulnerable populations have the chance to benefit from the rapid growth of the Internet. The digital divide within these countries can be bridged, and access to health information and health care can be improved; new forms of telecare also have begun to emerge [30].

There are, however, old and well-known problems that remain unsolved. In industrialized countries, organizational and sociotechnical factors are a core challenge, too. There have been statements that health care has remained relatively untouched by the ICT revolution that took place in the financial and industrial sectors during the past decade [31]. Health information systems still need improved functionality, flexibility, and adaptation to the health professionals' work practice. When a comprehensive health information system is to be built, the choice between holistic concepts, with broad but incomplete functionality, versus a combination of specialized and well-adapted niche products in a "best-of-breed" ensemble is still relevant. The ideal solution might be a component market allowing the composition of a system from independently deployable "plug-and-play" components from different vendors. Standardization efforts are aiming at this perspective, but it is far from realization today. Still, design of comprehensive systems is nontrivial, and costs are high, while at the same time it is difficult to demonstrate return on the necessary investment.

Return on Investment

To buy, deploy, and operate health information systems is cost-intensive. There is a great need to manage investments better and to justify them, so methods are needed to identify potential benefits and to quantify improvements in quality and cost savings. Reports exist on reduced waiting times, on reduction of office work, and on various types of possible cost savings [32,33]. Numerous investigations have also focused on the potential of information systems to reduce errors in medicine. The key idea has been to provide decision support at the point of care by presenting aggregated case-specific information from the patient database and combining it with domain-specific knowledge stored in knowledge bases. The spectrum of methods implemented to support health professionals is broad: reminders, alerts, structured ordering, prompts for consequent orders, and presentation of aggregated and goal-oriented information in typical decision situations have been used [34–40]. Decision support modules have been integrated into the users' work practice, so interactions take place when an order is entered, when a result is read, or when a report is written. Various modes of interactions have been investigated successfully, including conventional asynchronous interaction via e-mail [41] on one hand and rapid communication via pager in emergency situations on the other [42]. In this context, the relevance of analyzing the way health professionals interact and communicate has been identified [43], and excessive burdens on memory could possibly be reduced [44].

Effects of these IT-based decision support modules on outcomes and effects on the care process have been demonstrated [45,46]. A fundamental insight has emerged indicating that successful prevention efforts need to focus on root causes, that is, on errors in the design and implementation of systems, not on the errors themselves [47].

To identify potential benefits, clinical databases can be used as data mining repositories. Moreover, clinical databases can serve in the evaluation of past, unaided medical decisions and also to deliver baseline data against which the success of an intervention can be measured [48].

During the IMIA working conference, the challenges and questions of how to verify and demonstrate the outcomes of health information systems have been discussed intensively. It has been recommended that "packaged" approaches be developed, including a set of validated instruments and a library of study results [49]. In the conference proceedings, practical solutions have been suggested. These include addressing the complexity of health information systems by carrying out pragmatic studies; by questioning different personnel groups separately; by weighing and summing up separate impacts; by isolating important functions; by exploiting natural experiments, that is, measuring workloads or help line calls; and by utilizing typical incremental deployment for before–after measurements [50].

Integration and Interoperability

System integration is still a challenge, both between and within institutions. The development and use of standards, especially HL7 and DICOM, have substantially reduced this problem, typically by facilitating the construction of interfaces. Dedicated tools for EAI (Enterprise Application Integration), such as interface engines, have been helpful in managing interfaced systems. Yet, interfaces still have to be implemented and maintained, and the mapping between different interfaces is still cumbersome and error prone.

Compared to holistic approaches, additional efforts are needed to provide workflow over the module and subsystem borders, whereas generalist vendors, who are trying to build all-in-one solutions, are providing mechanisms to support workflow within their holistic environment. Today's systems tend to be a combination of some "leading" system combined with a number of interfaced subsystems; workflow support across the borders of these subsystems is limited. Workflow engines, which have been quite successful in business branches like banking, are beginning to be introduced in health information systems [51]; their positive effect on the healthcare environments is yet to be proven.

Real interoperability in the sense of seamless interaction and cooperation between system modules from different vendors is still not within reach. Component technology is considered a promising approach toward increased openness and interoperability [52]. The basic idea is to build well-structured systems out of independently understandable and reusable building blocks [53]. One ideal, a component market with "plug-and-play" connection of previously unrelated components playing together in a global solution, has been mentioned above. A somewhat less ambitious, but still helpful, perspective would be the existence of "modify-and-reuse" components. There is no straightforward solution to realizing these ideas, however, because components require technical, syntactical, and semantic compatibility to be seamlessly integrated into a comprehensive system.

Although standards for technical and syntactical compatibility are beginning to consolidate (e.g., CORBA, XML), semantic compatibility is still the biggest challenge since it encompasses more than the domain-specific standards that HL7 currently addresses. Major questions have to be solved: Common ontologies, including standard terminologies and clinical models, are needed as a basis for a common understanding of shared concepts [54,55]. The fact that every model and terminology in medicine keeps evolving over time makes this problem even more difficult. In addition, components need to be mapped into a common context, that is, into an application framework describing health information systems functionality and basic services. The discussion group on open architectures provided a description during the Heidelberg conference. Among the recommendations of this group were to comply with existing standards, to implement first and standardize next, to pursue open source solutions, and to pursue common infrastructures [56].

The availability of Web technologies helps to solve the integration problem: on the human–computer interaction level, homogeneity can be reached much easier now. Yet, the fundamental problems of autonomy and semantic heterogeneity of underlying components remain and need complex solutions, which enforce consensus on different levels of interaction. The predominant approach of today is still to use a physical repository to collect data from different, often heterogeneous and autonomous sources into one central database [57]. In addition to this conventional database for online transaction processing (OLTP), data warehouses for online analytical processing (OLAP) are becoming more prevalent. By providing multidimensional views of large amounts of data, warehouses assist in strategic decisions and support a shift toward cost- and outcome-oriented information management [58].

Sociotechnical Issues and System Design

The central role of sociotechnical and organizational issues for health information management systems has been identified early, and many new and important aspects have been identified during the past years. Lorenzi and Riley have pointed out that not considering various organizational issues bears the risk of system failures [59]. Sauer has presented an overview of about 50 factors associated with failures. These factors can be assigned to factor classes, which comprise management commitment, user involvement, value/benefit, mutual understanding between involved groups, design quality, technical quality, and management processes [60].

The need of user participation in analyzing and modeling the application domain and in developing and introducing systems has been identified under various perspectives. Coiera has criticized a lack of common ground between system designers and users [61]. Anderson has observed that medical records reflect both the clinical reasoning process and an individual's practice style, whereas computerized systems tend to lose these individual characteristics [62]. Berg has warned of replacing a "seemingly messy work culture" by the "rationality" of computer-based systems, which may obstruct work by too much prefixed structure [63]. Moreover, Berg and Toussaint found that the models underlying conventional paper information systems, which have evolved over a long period of time, form a perfect match with the working needs of healthcare professionals [64]. Replacing them inadequately and introducing IT systems with wrongly designed workflow will increase workload and may cause failures.

The complete process of designing, implementing, and deploying a health information system consists of different project phases with different groups of persons involved. IT staff in healthcare institutions, together with the institutions' health professionals, have to perform tasks like identifying goals, analyzing the existing IT environment and planning change, selecting solutions, organizing training and managing change, and deploying new modules. The latter typically includes intensive customization, interfacing, organization of a help desk, and communication of problems with a vendor, which results in a long-lasting, iterative, and incremental task. At the vendors' side, typical software engineering processes are performed, which also consist of several phases, from analyses and modeling to implementation and iterative refinement [65].

In these complicated processes, failures are common. The problem is not specific to the health environment; the term "software crisis" refers to enormous losses in IT development in general. In 1995, the Standish Group reported investments in the U.S. of $81 billion for software projects that did not end successfully, and only 9 percent of major U.S. software projects were finished on time and budget [66]. A recent study by the U.S. National Institute of Standards and Technology [67] also reported losses of $59 billion due to inadequate testing of software. Health care is one of the most difficult domains, if not the most difficult of all, for applying ICT. Moreover, in health information systems development, software engineering methods may lag behind those used in other safety-critical environments [68].

To cope with the problem of inadequate IT solutions, which are at risk for failure, several approaches are needed, notably consistent project management, including adequate change management, as well as improved software engineering and system development processes. Risk management with a focus on robustness may be the most important prerequisite.

Fundamental aspects of *project management* and of *change management* were described and analyzed during the Heidelberg IMIA conference. Besides technical skills, project management skills are needed to plan, direct, control, motivate, and staff. Organizational skills are needed to interface with the information system stakeholders [69]. It is helpful in this context to know the different roles of people who are involved in a project [70]. Managing change requires knowledge about an organization's milieu; it needs to start at the conceptual level, to proceed toward commitment, and to understand what is needed to make the outcome happen [71]. Health information systems development and deployment will increasingly focus on communication and human factors, resulting in a more consistent interaction design [72].

Software Engineering Concepts

Software engineering concepts are changing from the classic model ("waterfall") to iterative approaches. This is an appropriate fit for the healthcare work environment, where rapid prototyping is helpful to better adapt information systems to health professionals' work practice. To analyze and model workflow, simple and robust techniques are needed, that is, use cases and graphic tools [73]. Graphic models need to be easily understood by health professionals to support participatory design process. As participation may be time consuming, it is important to come to practical solutions quickly, at least in prototype, and not to lose momentum in the project [74]. Finally, project experiences have confirmed the need to adapt running systems to changing requirements [75]. Berg and Toussaint have even pointed out that, during deployment phase, "the information system's 'requirements' . . . will *necessarily* evolve" [76].

Risk

Risk should be considered under several perspectives: Risk categories may range from complete failure to different levels of additional costs. Risk types comprise aspects such as insufficient reaction to the socioeconomic context and to external dependencies, inadequate planning and identification of requirements and scope, technical problems, insufficient management, and lack of ownership. These categories and types have to be identified and considered. Sauer has pointed out that factors associated with failure cannot be controlled in a simplistic way. Information system (IS) development is faced with a variety of failure phenomena, and with a multitude of human, organizational, and technical characteristics and a spectrum of limiting factors [77]. The choices Sauer has identified are risk containment, typically by buying a package to reduce self-development or by outsourcing, or risk control, which includes the identification of organizational structural causes of failure, or a compromise between the two approaches, which could mean selective outsourcing or partitioning into subprojects.

In summary, the complete processes of project management and software development deserve more attention, and a consequent use of sound and robust methodologies is needed. Software engineering and IS development processes need to be based on a deeper understanding of the social and cognitive context and on exploration of the "communication space" [78]. A change in the process of health information systems development can be expected toward a more participatory and evolutionary approach, focusing on communication behavior and on cooperative work practices. In this process, the roles and needed skills of the people involved need to be identified and defined more clearly, for example, the distribution of competence and responsibility of users and IT staff of the healthcare institution, on the one hand, and of vendors on the other. The potential for a system to evolve and to be effectively adaptable to changing needs may be more important than sophisticated but hard-coded health information systems functionality [79]. A look at the complexity of health information systems and at IT failure rates shows the vital importance of keeping the software engineering process and the software product as robust and simple as possible. In this sense, Sauer has argued for the need to apply not only "best practices" but to develop "minimum practices" [80].

Global Challenges and Outlook

Successful Systems and Projects Exist Worldwide

ICT development in the healthcare domain is making progress worldwide. Conferences from around the world show growing interest in health information systems and give an indication of the broad spectrum of successful IT projects. The following examples illustrate this:

- MEDITEL 2002, a conference of the Medical Computer Society of India in August 2002, focused on the topics telemedicine, e-healthcare, information technology in hospitals, business process outsourcing in health care, information technology, and medical education [81].
- Topics of the First Middle East Conference on Healthcare Informatics, October 2002, included e-health, teaching and learning in the information age, healthcare informatics training, social shaping of medical informatics, and management of information [82].
- Informedica 2002, the 2nd Ibero-American Congress of Medical Informatics on the Internet, chose the motto "paving the way to global e-health" [83].
- MIST 2002, the Medical Informatics Symposium in Taiwan, in October 2002, was directed at "Achieving a knowledge-based economy in biomedicine through informatics" and covered topics such as the paperless hospital, bioinformatics, and free software [84].

Significant IT efforts to build national IT infrastructures supporting health care are taking place worldwide, and there are numerous reports of successful projects [85–89]. National and international training programs also help to foster the needed skills.

As mirrored in these conference topics, there is a growing awareness of the potential of IT systems in health care, of the potential of the Internet, and of all forms of telehealth. e-healthcare applications also have been realized in many countries around the world. The growth of the Internet is a significant factor influencing global health care, presenting an opportunity to make medical information and knowledge available worldwide. While the predicted "global village" of the 21st century [90,91], with global empowerment and diversification of healthcare information, seems technically feasible, the basic problems outlined in the first section of this chapter and the difficulties in making high-quality information globally available [92] are still raising significant questions.

Sociotechnical Issues Are of Central, Worldwide Importance

To a remarkable degree, sociotechnical aspects are of relevance to the design, development, and deployment of health information systems worldwide. Health information systems are dependent on their socioeconomic context, and the challenges in transferring successful solutions into environments with varying socioeconomic factors have been documented [93].

Adequate software development and deployment processes are of relevance in all environments worldwide, and most of the challenges and perspectives described in the foregoing section do exist worldwide. A clear description of goals, consistent project management, and adequate change management are needed. More attention to identifying benefits and risks, to quantifying return on investment, and to fitting systems into the organizational context is expected to evolve in the near future. A sound methodology should help ask the right questions during all phases of the health information systems development process. Potential answers to these questions could become a library of evaluation results and of project reports, helping to direct systems design. A component market as described above could facilitate the implementation of concepts.

In general, technology should be the enabler, not the driver [94]. The Internet and new technologies, such as wireless local area networks (LANs), satellite communication, smart cards, handheld computers, improved speech recognition, and robotics, offer opportunities. However, technologies have to meet the challenges as well: improved tools to support the analysis and modeling of processes, more robust software engineering approaches, increased openness, and better adaptability of systems are needed.

Bioinformatics: A New Perspective for Health Information

The bioinformatics revolution represents significant potential and impact for the design of future health information systems. The Human Genome Project has massively influenced our understanding of the molecular cause of diseases, and it will create new diagnostic and therapeutic methods. To reach this goal, researchers are following a bottom-up approach: from DNA and protein sequences to biological function, physiology, and pathophysiology; from molecules to cells, tissues, and organs; and further up to patients and diseases. The genetic code is simple and elegant, but an enormous amount of (faulty) data has to be handled in bioinformatics. The challenges ahead are to understand pathophysiology and its variations, to develop diagnostic and therapeutic methods, and to finally support clinical practice. For this goal, gene and structure data will have to be correlated with clinical data, that is, with phenotypes and with functions, which will result in another massive increase of complexity [95–100]. The spectrum for future information system types is broad: genetic data can be added to the patient record, and new types of databases will develop, such as genome epidemiology databases, tumor databases, and databases for pharmacogenomics. Projects like the Stanford PharmGKB [101] project and the Human Genome Epidemiology Network HuGeNet [102,103] by the Centers for Disease Control are remarkable examples of integrating genome information with clinical and epidemiological data.

Conclusions

Problems, potential, and perspectives of health information systems worldwide have been outlined in this chapter. There are indicators that IS can support a revolutionary change toward a globally transformed health system with equitable access to information and to health care worldwide. Foundations are new or improved technologies and a much better understanding of the principles of IS design, development, and deployment. On the other hand, pessimistic comments have criticized the poor effects of IT on health care. Causes of IT failures have been investigated for decades; however, further problems or even failures have not been prevented. Moreover, many countries of the world suffer from poverty, and their IT infrastructure is weak: IT investment needs a clear vision and justification. Some major aspects can be summarized as follows:

- While problems of limited access and of quality deficits have to be solved, the Internet will influence health care worldwide. Collaboration and dissemination of information and knowledge may be dramatically improved, and e-healthcare can bring significant benefits.
- Standards and technology have made progress. To an increasing extent, health professionals' work practice can be supported in distributed environments.
- A significant prerequisite for this goal has been fulfilled: worldwide, the understanding of the multidimensional sociotechnical foundations of health information systems has dramatically improved, and attention has been directed toward goals, benefits, and outcomes. Managing risk and pursuing simple, robust solutions should be among the fundamental axes of projects.
- Numerous strategic IT applications in health care exist, and further breakthroughs can be predicted. In the evolving distributed healthcare environment, questions of patient privacy, data confidentiality, and security arise and have to be answered.
- Integrating the bioinformatics perspective into information systems design will significantly contribute to the transformation of health care.

The most important factor for future action may be that our understanding of health information systems as complex sociotechnical systems has deepened. Health information systems design and development is a multidimensional process, with a multitude of influencing factors of high interdependence. A successful transformation of health care, while proceeding from step to step incrementally, will have to consider the complete system in its multidimensional structure and its complexity [104].

References

1. Kuhn KA, Giuse DA, Talmon JL. The Heidelberg Conference—setting an agenda for the IMIA Working Group on Health Information Systems. Editorial. Int J Med Inform 2003; 69:77–82.

2. Kuhn KA, Giuse DA, Haux R. IMIA Working Conference on Health Information Systems 2002 in Heidelberg. Practical HIS Experiences. Methods Inform Med 2003;42: VI–VIII.
3. World Bank. World development indicators database (PC and Internet data from the International Telecommunication Union's ITU World Telecommunication Development Report 2001). www.worldbank.org/data/dataquery.html; last access Dec. 10, 2002.
4. Oliveri N, Lindsay J, Layzell BR, et al. IMIA Working Group 9: Health Informatics for developing countries. Workshop: globalization and development. In: Patel VL, Rogers R, Haux R, editors. Medinfo 2001. Proceedings of 10th World Congress on Medical Informatics. p. 1538.
5. Parent F, Coppieters Y, Parent M. Information technologies, health, and "globalization": anyone excluded? J Med Internet Res 2001;3(1):e11. http://www.jmir.org/2001/1/e11/; last access Dec. 4, 2002.
6. Mbarika V, Jensen M, Meso P. Cyberspace across Sub-Saharan Africa. Commun ACM 2002;45:17–21.
7. Chandrasekhar CP, Gosh J. Information and communication technologies and health in low income countries: the potential and the constraints. Bull WHO 2001;79:850–853.
8. Braa J. A study on the actual and potential usage of information and communication technology at district and provincial levels in Mozambique with a focus on the health sector. EJISDC 5 2001;2:1–29; http://www.ejisdc.org; last access Nov. 27, 2002.
9. Soriyan HA, Akinde AD, Korpela M, et al. Preconditions for information system development for African healthcare institutions: the MINPHIS experience and a software industry survey in Nigeria. In: Patel VL, Rogers R, Haux R, editors. Medinfo 2001. Proceedings of 10th World Congress on Medical Informatics, p. 74.
10. Soriyan HA, Korpela MJ, Mursu AS et al. Information systems development for healthcare in Africa: the INDEHELA-Methods project. http://www.uku.fi/atkk/indehela/inde-h99.pdf; last access Nov. 27, 2002.
11. Sahay S. Special issue on "IT and health care in develping countries." EJISDC 5 2001;0:1–6; http://www.ejisdc.org; last access Nov. 27, 2002.
12. Heywood AB, Campbell BC. Development of a primary health care system in Ghana: lessons learned. Methods Inform Med 1997;36:63–68.
13. Braa J, Heywood A, Shung King M. District level information systems: two cases from South Africa. Methods Inform Med 1997;36:115–121.
14. Braa J. A study on the actual and potential usage of information and communication technology at district and provincial levels in Mozambique with a focus on the health sector. EJISDC 5 2001;2:1–29; http://www.ejisdc.org; last access Nov. 27, 2002.
15. Karras BT, Kimball AM, Gonzales V, et al. Informatics for Peru in the new millennium. In: Patel VL, Rogers R, Haux R, editors: Medinfo 2001. Proceedings of 10th World Congress on Medical Informatics. p. 1033–1037.
16. Chandrasekhar CP, Gosh J. Information and communication technologies and health in low income countries: the potential and the constraints. Bull WHO 2001;79:850–853.
17. Soriyan HA, Korpela MJ, Mursu AS, et al. Information systems development for healthcare in Africa: the INDEHELA-Methods project. http://www.uku.fi/atkk/indehela/inde-h99.pdf; last access Nov. 27, 2002.
18. Seror A. The Internet, global healthcare management systems, and sustainable development: future scenarios. EJISDC 5 2001;1:1–18.
19. Mbarika V, Jensen M, Meso P. Cyberspace across Sub-Saharan Africa. Commun ACM 2002;45:17–21.
20. Krishna S, Madon S. Conference Report: 7th International Working Conference of International Federation for Information Processing (IFIP) WG 9.4, 2002; Bangalore, India. http://www.iimahd.ernet.in/egov/ifip/aug2002/article5.htm. See also http://is.lse.ac.uk/ifipwg94/. Accessed Dec. 4, 2002.
21. Parent F, Coppieters Y, Parent M. Information technologies, health, and "globalization": anyone excluded? J Med Internet Res 2001;3(1):e11; http://www.jmir.org/2001/1/e11/; last access Dec. 4, 2002.

22. Clayton PD, Narus SP, Huff SM, et al. Building a comprehensive clinical information system from components: the approach at Intermountain Health Care. Methods Inform Med 2003; 42:1–7.
23. Degoulet P, Marin L, Lavril M, et al. The HEGP component-based clinical information system. Int J Med Inform 2003;69:115–126.
24. Giuse DA. Provider order entry with integrated decision support: from academia to industry. Methods Inform Med 2003;42:45–50.
25. Kuhn KA, Lenz R, Elstner T, et al. Experiences with a generator tool for building clinical application modules. Methods Inform Med 2003;42:37–44.
26. Lechleitner G, Pfeiffer KP, Wilhelmy I, et al. Cerner Millennium: the Innsbruck experience Methods Inform Med 2003;42:8–15.
27. Gell G, Schmücker P, Pedevilla M, et al. SAP and Partners: IS-H & IS-H*MED. Methods Inform Med 2003;42:16–24.
28. Flatley Brennan P, Safran C. Recommendations of Conference Track 3: patient empowerment. Int J Med Inform 2003;69:301–304.
29. Safran C. The collaborative edge: patient empowerment for vulnerable populations. Int J Med Inform 2003;69:185–190.
30. Raghupathi W, Tan J. Strategic IT applications in health care. Commun ACM 2002;45:56–61.
31. Committee on Quality of Healthcare in America, Institute of Medicine. Crossing the quality chasm: a new health system for the 21st century. Washington, DC: National Academic Press; 2001.
32. Haruki Y, Ogushi Y, Okada Y, Kimura M, Kumamoto I, Sekita Y. Status and perspective of hospital information systems in Japan. Methods Inform Med 1999;38:200–206.
33. Raghupathi W, Tan J. Strategic IT applications in health care. Commun ACM 2002;45:56–61.
34. Bates DW, Cohen M, Leape LL, et al. Reducing the frequency of errors in medicine using information technology. J Am Med Inform Assoc 2001;8:299–308.
35. Haug PJ, Rocha BH, Evans RS. Decision support in medicine: lessons from the HELP system. Int J Med Inform 2003;69:273–284.
36. Evans RS, Pestotnik SL, Classen DC, et al. A computer-assisted management program for antibiotics and other antiinfective agents. N Engl J Med 1998;338:232–238.
37. Teich JM, Glaser JP, Beckley RF, et al. The Brigham integrated computing system (BICS): advanced clinical systems in an academic hospital environment. Int J Med Inform 1999;54: 197–208.
38. Classen DC, Pestotnik SL, Evans RS, et al. Computerized surveillance of adverse drug events in hospital patients. JAMA 1991;266:2847–2851.
39. Tierney WM, Miller ME, Overhage JM, McDonald CJ. Physician inpatient order writing on microcomputer workstations. Effects on resource utilization. JAMA 1993;269:379–383.
40. Overhage JM, Tierney WM, Zhou X, McDonald CJ. A randomized trial of "corollary orders" to prevent errors of omission. J Am Med Inform Assoc 1997;4:364–375.
41. Rind DM, Safran C, Phillips RS, et al. Effect of computer-based alerts on the treatment and outcomes of hospitalized patients. Arch Intern Med 1994;154:1511–1517.
42. Kuperman GJ, Teich JM, Bates DW, et al. Detecting alerts, notifying the physician, and offering action items: a comprehensive alerting system. In: Cimino JJ, editor. Proc AMIA Annu Fall Symp 1996;704–708.
43. Coiera E. When conversation is better than computation. J Am Med Inform Assoc 2000; 7:277–286.
44. Parker J, Coiera E. Improving clinical communication: a view from psychology. J Am Med Inform Assoc 2000;7:453–461.
45. Bates DW, Cohen M, Leape LL, et al. Reducing the frequency of errors in medicine using information technology. J Am Med Inform Assoc 2001;8:299–308.
46. Ball MJ, Douglas JV. Redefining and improving patient safety. Methods Inform Med 2002; 41:271–276.
47. Leape LL. A systems analysis approach to medical error. J Eval Clin Pract 1997;3:213–222.

48. Haug PJ, Rocha BH, Evans RS. Decision support in medicine: lessons from the HELP system. Int J Med Inform 2003;69:273–284.
49. Friedman CP, Haug PJ. Report of Conference Track 5: HIS outcomes and metrics. Int J Med Inform 2003;69:307–309.
50. Wyatt JC, Wyatt SM. When and how to evaluate health information systems? Int J Med Inform 2003;69:251–259.
51. Haux R, Seggewies C, Baldauf-Sobez W et al. Soarian—workflow management applied for health care. Methods Inform Med 2003;42:25–36.
52. Lenz R, Huff SM, Geissbühler A. Report of Conference Track 2: pathways to open architectures. Int J Med Inform 2003;69:297–299.
53. Szyperski C. Component software: beyond object oriented programming. Reading: Addison Wesley; 1998.
54. Stead WW, Miller RA, Musen MA, et al. Integration and beyond: linking information from disparate sources and into workflow. J Am Med Inform Assoc 2000;7:135–145.
55. Lenz R, Kuhn KA. Intranet meets hospital information systems—the solution to the integration problem? Methods Inform Med 2001;40:99–105.
56. Lenz R, Huff SM, Geissbühler A. Report of Conference Track 2: pathways to open architectures. Int J Med Inform 2003;69:297–299.
57. Kuhn KA, Giuse DA. From hospital information systems to health information systems—problems, challenges, perspectives. Methods Inform Med 2001;41:275–287.
58. Raghupathi W, Tan J. Strategic IT applications in health care. Comman ACM 2002;45:56–61.
59. Lorenzi NM, Riley RT. Managing change: an overview. J Am Med Inform Assoc 2000; 7:116–124.
60. Sauer C. Deciding the future for IS failures: not the choice you might think. In: Currie W, Galliers R, editors. Rethinking management information systems. Oxford: Oxford University Press; 1999. p. 279–309.
61. Coiera E. When conversation is better than computation. J Am Med Inform Assoc 2000; 7:277–286.
62. Anderson JG. Clearing the way for physicians' use of clinical information systems. Commun ACM 1997;40:83–90.
63. Berg M. Patient care information systems and health care work: a sociotechnical approach. Int J Med Inform 1999;55:87–101.
64. Berg M, Toussaint P. The mantra of modeling and the forgotten powers of paper: a sociotechnical view on the development of process-oriented ICT in health care. Int J Med Inform 2003;69:223–234.
65. Versteegen G. Projektmanagement mit dem Rational Unified Process. Berlin: Springer; 2000.
66. The Standish Group "Chaos." 1995. (Cited in Versteegen 2000; ref. [65].)
67. National Institute of Standards and Technology. Planning Report 02-3. The economic impacts of inadequate infrastructure for software testing. U.S. Dept of Commerce, Washington, DC; 2002.
68. Wyatt JC, Wyatt SM. When and how to evaluate health information systems? Int J Med Inform 2003;69:251–259.
69. Lorenzi NM, Riley RT. Organizational issues = change. Int J Med Inform 2003;69:197–203.
70. Ash JS, Stavri PZ, Dykstra R, Fournier L. Implementing computerized physician order entry: the importance of special people. Int J Med Inform 2003;69:235–250.
71. Lorenzi NM, Riley RT. Organizational issues = change. Int J Med Inform 2003;69:197–203.
72. Coiera E. Interaction design. Int J Med Inform 2003;69:205–222.
73. Versteegen G. Projektmanagement mit dem Rational Unified Process. Berlin: Springer; 2000.
74. Heywood AB, Campbell BC. Development of a primary health care system in Ghana: lessons learned. Methods Inform Med 1997;36:63–68.
75. Kuhn KA, Lenz R, Elstner T, et al. Experiences with a generator tool for building clinical application modules. Methods Inform Med 2003;42:37–44.

76. Berg M, Toussaint P. The mantra of modeling and the forgotten powers of paper: a sociotechnical view on the development of process-oriented ICT in health care. Int J Med Inform 2003; 69:223–234.

77. Sauer C. Deciding the future for IS failures: not the choice you might think. In: Currie W, Galliers R, editors. Rethinking management information systems. Oxford: Oxford University Press; 1999. p. 279–309.

78. Coiera E. Interaction design. Int J Med Inform 2003;69:205–222.

79. Kuhn KA, Lenz R, Elstner T, et al. Experiences with a generator tool for building clinical application modules. Methods Inform Med 2003;42:37–44.

80. Sauer C. Deciding the future for IS failures: not the choice you might think. In: Currie W, Galliers R, editors. Rethinking management information systems. Oxford: Oxford University Press; 1999. p. 279–309.

81. www.medindia.net/meditel/2002; last access Nov. 27, 2002.

82. www.ifhi.org; last access Nov. 27, 2002.

83. www.informedica.org/2002; last access Nov. 27, 2002.

84. http://mist.med.org.tw; last access Nov. 27, 2002.

85. Din B-F, Wu L-P, Zhang Y. Community health information and its management system: a new form for the next century. In: Patel VL, Rogers R, Haux R, editors. Medinfo 2001. Proceedings of 10ᵗʰ World Congress on Medical Informatics. p. 724–726.

86. De F Leao B, Bernardes MM, Levin J. The Brazilian National Health Informatics strategy. In: Patel VL, Rogers R, Haux R, editors. Medinfo 2001. Proceedings of 10ᵗʰ World Congress on Medical Informatics. p. 38–42.

87. Eltchiian R, Mironov S, Emelin I. Russian telemedicine project. In: Patel VL, Rogers R, Haux R, editors. Medinfo 2001. Proceedings of 10ᵗʰ World Congress on Medical Informatics. p. 870.

88. Raza Abidi SS, Han CY, Raza Abidi S. Patient empowerment via "pushed" delivery of personalised healthcare educational content over the Internet. In: Patel VL, Rogers R, Haux R, editors. Medinfo 2001. Proceedings of 10ᵗʰ World Congress on Medical Informatics. p. 1425–1429.

89. Ball MJ, Peterson H, Douglas JV. The computerized patient record: a global view. MD Comput 1999;16:40–46.

90. Mullins HC, Higgins R, Kidd M, et al. It is time for a global strategy for use of IT in primary care? In: Patel VL, Rogers R, Haux R, editors. Medinfo 2001. Proceedings of 10ᵗʰ World Congress on Medical Informatics. p. 1523.

91. Seror A. The Internet, global healthcare management systems, and sustainable development: future scenarios. EJISDC 5 2001;1:1–18.

92. Geffen L, Hanmer L, Isaacs S. Developing world access to information—entrenching poverty of enhancing knowledge? In: Patel VL, Rogers R, Haux R, editors. Medinfo 2001. Proceedings of 10ᵗʰ World Congress on Medical Informatics. p. 1525.

93. Southon FC, Sauer C, Dampney CN. Information technology in complex health services: organizational impediments to successful technology transfer and diffusion. J Am Med Inform Assoc 1997;4:112–124.

94. Ball MJ, Peterson H, Douglas JV. The computerized patient record: a global view. MD Comput 1999;16:40–46.

95. Altman RB. The interaction between clinical informatics and bioinformatics: a case study. J Am Med Inform Assoc 2000;7:439–443.

96. Martin-Sanchez F, Maojo V, Lopez-Campos G. Integrating genomics into health information systems. Methods Inform Med 2002;41:25–30.

97. Kulikowski CA. The micro-macro spectrum of medical informatics challenges: from molecular medicine to transforming health care in a globalizing society. Methods Inform Med 2002;41:20–24.

98. Maojo V, Iakovidis I, Martin-Sanchez F, et al. Medical informatics and bioinformatics: European efforts to facilitate synergy. J Biomed Inform 2001.

99. Miller PL. Opportunities at the intersection of bioinformatics and health informatics: a case study. J Am Med Inform Assoc 2000;7:431–438.

100. Kohane IS. Bioinformatics and clinical informatics: the imperative to collaborate. J Am Med Inform Assoc 2000;7:511–516.
101. Hewett M, Oliver DE, Rubin DL et al. PharmGKB: the pharmacogenetics knowledge base. Nucleic Acids Res 2002;30:163–165.
102. Khoury MJ. Human genome epidemiology: translating advances in human genomics into population-based data for medicine and public health. Genet Med 1999;1(3):71–73.
103. http://www.cdc.gov/genomics/hugenet/about/translate.htm; last accessed Dec. 4, 2002.
104. Ball MJ. Hospital information systems: perspectives on problems and prospects, 1979 and 2002. Int J Med Inform 2003;69:83–89.

Index

Health Informatics Series
(formerly Computers in Health Care)

(continued from page ii)

Introduction to Clinical Informatics
P. Degoulet and M. Fieschi

Behavioral Healthcare Informatics
N.A. Dewan, N.M. Lorenzi, R.T. Riley, and S.R. Bhattacharya

Patient Care Information Systems
Successful Design and Implementation
E.L. Drazen, J.B. Metzger, J.L. Ritter, and M.K. Schneider

Introduction to Nursing Informatics, Second Edition
K.J. Hannah, M.J. Ball, and M.J.A. Edwards

Strategic Information Management in Hospitals
An Introduction to Hospital Information Systems
R. Haux, A. Winters, E. Ammenwerth, and B. Brigl

Information Retrieval
A Health and Biomedical Perspective, Second Edition
W.R. Hersh

The Nursing Informatics Implementation Guide
E.C. Hunt, S.B. Sproat, and R.R. Kitzmiller

Information Technology for the Practicing Physician
J.M. Kiel

Computerizing Large Integrated Health Networks
The VA Success
R.M. Kolodner

Medical Data Management
A Practical Guide
F. Leiner, W. Gaus, R. Haux, and P. Knaup-Gregori

Organizational Aspects of Health Informatics
Managing Technological Change
N.M. Lorenzi and R.T. Riley

Transforming Health Care Through Information, Second Edition
N.M. Lorenzi, J.S. Ash, J. Einbinder, W. McPhee, and L. Einbinder

Trauma Informatics
K.I. Maull and J.S. Augenstein

Consumer Informatics
Applications and Strategies in Cyber Health Care
R. Nelson and M.J. Ball

Public Health Informatics and Information Systems
P.W. O'Carroll, W.A. Yasnoff, M.E. Ward, L.H. Ripp,
and E.L. Martin

Advancing Federal Sector Health Care
A Model for Technology Transfer
P. Ramsaroop, M.J. Ball, D. Beaulieu, and J.V. Douglas

Medical Informatics
Computer Applications in Health Care and Biomedicine, Second Edition
E.H. Shortliffe and L.E. Perreault

Filmless Radiology
E.L. Siegel and R.M. Kolodner

Cancer Informatics
Essential Technologies for Clinical Trials
J.S. Silva, M.J. Ball, C.G. Chute, J.V. Douglas, C.P. Langlotz, J.C. Niland,
and W.L. Scherlis

Clinical Information Systems
A Component-Based Approach
R. Van de Velde and P. Degoulet

Knowledge Coupling
New Premises and New Tools for Medical Care and Education
L.L. Weed

Healthcare Information Management Systems
Cases, Strategies, and Solutions, Third Edition
M.J. Ball, C.A. Weaver, and J.M. Kiel

Organizational Aspects of Health Informatics, Second Edition
Managing Technological Change
N.M. Lorenzi and R.T. Riley